Environmental Biotechnology

Environmental Biotechnology

K ALLEN

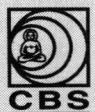

CBS Publishers & Distributors Pvt Ltd

New Delhi • Bengaluru • Chennai • Kochi • Kolkata • Mumbai • Pune
Hyderabad • Nagpur • Patna • Vijayawada

Environmental Biotechnology

ISBN: 978-81-239-2832-6

Copyright © Publisher

First Edition: 2016

Published by Satish Kumar Jain and produced by Varun Jain for

CBS Publishers & Distributors Pvt Ltd

4819/XI Prahlad Street, 24 Ansari Road, Daryaganj, New Delhi 110 002, India.

Ph: 23289259, 23266861, 23266867   Website: www.cbspd.com

Fax: 011-23243014   e-mail: delhi@cbspd.com; cbspubs@airtelmail.in.

Corporate Office: 204 FIE, Industrial Area, Patparganj, Delhi 110 092

Ph: 4934 4934   Fax: 4934 4935   e-mail: publishing@cbspd.com; publicity@cbspd.com

Branches

- **Bengaluru:** Seema House 2975, 17th Cross, K.R. Road,
  Banasankari 2nd Stage, Bengaluru 560 070, Karnataka
  Ph: +91-80-26771678/79   Fax: +91-80-26771680   e-mail: bangalore@cbspd.com

- **Chennai:** 7, Subbaraya Street, Shenoy Nagar, Chennai 600 030, Tamil Nadu
  Ph: +91-44-26680620, 26681266   Fax: +91-44-42032115   e-mail: chennai@cbspd.com

- **Kochi:** Ashana House, No. 39/1904, AM Thomas Road, Valanjambalam, Eranakulam 682 018,
  Kochi Kerala
  Ph: +91-484-4059061-65   Fax: +91-484-4059065   e-mail: kochi@cbspd.com

- **Kolkata:** 6/B, Ground Floor, Rameswar Shaw Road, Kolkata-700 014, West Bengal
  Ph: +91-33-22891126, 22891127, 22891128   e-mail: kolkata@cbspd.com

- **Mumbai:** 83-C, Dr E Moses Road, Worli, Mumbai-400018, Maharashtra
  Ph: +91-22-24902340/41   Fax: +91-22-24902342   e-mail: mumbai@cbspd.com

- **Pune:** Bhuruk Prestige, Sr. No. 52/12/2+1+3/2 Narhe, Haveli
  (Near Katraj-Dehu Road Bypass), Pune 411 041, Maharashtra
  Ph: +91-20-64704058, 64704059, 32392277   Fax: +91-20-24300160 e-mail: pune@cbspd.com

Representatives

- **Hyderabad**   0-9885175004   • **Nagpur**   0-9021734563
- **Patna**   0-9334159340   • **Vijayawada**   0-9000660880

Printed at India Binding House, Noida, UP

Preface

Environmental biotechnology is the application of biotechnology to all aspects of the environment. In the recent past, ample attention has been focused on environmental quality, and environmental biotechnology has emerged at a time when deterioration of environmental health has come to an all time high. It is a specific application of biotechnology to the management of environmental problems.

The emerging areas of environmental biotechnology are: (i) development of novel and environmentally improved production technologies with good quality end-products, but fewer by-products (or wastes), (ii) use of less purified substrates (and wastes) for the production of required products of good quality with acceptable costs without causing any problems to the environment, (iii) improved methods of resource use with substantial reduction of waste generation, (iv) controlled production of very specific biocatalysts, (v) planned and efficient consumption of bioresources to get maximum benefit from the limited biomass, (vi) development of technology for the protection and continuance of the existing local as well as global biodiversity, (vii) recycling of the industrial by-products to reduce the problem of pollution, and (viii) use of biological organisms to reclaim the contaminated habitats.

Environmental biotechnology has emerged as an associated technology of the industrial production processes so as to make the latter environment friendly. Environmental biotechnology, initially started with waste-water treatment in urban areas, has been extended, among others to soil remediation, off gas purification, pesticide degradation, heavy metal removal, surface and groundwater cleaning, industrial waste-water purification, deposition techniques of waste in sanitary landfills, composting of bioorganic residues, environmental risk analysis and biopesticide developments. Each chapter covers an important aspect of environmental biotechnology with an accurate up-to-date account of each topic.

This book is divided into six sections. Section I is devoted to general considerations. Chapter 1 is the introducing chapter and gives a review of environmental biotechnology. To design pollution control devices, knowledge of the nature of pollutants, the micro-organisms involved in the biodegradation of waste material, biochemical pathways, etc. is a prerequisite. To utilise this information it is equally necessary to know about the stoichiometry (material and energy balances) as well as the reaction kinetics of the processes involved. Considering this chapters 2 and 3 are devoted to stoichiometry and bacterial energetics. Chapter 4 deals with bioreactor design. Stoichiometry and reaction kinetics together provide the quantitative approach essential for the design of bioreactors and design calculations. Chapter 5 tackles microbes and metabolism. Microbes, which widely occur in nature (air, water and soils), play various roles in matter cycles. Though they pollute the environment (biological pollution), they also can help to improve upon its quality.

Section II explains the role of environmental biotechnology in waste-water treatment. The water that is released after use by the domestic and industrial sectors into the environment is usually termed as waste-water. The main function of domestic waste treatment systems is to reduce the organic content, pathogenic micro-organisms, and suspended solids as far as possible in order to be able to return to rivers and coastal waters without causing pollution, especially those rivers used as a source of drinking water. Chapter 6 points the biological treatment fundamentals. Chapters 7 and 8 encompass biological treatment of waste-water and solid wastes. Chapter 9 discusses biomethanation systems for energy recovery from urban and industrial waste-waters.

Section III deals with environmental biotechnology in soil and landfill. Chapters 10 and 11 concentrate on biological soil treatment and life cycle assessment in soil bioremediation planning. Chapter 12 is devoted to slurry decontamination process and explain the broad spectrum technologies, focusing on treatment and recycling of contaminated soils, sediments and sludges. Chapter 13 tackles immobilisation of pesticides in soil through enzymatic reactions. Immobilisation phenomena occurring in soil are of great importance because they may lead to a considerable reduction in bioavailability of pesticides. Both enzymes and abiotic catalysts can mediate the immobilisation process.

Section IV discusses applications of environmental biotechnology in various industries such as chemical, food processing and metal and mining. Chapter 14 deals with chemical industries. With advent of new technologies and better bioprocesses, environmental biotechnology is acquiring new meaning to the chemical industry. In several instances bioprocess seem to be cleaner and efficient than existing chemical processes. Drugs and pharmaceuticals, fine chemicals, new molecules synthesis, petroleum refining and petrochemicals, pulp and paper, sugar and distillery, leather and tannery, paint and dyes, pesticides and insecticides are some of the areas which are becoming more and more biotechnology driven. Chapter 15 explains various food processing industries such as dairy, starch, vegetable oil, meat processing, etc. Chapter 16 is devoted to metal and mining industries. Toxic heavy metals have adverse effects on aquatic and terrestrial ecosystems. Despite this, micro-organisms are commonly found in polluted habitats and possess a range of morphological and physiological attributes that enable survival. Section V discusses biodegradation and biotransformation. Biodegradation is generally considered as a phenomenon of biological transformation of organic compounds by living organisms, particularly microbes. Chapter 17 concentrates on bioremediation and discusses characteristics of contamination their biodegradability, and engineering studies of bioremediation. Chapter 18 tackles methods for biocatalysis and biotransformation. Concepts and general features of biotransformation, etc. are discussed in detail. Chapter 19 is devoted to bioremediation—an advanced strategy to restore health of aquaculture pond ecosystems. Chapter 20 explains the biodegradation of organic pollutants. The chapter discusses biodegradation of important organic pollutants such as polymers, hydrocarbons, pesticides, etc. Section VI focuses on special topics. Chapter 21 deals with environmental monitoring. To effectively monitor the environment as well as devise pollution abatement methods, it is necessary to know the quality of the environment-quantitatively. Chapter 22 concentrates on microbial biodiversity: strategies for its recovery.

This reference textbook on *Environmental Biotechnology* is designed to fulfil the requirements of undergraduates and postgraduates in the disciplines of environmental biotechnology, microbial ecology, biotechnology, biochemical engineering. The book will also be useful for scientists, researchers, and professionals interested in exploring the role of micro-organisms in public health and waste-water engineering.

Glossary and index have been provided at the end for quick reference. Diagrams, figures and tables supplement the text. All the topics have been covered into a cogent and lucid style to help the reader grasp the information quickly and easily.

K Allen

Contents at a Glance

SECTION V

SECTION VI

Contents

SECTION I

SECTION II

SECTION III

SECTION IV

SECTION V

SECTION I

General Considerations

Chapter 1

Environmental Biotechnology: A Review

INTRODUCTION

The term environment means surroundings. Once qualified with specific reference, the term acquires more definite meaning. Earth's environment is endowed with atmosphere, hydrosphere, lithosphere, cryosphere and biosphere. All these components are distinguished on the basis of their respective distinct physical properties and they represent dynamic interacting subsystems of the environment. Interaction between the subsystems implies flow of material and energy whereby diverse life forms (plants, animals and microbes) reproduce, evolve and live. Energy requirements, to sustain the dynamic exchange of material and energy between these subsystems, primarily come from sun.

Environment is a combination of physical (solar radiation, Earth's atmosphere, hydrosphere, cryosphere and lithosphere) and biotic (plants, animals and microbes) components which surround us (man). One aspect common to all subcomponents is that we can see, hear, smell, feel and taste them.

Environmental biotechnology, an important branch of biotechnology, deals with the detection of environmental contaminants contained in industrial, agricultural, and domestic wastes and the remediation of the pollution caused by this contamination. The study of this discipline primarily spans two main areas: (i) environment science, and (ii) biotechnology. Environmental biotechnology involves applying the knowledge of biotechnology to solve environmental problems.

Environmental biotechnology is one of the several areas of biotechnology, which applies the principles of microbiology to various environmental issues such as treatment of industrial and municipal wastewater; improvement in the quality of drinking water; restoration of commercial, archaeological, and other sites which are being destroyed by hazardous materials; protection of rivers, lakes, and coastal waters from environmental contaminants; prevention of the spreading of pathogens through water or air; production of environmentally benign chemicals such as ethanol, methanol, methane, etc. and reduction of industrial residuals in order to check the production of pollutants requiring disposal.

Environmental biotechnology employs a diverse set of methodological approaches to explore and exploit the natural biodiversity of micro-organisms and their enormous metabolic capacities. This field includes the application of micro-organisms for improvement of environmental quality, the discovery of micro-organisms with metabolic potentials that can be employed for industrial applications, and the use of molecular methods for assessing the natural distributions of micro-organisms in the environment and the ecological functions they perform. The characteristics that distinguish environmental biotechnology from other fields of biotechnology are the necessity of achieving microbial functions in complex environments that are not subject to the precise experimental control that can be achieved in

3

bioreactors and the examination of individual micro-organisms and their functions in complex diverse microbial communities.

ISSUES FOR ENVIRONMENTAL BIOTECHNOLOGY

International Issues

Concept of greenhouse effect is associated with significant increase in the concentration of global warming gases (GWGs) responsible for this effect or the introduction of new compounds having similar effect. They cause serious shift in the radiation balance and increase GWGs which results in an increase in the average surface temperature of the earth. Consequently, it is evident that this shift will have serious implications on the global climate regime. The ensuing effects will be felt on food security, erratic rainfall pattern, sea level rise and displacement of communities from coastal areas.

The greatest degree of pollution has been noted in the coastal oceans which contribute most of the biomass to the terrestrial and oceanic food chain. Entry of the nutrient loaded freshwater from the land is the major cause of changes in the density and diversity of life forms in the coastal oceans. Eutrophication, appearance of toxic algal bloom and sedimentation are the major threats to the aquatic flora and fauna of coastal oceans. There are reports that in many coasts of the world there is a higher rate of sedimentation due to the entry of colloidal clay particles through freshwater inflow from the land. More amounts of biomass are being added to the sediment and there is a greater degree of anaerobic activity in the sediment, than in the past. Significant emission of methane has been reported not only in the coastal habitat, but also from the floor of the deep ocean.

Air pollution

Air is a natural resource and is fundamental to human life as it makes breathing possible. It is the basis for the existence of all forms of terrestrial and two-thirds of all biological species, and is also one of the important sources for economic development like agricultural and industrial production, energy generation, heating, cooling and so on.

Air becomes damaging to nature and human health when there is an excess of polluting elements in it. Air pollution has become an important factor of environmental degradation all over the world. The increasing agglomeration, in particular, industrialisation, manufacturing units, urbanisation, motorisation and burning of fuel material in households produce a large amount of air polluting substances which have a harmful effect, especially on human health, animal and plant life, and even on the buildings and works of art.

Air pollution may be defined as that quantity of pollutants which is sufficient to cause injury to human beings and other living creatures, and damage to objects. It has been observed that under due to increased concentration of air pollutants, human deaths have also increased. Diseases like bronchial asthma, lung cancer, irritation reaction, heart and brain damages, etc. are probably due to the adverse effects of high concentration of air pollutants.

Air pollution can be categorised into two groups; first the release of pollutants into the atmosphere from a specific source, and the second from pollutants resulting from chemical changes that take place in the atmosphere. When the amount of such pollutants in the air exceeds a certain level, then the air pollution is created. Pollutants may be in the form of dust, odours or vapours. The quantities of pollutants which are dangerous to nature have been determined both by national and international organisations.

Atmosphere represents the most dynamic subsystem of the environment. Any material introduced at a specific location in atmosphere can spread to other locations in the direction of wind flow or through passive diffusion/dispersion.

Air pollution has regional and global dimensions. Global dimensions of air pollution are associated with the presence of pollutants in air having long residence time (> 1 year) and they acquire homogeneous global atmospheric concentration per unit volume of air. It is of course, obvious that their impact will also have global dimensions. Presence of CO_2, CH_4, CFCs in atmosphere represents global dimension of air pollution.

On the other hand, pollutants having short residence time (<30 days) when present at specific location in atmosphere will have local or regional impact. The differences in the short and long residence time of a pollutant are a function of its chemical and photochemical activities. More activity implies short residence time. Chemically stable pollutants (e.g. CO_2, CH_4, etc.) have longer residence time. NO_x, SO_2, etc. in air are chemically active and cause acid rain which has regional impact; they have short residence time.

Energy crisis

Of late it has been realised that conventional energy sources cannot support human activities for an indefinite period and, more or less, a global crisis is being felt in the energy sector. The crude oil price has gone to an all time high in the recent past. There is also a proportionate decrease in the coal and mineral reserves and a decline of forest cover in the developing countries, due to the collection of firewood.

There is a search to reduce energy consumption through efficient technology and to generate as much energy as possible, from non-conventional sources, so as to reduce the burden on the traditional energy reserves. There is a search for and attempt to develop an environment friendly technology for the production of energy to satisfy energy demands, which are increasing exponentially everyday.

Oil spills

Oil spills have also been considered as a major threat to the world environment, in general and the marine ecosystem, in particular. The alarming rate of decline in the mangrove forests in the West Asian countries is due to oil withdrawal and oil spills in the coastal soil and ocean. There are also accidental releases of oil into the ocean environment during exploration, removal and/or transport.

Decline and loss of species

There is an unprecedented change in global biodiversity due to a variety of ecosystem unfriendly events. The most important amongst them are land conversion, pollution, unsustainable harvesting of natural resources and the introduction of exotic species. The relative importance of these driver events differs between ecosystems. For example, land conversion is more intensive in tropical forests, but less intensive in temperate, boreal and Arctic regions. Atmospheric nitrogen deposition is more in northern temperate areas close to cities, but it has less impact on diversity in inner forests. Introduction of exotic species is related to patterns of human activity—those areas away from human intervention generally receive fewer introduced species.

The ultimate causes of species loss are human population growth, together with the unsustainable pattern of consumption, increasing production of wastes and pollution, urban development and inequities in the distribution of wealth and resources.

National Issues

Water pollution

Water covers 70 per cent of earth's surface and its importance to all types of life on earth is vital. Water present in oceans, rivers and lakes is cycled through hydrological cycle in the form of rainfall. Physical and chemical properties of water make it a good solvent (water dissolves more substances than any other known solvent and acts as a carrier of material and energy exchange between different subsystems of the environment).

Generally, water pollution is a state of deviation from the pure condition, whereby its normal functions and properties are affected. Water is said to be polluted when it is contaminated with:
1. Dissolved gases like H_2S, CO_2, NH_3 and N_2.
2. Dissolved minerals like sodium, calcium and magnesium salts.
3. Suspended impurities like clay, sand, mud and organic matter.
4. Micro-organisms like bacteria, viruses, protozoas and worms.
5. Contamination of isotopes (radiologically active substances).

Pollution of water is defined as the presence of some foreign organic, inorganic, biological, radiological and physical substance or property that tends to degrade its quality and either constitutes a health hazard or otherwise decreases its utility.

Thus, water pollution may be defined as the addition of any foreign material or any physical change in natural water which may adversely affect living life directly or indirectly, either in the short run or in the long run.

Water pollution mainly occurs due to sewage, industrial and trade waste, agricultural pollutants and physical pollutants like heat and radioactive materials. The sources of water pollution can be classified controllable and uncontrollable depending upon their nature, and can be divided into two parts: (i) natural sources, and (ii) man-made sources.

Oxygen-demanding waste

Presence of oxygen in water bodies, also known as dissolved oxygen (DO), is crucial to the survival of lifeforms in water (fish, organisms, micro-organisms, plants, phytoplanktons, etc.). Oxygen exchange in water bodies, from air to water, takes place from surface but its low solubility in water limits its concentration (maximum solubility 14.7 mg l^{-1}). Low oxygen levels (<3 mg l^{-1}) disrupt the food chain in water and indicate pollution.

Solid waste

To maintain quality of environment and life it is essential that solid waste generated at every point be disposed properly. Untreated waste, disposed carelessly is breeding ground for disease vectors: mosquitoes, flies, rats, etc. Organisms disperse solid waste and this makes it easier for pathogens to infect children. Effective way to handle solid waste requires action starting from household to neighbourhood, community and municipality. In theory the task seems easy, but simple calculation done on the daily solid waste generated at city level turns out to be a huge number. Effective handling of solid waste becomes easier if participation starts from individual level onwards. This requires awareness towards the perils of mishandling solid waste. Number of episodes concerning the spread of a disease in cities in recent times are linked with unconcern towards handling of solid waste problem.

Sources of solid waste

Home is the smallest unit where daily waste of diverse kinds is generated. Types of waste generated consist of nonusable part of vegetables, fruits and other related constituents linked with daily cooking and is classified as degradable organic waste. Part of the solid waste also consists of nondegradable plastics — plastic bags, toys and other articles (paper, cardboard boxes, old clothes, polyesters, cotton, etc.) — broken glass, chemicals and metals. As we go up, beyond home to community level activities, the amount of waste produced multiplies, but overall pattern of the type of waste generated remains similar, only respective proportion of the kind of waste varies. Waste generated at industrial outlets varies significantly as it depends on the type of products being produced in respective units. Proper handling of waste requires well thought out management steps initiated at each level in the community where awareness toward the need to handle solid waste is inculcated.

Strategy for solid waste management

Key strategy before handling solid waste and managing it involves two central features: (i) minimising the waste generation at each point, and (ii) recycling the waste, whenever it is possible to do so. These two steps decrease the overall burden of solid waste management significantly. Both steps, simple in concept, involve conscious decision to reduce the waste by taking steps involving use of reusable bags to carry goods.

Sorting and management of solid waste

To maximise the role of recycling of solid waste it is essential to sort the waste at the waste generating point in different categories to facilitate the recycling in practice easily. Recycling solid waste can be achieved under following heads. Organic waste can be recycled through process of composting. Fruits and vegetable waste, animal dung and fallen leaves from plants form excellent soil conditioner and fertiliser (compost). Implementation to make compost at home level can be achieved by using a suitable container. The contents of the container after few weeks can be used as fertiliser. Vegetable waste and dried weeds can be chopped and compressed into small bricks and dried in sun. Like dried cow dung, they can be used to replace charcoal or wood as cooking fuel.

Glass and plastic waste can be reused in plastic and glass industries to reproduce wares for reuse. The task of collecting these waste items under different heads makes the recycling task more efficient and convenient. Construction debris and other waste building material can also be reused. Often the construction of new house or a building involves razing old structures. The debris produced in this manner can be used very effectively as filling material under floors.

Used tyres can be recycled by establishing appropriate recycling units. In the absence of this facility it is advisable to burry them to avoid collection of water during rainy season which encourages mosquito breeding. Burning of tyres should be avoided as the process leads to the emission of toxic fumes.

Soil pollution

The contamination of soil (or) land with acid rain, excess of fertilisers, wrong fertilisers, insecticides and herbicides is termed as 'soil pollution'.

The following are some of the important sources which pollute the soil:
1. Repeated and excess use of fertilisers and pesticides at random cause soil pollution. For example, due to excess use of $(NH_4)_2SO_4$ chemical fertiliser for several times, the SO_4^{-2} ion present in it gets accumulated into the soil. The soil then becomes infertile to plant growth due to acidity.

Similarly, due to repeated and excess use of fertilisers containing KNO_3 (or) $NaNO_3$, plant growth will be retarded due to the accumulation of Na^+, K^+ ions in the soil which makes it alkaline.

2. Soil pollution arises due to the application of defective methods in the cultivation processes.
3. Soil gets polluted due to the release of the cysts from antameba, ascaris, pigworm, etc. which enters into the human body through food chain.
4. Acid rain is another source of soil pollution. Sulphur and nitrogen oxides in the air undergo photo, chemical and catalytic oxidation followed by the interaction with rainy water or moisture to form H_2SO_4 and HNO_3.

When compared with atmosphere and hydrosphere, soil, the uppermost layer of earth's surface, has very different physical properties. Mixing and movement of pollutants is very slow within the soil matrix. Any deposition on soil that cannot be processed by the natural inorganic and organic forces will accumulate. When such materials become concentrated in a given area, they interfere with the growth in soil organic life. Such conditions pertain to the pollution of soil. Top soil surface will receive material sediments under gravity from atmosphere, through rainfall, water runoff or human centered activities. Some of the reasons leading to soil pollution are given below.

Acid rain

Rain tends to be naturally acidic with a pH of 5.6 to 5.7 due to the reaction of atmospheric CO_2 with water to produce carbonic acid. This small amount of acidity is sufficient to dissolve minerals in the earth's crust and make them available to plant and animal life, but it is not acidic enough to inflict any major damage. Other atmospheric substances from volcanic eruptions, forest fires and other similar natural phenomena also contribute to the acidity in rain. Thus, even with the enormous amounts of acids created by nature annually, normal rainfall is able to assimilate them to the point where they cause little, if any, known damage. But, it is the contributions of SO_x, NO_x, etc. from anthropogenic activities that disturb this acid balance and convert natural and mildly acidic rain into precipitation with far reaching environmental consequences.

Acid rain represents one of the major consequences of air pollution, because of large SO_x and NO_x emissions from big industrial areas. The longer the SO_x and NO_x remain in the atmosphere, the greater are the chances of their oxidation to H_2SO_4 and HNO_3 due to photochemical and catalytic chemical reactions. Acid rains may cause extensive damage to materials and terrestrial ecosystems, such as water, fish, vegetation, stone, steel, paint, soil and mankind.

The only practical approach to counter the problem of acid rain is to reduce SO_x and NO_x emissions. The following three general options are considered for this purpose:

1. Energy conservation resulting in reduced fuel consumption and hence slower emissions of SO_x and NO_x. Conservation via more efficient fuel use and through improved thermal insulation is also being studied.
2. Desulphurisation and denitrification of fuels of stack gases and increased use of fuels naturally low in sulphur content or use of technologies that reduce SO_x and NO_x emissions. Desulphurisation and use of low NO_x-producing technologies are the only viable control options today and will perhaps continue to be so for some more time.
3. Substitutions for fossil fuels by other alternative energy forms may offer future solutions to this problem.

Reduction of SO_x emissions can be accomplished by: (i) removing the sulphur content before the fuel is burnt with the help of techniques such as coal cleaning, coal gasification and desulphurisation of liquid fuels; (ii) removing the sulphur content during combustion, as in fluidised-bed combustion; and (iii) removal of sulphur emissions after combustion, as in stack or flue gas desulphurisation systems or scrubbers. The future of SO_x control from traditional fuel sources lies in the perfection of these techniques.

Reduction of NO_x emissions from stationary combustion sources can be achieved by modification of furnace and burner design, and/or modification of operating conditions. The combustion modification techniques available now include using two-stage combustion, precisely controlling air, injecting water during combustion, recirculating flue gases, and/or by altering design of firing chambers. Reductions in NO_x emissions from mobile combustion sources may be achieved by lowering the combustion temperatures in the engine and catalytic removal of NO_x from exhaust gases using devices such as a three-way system that simultaneously reduces carbon monoxide, hydrocarbons and NO_x.

Acid-forming precursors in atmosphere eventually are removed through rainfall. Deposition of acid rain on soil decreases the soil pH below 4.0. Such conditions deter any organic activity and soil is excluded from its normal use.

Pesticides and herbicides

Prevalent agriculture practices use pesticides to minimise the crop damage due to insects and pests. In developing countries, they are also used to control vector-borne diseases. Herbicides are used to eliminate unwanted plants growing with the desired crop. Ultimately, all these chemicals build up in areas adjacent to agriculture fields. Eventually they leach into the ground water and enter the food chain. These conditions threaten human health.

Landfills

Urban areas produce enormous daily waste from diverse activities. Disposal of this waste, if not managed in systematic manner, can cause serious problems by contaminating the land surrounding the disposal site. Presence of nonbiodegradable materials (polymers and plastics) adds to the problem. Groundwater contamination and spread of pathogenic organisms from such contaminated sites can pose serious health problems.

SCOPE OF ENVIRONMENTAL BIOTECHNOLOGY

Biotechnology for a Safer Environment

Different industrial processes and agricultural practices have damaged the environment considerably, till date. It is now required to modify the present technologies for minimising the extent of degradation of the environment by these processes. This has prompted researchers to develop technologies that have scope for the utilisation of biological organisms, to generate bioresources and to reduce the impact on the existing natural resources. Such technologies are aimed at producing products without causing a significant damage to the environment. Environmental biotechnology aims at the protection of the environment, purification of the environment from toxicants and contaminants and prevention of the degradation of valuable natural resources—soil, air, water and mineral resources. The most important environment friendly processes are: (i) study of the rate and effects of agricultural pesticide application and enhancement of the biodegradation of pesticides; (ii) minimisation of waste-water generation and treatment processes for urban and industrial waste-water; (iii) removal of nutrients for the prevention of eutrophication in surface waters; (iv) degradation of organic pollutants and xenobiotics in waste-water and solid wastes; (v) aerobic and anaerobic composting technology for the degradation of solid wastes; (vi) biological transformation and bioremediation of heavy metals for the reclamation of mine waste soil; (vii) experimental design for assessing the effect of pollutants in the ecosystem; and (viii) development of environment friendly biopesticides as a replacement of organosynthetic chemicals.

Bioremediation, which exploits the metabolic capacities of micro-organisms remove pollutants from the environment, is among the most heralded applications of environmental biotechnology. It has successfully been applied to major oil spills and numerous contaminated sites, thereby reducing the environmental damage caused by those pollutants and decreasing the risks they pose to human health. Most applications of bioremediation have been based on biostimulation, relying on the natural activities of indigenous micro-organisms and using environmental modifications, such as addition of mineral nutrients, to stimulate the rates at which micro-organisms metabolise pollutants. Such approaches are particularly effective in the remediation of petroleum hydrocarbon-polluted environments. Additionally, some applications of bioremediation of contaminated soils and waters involve bioaugmentation, in which cultures of micro-organisms with specific pollutant-degrading capabilities are added to a polluted site.

Compared to the bioremediation of petroleum hydrocarbons, greater complexities occur with regard to metal and chlorinated xenobiotic-contaminated environments. Many chlorinated xenobiotic compounds are resistant to microbial attack and persist in the environment. In some cases cometabolism can be employed for the remediation of environments polluted with such compounds, as this approach enables micro-organisms growing on one growth substrate to gratuitously biotransform a recalcitrant pollutant. Recombinat DNA methodologies can also be used to genetically engineer micro-organisms with the capacity to degrade many of these compounds, and many research efforts have been examining this methodological approach.

Concern about the environmental impact of genetically engineered micro-organisms has greatly constrained the possibility of deliberately releasing recombinant micro-organisms for environmental remediation. Using such recombinat micro-organisms may be possible within contained bioreactors, but their broader environmental applications will depend upon new understanding of ecological functions and risk assessments related to populations of introduced organisms.

As greater emphasis is being placed on pollution prevention than on remediation, micro-organisms are also being considered for their potential uses as biocatalysts. Biotechnology can play an important role because of its environmental advantages and its economic competitiveness in a number of industrial sectors. At an equivalent level of production, biocatalysts can reduce materials and energy consumption, as well as pollution and waste. A wide range of 'environmentally friendly chemicals' can be made from biomass, including biodegradable plastics and other novel biopolymers that do not accumulate and cause environmental damage. Biotechnology may also be used to produce cleaner fuels (for example, by selectively removing sulphur from diesel fuel and gasoline) that reduce the release of atmospheric pollutants. Alternative biomass-based fuels, such as bioethanol also can reduce the build-up of atmospheric carbon dioxide, thereby reducing global warming.

Biomining and biological control are additional important commerical applications of environmental biotechnology. Biomining is used for the recovery of copper and uranium; it is based upon the oxidation of metal sulphides so as to increase the solubility of the metal and its recovery by leaching. In biological control, micro-organisms are used as pesticides and herbicides. The effectiveness of microbial pesticides and herbicides is based on the natural antagonism or pathogenicity of specific micro-organisms toward particular plants and animals. Biological control is considered an environmentally more friendly method for controlling weeds, insects, and other pests populations than are applications of chemicals for controlling these unwanted nuisance populations.

Besides the applications of micro-organisms to reduce pollution and to support recovery of materials from the environment, environmental biotechnology is playing an important role in exploring natural ecological function. In many instances molecular approaches are providing new avenues for understanding the roles of micro-organisms within soils and waters that contribute to the maintenance of environmental quality and ecological productivity. Modern molecular techniques are facilitating studies on complex natural communities. Analyses of microbial communities often depend upon nucleic acid amplification techniques such as the PCR to make rare populations detectable, gene probes and hybridisation to detect specific genes and diagnostic nucleic acid sequences, and additional methods such as restriction digestion and electrophoretic separation to detect polymorphisms and specific strain characteristics.

Molecular methods are especially useful in assaying the diversity of complex microbial communities in their natural habitats, such as within biofilms. By revealing the natural functions of micro-organisms in the environment, it is possible to control some of those microbial activities, for example, to limit biocorrosion. It is also possible to carry out bioprospecting for micro-organisms with specific metabolic functions that are useful for industrial processes or that produce natural products that have commercial value, for example, as medicinals. In this manner the exploration of the natural microbial world can be exploited by environmental biotechnology.

Chapter 2

Stoichiometry and Bacterial Energetics

INTRODUCTION

The growth of micro-organisms occurs within a wide range of pHs and temperatures, and on a wide variety of nutrients. Figure 2.1 shows a typical batch experiment where a substrate (starting at concentration C_{so}) is converted by a micro-organism (C_{xo} at $t = 0$). The micro-organism grows exponentially at a specific growth rate μ^{max} and with yield Y_{Dx}^m. After depletion of the substrate, which is characterised by the substrate affinity constant K_s and a threshold concentration, the biomass concentration reaches $C_x = C_{xo} + Y_{Dx}^m C_{so}$. Subsequently the biomass concentration decreases due to maintenance and/or biomass decay, which is characterised by the maintenance coefficient m_D (or the decay coefficient k_d). The relevant substrate always acts as electron donor, and, therefore, it is proper to define the biomass yield and maintenance on donor (D).

In the design of processes with growing micro-organisms (fermentation processes and biological waste-treatment processes) the key parameters that need to be considered are the maximal biomass yield on substrate (Y_{Dx}^m), the substrate maintenance coefficient m_D, the maximal growth rate (μ_{max}), and the substrate affinity constant (K_s).

These four key parameters are sufficient to describe growth of micro-organisms in a standard mathematical model. A practical problem is, however, that the values of these parameters can vary by more than two orders of magnitude for different electron donors or acceptors used by different micro-organisms, as indicated in Fig. 2.1. It should be realised that conventionally stoichiometric parameters are expressed with C-mol of biomass, C-mol of electron donor for organic, and mol of donor for inorganic donors (C-mol X/(C)-mol D). It is, therefore, of interest to provide a general method to estimate values of these parameters for any chemotrophic growth system. Such methods have been provided by, for example, Battley, Roels, and Westerhoff. Recently, these methods have been critically evaluated with respect to general applicability and internal consistency. It was concluded that none of these methods was satisfying. However, a new method was proposed that is generally applicable and lacks the mentioned problem. Further, it should be recognised that in growth processes not only biomass production (r_x in C-mol biomass per m^3 reactor/hr) and electron donor (substrate) consumption r_D in C-mol substrate (for carbon compounds), or mol substrate (for noncarbon compounds) per m^3 reactor/hr are important. Also, the other conversions, such as O_2 consumption, N source consumption, heat production, and CO_2 production are highly relevant for the process design to calculate, for example, the required O_2 and heat transfer. Clearly, the full stoichiometry of the growth process should also be calculated and methods to achieve this are of major interest.

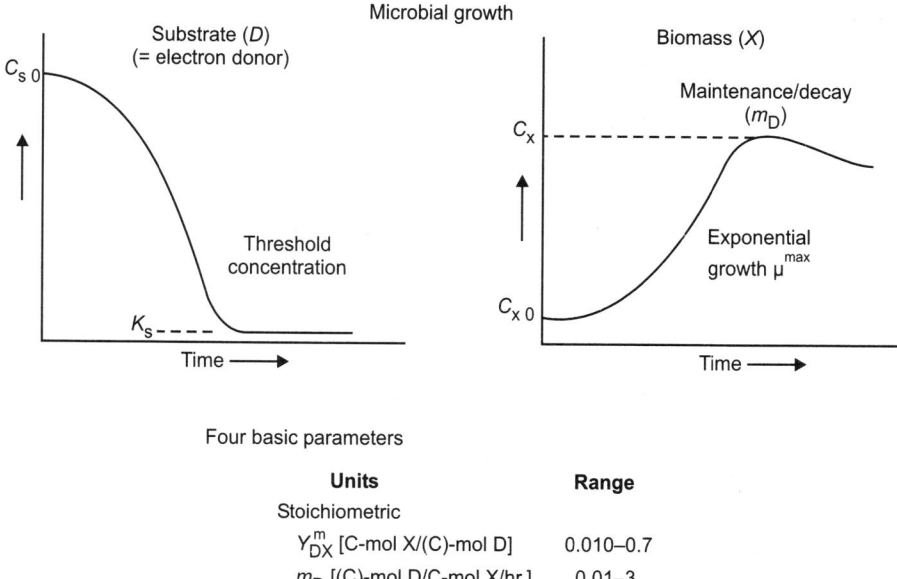

Microbial growth

Fig. 2.1. A typical microbial growth batch profile of biomass concentration and substrate concentration.

STANDARD DESCRIPTION OF MICROBIAL GROWTH STOICHIOMETRY

The stoichiometry of microbial growth is most easily understood from Fig. 2.2. Figure 2.2a introduces the biomass composition of 1 C-mol biomass (the ash-free organic fraction). The composition shown is fairly typical and is taken from Roels. One C-mol ash-free organic biomass is the amount of organic dry biomass that contains 12 grams of carbon.

The indicated biomass organic fraction corresponds to an elemental composition of 48.8 per cent carbon, 7.3 per cent hydrogen, 32.5 per cent oxygen, and 11.4 per cent nitrogen (w/w).

In practice, total dry biomass, which includes the organic fraction and the ash fraction (S, P, K, Mg, etc.), is measured. In general, the organic and ash fraction are obtained by combusting the organic biomass at 500° to 600°C and weighing the ashes. Recently, Battley has indicated that this simple procedure underestimates the real organic biomass weight by 5 to 6 per cent. This is due to the formation of P, S, and metal oxides in the ash during combustion, whereas such oxides are not present in the dry biomass. The composition formula follows directly from the elemental analysis of the biomass. In Fig. 2.2a only the four major elements (C, H, O, N) are shown; however, it is straightforward to include P, S, and metals such as K or Mg in this composition formula, and also in the stoichiometric/energetic calculation. Figure 2.2a also shows that in the formation of biomass for all chemotrophic growth systems a C source, N source, H_2O, CO_2, and H^+ are always involved. These five compounds provide the building elements for making biomass. This is also called anabolism. For heterotrophic organisms the C source is organic; for autotrophic organisms the C source is CO_2.

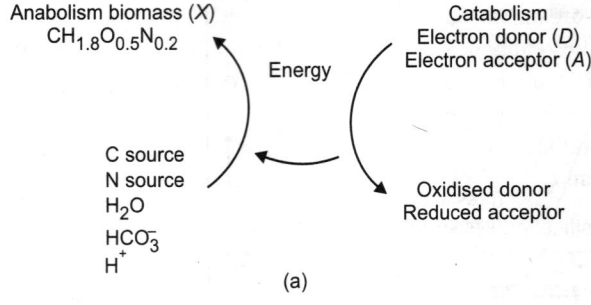

Microbial growth system

Anabolism biomass (X)
$CH_{1.8}O_{0.5}N_{0.2}$

Energy

Catabolism
Electron donor (D)
Electron acceptor (A)

C source
N source
H_2O
HCO_3^-
H^+

Oxidised donor
Reduced acceptor

(a)

Relevant stoichiometry

$-\dfrac{1}{Y_{DX}}$ (C)-mol electron donor $-$ (...) N-source

$-\dfrac{1}{Y_{AX}}$ mol electron acceptor $+$ 1 C-mol biomass

$+\dfrac{1}{Y_{QX}}$ (heat) $+\dfrac{1}{Y_{GX}}$ Gibbs energy

$+$ (...) H_2O $+$ (...) HCO_3^+ $+$ (...) H^+

Many different possibilities

Donor	Acceptor	C-source
Organic	Organic	Organic
Inorganic	Inorganic	Inorganic

$Y_{DX}0.01 - 0.7$ C-mol$X$/(C)mol donor

(b)

Fig. 2.2. (a) System definition of microbial growth. (b) Macrochemical reaction equation of microbial growth.

Although it is possible to establish a stoichiometrically correct description to make biomass from these five building compounds, it is easily shown that this is not acceptable from the point of view of the second law of thermodynamics. It has been calculated that the Gibbs energy of such a hypothetical reaction, depending on the C source used, is often positive, although sometimes small negative values can also be calculated. In addition, it is known that to convert the five compounds into biomass, micro-organisms use a large amount of biochemical energy in the form of ATP. Clearly the production of biomass from the five building compounds requires input of large quantities of Gibbs energy. The amount of energy needed to make biomass depends on the type of C source used. Intuitively, one expects that making 1 C-mol biomass from CO_2 requires more Gibbs energy than making 1 C-mol biomass from an organic compound. A quantitative relation for this energy need is presented later (Eqs 2.2, 2.3a, and 2.3b). The required energy, which must be taken as Gibbs energy and not as enthalpy, is delivered by a redox reaction between an electron donor and an electron acceptor. This redox reaction is called catabolism (Fig. 2.2a). Examples are the aerobic combustion of glucose ($C_6H_{12}O_6 + 6O_2 \rightarrow 6HCO_3^-$ $+ 6H^+$) and the anaerobic formation of ethanol from glucose ($C_6H_{12}O_6 + 2H_2O \rightarrow 2HCO_3^- + 2H^+ +$ $2C_2H_5OH$). Obtaining the required Gibbs energy is as essential for micro-organisms as it is for higher organisms, and even for human society. Therefore, it should not be surprising that during evolution a wide diversity of micro-organisms developed that are mainly different in the applied redox reaction for catabolism to obtain Gibbs energy (Fig. 2.2b). Electron donor or acceptor couples can be organic and inorganic compounds. This microbial variety in catabolic possibilities for generating Gibbs energy has led to the use of a classification system for naming micro-organisms (Table 2.1). This system is understandably based on the source of Gibbs energy (light or chemical energy), the source of electron donor (inorganic or organic), and the source of biomass carbon (CO_2 or organic).

Table 2.1. Microbial classification system.

Source of Gibbs energy	Source of electron donor	C-source
Light (phototrophic)	Inorganic (lithotrophic)	CO_2 (autotrophic)
Chemical (chemotrophic)	Organic (organotrophic)	Organic (heterotrophic)

In addition, micro-organisms may employ a wide variety of electron acceptors, as reflected in their class names. These class names are related to the electron acceptor used in catabolism (O_2, aerobic; NO_3^-, denitrification; SO_4^{2-}, sulphate reduction) fermentation (absence of external electron acceptor), or to the product of the catabolic reaction (CH_4, methanogenic; acetate, acetogenic; H_2S, sulphidogenic, etc.). The C source also functions often as electron donor, except in autotrophic micro-organisms, where the C source is CO_2. For example, a micro-organism growing aerobically in the dark on H_2S as the electron donor (inorganic compound) using CO_2 as the C source is called an aerobic chemolithoautotrophic organism. In summary, in each realistic chemotrophic microbial growth system there must be present the five compounds of anabolism and an electron donor/acceptor combination for catabolism.

These considerations bring us then to Fig. 2.2b, which shows the macrochemical reaction equation containing all the stoichiometric information of the growth process. The macrochemical equation of Fig. 2.2b should not be considered a mathematical equation but is a chemical reaction where substrates and products have negative and positive stoichiometric coefficients, respectively. Therefore, for $a = 0$, sign is absent. In addition, the stoichiometric involvement of enthalpy and Gibbs energy is expressed in their respective stoichiometric coefficients (Y_{QX}, and Y_{GX}, which have units of C-mol X/kJ). The macrochemical reaction equation is, therefore, a compact, but exact form of notation of the relevant stoichiometry of growth. This macrochemical equation shows that for the formation of +1 C-mol of biomass an amount of $-1/Y_{DX}$ of electron donor is required.

The minus sign shows that the electron donor is consumed. Y_{DX} is in C-mol biomass per C-mol electron donor (in case of an organic donor) or per mol donor (in case of an inorganic donor). Its units are written as C-mol X/(C) mol D. An amount of $-1/Y_{AX}$ mol electron acceptor is consumed (minus sign) per 1 C-mol biomass produced and, in addition, $1/Y_{QX}$ kJ of heat and $1/Y_{GX}$ kJ of Gibbs energy are involved in the production of 1 C-mol of biomass. $1/Y_{QX}$ and $1/Y_{GX}$ are found as the conventionally calculated enthalpy of reaction and Gibbs energy of reaction of the macrochemical reaction equation, which produces 1 C-mol of biomass. Finally, certain amounts of H_2O, CO_2, (or HCO_3^-), H^+, and N source are involved. It is important that in each macrochemical reaction equation in which biomass is grown, HCO_3^-, H_2O, H^+, and N source be present. The differences between different organisms occur mostly in the electron acceptor/donor combinations used. The N source is often NH_4^+ and sometimes NO_3^-, N_2, or something else.

The most important point in stoichiometry is to recognise that it is nearly always sufficient to measure one stoichiometric coefficient, that is, Y_{DX}, which is the traditional biomass yield on substrate (equal to carbon source and electron donor). All the other stoichiometric coefficients then follow from the so-called conservation equations (elements, electric charge, and enthalpy).

Example 2.1a: Calculation of stoichiometric coefficients in the macrochemical equation.

Consider the aerobic growth of *Pseudomonas oxalaticus* on oxalate using NH_4^+ as the N source. The relevant chemical compounds in this growth system are the five compounds [biomass ($CH_{1.8}O_{0.5}N_{0.2}$), NH_4^+, HCO_3^-, H^+, H_2O], the electron donor oxalate ($C_2O_4^{2-}$), and the electron acceptor O_2. In total, there are seven compounds and four elements (C, H, O, N). The conversion rates of these compounds are mathematically related by the conservation relations of C, H, O, N, and electric charge. In total there are five independent relations. This means that seven conversion rates are related by five conservation equations, and that the measurement of two rates (e.g. biomass production r_X and consumption of the electron donor oxalate r_D), which is equivalent to the measurement of $Y_{DX} = r_X/-r_D$, allows the calculation of all other yields.

Suppose that from measurement the biomass yield Y_{DX} is found to be $+0.086$ C-mol biomass produced per C-mol oxalate consumed. The proper macrochemical reaction equation can be written in a general form, without knowing all the stoichiometric coefficients but one ($+1$ for biomass), as:

$$fC_2O_4^{2-} + aNH_4^+ + bH^+ + cO_2 + dH_2O + 1CH_{1.8}O_{0.5}N_{0.2} + eHCO_3^-$$

The following conservation equations can now be written:

C conservation	$2f + 1 + e = 0$
H conservation	$4a + b + 2d + 1.8 + e = 0$
O conservation	$4f + 2c + d + 0.5 + 3e = 0$
N conservation	$a + 0.2 = 0$
Charge conservation	$-2f + a + b - e = 0$

Clearly there are six unknown stoichiometric coefficients (a–f) that are related by five conservation equations. (Biomass has been assigned a convenient, yet arbitrary coefficient $+1$.) Having one measured coefficient allows the calculation of all other coefficients. Y_{DX} was measured as 0.086. This means that $1/0.086 = 11.63$ C-mol oxalate are consumed to produce 1 C-mol biomass. The previously defined macrochemical equation contains f mol of oxalate, which was two carbon atoms. The stoichiometric coefficient f therefore has the value $-1163/2 = -5.815$ (remember the minus sign). Using this f value and the five conservation equations, one can calculate the whole chemical growth stoichiometry. The result is:

$$-5.815C_2O_4^{2-} - 0.2NH_4^+ - 0.8H^+ - 1.857O_2 - 5.42H_2O + 1CH_{1.8}O_{0.5}N_{0.2} + 10.63HCO_3^-$$

All the different biomass yields can be read from this reaction equation; thus, $Y_{AX} = 1/1.857 = 0.538$ C-mol biomass/mol O_2 or $Y_{CX} = 1/10.63 = 0.094$ C-mol biomass per mol CO_2.

In the Example 2.1a, only the chemical stoichiometry was calculated. However, there are two additional biomass yields of interest that relate the heat production and Gibbs energy dissipation occurring during the growth process to biomass production. These yields can be simply calculated if the full chemical stoichiometry is known by using tabulated ΔH_f^0 and ΔG_{f-}^{01} values (at pH = 7 and standard conditions) and calculating the enthalpy and Gibbs energy of reaction (Example 2.1b).

Table 2.2 contains all the required thermodynamic information as taken from Thauer and others. The values for biomass are taken from Roels. Although there is some discussion about the value of ΔG_f^{01} for biomass, its value is not very important in thermodynamic calculations, as shown by Heijnen.

Table 2.2. Standard Gibbs energy and enthalpy of formation.

Compound name	Composition	ΔG_f^{01} (kJ/mol)	ΔH_f (kJ/mol)
Biomass	$CH_{1.8}O_{0.5}N_{0.2}$	−67	−91
Water	H_2O	−237.18	−286
Bicarbonate	HCO_3^-	−586.85	−692
$CO_2(g)$	CO_2	−394.359	−394.1
Ammonium	NH_4^+	−79.37	−133
Proton	H^+	−39.87	0
$O_2(g)$	O_2	0	0
Oxalate^{2-}	$C_2O_4^{2-}$	−674.04	−824
Carbon monoxide	CO	−137.15	−111
Formate	CHO_2^-	−335	−410
Glyoxylate	$C_2O_3H^-$	−468.6	
Tartrate^{2-}	$C_4H_4O_6^{2-}$	−1010	
Malonate^{2-}	$C_3H_2O_4^{2-}$	−700	
Fumarate^{2-}	$C_4H_2O_4^{2-}$	−604.21	−777
Malate^{2-}	$C_4H_4O_5^{2-}$	−845.08	−843
Citrate^{3-}	$C_6H_5O_7^-$	−1168.34	−1515
Pyruvate$^-$	$C_3H_3O_2^-$	−474.63	−596
Succinate^{2-}	$C_4H_4O_4^{2-}$	−690.23	−909
Gluconate$^-$	$C_6H_{11}O_7^-$	−1154	
Formaldehyde	CH_2O	−130.54	
Acetate	$C_2H_3O_2^-$	−369.41	−486
Dihydroxyacetone	$C_3H_6O_3$	−445.18	−
Lactate	$C_3H_5O_3^-$	−517.18	−687
Glucose	$C_6H_{12}O_6$	−917.22	−1264
Mannitol	$C_6H_{14}O_6$	−942.61	−
Glycerol	$C_3H_8O_3$	−488.52	−676
Propionate$^-$	$C_3H_5O_{2+}$	−361.08	−
Ethylene glycol	$C_2H_6O_2$	−330.50	
Acetoine	$C_4H_8O_2$	−280	−
Butyrate	$C_4H_7O_2^-$	−352.63	−535
Propanediol	$C_3H_8O_2$	−327	−
Butanediol	$C_4H_{10}O_2$	−322	−
Methanol	CH_4O	−175.39	−246
Ethanol	C_2H_5O	−181.75	−288
Propanol	C_3H_8O	−175.81	−331
n-Alkane	$C_{15}H_{32}$	+60	−439
Propane	C_3H_8	−24	−104

(Contd ...)

Compound name	Composition	ΔG_f^{01} (kJ/mol)	ΔH_f (kJ/mol)
Ethane	C_2H_6	−32.89	−85
Methane	CH_4	−50.75	−75
$H_2(g)$	H_2	0	0
N_2 (g)	N_2	0	0
Nitrite ion	NO_2^-	−37.2	−107
Nitrate ion	NO_3^-	−111.34	−173
Iron II	Fe^{2+}	−78.87	−87
Iron III	Fe^{3-}	−4.6	−4
Hydrogen sulphide (g)	H_2S	−33.56	−20
Sulphide ion	HS^-	+12.05	−17
Sulphate ion	SO_4^{2-}	−744.63	−909
Thiosulphate ion	$S_2O_3^{2-}$	−513.2	−608

Note: pH = 7,1 atm, 1 mol/l 298 K.

Example 2.1b: Calculation of the yield of biomass on enthalpy and Gibbs energy (Y_{QX} and Y_{GX}).

The chemical stoichiometry from Example 2.1a and the appropriate ΔH_f^0 and ΔG_f^{01} values from Table 2.2 can be used to obtain the heat (enthalpy) and Gibbs energy of reaction.

The enthalpy of reaction, using ΔH_f^0 from Table 2.2, is calculated as:

$$(10.63)(-692) + 1(-91) - (5.42)(-286) - (1.857)(0) - (0.8)(0)$$

$$- (0.2)(-133) - (5.815)(-824) = -1078.7 \text{ kJ}$$

For the Gibbs energy of reaction using ΔG_f^{01} values there follows a value of −1052.4 kJ. Because in the macrochemical reaction 1 C-mol of biomass is produced, this means that for each 1 C-mol biomass produced there is a heat production of 1078.7 kJ and a Gibbs energy dissipation of 1052.4 kJ, showing that $Y_{QX} = 1/1078.7 = 0.00093$ C-mol biomass produced per kilojoule heat produced and that $Y_{GX} = 1/1052.4 = 0.0095$ C-mol biomass produced per kilojoule of Gibbs energy dissipated. The complete chemical and energetic stoichiometry now can be written as:

$$-5.815C_2O_4^{2-} - 0.2NH_4^+ - 0.8H^+ - 1.857O_2 - 5.42H_2O + 1CH_{1.8}O_{0.5}N_{0.2}$$

$$+ 10.63HCO_3^- + 1078.7 \text{ kJ heat} + 1052.4 \text{ kJ Gibbs energy}$$

Example 2.1 shows that the complete chemical and energetic stoichiometry of microbial growth can be calculated from one measured yield using conservation equations and the Gibbs energy and enthalpy balance (elements, charge, enthalpy, and the Gibbs energy balance). This means also that there must exist mathematical relations between Y_{DX}, Y_{AX}, Y_{CX}, Y_{QX}, and Y_{GX} (Fig. 2.2b). These relations are addressed in a later section (see Eqs 2.9a–2.9e). It is obvious that this knowledge of the complete growth stoichiometry provides essential engineering information with respect to reactor design on the amount of O_2 that must be transferred (aeration capacity), the amount of carbon dioxide that must be removed (ventilation), the amount of heat to be removed (cooling capacity), or the amount of fermentation products (in anaerobic growth).

The amounts of the required N source and HCO_3^- (autotrophic growth) also follow from these stoichiometric calculations.

MEASUREMENT OF GROWTH STOICHIOMETRY

As shown earlier, the measurement of one stoichiometric coefficient suffices, in general, to calculate all the other stoichiometric coefficients using the conservation relations. This measured stoichiometric coefficient requires the measurement of two conversion rates because, by definition, a stoichiometric coefficient is the ratio of two conversion rates. For example, $Y_{DX} = r_X/-r_D$. The most simple growth system contains eight conversion rates (biomass, N source, H^+, H_2O, CO_2, electron donor, electron acceptor, heat production) and six conservation equations (C, H, O, N, enthalpy, charge). Measurement of two conversion rates is then sufficient to calculate all other rates and, hence, the complete growth stoichiometry. Currently, the most common measurements are biomass production and substrate (equal to electron donor) consumption. For aerobic growth the on-line measurement of O_2 consumption and CO_2 production by the analysis of O_2 and CO_2 in the off-gas in air-sparged fermentors is becoming more and more routine. Especially for autotrophic growth, the on-line measurement of CO_2 consumption by off-gas analysis gives direct and highly accurate information on microbial growth (because all consumed CO_2 appears as biomass). This method was very successfully applied to study the growth stoichiometry and kinetics of solid pyrite oxidation by Fe^{2+}-oxidising bacteria and of *Methanobacrerium thermo-autotrophicum* on H_2/CO_2. Most recently, it was also shown that on-line measurement of heat production during microbial growth can be used to explore growth stoichiometry and kinetics.

However, such a simple approach of measuring only two conversion rates often makes certain assumptions:

1. Each chosen pair of measured conversion rates will allow the complete calculation of all other conversion rates.
2. All measurements are reliable within a certain statistical error but without a systematic deviation.
3. The assumed description of the growth system is correct, which means that by-products or additional substrates are assumed to be absent.

All these assumptions are subject to critical considerations. Here, simple examples are provided to illustrate the points of interest.

Noncalculability of Stoichiometry

Suppose that in Example 2.1a the chosen two conversion rates to be measured are biomass production (r_X) and NH_4^+ consumption (r_N). Measurement of these two rates would not lead to a calculation of the other rates because r_X and r_N occur in the nitrogen-conservation equation in such a way that r_X uniquely determines r_N, and vice versa. It is then said that r_X and r_N are redundant. The N balance gives a constraint for these two measured conversion rates that can be used to calculate the statistically best estimate of r_X and r_N, which also exactly satisfies the N balance. Clearly the choice of the two measured rates must be such that calculability of all other conversion rates is assured. In Example 2.1a, suitable combinations would be the oxygen consumption rate (r_O) and biomass production rate (r_X), r_O and the carbon dioxide production rate (r_C), or r_X and the heat production rate (r_Q).

Ill-Conditioned Calculability of Stoichiometry (Error Propagation)

It is well known that measured conversion rates have a certain measurement error. The subsequently calculated conversion rates, from combining the conservation relations and the two measurements, have an error due to error propagation. It is obviously of great practical importance to choose two measured conversion rates where this error propagation is minimal. A simple example to illustrate this problem is the aerobic growth of biomass on the donor glucose. If oxygen consumption ($-r_O$) and carbon dioxide production (r_C) are the measured rates, then the following relations (using conservation relations and the standard biomass composition) to calculate r_X and $-r_D$ (in C-mol glucose/m^3 hr) from the measured r_C and ($-r_O$) can be derived:

$$r_X = 20r_C - 20(-r_O)$$
$$(-r_D) = 20(-r_O) - 21r_C$$

Due to the large multiplication factors of 20 and 21 in these equations, the propagation of the measurement errors in r_C and r_O into r_X and $-r_D$ is enormous.

If the donor conversion rate ($-r_D$) and the carbon dioxide production rate (r_C) were chosen as the measured rates r_X and ($-r_O$) would be calculated as:

$$r_X = (-r_D) - r_C$$
$$(-r_O) = -0.05(-r_D) + 1.05r_C$$

The error propagation now is much lower and, therefore, from the measured ($-r_D$) and (r_C), r_X and ($-r_O$) can be calculated, as can be the other conversion rates involved. Clearly the aspect of error propagation is of major importance, and this propagation can be significantly decreased by a proper choice of the conversion rates to be measured.

Redundancy of Measurements

As stated earlier, in general two well-chosen measured conversion rates are usually sufficient to reliably calculate the complete stoichiometry. However, it is advantageous (Example 2.2) to measure more conversion rates than the minimum requirement of two. This leads to so-called redundant measurements, which can be used for two purposes error diagnosis and data reconciliation.

Error diagnosis

1. To check the validity of the defined growth systems with respect to the absence of by-products or possible second substrates.
2. To check the measured conversion rates for systematic errors.

Data reconciliation

To decrease the measurement error in the calculated and measured conversion rates, provided that the statistically based checks (error diagnosis) on the validity of the growth system and the systematic errors in the measured conversion rates are passed.

Example 2.2: Use of redundant measurements to establish the presence of errors in the definition of the growth system or in the measurements.

Consider the microbial growth system of Example 2.1a, where the following four conversion rates have been measured. The biomass has the standard elemental composition.

Biomass production	$r_X = +1$ C-mol/hr
O_2 consumption	$-r_O = 1.2$ mol/hr
HCO_3^- production	$r_C = 10.5$ mol/hr
Oxalic acid ($C_2O_4^{2-}$ consumption)	$-r_D = 5.8$ mol/hr

We know that a minimum of two rate measurements are needed to calculate the full stoichiometry. Therefore, there are two redundant measurements. We can now establish the conservation equations (with r_W, r_H, and r_N as the water, proton, and NH_4^+ conversion rates, respectively) based on conversion rates as:

C conservation	$2r_D + r_X + r_C = 0$
H conservation	$4r_N + r_H + 2r_W + 1.8r_X + r_C = 0$
O conservation	$4r_D + 2r_O + r_W + 0.5r_X + 3r_C = 0$
N conservation	$r_N + 0.2r_X = 0$
Charge conservation	$-2r_D + r_N + r_H - r_C = 0$

By eliminating the three non-measured rates (r_W, r_H, r_N) from these five conservation equations, one obtains $5 - 3 = 2$ equations, which relate the measured conversion rates only, The result is as follows:

$$2r_D + r_X + r_C = 0$$
$$2r_D - 4r_O + 4.2r_X = 0$$

The first relation can be recognised as the carbon balance, and the second is so-called electron balance or the balance of degree of reduction. With respect to the C balance, one finds from the measurements:

$$\text{C-in} = 2 \times 5.8(\text{oxalate}) = 11.6 \text{ C-mol/hr}$$
$$\text{C-out} = 1(\text{biomass}) + 10.5(CO_2) = 11.5 \text{ C-mol/hr}$$

Clearly the C balance seems satisfying (0.86 per cent gap). For the balance of degree of reduction one obtains:

$$\text{Electrons in} = 2 \times 5.8 = 11.6 \text{ mol electrons/hr}$$
$$\text{Electrons out} = -1.2(-4) + 1(4.2) = 9 \text{ mol electrons/hr}$$

Clearly there is a large gap of 2.6 mol electrons/hr

Because the C balance fits, it is reasonable to assume that the measured values of r_D, r_X, and r_C are reliable. The balance of degree of reduction can, therefore, be wrong for two reasons:

1. A very inaccurate measurement of r_O.
2. If the measurement of r_O is found to be correct, then the only other possibility is the presence of an additional electron acceptor (e.g. NO_3^-). This would be an error in the defined growth system.

Mathematically Complete Analysis of Calculability, Analysis of Redundancy, Error Diagnoses, and Data Reconciliation

In the preceding section simple examples were provided to highlight the problems in accurately establishing the full growth stoichiometry from measurements. Because all these calculations are based on linear conservation relations, it is highly appropriate to use matrix algebra. Basic to these calculations is the 'elemental' matrix, which specifies the element, charge, and enthalpy information for each compound in the growth system. Recently, an extensive and coherent mathematical description has been provided for calculability, redundancy analysis, error diagnosis, statistical aspects, and data reconciliation using involved matrix algebra. The developed mathematical theory has been put in a user-friendly computer program called Macrobal.

EFFECT OF GROWTH RATE ON GROWTH STOICHIOMETRY

Maintenance Energy Concept

In his pioneering work, Monod found that in exponential growth the amount of biomass formed increased in proportion to the amount of substrate consumed. This led to the definition of growth yield Y_{DX}

[amount of biomass produced per amount of electron donor (substrate) consumed]. We have seen that Y_{DX} usually determines the complete growth stoichiometry. With the introduction of the chemostat in the early 1950s, microbial growth could be studied at a range of growth rates, and it became clear that Y_{DX} decreased at lower growth rates μ, as shown in Fig. 2.3. This phenomenon was explained by two different concepts:

1. Endogenous respiration or microbial decay, determined by the parameter k_d.
2. Electron donor (substrate) requirements for maintenance, determined by the parameter m_D.

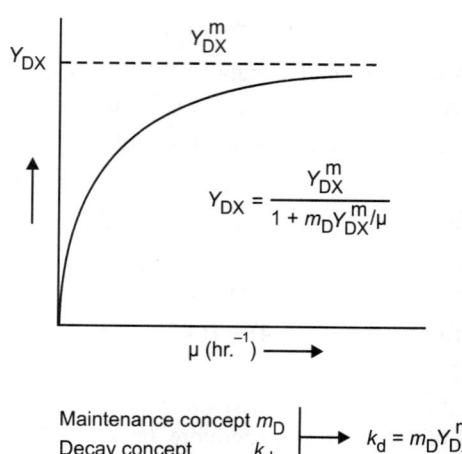

Fig. 2.3. Dependence of Y_{DX} on growth rate μ.

The basic idea is, however, similar in recognising that a micro-organism is a complex structure where the polymers (proteins, etc.) are subject to slow thermal denaturation and where there are numerous small leaks associated with the many transmembrane gradients (e.g. Na^+ leaking into the micro-organism). These leaking substances must be pumped out, and the degraded polymers must be rebuilt at the expense of Gibbs energy. This results in a small, but finite, need of Gibbs energy to maintain the biomass structure and the transmembrane gradients (maintenance Gibbs energy). In the concept of endogeneous respiration or microbial decay, this energy is produced by catabolism of biomass itself. In the concept of maintenance this energy is produced by catabolism of a part of the substrate (electron donor).

Mathematically, the dependence of Y_{DX} on growth rate μ is described by Eq. 2.1a and shown in Fig. 2.3.

$$1/Y_{DX} = 1/Y_{DX}^m + m_D/\mu \tag{2.1a}$$

This equation contains two model parameters, Y_{DX}^m and m_D, where m_D is the rate of consumption of electron donor (substrate) that is catabolised to generate the necessary Gibbs energy flow for maintenance in C-mol electron donor per C-mol biomass per hour. Y_{DX}^m is the maximal biomass yield. Figure 2.3 shows that Y_{DX}, using Eq. 2.1a, decreases with decreasing growth rate. Clearly, at higher growth rates Y_{DX} comes close to Y_{DX}^m. Using typical values for m_D it can be shown that only for $\mu < 0.01$ to 0.05 hr^{-1}, Y_{DX} starts dropping significantly below Y_{DX}^m. This means that in exponential growth, as occurs in batch fermentation where μ is high, the stoichiometry is properly covered by Y_{DX}^m. However, in many industrial-fed batch-production processes, maintenance is extremely important due to the low growth rates applied. For example, in penicillin fermentation $μ ≈ 0.01 \ hr^{-1}$ and about 70 per cent of all consumed glucose is spent for maintenance. Similarly, in waste-water-treatment processes, where low growth rates are also applied, the maintenance effects are very relevant. However, in this area one often uses the biomass decay coefficient k_d. This coefficient is, however, related to m_D according to $k_d = m_D \ Y_{DX}^m$. In general, it can be shown that all biomass yields, Y_{iX} as defined in Fig. 2.2a, decrease with decreasing growth rate μ.

Measuring m_D

Equation 2.1a shows that Y_{DX}^m and m_D can be obtained directly by measuring Y_{DX} at different growth rates μ. Using Eq. 2.1a to plot $1/Y_{DX}$ versus $1/μ$ as a straight line to obtain $1/Y_{DX}^m$ and m_D is, however, not desirable, because the error distribution of the measurements Y_{DX} and μ is completely distorted due to the use of $1/Y_{DX}$ and $1/μ$.

It is more proper to directly use the nonlinear Eq. 2.1a in combination with the measured Y_{DX} and μ, and to use an algorithm for nonlinear parameter estimation. It is stressed that for accurate m_D values one should measure Y_{DX} at low growth rates $(0.005–0.03 \ hr^{-1})$.

Example 2.3a: Calculating Y_{DX}^m and m_D from measured Y_{DX} as function of growth rate μ.

Consider aerobic growth on glucose and that there are two measurements available. At $μ = 0.5 \ hr^{-1}$, $Y_{DX} = 0.49$ C-mol biomass per C-mol glucose, and at $μ = 0.02 \ hr^{-1}$, $Y_{DX} = 0.33$. Applying equation 2.1a will show that $Y_{DX}^m = 0.50$ and $m_D = 0.02$ C-mol glucose/C-mol biomass/hr.

Other Maintenance Quantities

Micro-organisms require Gibbs energy for maintenance. This is obtained by catabolising the required amount of electron donor m_D. It is then obvious that other quantities, such as electron acceptor, heat, Gibbs energy, oxidised electron donor, and reduced electron acceptor, are also involved in maintenance, to catabolise the m_D electron donor. These maintenance-related quantities are directly obtained from the stoichiometry of the catabolic reaction (Example 2.3b).

Example 2.3b: Calculating other maintenance rates using the catabolic reaction.

In Example 2.3a it was found that $m_D = 0.02$ C-mol glucose/C-mol biomass/hr.

In the growth system being considered, the catabolic reaction is the aerobic oxidation of glucose according to:

$$C_6H_{12}O_6 - 6O_2 + 6HCO_3^- + 6H^+ + 2814 \ kJ \ heat + 2843 \ kJ \ Gibbs \ energy$$

Using the stoichiometry of this catabolic reaction and the known m_D, it is now easy to calculate the other maintenance rates:

Maintenance glucose m_D	= 0.02 C-mol glucose/C-mol Xh
	= 0.02/6 mol glucose/C-mol biomass/hr
Maintenance oxygen m_A	= 0.02/6 × 6 mol O_2/C-mol biomass/hr
Maintenance HCO_3^- m_C	= 0.02/6 × 6 mol CO_2/C-mol biomass/hr
Maintenance heat m_q	= 0.02/6 × 2814 kJ/C-mol biomass/hr
Maintenance Gibbs energy m_G	= 0.02/6 × 2843 kJ/C-mol biomass/hr

Complete Growth Stoichiometry as a Function of Growth Rate

Equation 2.1a shows how $1/Y_{DX}$ depends on the growth rate μ and the two parameters Y_{DX}^m and m_D. Completely similar equations can be derived for growth yields on acceptor (A), carbon dioxide (C), heat (Q), and Gibbs energy (G) according to Eq. 2.1b:

$$1/Y_{iX} = 1/Y_{iX}^m + \frac{m_i}{\mu}$$

... (2.1b)

Here i can be A, C, Q, or G. The maintenance coefficients for the different compounds are related to m_D according to Example 2.3b. The maximal yields Y_{AX}^m, Y_{CX}^m, Y_{QX}^m and Y_{GX}^m are related to Y_{DX}^m, and can be found by solving the macrochemical equation, using the available Y_{DX}^m value, according to Example 2.1.

THERMODYNAMICALLY BASED METHOD TO ESTIMATE GROWTH STOICHIOMETRY

In the previous paragraphs the methods for accurate measurement of a growth stoichiometric coefficient, as, for example, the biomass yield on electron donor Y_{DX} and the subsequent calculation of all the non-measured stoichiometric coefficients of the macrochemical equation (using the conservation principles) have been provided. In past decades, the value of Y_{DX} for many different micro-organisms, different electron donors, C sources, and electron acceptors has been measured under C- and energy-limited growth conditions. Many methods have been proposed to predict Y_{DX} because of its obvious importance. Recently, a critical evaluation of these methods has been performed. The following criteria were used for the evaluation:

1. The method should be generally applicable to all chemotrophic growth systems.
2. The method should relate directly to the second law of thermodynamics.
3. No detailed knowledge of metabolism is required; only the identity of the electron donor, C source, and electron acceptor is known.
4. Methodological problems are absent.

The conclusion of this evaluation was that none of the published methods satisfied these simple criteria. Therefore, an alternative method that satisfies the mentioned criteria has been proposed. This method is based on $1/Y_{GX}$, which is the amount of Gibbs energy (in kilojoules) that must be dissipated for the production of I C-mol biomass. The Gibbs energy stoichiometric parameter $1/Y_{GX}$ has already been introduced as one of the stoichiometric coefficients in the macrochemical reaction equation (Fig. 2.2b). Therefore, it is obvious that this energetic parameter can be calculated directly if only one of the chemical stoichiometric coefficients has been measured and if the electron donor, electron acceptor, and C source are known (see Example 2.1b, where $1/Y_{GX} = 1052$ kJ/C-mol biomass).

Furthermore, it is well known that the value of growth yields depends on the growth rate (μ) due to the Gibbs energy that must be used for maintenance. This means that the Gibbs energy needed to produce biomass should be divided into two parts:

1. A growth-related part.
2. A maintenance-related part.

Mathematically this can be expressed as:

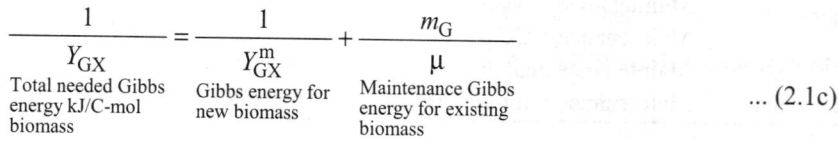

$$\underset{\substack{\text{Total needed Gibbs} \\ \text{energy kJ/C-mol} \\ \text{biomass}}}{\frac{1}{Y_{GX}}} = \underset{\substack{\text{Gibbs energy for} \\ \text{new biomass}}}{\frac{1}{Y_{GX}^m}} + \underset{\substack{\text{Maintenance Gibbs} \\ \text{energy for existing} \\ \text{biomass}}}{\frac{m_G}{\mu}}$$

... (2.1c)

where $1/Y_{GX}^m$ is the Gibbs energy needed to make 1 C-mol of biomass (kJ/C-mol X) and m_G is the Gibbs energy needed for biomass maintenance (kJ/C-mol biomass hr).

The biomass specific growth rate (hr^{-1}) is μ.

Clearly, at high growth rate μ, the m_G/μ term becomes negligible and $1/Y_{GX}$ becomes practically equal to Y_{DX}^m. At low growth rates Y_{GX} becomes much lower than Y_{GX}^m.

Equation 2.1c shows that in order to calculate Y_{GX} as a function of growth rate μ we need information about Y_{GX}^m and m_G. In the past years two simple correlations have been found with which to estimate Y_{GX}^m and m_G. These correlations were established using a very large body of experimental growth yields, which covered carbon- and energy-limited growth for the following:

1. Many different micro-organisms (bacteria, fungi, plant cells).
2. Many different C sources, including CO_2 and a wide variety of organic substrates.
3. Different electron acceptors (aerobic, anaerobic, denitrifying).
4. Electron donors that need reversed electron transport (RET).

The resulting correlations are given in Eqs 2.2 and 2.3. Figure 2.4 shows the m_G data used to establish Eq. 2.2; Fig. 2.5 shows the $1/Y_{GX}^m$ data used to establish the correlations 2.3a and 2.3b.

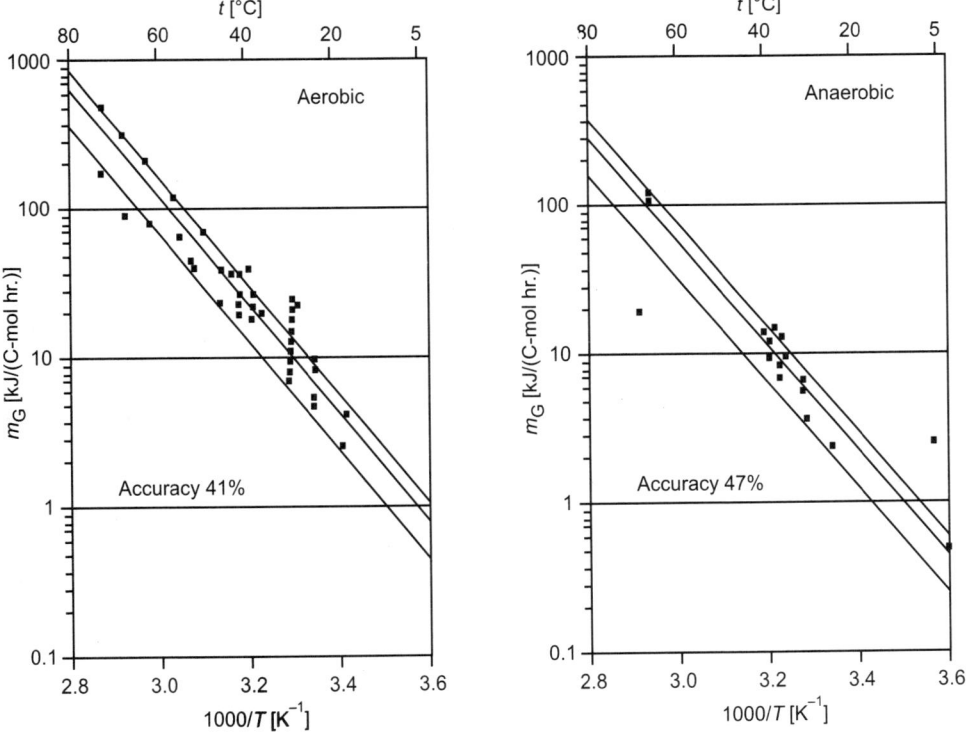

Fig. 2.4. Maintenance Gibbs energy m_G (in kJ/C-mol biomass hr) for aerobic (a) and anaerobic (b) growth shown as an Arrhenius function of temperature. The lines represent Eq. 2.2.

Maintenance Gibbs Energy Need m_G

The data for m_G as a function of temperature shown in Fig. 2.4 can be correlated with an Arrhenius type of relation:

$$m_G = 4.5 \ \exp\left[\frac{-69,000}{R}\left(\frac{1}{T} - \frac{1}{298}\right)\right] \qquad \text{... (2.2)}$$

This correlation was found to hold (with ±40 per cent accuracy) for a very wide variety of organisms, for different electron donors, for aerobic and anaerobic conditions, and for a temperature range of 5°–75°C. Obviously, the main influencing factor is the temperature, which behaves as an Arrhenius function with an activation energy of 69,000 J/mol.

The type of electron donor (organic or inorganic), the micro-organism, and the electron acceptor are of minor importance. This seems logical, because maintenance is a biomass-linked Gibbs-energy-requiring process that counteracts the biomass-deteriorating processes (protein degradation, leakage over cell membranes, etc.).

Gibbs Energy for Growth

The data for Y_{GX}^m shown in Fig. 2.5a (heterotrophic growth) and Fig. 2.5b (autotrophic growth) can be correlated by Eqs 2.3a and 2.3b. For autotrophic growth it was found to be important to distinguish electron donors for which reversed electron transport (RET) was necessary. Such electron donors (e.g. Fe^{2+}/Fe^{3+}, NH_4^+/NO_2^-) provide electrons that have insufficient Gibbs energy to reduce the C source CO_2 to biomass. Micro-organisms using such electron donors first have to increase the Gibbs energy level of the donor electrons by the biochemical process RET.

Heterotrophic growth/autotrophic growth (–RET)

$$1/Y_{GX}^m = 200 + 18(6 - C)^{1.8} + \exp[((3.8 - \gamma)^2)^{0.16} (3.6 + 0.4C)] \qquad \text{... (2.3a)}$$

Autotrophic growth (+RET):

$$1/Y_{GX}^m = 3500 \qquad \text{... (2.3b)}$$

It was found that the Gibbs energy dissipation required for the production of 1 C-mol biomass mainly depends on the C source used (Eqs 2.3a and 2.3b). The type of micro-organism and the type of electron acceptor have only minor effects, as shown in Figs 2.5a and 2.5b. The influence of the C source on Y_{GX}^m can be characterised by the following:

1. Its number C of carbon atoms (e.g. for CO_2 C = 1 and for glucose C = 6) as shown in Fig. 2.5a.
2. Its degree of reduction γ.

γ is a stoichiometric number of a chemical compound that represents the number of electrons in the compound. For organic compounds γ is per C-mol, for inorganic compounds y is per mol. For example, for CO_2 $\gamma = 0$, for CH_4 $\gamma = 8$, and for glucose $\gamma = 4$. The concept of degree of reduction will be further elucidated extensively later in this chapter. For organic compounds (Fig. 2.5a), γ has a value between 0 and 8.

For inorganic compounds (Fig. 2.5b), only a lower value of 0 holds; a maximal value does not exist because there is no normalisation per atom.

It is relevant to know that biomass has a degree of reduction of about 4.2. Equation 2.3a and Fig. 2.5a show that, in the situation that RET is not required for both hetero- and autotrophic growth, the Gibbs energy needed to produce biomass.

1. Increases if the number of C atoms in the carbon source (the parameter C in Eq. 2.3a) decreases.
2. Increases if the degree of reduction of the carbon source (the parameter γ in Eq. 2.3a) is smaller or larger than about 3.8.

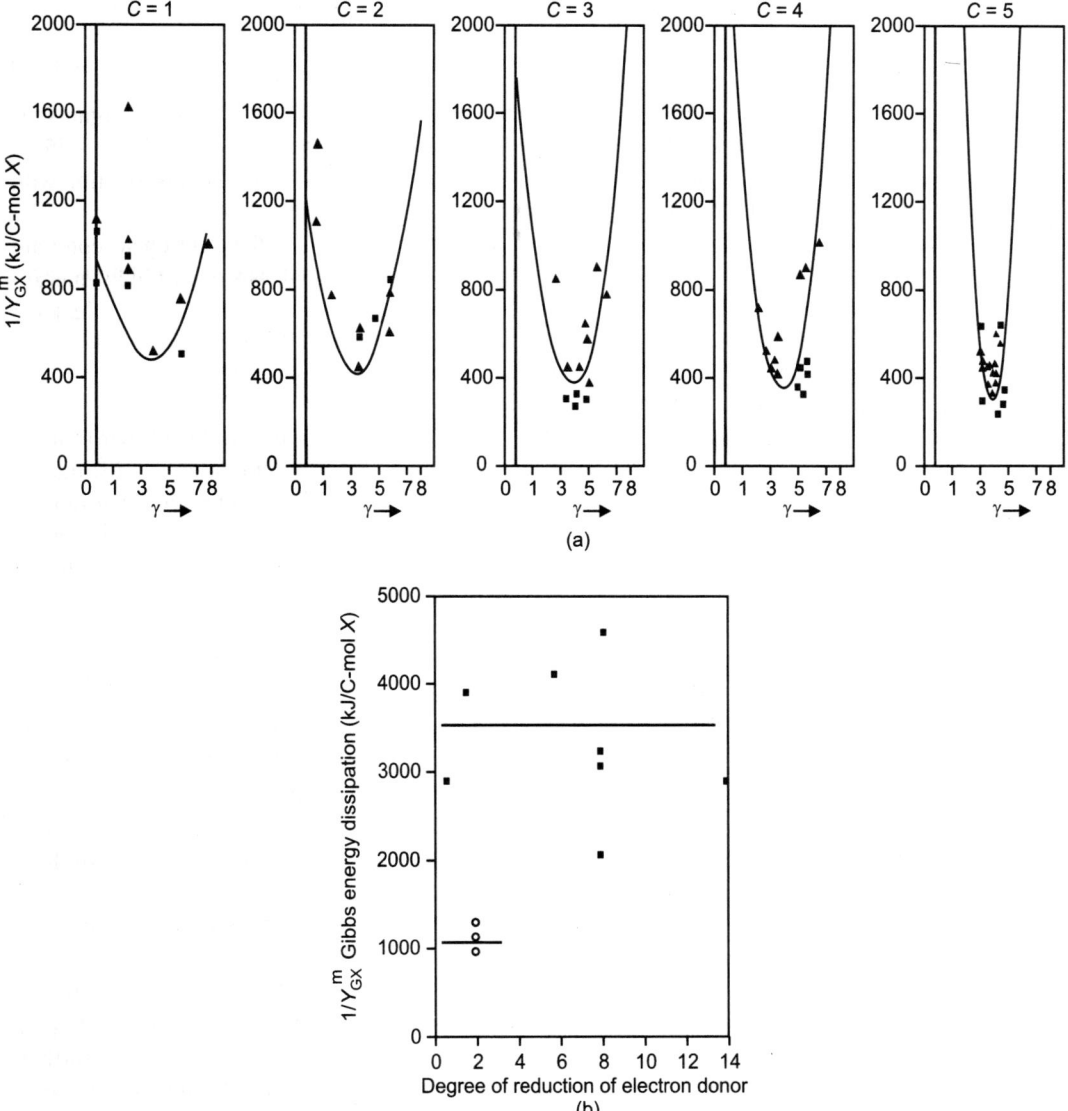

Fig. 2.5. Reciprocal maximal yield of biomass on Gibbs energy, $1/Y_{GX}^m$, (kJ/C-mol X); (a) Heterotrophic growth (triangles, aerobic; squares, fermentation, X's denitrifying systems); C is the number of carbon atoms in the carbon source; γ is the degree of reduction of the carbon source. (b) Autotrophic growth (squares, electron donors where reversed electron transport [RET] is needed; circles, donors without RET). The lines represent Eqs 2.3a and 2.3b.

Equation 2.3a further shows that for heterotrophic growth $1/Y_{GX}^m$ ranges between about 200 and 1000 kJ/C-mol biomass, for the C sources explored, for which:

1. The number of carbon atoms in the carbon source ranges between $C = 1$ (e.g. CO_2, formate, methane) and $C = 6$ (e.g. glucose, citrate).
2. The degree of reduction of the C source γ ranges between 0 (for CO_2) and 8 (for CH_4).

The effect of the number of C atoms (C) and degree of reduction (γ) of the C source can be simply understood as follows:

1. Biomass contains many polymers that contain monomers of four to six C atoms. If the C source contains fewer than four to six C atoms, the micro-organism must perform extra biochemical reactions to achieve C-C couplings. This requires extra Gibbs energy, compared to a C source that has six C-atoms, Hence $1/Y_{GX}^m$ increases for C-sources with less carbon atoms.

2. Biomass has $\gamma = 4.2$. If the C source is more reduced ($\gamma > 4.2$) or more oxidised ($\gamma < 4.2$), there is a need for additional oxidation reactions or reduction reactions, respectively, as compared to a carbon source (like glucose) with $\gamma = 4$. These additional reactions lead to extra Gibbs energy dissipation, leading to a higher value of $1/Y_{GX}^m$.

Simply stated, the more biochemical tinkering is needed to convert an organic C source into biomass, the more Gibbs energy is dissipated and the higher $1/Y_{GX}^m$ becomes. Obviously glucose ($C = 6, \gamma = 4$) is a nearly ideal C-source because it requires the least Gibbs energy dissipation for biomass production. According to Eq. 2.3a, for glucose $1/Y_{GX}^m = 200 + 0 + 36 = 236$ kJ/C-mol biomass. In contrast, CO_2 is a very poor C source, because it requires about four times as much Gibbs energy ($1/Y_{GX}^m = 200 + 236 + 460 = 986$ kJ/C-mol according to Eq. 2.3a). Equation 2.3b shows that for autotrophic growth, in the situation where RET is needed (which occurs for many inorganic electron donors), $1/Y_{GX}^m$ has a very high value of 3500 kJ/C-mol biomass. This value should be compared to autotrophic growth without RET as occurs with, for example, H_2 or CO as electron donor (for which $1/Y_{GX}^m \approx 1000$ kJ/C-mol according to Eq. 2.3a).

Obviously, the use of RET increases the Gibbs energy dissipation needed for biomass production tremendously. The explanation is that, using the RET process, the electrons of the electron donor are increased in energy level, up to the energy level of electrons in NADH in order to make CO_2 reduction to biomass thermodynamically feasible. This 'energy-pumping' process (RET) apparently requires a large amount of Gibbs energy, of about $3500-1000 = 2500$ kJ/C-mol biomass produced.

The effect that the type of the available C source has on the Gibbs energy needed for biomass synthesis is well known in biochemistry. Biochemists express the energy need in ATP. Figure 2.6 compares the calculated Gibbs energy dissipation needed for biomass synthesis ($1/Y_{GX}^m$, in kJ/C-mol X) with the theoretically calculated amount of ATP expenditure for biomass synthesis in mol ATP/C-mol X. The points shown are for different C sources, ranging from glucose to CO_2. The parenthetical numbers are the published biomass yields on ATP in gram-X/mol ATP. It is clear that there is a close correspondence, which is logical. Equations 2.3a and 2.3b provide the energy needed for biomass synthesis in kilojoules, whereas the biochemists use mol ATP as the energy measure. In conclusion, it should be realised that Eqs 2.2, 2.3a and 2.3b are completely sufficient to estimate a biomass yield and the full macrochemical equation for any arbitrary chemotrophic growth system. The predictive accuracy of this correlation for chemotrophic growth has been shown to be ± 10 to 20 per cent relative error in a yield range of nearly two orders of magnitudes of 0.01–0.70 C-mol biomass per C-mol organic electron donor or per mol inorganic donor while covering aerobic, anaerobic, denitrifying, autotrophic microbial systems with and without RET (Fig. 2.7).

Example 2.4. Calculation of the full macrochemical reaction equation using the correlations of Eqs 2.2, 2.3a, and 2.3b.

It is assumed that a micro-organism grows anaerobically on methanol as C source and electron donor with NH_4^+ as the N source and acetate is produced. The growth system contains biomass, NH_4^+, H^+,

HCO_3^-, H_2O, methanol, and acetate as the seven compounds. The general macrochemical reaction equation for the production of 1 C-mol biomass can be written as follows:

$$f CH_3OH + aNH_4^+ + bH^+ + cC_2H_3O_2^- + dH_2O + 1CH_{1.8}O_{0.5}N_{0.2} + eHCO_3^-$$

Clearly there are six unknown stoichiometric coefficients (a-f). However, using Eq. 2.3a we can calculate that ($C = 1$, $\gamma = 6$ for methanol, maintenance has been neglected) $1/Y_{GX}^m = 200 + 326 + 172 = 698$ kJ/C-molX. This means that we know that the Gibbs energy of reaction of the macrochemical reaction equation equals –698 kJ.

We can now write the conservation equations for C, H, O, N, electric charge, and the Gibbs energy balance (taking values of ΔG_f^{01} from Table 2.2):

C balance	$f + 2c + 1 + e = 0$
H balance	$4f + 4a + b + 3c + 2d + 1.8 + e = 0$
O balance	$f + 2c + d + 0.5 + 3e = 0$
N balance	$a + 0.2 = 0$
Charge balance	$a + b - c - e = 0$

Gibbs energy balance $(-175.39)f + (-79.37)a + (-39.87)b + (-369.41)c$

$$+ (-237.18)d + (-67)1 + (-586.85)e + 698 = 0$$

Solving these six equations gives, for a to f,

$$a = -0.2;\ b = 2.866;\ c = 8.898;\ d = 12.964;\ e = -6.232;\ f = -12.564$$

This gives a biomass yield on methanol of $1/12.564 = 0.08$ C-mol biomass/C-mol methanol. The stoichiometric result also shows that the acetate production is $8.898/12.564 = 0.70$ mol acetate/mol methanol, showing a C yield of 1.4 acetate carbon/methanol-carbon. This is, of course, due to the CO_2 fixation that occurs (6.232 mol HCO_3^- per 12.564 mol methanol).

If maintenance is not allowed to be neglected m_G must be taken into account. For example, the temperature is assumed to be 50°C. Equation 2 then shows that $m_G = 38.8$ kJ/C-mol biomass hr. If the growth rate $\mu = 0.03$ hr^{-1}, then we can calculate, using Eq. 2.1c that $1/Y_{GX} = 698 + 38.8/(0.03) = 1991$ kJ/C-mol biomass. Using this number one can solve the six equations to obtain the complete stoichiometry, which holds under these conditions.

Before ending this chapter, a final warning is relevant. The described thermodynamic method of predicting growth stoichiometry is based on a very wide database of experimentally measured growth systems. No detailed biochemical information is required, because intrinsically a kind of average biochemistry used by most organisms is assumed.

This is an attractive feature, but in the end we should consider that, of course, the biochemistry used by micro-organisms does have a significant influence. For example, for the anaerobic ethanol fermentation on glucose the mentioned method will give $Y_{DX} = 0.15$ C-mol biomass/C-mol glucose. This is indeed found for *Saccharomyces cerevisae*. However, another organism, *Zymomonas mobilis*, does the same glucose/ethanol process, but with $Y_{DX} = 0.07$. The explanation is that *Z. mobilis* uses a completely different biochemical pathway for glucose catabolism than *S. cerevisae*. From this example we can also learn that if the predicted biomass yield differs very substantially from the actually measured yield, it might be possible that the micro-organism being studied uses a novel pathway for catabolism or anabolism.

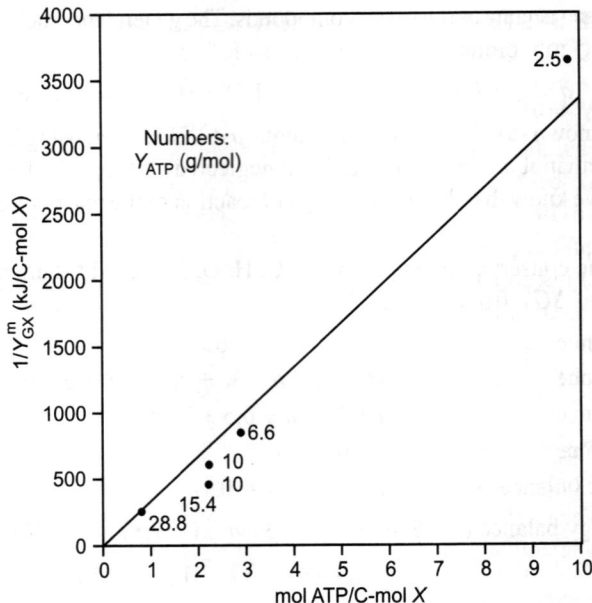

Fig. 2.6. Comparison of energy needed for biomass synthesis on different carbon sources in mol ATP/C-mol biomass and in kJ/C-mol biomass $(1/Y_{GX}^m)$. The numbers refer to the conventional biomass yield on ATP in gram biomass/mol ATP for different carbon sources.

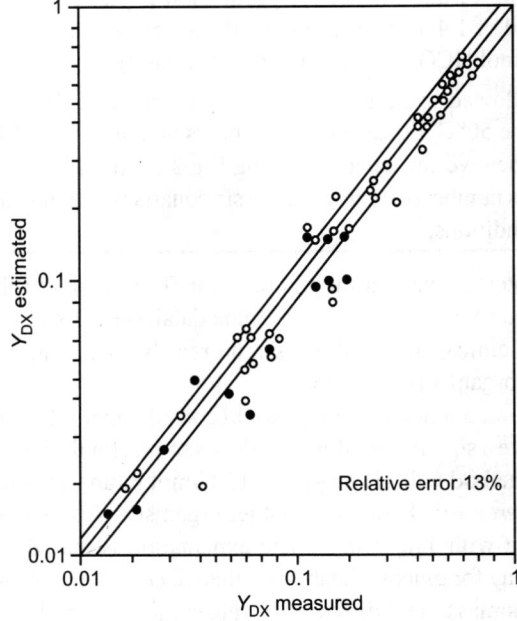

Fig. 2.7. Comparison of measured and predicted biomass yield Y_{DX} (solid circles, fermentative; open circles, aerobic growth systems).

USEFUL REFERENCE SYSTEM TO SIMPLIFY GROWTH STOICHIOMETRIC AND ENERGETIC CALCULATIONS AND TO GAIN INSIGHT

Growth Reference System

In the preceding sections, the stoichiometric coefficients for the macrochemical reaction equation of biomass formation have been solved by setting up the proper conservation equations (C, H, O, N, charge, enthalpy) and the Gibbs energy balance. Although this is a sufficient and straightforward method, solving these linear equations remains unattractive and does not provide insight. To simplify these calculations and to gain insight, a special reference system has been designed—the growth reference system. This reference system is based on the observation that, in all chemotrophic growth systems, H_2O, HCO_3^-, H^+, and N source (mostly NH_4^+) occur as chemical compounds (see earlier section on growth system definition). In this special reference system each chemical compound is assigned three new numbers.

γ The degree of reduction, which represents the electron content per C-mol (for organic compounds) or per mol (for inorganic compounds).

ΔG_e The Gibbs energy per electron present in the compound.

ΔH_e The enthalpy per electron present in the compound.

Clearly γ is a stoichiometric quantity and ΔG_e and ΔH_e are energetic parameters.

The reference system is designed such that for H_2O, HCO_3^-, H^+ (pH = 7), N source for growth, HPO_4^{2-}, NO_3^-, SO_4^{2-}, and Fe^{3+}, the values of γ, ΔG_e, and ΔH_e are zero. For ΔG_e, the biochemical standard conditions (1 mol/l, 1 bar, pH = 7298 K) are assumed, ΔH_e is calculated for CO_2 (gas) because of the large heat effect of HCO_3^- (liq) $\Leftrightarrow$ CO_2 (gas) transfer. The calculation of γ, ΔG_e, and ΔH_e follows from the reference redox half reaction where 1 C-mol of organic or 1 mol of inorganic compound is converted into the reference chemicals and a number of electrons. The number of electrons is by definition equal to γ (Example 2.5). From the Gibbs energy and enthalpy of this reference reaction, called ΔG_{ref} and ΔH_{ref} (calculated with the usual thermodynamic ΔG_f^{01}, and ΔH_f^{01} values, see Table 2.2), the values of ΔG_e and ΔH_e follow from equations 2.4a and 2.4b.

$$\Delta G_e = \frac{-\Delta G_{ref}}{\gamma} \qquad \text{... (2.4a)}$$

$$\Delta H_e = \frac{-\Delta H_{ref}}{\gamma} \qquad \text{... (2.4b)}$$

Example 2.5. The reference redox half reaction and calculation of γ and ΔG_e for chemical compounds.

For methanol the following reference redox half reaction can be set up according to the preceding definition by converting methanol to the reference compounds HCO_3^-, H_2O, and H^+

$$-1CH_4O - 2H_2O + HCO_3^- + 7H^+ + 6e^-$$

In this reference redox half reaction, 1 C-mol methanol is converted and six electrons are produced, hence $\gamma = +6$ for methanol. Using the ΔG_f^{01} values from Table 2.2, the ΔG_{ref} for the methanol-reference redox half reaction follows as (standard conditions)

$$\Delta G_{ref}^{01} = (7)(-39.87) + 1(-586.85) - (2)(-237.18) - (1)(-181.75) = -216.192 \text{ kJ}$$

This gives for the ΔG_e^{01} value of methanol by Eq. 2.4a

$$\Delta G_e^{01} = -\left(\frac{-216.192}{6}\right) = +36.032 \text{ kJ/e-mol}$$

Obviously ΔH_e can be calculated in a similar way by calculation of ΔH_{ref}.

For biomass the following redox half reaction can be set up, assuming that NH_4^+ is the N source:

$$-1CH_{1.8}O_{0.8}N_{0.2} - 2.5H_2O + HCO_3^- + 0.2NH_4^+ + 5H^+ + 4.2e^-$$

Obviously, the degree of reduction for biomass is 4.2. The ΔG_{ref}^{01} value is obtained similarly as earlier for methanol. ΔG_{ref}^{01} can be calculated to be -142.128 kJ, giving

$$\Delta G_e = -(-142.128)/(4.2) = +33.840 \text{ kJ/e-mol}$$

In a similar way as shown in Example 2.5 for each chemical compound, the values of γ, ΔG_e, and ΔH_e can be calculated for a large number of relevant compounds. Table 2.3 contains all relevant stoichiometric and energetic information for growth systems, clearly shown in the following. A point of attention is the finding (Table 2.3) that for biomass the degree of reduction depends on the N source used in the growth system. For example $\gamma = 4.2$ for NH_4^+ and 5.8 for NO_3^- as N source. This is a consequence of the reference definition. The advantage is that the N source disappears from the stoichiometric calculations using γ, ΔG_e, and ΔH_e. The defined reference system is closely related to the generalised degree of reduction as defined by Roels and Erickson. It can be seen that for reduced organic compounds γ is between 0 and 8 (per C-mol). For inorganic compounds, such an upper limit does not exist (because there is not a normalisation per atom). For O_2, γ is negative (-4), which is logical for an acceptor. ΔG_e is related to the conventional redox potential of redox half reactions ($\Delta G_e^{01} = -FE_0^1$). ΔG_e is calculated using HCO_3^- (the most abundant form of carbon dioxide at pH = 7); ΔH_e has been calculated using CO_2 (gas) as reference, to take the large heat effect of $HCO_3^- \rightarrow CO_2$ (gas) into account.

Table 2.3. Calculated γ, ΔG_e^{01}, and ΔH_e^0 values for chemical compounds under standard conditions.

Compound	γ Degree of reduction per C-mole for organic and per mole for inorganic compounds in electrons/(C)-mole	ΔG_e^{01} (kJ/e-mol)	ΔH_e^0 (kJ/e-mol)
Biomass/NH_4^+ – N source	+4.2	+33.480	−26.1
Biomass/NO_3 – N source	+5.8	+14.820	−44.2
Biomass/N_2 – N source	+4.8	+32.948	·−26.3
N source for growth	0	0	0
HCO_3^-	0	0	0
Oxalate	+1	+52.522	−20
Formate	+2	+39.186	−15.50
Glyoxylate	+2	+48.229	–
Tartrate	+2.5	+39.577	–
Malonate	+2.67	+28.976	–
Fumarate	+3	+33.662	−31.60
Malate	+3	+33.354	−32.20
Citrate	+3	+32.282	−33.90
Pyruvate	+3.33	+34.129	−23.60
Succinate	+3.50	+28.405	−36.30

(Contd ...)

Compound	γ Degree of reduction per C-mole for organic and per mole for inorganic compounds in electrons/(C)-mole	ΔG_e^{01} (kJ/e-mol)	ΔH_e^0 (kJ/e-mol)
Gluconate	+3.67	+39.106	–
Formaldehyde	+4	+45.326	–0.10
Acetate	+4	+26.801	–33.50
Lactate	+4	+31.488	–28.90
Glucose	+4	+39.744	–25.75
Mannitol	+4.33	+38.777	–
Glycerol	+4.67	+37.625	–24.30
Propionate	+4.67	+26.939	–33.80
Ethylene glycol	+5	+37.292	–
Acetoin	+5	+32.625	–
Butyrate	+5	+27.000	–33.30
Propanediol	+5.33	+33.177	–
Acetone	+5.33	+28.718	–30.90
Butanediol	+5.50	+31.374	–
Methanol	+6	+36.032	–23
Ethanol	+6	+30.353	–28.90
Propanol	+6	+29.144	32.50
n-Alkane	+6.13	+26.694	–
Propane	+6.66	+25.948	–31.90
Ethane	+7	+25.404	–31.40
Methane	+8	+22.925	–31.50
CO	+2	+47.477	–1.5
H_2	+2	+39.870	0
SO_4^{2-}	0	0	0
SO_3^{2-}	+2	+50.296	–
S^0	+6	+19.146	–55.2
$S_2O_3^{2-}$	+8	+23.584	–27.5
HS^-	+8	+20.850	–43.9
NO_3^-	0	0	0
NO_2^-	+2	–41.650	–108.5
NO(g)	+3	–96.701	–
$N_2O(g)$	+8	–57.540	–124.55
NH_4^+	+8	–35.109	–101.9
N_2	+10	–72.194	–136.4
Fe^{3+}	0	0	0
Fe^{2+}	+1	–74.270	–46.8
H_2O	0	0	0
O_2	–4	–78.719	–143

Note: pH = 7, 1 mol/l, 1 atm, 298 K.

Balance of Degree of Reduction, Atomic Degrees of Reduction and the COD Balance

In the previously defined 'growth reference' system, γ_i was introduced as the degree of reduction of compound i. This parameter is important in stoichiometric calculations, because due to the principle of electron conservation, an electron balance can be defined. This is the so-called balance of degree of reduction. This is not an additional conservation principle (in addition to C, H, O, N, and charge conservation). The balance of degree of reduction can be obtained from the usual C, H, O, N, and charge balances by eliminating (by suitable substitutions) H^+, H_2O, HCO_3^-, and the N source. Hence, the balance of degree of reduction is a suitable linear combination of already available conservation equations. The importance of the balance of degree of reduction is that, by definition, in this balance, only biomass formation, consumption of electron donor, and consumption of electron acceptor are related. Based on the previous definition of the reference set of compounds in the growth reference system it is also possible to calculate the degree of reduction of atoms and of electric charge (Table 2.4).

Table 2.4. Degree of reduction of atoms and electric charge according to the definition of the growth reference system.

Atom or charge	Degree of reduction of atoms
H	+1
O	−2
C	+4
Charge +1	−1
Charge −1	+1
S	+6
P	+5
N	+5
N in N index in biomass	+ 3 for NH_4^+ or NH_3 as N source 0 for N_2 as N source
	+ 5 for NO_3^- or HNO_3 as N source

It should be noted that the atomic degree of reduction for the N atom in biomass depends on the applied N source as a consequence of the defined growth reference system as explained earlier. Using the γ values of atoms and electric charge in Table 2.4, it is straightforward to calculate the γ values for any chemical compound for which the elemental composition is known (Example 2.6a). This is an equivalent alternative to writing the reference redox half reaction to obtain γ (Example 2.5).

Example 2.6a. Direct calculation of γ from elemental composition.

Using the atomic degrees of reduction (Table 2.4) it can easily be checked that indeed for the reference chemicals $\gamma = 0$:

H_2O	$\gamma = 2 \times 1 + 1(-2) = 0$
CO_2	$\gamma = 1 \times 4 + 2(-2) = 0$
HCO_3^-	$\gamma = 1 \times 1 + 1 \times 4 + 3(-2) + 1 = 0$
H^+	$\gamma = 1 \times 1 + 1(-1) = 0$

For the degree of reduction of biomass (γ_X) it is easy to show that this is a function of the N source used. Using the standard elemental biomass composition $CH_{1.8}O_{0.5}N_{0.2}$ and using the N degree of reduction for the different N sources (Table 2.4) one obtains

$$-NH_4^+ \text{ as N-source } \gamma_X = 1 \times 4 + 1.8 \times 1 + 0.5(-2) + 0.2(-3) = 4.2$$

$-NO_3^-$ as N-source $\gamma_X = 1 \times 4 + 1.8 \times 1 + 0.5 \times (-2) + 0.2(5) = 5.8$

For the electron content of an organic substrate (e.g. acetate ion, $C_2H_3O_2^-$) the amount of electrons is $2 \times 4 + 3 \times 1 + 2(-2) + 1(+1) = 8$. Because for organic compounds γ is defined as the number of electrons per C atom, we obtain for acetate with 2 carbon atoms $\gamma = 8/2 = 4$.

The degree of reduction balance is also called chemical oxygen demand (COD) balance in wastewater engineering. The COD balance is equivalent to the balance of degree of reduction. COD is a number assigned to each chemical and represents the consumed O_2 on total oxidation in g O_2/g compound. There is a direct link with degree of reduction. Each mole of electrons represents 8 grams COD. This is easily understood, because the consumption of 1 mol O_2 represents the acceptance of 4 mol electrons ($\gamma = -4$; see Table 2.3). One mol O_2 represents -32 g COD and therefore 1 mol electrons = 8 g COD.

Example 2.6b: Calculation of COD values.

Consider glucose, in which 1 mol (= 180 grams) represents (according to Table 2.3) a total of 6×4 electrons = $6 \times 4 \times 8 = 192$ g O_2. Clearly glucose has a COD value of 192/180 = 1.0667 g COD/g glucose. The NO_3^-/N_2 acceptor couple has $\gamma_A = -5$ electrons. The COD value of $NO_3^- - N$ is then $-5 \times 8/14 = -2.857$ g COD per gram nitrate-nitrogen.

The values of γ, ΔG_e, and ΔH_e from Table 2.3 can be used for very easy stoichiometric and energetic calculations as shown in Examples 2.7a and 2.7b.

Example 2.7a: Calculation of the stoichiometry of Example 2.1a using γ values.

In Example 2.1a, five equations were solved to calculate the full macrochemical equation. Using the γ values of Table 2.3 we can first make the balance of degree of reduction. For the electron donor oxalate $\gamma_D = 1$ per carbon or 2 per mole oxalate; for biomass $\gamma_X = 4.2$ and for the electron acceptor $O_2 \gamma_A = -4$ (Table 2.3). For all the other chemicals (N source, H^+, H_2O, HCO_3^-) $\gamma = 0$ by definition. The γ balance is now:

$$2f - 4c + 4.2 = 0$$

Because $f = -5.815$ we obtain $c = -1.857$ directly.

From the C balance we then obtain $e = +10.63$. From the N balance $a = -0.20$, from the charge balance $b = -0.8$, and from the O or H balance we finally find $d = -5.42$. This is, as expected, the same result as before in Example 2.1a.

Example 2.7b. Calculation of Gibbs energy of reaction in Example 2.1b using ΔG_e values.

Using the now-available full macrochemical stoichiometry, it is possible to calculate the, Gibbs energy of reaction using the Gibbs energy balance.

For each chemical compound the Gibbs energy contribution follows from the product of its number of electrons and its ΔG_e number. For example (using Table 2.3), the Gibbs energy contribution for oxalate, O_2, and biomass in the growth reference system follows as:

Oxalate $= 2 \times 1 \times 52.522 = +105.04$ kJ
$O_2 = -4 \times (-78.719) = 314.876$ kJ
Biomass $= 4.2 \times 33.840 = 142.128$ kJ

For all other reactants the Gibbs energy contribution in the growth reference system is zero. For the Gibbs energy of the macrochemical-reaction equation we obtain then from the available full stoichiometry:

$$-5.815(105.04) - 1.857(314.876) + 142.128 = -1053 \text{ kJ}$$

This is the same as obtained before, but now the calculation has only three terms.

Energetics of Redox Couples, Catabolic Redox Reactions, RET and Energetic Regularities

It was pointed out earlier that for each microbial growth system a catabolic redox reaction is needed where an electron donor couple reacts with an electron acceptor couple. For the generation of maintenance energy the catabolic reaction is also required. For example, in aerobic growth on glucose the electron donor couple is glucose/HCO_3^- (glucose is oxidised to HCO_3^-) and the electron acceptor couple is O_2/H_2O (O_2 is reduced to H_2O). However, for anaerobic growth on glucose, where the catabolic reaction is the conversion of glucose into ethanol, the electron donor couple is glucose/HCO_3^- and the electron acceptor is the HCO_3^-/ethanol couple. To be able to quickly calculate the catabolic energy production, it is relevant to define the ΔG_e, ΔH_e, and γ values of redox couples i/j. These can be calculated from γ, ΔG_e, and ΔH_e, values (Table 2.3) using Equations 2.5a–2.5c.

$$\gamma_{couple} = \gamma_i - \gamma_j \qquad \qquad \text{... (2.5a)}$$

$$\left(\Delta G_e\right)_{couple} = \frac{(\gamma \Delta G_e)_i - (\gamma \Delta G_e)_j}{\gamma_i - \gamma_j} \qquad \qquad \text{... (2.5b)}$$

$$\left(\Delta H_e\right)_{couple} = \frac{(\gamma \Delta H_e)_i - (\gamma \Delta H_e)_j}{\gamma_i - \gamma_j} \qquad \qquad \text{... (2.5c)}$$

Equations 2.5a–2.5c have the following properties:
1. If we invert the redox couple, for example, i/j into j/i, we are in fact inverting the redox half reaction of the redox couple. The value of γ changes sign, which is logical because produced electrons become consumed electrons. The value of ΔG_e and ΔH_e does not change, which is logical because the energetics of the reaction do not change.
2. If the redox couple i/j contains a biological reference compound (e.g. $j = HCO_3^-$, H_2O, H^+, NO_3^-, SO_4^{2-}) then for compound j the value of γ, ΔG_e, and ΔH_e is zero. Equations 2.5a–2.5c then show that the value of γ, ΔG_e, and ΔH_e of the redox couple i/j becomes equal to the tabulated values of the i component in Table 2.3. For example, if the redox couple is an organic compound/HCO_3^-, then the γ, ΔG_e, and ΔH_e value of the organic compound follow directly from Table 2.3.
3. If the redox couple does not contain a reference chemical then Eqs 2.5a–2.5c must be used to calculate γ, ΔG_e, and ΔH_e. Table 2.5 shows some examples.

It can be seen from Table 2.5 that electron donor couples are characterised by positive γ values and electron-acceptor couples by negative γ values (which is logical). As stated earlier, in each microbial growth system there functions a catabolic reaction between an electron donor and an electron acceptor, which generates the required (for anabolism and maintenance) Gibbs energy. It is noted (Eq. 2.6c) that in a full catabolic redox reaction, the redox couple with the highest ΔG_e value must be the electron donor; the redox couple with the lowest ΔG_e value is the acceptor (Example 2.8a).

Table 2.5. ΔG_e, and ΔH_e values of redox couples under standard conditions.

Redox couple	γ [per (C-)mol]	ΔG_e (kJ/e-mol)	ΔH_e (kJ/e-mol)
$NH_4^+/\frac{1}{2}N_2$	3	+26.703	−44.3
$NH_4^+/\frac{1}{2}N_2^-$	6	−32.928	−99.665
NO_2^-/NO_3^-	2	−41.647	−108.5
Lactate/pyruvate	2	+18.283	−55.4
Fumarate/succinate	−2	−3.137	−64.5

(Contd ...)

Redox couple	γ (per (C-)mol)	ΔG_e (kJ/e-mol)	ΔH_e (kJ/e-mol)
$NO_3^-/\tfrac{1}{2}N_2$	-5	-72.194	-136.4
$NO_2^-/\tfrac{1}{2}N_2$	-3	-92.559	-155
$NO(g)/\tfrac{1}{2}N_2$	-2	-35.434	$-$
$N_2O(g)/N_2$	-2	-130.809	-183.8
Glucose/HCO_3^-	4	$+39.744$	-25.75

Example 2.8a: Recognising electron donor and acceptor.

Consider the following catabolic reaction: $C_6H_{12}O_6 + 6O_2 \rightarrow 6HCO_3^- + 6H^+$. The two redox couples are $C_6H_{12}O_6/HCO_3^-$ and O_2/H_2O. According to Table 2.3, the glucose couple has $\Delta G_e = +39.744$ kJ/e-mol and the O_2 couple has $\Delta G_e = -78.719$ kJ/e-mol. Clearly glucose is the electron donor and O_2 is the acceptor. Consider now the catabolic reaction $C_6H_{12}O_6 + 2H_2O \rightarrow 2HCO_3^- + 2H^+ + 2C_2H_5OH$. This is the catabolic reaction in the ethanol fermentation. The redox couples are $C_6H_{12}O_6/HCO_3^-$ and HCO_3^-/C_2H_5OH. From Table 2.3 we read for the glucose couple that $\Delta G_e = +39.744$ and for the ethanol couple $\Delta G_e = +30.353$. Now glucose is the donor and HCO_3^-/ethanol is the acceptor.

Because the catabolic reaction liberates the Gibbs energy required for the anabolism, it is important to calculate this amount of energy. Using the ΔG_e approach, we can then write directly Eqs 2.6a and 2.6b to calculate the Gibbs energy of reaction (ΔG_{CAT}) of the catabolic reaction. ΔG_{ED} and ΔG_{EA} are the electron Gibbs energy of the acceptor and donor couples:

$$-\Delta G_{CAT} = \gamma_D(\Delta G_{ED} - \Delta G_{EA}) \qquad \text{... (2.6a)}$$

The enthalpy of reaction ΔH_{CAT} of the catabolic reaction can be calculated similarly:

$$-\Delta H_{CAT} = \gamma_D(\Delta H_{ED} - \Delta H_{EA}) \qquad \text{... (2.6b)}$$

ΔG_{CAT} and ΔH_{CAT} represent the Gibbs energy and enthalpy of reaction of the catabolic reaction consuming 1 C-mol organic or 1 mol inorganic compound of electron donor. Dimensions are kJ/(C)-mol donor. γ_D is the degree of reduction of the donor couple in mol electrons/(C)-mol donor, which is always positive. According to the second law of thermodynamics ΔG_{CAT} must be negative. Therefore, Eq. 2.6c, the second law of thermodynamics, holds:

$$\Delta G_{ED} > \Delta G_{EA} \qquad \text{... (2.6c)}$$

This shows that indeed the electron donor couple always has the highest ΔG_e value.

Example 2.8b: Calculation of catabolic Gibbs energy production using ΔG_e.

Consider the catabolic reactions in Example 2.8a. For aerobic glucose oxidation we can calculate, using Eq. 2.6a and Table 2.3

$$(-\Delta G_{CAT}) = 4 \times [39.644 - (-78.719)] = 473.852 \text{ kJ, so that } \Delta G_{CAT} = -473.852 \text{ kJ}$$

This is the Gibbs energy released for the aerobic combustion of 1 C-mol glucose. For 1 mol of glucose (6 C-atoms) the Gibbs energy of the catabolic reaction is $6 \times (-473.852) = -2843$ kJ.

For anaerobic ethanol fermentation of glucose we can calculate for the catabolic reaction $(-\Delta G_{CAT}) = 4 \times (39.744 - 30.353) = 37.564$ kJ per C-mol glucose. For 1 mol glucose the catabolic Gibbs energy of the catabolic reaction becomes $6 \times (-37.564) = -225.34$ kJ. This is the same as calculated in Example 2.3b.

The use of ΔG_e and ΔH_e now also reveals some interesting energetic regularities. Table 2.3 shows that for many organic donor compounds, the ΔH_e and ΔG_e values are rather close, with an average $\Delta G_e = +32 \pm 8$ kJ/e-mol and average $\Delta H_E = -28 \pm 5$ kJ/e-mol. These values are also close to the ΔG_E and ΔH_E value of biomass. Hence we can write for organic electron donors the important regularity

$$\Delta G_{ED} \approx \Delta G_{EX} \qquad \ldots (2.7a)$$

$$\Delta H_{ED} \approx \Delta H_{EX} \qquad (2.7b)$$

For autotrophic growth using inorganic electron donors, the ΔG_{ED} values are, in general, much lower than ΔG_{EX} (consider NH_4^+/NO_2^-, F_e^{2+}/F_e^{3+}, etc. in Table 2.4). For autotrophic growth (CO_2 as C source), this means that for these electron donors there is a need for Gibbs energy input in order to realise CO_2 reduction to biomass. This is achieved by RET. Knowing this we can write Eq. 2.7c to recognise RET.

$$\Delta G_{EX} > \Delta G_{ED} \qquad \ldots (2.7c)$$

Finally, it is now easy to calculate the heat production and Gibbs energy dissipation in oxidative catabolism of organic compounds. As stated earlier, for organic compounds the average $\Delta G_{ED} = 32$ kJ/e-mol and for O_2 as acceptor $\Delta G_{EA} = -78.719$ kJ/e-mol. Hence, per mole of electron transferred between donor and acceptor, the available Gibbs energy is $32 - (-78.719) = 110.72$ kJ. Per mole of consumed O_2 (which accepts four electrons, $\gamma_A = -4$) in the combustion of any organic compound, the Gibbs energy made available by combustion of the organic compound is then $4 \times 110.72 = 443$ kJ per consumed mol O_2. Analogously, one can find for the produced heat per mole of O_2 in the combustion of organic compounds a value of 460 kJ per mole O_2. It is also obvious that the mentioned inaccuracy in the average ΔG_E or ΔH_E values for organic compounds only results in a minor error of 5 to 8 per cent in the calculated Gibbs energy dissipation and heat production. These are very important rules of thumb for the fermentation industry.

MATHEMATICAL EQUATIONS TO CALCULATE THE GROWTH STOICHIOMETRY FROM KNOWN GIBBS ENERGY DISSIPATION

Deriving the Equations

In Example 2.1, it was shown that one suitably measured stoichiometric coefficient, for example, Y_{DX}, allows the calculation of all other stoichiometric coefficients, including the dissipated Gibbs energy $1/Y_{GX}$. This means that knowledge of $1/Y_{GX}$ should enable the calculation of all stoichiometric coefficients, as shown in Example 2.4.

It has also been shown that Y_{GX} can be estimated for arbitrary growth systems under different growth rates and temperatures using the correlations (Eqs 2.2 and 2.3). Here we show that particularly simple equations to calculate all yields from Y_{GX} can be obtained by using the γ, ΔG_e, and ΔH_e parameters introduced in the previous section.

The general macrochemical reaction equation can be written as shown in Fig. 2.2b. In this macro-chemical equation, the electron donor and acceptor are written in C-mol (for organic compounds) or in mol (for inorganic compounds). The (. . .) stoichiometric coefficients are not given separate symbols. They follow easily from the charge balance (for H^+), N balance (for N source), from O or H balance (for H_2O), and the carbon balance (for HCO_3^-). For autotrophic growth, the HCO_3^- stoichiometric coefficient is -1. Three balances can be written based on the conservation principles of electrons and enthalpy and the Gibbs energy balance.

Balance of degree of reduction

$$-\gamma_D/Y_{DX} - \gamma_A/Y_{AX} + \gamma_X = 0 \qquad \dots (2.8a)$$

Enthalpy balance

$$-\gamma_D\Delta H_{ED}/Y_{DX} - \gamma_A\Delta H_{EA}/Y_{AX} + \gamma_X\Delta H_{EX} + 1/Y_{QX} = 0 \qquad \dots (2.8b)$$

Gibbs energy balance

$$-\gamma_D\Delta G_{ED}/Y_{DX} - \gamma_A\Delta G_{EA}/Y_{AX} + \gamma_X\Delta G_{EX} + 1/Y_{QX} = 0 \qquad \dots (2.8c)$$

From equation 2.8a it follows that Y_{AX} is directly related to Y_{DX} (equation 2.9a):

$$\frac{1}{Y_{AX}} = \frac{\gamma_D}{(-\gamma_A)Y_{DX}} - \frac{\gamma_X}{(-\gamma_A)} \qquad \dots (2.9a)$$

The degree of reduction of the acceptor γ_A is (by definition) a negative number. Using Eqs 2.8a–2.8c, it is also possible to calculate directly Y_{DX}, Y_{AX}, and Y_{QX} as function of Y_{GX}. If we further use the found energetic regularity that $\Delta G_{EX} \approx \Delta G_{ED}$ (Eq. 2.7a) and replace $(\Delta G_{ED} - \Delta G_{EA})$ by $(\Delta G_{CAT})/\gamma_D$ using Eq. 2.6a, it is possible to derive the simple Eqs 2.9b–2.9e. It is noted that ΔG_{CAT} is the Gibbs energy of the catabolic reaction of 1 C-mol organic or 1 mol inorganic compound, and that therefore $(-\Delta G_{CAT})$ is the Gibbs energy released in the catabolic reaction of 1 C-mol of organic or 1 mol of inorganic electron donor. (ΔG_{CAT}) is then by definition >0 and its units are kJ/(C)-mol donor. ΔG_{CAT} and ΔH_{CAT} follow from Eqs 2.6a and 2.6b using ΔG_{EA} and ΔG_{ED} values (Tables 2.3 and 2.5).

$$Y_{DX} = \frac{(-\Delta G_{CAT})}{1/Y_{GX} + \gamma_X/\gamma_D(-\Delta G_{CAT})} \qquad \dots (2.9b)$$

$$Y_{AX} = \frac{(-\gamma_A/\gamma_D)(-\Delta G_{CAT})}{1/Y_{GX}} \qquad \dots (2.9c)$$

$$1/Y_{QX} = \frac{(-\Delta H_{CAT})}{(-\Delta G_{CAT})}1/Y_{GX} \qquad \dots (2.9d)$$

Furthermore, it is often interesting to study Y_{DA}, which is the amount of electron acceptor couple consumed relative to the amount of electron donor consumed. For micro-organisms growing aerobically on organic matter, this would be the mole of O_2 consumed per C-mole of organic compound consumed. For anaerobic growth this would be the amount of anaerobic products per amount of organic substrate in C-mole product per C-mole substrate. Because $Y_{DA} = Y_{DX}/Y_{AX}$ we obtain

$$Y_{DA} = [\gamma_D/(-\gamma_A)]\frac{1/Y_{GX}}{1/Y_{GX} + \gamma_X/\gamma_D(-\Delta G_{CAT})} \qquad \dots (2.9e)$$

Applications of the Mathematical Stoichiometry Relations

The obtained stoichiometric relations (Eqs 2.9a–2.9e) can now easily be applied. In this section, their use is demonstrated with the following subjects:

1. Calculation of the complete growth stoichiometry.
2. Calculation of maintenance coefficients and maximal growth yields.
3. Calculation of the limit to growth yield posed by the second law.
4. Calculation of COD-based growth yields.
5. Calculation of the relation between heat production and Gibbs energy dissipation.
6. Calculation of maximal product yields in anaerobic metabolism.

Calculation of the complete growth stoichiometry

If for a given growth system the C source, the electron donor (ΔG_{ED} to decide on RET using Eq. 2.7c), the temperature, and the growth rate are known, then Eqs 2.2 and 2.3 allow a direct calculation of the required Gibbs energy $1/Y_{GX}^m$ to produce 1 C-mol of biomass at high growth rates μ. Knowing the electron donor couple and acceptor couple, and using Table 2.3 and Eqs 2.5a–2.5c, the values of ΔG_{ED}, ΔG_{EA}, ΔH_{ED}, ΔG_{EA}, γ_D, and γ_A can be calculated and from this $(-\Delta G_{CAT})$ and $(-\Delta H_{CAT})$ using Eqs 2.7a and 2.7b. Using Eqs 2.9b–2.9e subsequently allows the complete stoichiometric calculation where H^+, N source, H_2O, and HCO_3^- must be calculated using the conservation equations of electric charge, N, O or H, and carbon.

Example 2.9a: Calculation of stoichiometry using Eqs 2.9b–2.9e.

Consider Example 2.4, where a micro-organism is grown anaerobically on methanol, producing acetate. Assume first that the growth rate is high, such that maintenance can be neglected. Equation 2.3a then shows that $1/Y_{GX}^m = 698$ kJ Gibbs energy per C-mol biomass. Methanol is the C-source, methanol/HCO_3^- is the electron donor, and HCO_3^-/acetate is the electron acceptor.

From Table 2.3 and using Eqs 2.5a–2.5c, we can then find that $\Delta G_{ED} = 36.032$ kJ/e-mol, $\Delta H_{ED} = -23$ kJ/e-mol; $\Delta G_{EA} = 26.801$ kJ/e-mol; $\Delta H_{EA} = -33.5$ kJ/e-mol. Also, $\gamma_D = 6$, $\gamma_A = -4$, and $\gamma_X = 4.2$. This provides that $-\Delta G_{CAT} = 6(36.032 - 26.801) = 55.386$ and $-\Delta H_{CAT} = -23 - (-33.5) = 63$ kJ/C-mol methanol. Using Eqs 2.9b–2.9e, we obtain the maximal growth yields (maintenance neglected).

$$
\begin{aligned}
1/Y_{DX}^m &= 13.3 \text{ mol methanol/C-mol biomass} \\
1/Y_{AX}^m &= 18.9 \text{ C-mol acetate/C-mol biomass} \\
&= 9.45 \text{ mol acetate/C-mol biomass} \\
1/Y_{QX}^m &= 794 \text{ kJ heat/C-mol biomass} \\
Y_{DA}^m &= 1.42 \text{ C-mol acetate/C-mol methanol} \\
&= 0.71 \text{ mol acetate/mol methanol}
\end{aligned}
$$

Using the C-balance $1/Y_{CX}^m$ is calculated as 6.6 mol HCO_3^- consumed/C-mol biomass produced. This overall stoichiometric result is very close to the exact solution obtained in Example 2.4. The small deviation arises from the assumption that $\Delta G_{EX} \approx \Delta G_{ED}$ (as discussed before). In general it be shown that the simple set of Eqs 2.9b–2.9e seldom deviates more than 5 per cent from the exact solution.

Maintenance coefficients and maximal yield coefficients

As indicated previously, relations between the maintenance coefficients follow from the catabolic reaction. The following relations can now be written to link the various maintenance coefficients to the maintenance Gibbs energy m_G using $-\Delta G_{CAT}$ (see also Example 2.9b). It is noted that m_G follows from the correlation (Eq. 2.2) and that ΔG_{CAT} is calculated for the catabolism of 1 (C)-mol of electron donor.

$$m_D = m_G/(-\Delta G_{CAT}) \qquad \dots (2.10a)$$

$$m_A = (\gamma_D/-\gamma_A)m_G/(-\Delta G_{CAT}) \qquad \dots (2.10b)$$

$$m_Q = m_G \frac{(-\Delta H_{CAT})}{(-\Delta G_{CAT})} \qquad \dots (2.10c)$$

$$m_C = m_G/(-\Delta G_{CAT}) \qquad \dots (2.10d)$$

Using Eqs 2.10a–2.10d, the value of the maintenance Gibbs energy requirement m_G can be calculated from either measured maintenance coefficients (for electron donor m_D, electron acceptor m_A, heat production m_Q, or carbon dioxide production m_C). Furthermore, it can easily be understood that the maximal biomass yields for electron donor, acceptor, and heat are found from Eqs 2.9b–2.9e by substitution of $1/Y_{GX}^m$ (instead of $1/Y_{GX}$) because the maintenance contribution is then neglected.

Example 2.9b: Effect of maintenance on stoichiometry.

In Example 2.9a the maintenance contribution was neglected. Assume that the micro-organism is growing at 37°C. Equation 2.2 then leads to $m_G = 13$ kJ/C-mol biomass hr. Using Eqs 2.10a–2.10c and using ΔG_{CAT} and ΔH_{CAT} (Example 2.9) we obtain:

$$m_D = 0.2347 \text{ mol methanol/C-mol biomass/hr}$$
$$m_A = 0.3521 \text{ C-mol acetate/C-mol biomass/hr}$$
$$m_Q = 14.787 \text{ kJ/C-mol biomass/hr}$$

Further assume that the growth rate $\mu = 0.02$ hr^{-1}. Using Eq. 2.1b, the Y_{iX}^m values obtained in Example 2.9a, and the m_i values obtained here, one obtains for the stoichiometry:

$$\text{Electron donor}(D)\ 1/Y_{DX} = 13.3 + \frac{0.2347}{0.02}$$
$$= 25.03 \text{ mol methanol/C-mol X}$$

$$\text{Electron donor}(A)\ 1/Y_{AX} = 18.9 + \frac{0.3521}{0.02}$$
$$= 36.50 \text{ C-mol acetate/C-mol X}$$

$$\text{Heat } 1/Y_{QX} = 794 + \frac{14.787}{0.02} = 1533 \text{ kJ heat/C-mol X}$$

$$Y_{DA} = 36.50/25.03 = 1.46 \text{ C-mol acetate/mol methanol}$$

These values can also be obtained directly from Eqs 2.9b–2.9e by substituting the complete Gibbs energy of growth and maintenance according to Eq. 2.1c:

$$1/Y_{GX} = 1/Y_{GX}^m + \frac{m_G}{\mu} = 698 + \frac{13}{0.02}$$
$$= 1348 \text{ kJ Gibbs energy/C-mol X}$$

Clearly, comparing Examples 2.9a and 2.9b, one observes that the yield of biomass Y_{DX} drops from 0.077 to 0.04 due to maintenance, but the acetate/methanol yield Y_{DA} increases from 1.42 to 1.46 C-mol acetate/mol methanol.

Second law limit of growth yield

As for any chemical reaction, the microbial growth yield is also limited by the second law of thermodynamics. This limit is achieved if $1/Y_{GX} = 0$, because this defines equilibrium. Equations 2.9c–2.9f then show that for the thermodynamic limits we can write the following:

Thermodynamic limits for growth yields:
$$Y_{DX} = \gamma_D/\gamma_X$$
$$1/Y_{AX} = 0$$
$$1/Y_{HX} = 0$$

Clearly, the more reduced electron donors (γ_D higher) have a higher Y_{DX} limit. This limit has already been determined.

COD-based yields

In waste-water treatment, the biomass yield is calculated on COD basis. Y_{COD} is the gram biomass COD over gram-substrate COD. Based on the COD definition we can write:

$$Y_{COD} = \frac{\gamma_X}{\gamma_D} Y_{DX} \qquad \ldots (2.11a)$$

This allows the following relation for Y_{COD} from equation 2.9b:

$$Y_{COD} = \frac{(-\Delta G_{CAT})}{(-\Delta G_{CAT}) + (\gamma_D / \gamma_X) 1 / Y_{GX}} \qquad \ldots (2.11b)$$

For aerobic growth on organic substrate $-\Delta G_{CAT} = \gamma_D[32 - (-78.719)] \approx \gamma_D \times 110$ kJ/C-mol. Here the average value of $\Delta G_{ED} = +32$ kJ/e-mol for organic matter was used as shown before. Substitution of $-\Delta G_{CAT}$ gives Y_{COD} for aerobic growth on organic substrate:

$$Y_{COD} = \frac{110}{110 + (1 / Y_{GX}) \gamma_X} \qquad \ldots (2.11c)$$

This equation shows that Y_{COD} for aerobic growth is not a constant, as often assumed with $Y_{COD} \approx 0.50$–0.67, but it depends also on the type of C source, because this determines $1/Y_{GX}$ (Eqs 2.3a and 2.3b). Also, to decrease the Y_{COD} leading to lower surplus-sludge production, one must, according to Eqs 2.11b and 2.11c:

1. Decrease $(-\Delta G_{CAT})$, by, for example, using anaerobic metabolism producing CH_4.
2. Increase $1/Y_{GX}$ by increasing temperature or decreasing the growth rate according to Eq. 2.1.

These predicted phenomena are well known and applied in waste-treatment processes.

Relation between heat production and Gibbs energy dissipation

According to Eq. 2.9d, the heat production $(1/Y_{QX})$ is related to Gibbs energy need $(1/Y_{GX})$ by the enthalpy and Gibbs energy of the catabolic reaction $(\Delta G_{CAT}$ and $\Delta H_{CAT})$. Table 2.6 shows some examples of growth systems to illustrate the relation between heat production and dissipated Gibbs energy for growth. From Table 2.6 we can conclude the following rules of thumb:

1. For aerobic (or denitrifying) growth systems on organic substrate, the Gibbs energy dissipation and heat production are nearly equal. The entropy contribution in the catabolic reaction is minimal (see glucose and acetate aerobic growth).
2. For anaerobic growth, heat production and Gibbs energy dissipation can be substantially different, due to entropic effects.

Obviously, if in the catabolic reaction there is a net decrease of molecules or a consumption of gaseous molecules, then there is a strong negative entropy contribution (see H_2/CO_2 aerobic and anaerobic) and there is a much higher heat production than Gibbs energy dissipation. If, however, in the catabolic reaction there is a net production of the amount of molecules and/or production of gaseous molecules (e.g. the glucose/ethanol fermentation or the methane production from acetate), then there is a very large positive entropy contribution, leading to a much lower heat production than the Gibbs energy dissipation. The entropic effect can even be so large that there is a calculated heat uptake during growth (e.g. methanation of acetate). This is obviously endothermic growth. So, contrary to a common belief, growth of micro-organisms is not necessarily related to heat production; there can be heat uptake as well. Experimental proof is, however, still lacking.

Table 2.6. Relation between heat production and Gibbs energy need.

Micro-organism	Growth condition	Y_{DX} (C-mol/(C)-mol)	$1/Y_{GX}$ Gibbs energy (kJ/C-mol biomass)	$1/Y_{QX}$ heat (kJ/C-mol biomass)	Entropy contribution (kJ/C-mol biomass)
Saccharomyces cerevisae	Glucose aerobic	0.57	332	+339	−7
Saccharomyces cerevisae	Glucose anaerobic	0.14	270	+95	+175
Hydrogenotroph	$H_2 + CO_2$ aerobic	0.13	1265	+1686	−421
Methanobacterium arborophilus	$H_2 + CO_2$ anaerobic	0.015	1035	+3923	−2888
Pseudomonas oxalaticus	Acetate aerobic	0.406	562	+593	−31
Methanobacterium soehngenii	Acetate anaerobic	0.024	597	−90	+687

Note: Heat production and Gibbs energy dissipation for (an)aerobic growth on glucose, H_2, and acetate; relative contribution of heat- and entropy-related dissipation.

Maximal product yields in anaerobic metabolism

In many microbial processes the valuable product (e.g. ethanol or lactic acid) is related to catabolism. The relevant stoichiometric coefficient is then the yield of the electron acceptor couple to electron donor Y_{DA}.

Equation 2.9e shows how this coefficient is determined by various factors and it appears that Y_{DA} is maximised.

1. For high Gibbs energy dissipation $1/Y_{GX}$. This means that high catabolic product yields are achieved for poor carbon sources, low growth rate, and high temperature, because $1/Y_{GX}$ is then maximised.
2. For catabolic reactions with low ΔG_{CAT}. This is understandable, because then the growth yield is minimised, which leads directly to higher product yield.
3. For highly reduced electron donors (γ_D high) and highly oxidised products (γ_A low). It is then even possible to achieve C yields larger than 1. An excellent example is the anaerobic production of acetate from methanol, where $Y_{DA} \approx 1.4$ C-mol acetate/C-mol methanol (Example 2.4).

GROWTH STOICHIOMETRY

The quantitative studies in microbiology often involve the assessment of growth stoichiometry. Stoichiometry is the quantitative relationship between reactants and products in a chemical reaction. In microbiology, stoichiometry stands for a quantitative relationship between substrates and products of microbial processes, including biomass formation (the consequence of complying with mass and energy conservation laws). In practical terns, kinetic and stoichiometry are tightly linked to each other, but stoichiometry mainly addresses problems of a static nature, whereas kinetics considers the dynamics questions.

Macrostoichiometry of Microbial Growth

By analogy to simple chemical reactions, we can represent growth as a conversion of a number of substrates (medium components) into cell mass and products. Growth of aerobic heterotrophic micro-organisms can be approximated by the following stoichiometric equation (substrates = biomass + products):

$$CH_mO_1 + a_1NH_3 + a_2HPO_4^{2-} + a_3K^+ + \ldots + bO_2 = YCH_pO_nN_qP_oK_v \ldots + a_4CO_2 + a_5H_2O \quad \ldots (2.12)$$

Here, microbial biomass is empirically expressed by the gross formula $CH_pO_nN_qP_oK_v...$, for example, if some average microbial cell contains per dry cell weight per cent C 46, H 7.5, O 31, N 11; and P, 1.3, then the biomass formula is $CH_{1.9}O_{0.5}N_{0.2}P_{0.01}$. The stoichiometric quotients $a_1-a_5 \ldots$, b and Y (biomass yield) specify quantities of substrate and products of microbial growth. If we know biomass yield and gross formulas of all substrates and products, then quotients $a_1-a_6 \ldots$ are easily calculated from conservation conditions.

There are at least two such conditions. First, the mass of each element (C, H, O, N, P, K, . . .) on the left side of equation 1 should be equal to that on the right side (mass balance). Second, if ionised substances are involved, we should take into account the balance of charges to satisfy the condition of electroneutrality. Table 2.7 demonstrates some examples of stoichiometric growth reactions relevant to biotechnology.

Described formalism is useful as a first step in biotechnological studies aimed at planning and optimising microbial growth.

Table 2.7. Selected macrostoichiometric equations describing growth of micro-organisms with different types of energy generation.

Microbial process	Substrates	Biomass	Products	Stoichiometric parameters	
Heterotrophic growth and by-product formation	$CH_mO_1 + a_1O_2 + a_2NH_3$	$= YCH_pO_nN_q$ +	$Y_pCH_rO_sN_t + a_3CO_2 + a_4H_2O$	$a_1 = 0.5(Yn + Y's - l + a_4) + a_3$ $a_2 = Yq + Y't, \; a_3 = 1 - Y - Y'$ $a_4 = 0.5\,[m + Y(3q - p) + Y'(3t - r)]$	A
Phototrophic growth (algae or plant cells)	$CO_2 + a_1H_2O + a_2NH_3$	$= YCH_pO_nN_q$ +	$a_3CH_rO_sN_t + a_4O_2$	$a_1 = 0.5\,[Y(p - 3n) + (r - 3t)(1 - Y)]$ $a_2 = Y(n - t) + t, \; a_3 = 1 - Y$ $a_4 = 0.5(2 + a_1 - Yn - a_3s)$	B
Methanogenesis[a]	$CO_2 + a_1H_2 + a_2NH_3$	$= YCH_pO_nN_q$	$a_3CH_4 + a_4H_2O$	$a_1 = 4 - 0.5Y(4 + 2n + 3q - p)$ $a_2 = Yq, \; a_3 = 1 - Y$ $a_4 = 2 - Yn$	C
Nitrification[b]	$YCO_2 + a_1O_2 + a_2NH_4^+$	$= YCH_pO_nN_q$ +	$a_3NO_3^- + a_4H^+ + a_5H_2O$	$a_1 = 2Y^{-1} - Y[1 + 0.25\,(p - 2n - 3q)]$ $a_2 = Y^{-1} + Yq, \; a_3 = Y^{-1}$ $a_4 = 2Y^{-1} + Yq, \; a_5 = Y^{-1} - 0.5Y(p - 3q)$	D

[a] Particular example of H_2-utilising methanogenic bacteria.

[b] The total growth balance for two phases of nitrification: oxidation of ammonium to nitrite and subsequent oxidation of nitrite to nitrate. Y is growth yield of bacterial maas per mass unit of oxidised N.

It estimates how much nutrient should be supplied to the fermenter to obtain the required amount of biomass or target product. However, it should be absolutely clear that stoichiometric equations like Eq. 2.12 are no more than an approximation to reality. The most severe deviation stems from the fact that unlike chemical reagents, microbial cells are characterised by changeable composition, and stoichiometric coefficients are not true constants. One task of contemporary microbial stoichiometry is to find out the functional relationships between stoichiometric parameters and internal (physiological) and external (environmental) factors.

Growth Yield: Catabolic and Conserved Substrates

The growth yield is one of the main stoichiometric parameters. It is defined as follows:

$$Y = -\frac{\delta x}{\delta s} \approx -\frac{\Delta x}{\Delta s} \qquad \ldots (2.13)$$

where Δx is the increase in microbial biomass consequent on utilisation of the amount Δs of substrate, and δx and δs are respective infinitely small increments. Rigorous definition of Y as derivative $\delta x/\delta s$ stems from the fact that Y can vary in time, the negative sign being introduced because x and s vary in opposite senses. Sometimes, it is used as the reciprocal of Y: $\alpha = 1/Y$, which is called the economic coefficient. It expresses explicitly the nutrient requirements for growth: how many mass units of a particular substrate should be consumed to produce one unit mass of cell material.

The growth efficiency depends generally on the partitioning of consumed element between new cell biomass and extracellular products. The mass balance (total element consumed = amount incorporated into cell plus amount incorporated into extracellular products) is as follows:

$$\delta E_s = \delta E_x + \delta E_p \qquad \ldots (2.14)$$

There are two groups of substrates for microbial growth: (i) catabolic substrates, which are sources of energy; and (ii) anabolic or conserved substrates, which are sources of biogenic elements forming cellular material. Catabolic substrates include H_2 for lithotrophic hydrogen bacteria, NH_4^+ and NO_2^- for nitrifying bacteria, S^0 for sulphur-oxidising bacteria, oxidisable or fermentable organic substances for heterotrophic bacteria and fungi, and so on.

Their consumption is accompanied by oxidation and dissipation of chemical substances into extracellular waste products that are no longer reusable as an energy source (Fermentation products such as acetate, ethanol, butyrate, and H_2 seem to be an exception because they do contain reusable oxidation potential, but it is not available under anaerobic conditions supervising fermentation.) (H_2O, NO_3^-, SO_4^{2-}, CO_2, etc.) The anabolic substrates after uptake are incorporated into *de novo* synthesised cell components, being conserved in biomass (that is why they are called conserved). Contrary to catabolic substrates, they can be reused (e.g. after cell lysis to be taken up by survived cells). The conserved substrates include nearly all the noncarbon sources of biogenic elements (N, P, K, Mg, Fe, and trace elements), CO_2 for autotrophs, and the indispensable amino acids and growth factors. Most catabolic substrates are used also as a source of biogenic elements. We can assess both these components separately in terms of respective yields, Y_E (biomass yield per mass unit of oxidised substrate) and Y_A (biomass yield per mass unit of assimilated substrate), from the experimentally measured yield Y. For C substrate, equation 2.15 can be specified as follows (total carbon consumed equals C incorporated into cell plus C oxidised to CO_2 to provide energy plus C incorporated into by-products):

$$\delta C_s = \delta C_x + \delta C_{CO_2} + \delta C_P \qquad \ldots (2.15)$$

Let us neglect the last term δC_P (by assuming that extracellular by-products can be reused and functionally are equivalent to C substrate) and divide the substrate balance by δC_x, which is the amount of biomass C produced, then:

$$\frac{1}{Y} = 1 + \frac{1}{Y_E} \qquad \qquad \dots (2.16)$$

where, Y = g biomass C g^{-1} substrate C and Y_E = g biomass C g^{-1} CO_2-C

$$\frac{1}{Y} = \frac{\sigma_x}{\sigma_s} + \frac{12}{Y_E \sigma_s} \qquad \qquad \dots (2.17)$$

where, Y = g CDW g^{-1} substrate, Y_E = g CDW $mmol^{-1}$ CO_2, and σ_x and σ_s are fractions of carbon in biomass and substrate, respectively. For example, if total measurable yield Y_j is 0.6 g biomass C g^{-1} glucose C, it means that from each g of consumed C, 0.6 g is incorporated into biomass (assimilated), and 0.4 g is dissimilated (oxidised to CO_2), then $Y_E = 0.6/0.4 = 1.5$. To calculate oxygen demand for aerobic growth (or biomass yield on O_2) we have a balance (oxygen required to produce 1 g CDW equals oxygen required to burn substrate consumed to produce 1 g CDW minus oxygen required to burn 1 g CDW):

$$1/Y_{O_2} = A/Y - B \qquad \qquad \dots (2.18))$$

where, A and B are constants estimated from stoichiometry of their respective combustion reactions (see Eq. 2.21 later), for example, the value of A is 33.33 mmol O_2 g^{-1} glucose and B is about 42 mmol O_2 g^{-1} CDW. The relationship between biomass yields on O_2 and CO_2 is derived from comparison of Eqs 2.17 and 2.18:

$$\frac{Y_{CO_2}}{Y_{O_2}} = \frac{A - BY}{\sigma_s - \sigma_x Y} \qquad \qquad \dots (2.19)$$

Now we will go back to the general substrate balance (Eq. 2.14) and derive an expression for conserved substrate. Again, we neglect term δE_P (because extracellular products are assumed to be reusable) and divide the balance by δx, which is the amount of biomass produced:

$$\frac{1}{Y} = \frac{\delta E_x}{\delta x} \approx \sigma_x \qquad \qquad \dots (2.20)$$

where, σ_x is the intracellular content of element incorporated into biomass from consumed substrate. Sometimes σ_x is called the cell quota. The values $1/Y$ and σ_x are not identical although they have the same dimension (e.g. milligram N per gram biomass) and very close numeric value. The reciprocal $1/Y$ is characterising the process (the expenditure of conserved substrate to synthesise biomass unit), whereas σ_x is an index of cell composition (the content of intracellular N per biomass unit). Formally, $1/Y$ is equal to the σ_x value of an infinitely small increment of cell biomass, and σ_x is the averaged value for entire cell. Notice that although σ_x is a slow and $1/Y$ is a rapid variable, their numerical values are exactly the same for balanced steady-state growth and can differ considerably during transients.

Yield Variation as Dependent on the Chemical Nature of Organic Substrates

In this section, we will discuss why biomass yield varies when micro-organisms are grown on different C substrates. This problem was best solved within the framework of the theory of mass and energy balance (TMEB). Evidently, the fraction of C in dry biomass is almost constant. By contrast, the content of carbon in utilised substrates, σ_s, and energetic quality of substrate vary over a broad range (e.g. compare methane versus oxalic acid). To characterise substrate and biomass by a single common measure, TMEB uses an index of degree of carbon reduction, γ related to the internal energy of organic compounds.

The heat liberated by biological or chemical oxidation is proportional to oxygen uptake or equally to the number of electrons gained by oxygen from oxidised substrates, according to Payne's term available electrons (ae). The heat production from an oxidation reaction averages at 27 kcal per ae equivalent. A carbon reduction degree, γ is defined as the number of ae per one carbon atom.

Its numeric value can be determined from the stoichiometry of the oxidation reaction:

$$CH_pO_nN_q + bO_2 = CO_2 + 0.5(p - 3q)H_2O + qNH_3 \qquad \text{... (2.21)}$$

$$\gamma = 4b = 4 + p - 2n - 3q \qquad \text{... (2.22)}$$

The ae balance for Eq. 2.12 can be written as:

$$\gamma_s + b(-4) = Y\gamma_x + Y_P\gamma_p \qquad \text{... (2.23)}$$

where, γ_s, γ_x, and γ_p are the carbon reduction degree of, respectively, substrate, biomass, and extracellular product. Dividing both sides of Eq. 2.12 by γ_s we obtain the relationship delineating the ae distribution between oxygen (ae used for respiration), biomass, and the intracellular product:

$$\frac{4b}{\gamma_s} + \frac{Y\gamma_x}{\gamma_s} + \frac{Y_P\gamma_p}{\gamma_s} = 1 \qquad \text{... (2.24)}$$

The second term in this equation is the fraction of ae transferred to biomass from utilised substrate, termed the energetic growth yield.

$$\eta = Y_C\gamma_x/\gamma_s \qquad \text{... (2.25)}$$

The third term designates that fraction of total substrate internal energy that is transferred to the product. It is called the energetic product yield.

$$\zeta = Y_P\gamma_p/\gamma_s \qquad \text{... (2.26)}$$

Energetic yield η is related to other stoichiometric parameters as follows:

$$\eta = Y\sigma_x\gamma_x/(\sigma_s\gamma_s)$$

$$\eta = Y_C\gamma_x/\gamma_s$$

where, Y is g CDW/g substrate and Y_C is g CDW-C/g substrate C.

The advantage of using η is that it varies within a much smaller range than other yield expressions. At one and the same efficiency of energy utilisation (η), the conventional biomass C yield Y_C is proportional to substrate reduction degree γ_s and, for example, it is four times higher on glucose ($\gamma_s = 4$) than on oxalate ($\gamma_s = 1$), 0.48 and 0.12 g C g^{-1} C, respectively (assuming $\eta = 0.5$ and $\gamma_x = 4.2$). The energetic growth yield η is more or less constant (0.5 to 0.7) for substrates with $\gamma_s \leq 4.2$ (4.2 corresponds to average reduction degree of microbial biomass), and it declines at higher γ_s. The attractiveness of macrostoichiometry and TMEB is that all growth coefficients are interrelated and could be measured from any available components of the culture mass balance.

For example, if you cannot record microbial growth by conventional routine as dry weight biomass (because of presence of solids in broth liquid), you may still calculate it from N or O_2 uptake, CO_2 evolution, pH titration rate, and so on.

Variations in Yield from Energy Source, Maintenance Requirements

To multiply and grow cells requires energy, but the opposite is not true: cells do not require growth to spend energy. Sometimes catabolic machinery is entirely wasteful (respiration without cell growth) and always at least some minor part of energy consumption is diverted from growth. To account for this phenomenon, it was postulated that microbes and cells require energy not only for growth but also for other maintenance purposes. Certain specific maintenance functions recognised now are turnover of cell material, osmotic work to maintain concentration gradients between the cell and its exterior, and cell motility.

According to conventional definition of maintenance, the balance of energy source is total energy source consumed equals consumption for cell growth plus consumption for maintenance:

$$\delta S_E = \delta S_G + \delta S_M \qquad \qquad ...(2.27)$$

Let us divide it by δx, the amount of biomass produced, then

$$\frac{1}{Y} = \frac{\delta S_G}{\delta x} + \frac{\delta S_M}{\delta x} = \frac{1}{Y^{max}} + \frac{m}{\mu} \qquad \qquad ...(2.28)$$

Here, $Y^{max} = \delta x/\delta S_G$ is true growth yield, that is, yield under imaginary conditions of maintenance being zero. The maintenance coefficient, m, is introduced as the specific (i.e. expressed per unit of biomass) rate of energy consumption for maintenance functions: $m = (1/x)(\delta S_M/\delta t)$. The ratio m/μ on the right side of Eq. 2.28 was derived as follows: $m/\mu = [(1/x)(\delta S_M/\delta t)]/[(1/x)(\delta x/\delta t)] = \delta S_M/\delta x$.

If we divide Eq. 2.27 by $x\delta t$ (note that the second term is $\delta S_G/(x\delta t) = [\delta x/x\delta t)]/[\delta x/\delta S_G)] = \mu/Y^{max}$), then we have:

$$q = \mu/Y^{max} + m \qquad \qquad ...(2.29)$$

where, q is specific rate of energy source consumption, $q = (1/x)(\delta S_E/\delta t)$.

It should be noticed that Y^{max} is a parameter, but not the yield of a real culture that always has some nonzero maintenance requirements. It is a very common mistake in the application of the maintenance concept to a particular organism: to take the real measured Y value and pick up from literature some average m coefficient. The correct way would be either to borrow concurrently two parameters Y^{max} and m or to treat actually observed Y as a variable that is altered along with specific growth rate μ according to Eq. 2.28:

$$Y = \frac{\mu Y^{max}}{\mu + m Y^{max}} \qquad \qquad ...(2.30)$$

There is another way to formulate maintenance requirements by stating that the net growth of cells μ is the difference between true growth (μ_{true}) and endogenous decay of cellular components (specific rate, a):

$$\mu = \mu_{true} - a$$

$$\mu_{true} = \mu + a$$

Then, for the rate of energy source uptake, we have,

or

$$\frac{\mu x}{Y} = \frac{\mu_{true} x}{Y^{max}} = \frac{(\mu + a)x}{Y^{max}}$$

$$\frac{1}{Y} = \frac{1}{Y^{max}} + \frac{a}{\mu Y^{max}}$$

... (2.31)

Comparing Eqs 2.28 and 2.31, we see that $a = mY^{max}$.

Experimental Determination of m

To practically determine the maintenance coefficient, the micro-organisms are grown in chemostat culture limited by energy sources at several dilution rates D (numerically D is equal to specific growth μ if steady state is achieved). At each D, we have to measure steady-state biomass $\tilde{x}$ and at least one of the following quantities residual substrate, $\tilde{s}$ to calculate $Y = \tilde{x}/(s_0 - \tilde{s})$; and the rate of respective energy-yielding process, such as respiration rate, v_{resp}, from O_2 uptake or CO_2 production rates to calculate specific metabolic activity, $q = v_{res}/\tilde{x}$. These data are fitted to Eqs 2.28 or 2.29, m and Y^{max} being found as nonlinear regression parameters. An example is presented in Fig. 2.8. Most available experimental data do obey this relationship. However, considerable deviation occurs at very low growth rates usually attained in chemostat with biomass retention or in dialysis culture. The experimental Y values for slowly growing cells are higher than predicted by Eqs 2.28 and 2.29 (see inset on Fig. 2.8). The explanation is very simple: the maintenance coefficient varies in response to nutritional status and could not be taken as an absolute constant; under substrate deficiency, the cells adjust their maintenance requirements to lower values by reducing turnover rate, osmotic work, and motility.

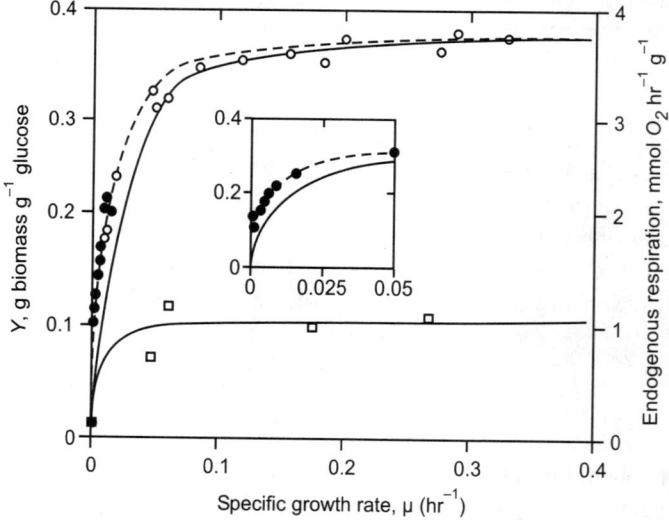

Fig. 2.8. Variation of growth yield (circles) and endogenous respiration (squares) as dependent on specific growth rate in chemostat (open symbols) and continuous dialysis culture (closed symbols). Solid curves were calculated from the synthetic chemostat model. The dotted curve was derived from the Pirt-Herbert model (equations 2.28 to 2.31), which predicts quite well intensive growth but fails in the region of extremely low growth rates.

The described experimental technique is indirect because it is based on measurements of μ-dependent Y variation rather than m itself, and there are some assumptions needed to be confirmed (e.g. that m is constant and that maintenance requirements are the only reason of Y variation). However, some components of maintenance requirements are available for direct estimation. In particular, we can assess the total turnover rate of cellular material a which is one of the main components of maintenance requirements (Eq. 2.31). The principal cell constituents that are turned over are proteins, nucleic acids, and cell wall polymers. The turnover rate is very close to endogenous respiration, which is the oxidation of those compounds produced from the turnover (breakdown) of cellular macrocomponents. Accurate measurements of endogenous respiration need to be made under normal growing conditions. It is known that the simple removal of cells from nutrient broth by filtration with subsequent washing and incubation in buffer renders strong stress and may alter the normal turnover rate. To avoid artifacts, we can use a label-substitution technique (Fig. 2.9). The chemostat culture is fed alternately from two bottles containing unlabelled and labelled $^{14}C(U)$ substrate respectively. The $^{14}CO_2$ evolution rate is recorded after switching to unlabelled substrate, when the main source of $^{14}CO_2$ are cell components. The calculated a value was found to be rather high, accounting for the major part of total maintenance determined by the indirect method. The endogenous respiration declined at the low growth rate (Fig. 2.8), indicating that under starving conditions, self-adjustment of the maintenance requirement occurs mainly as a reduction in the turnover rate of macromolecules.

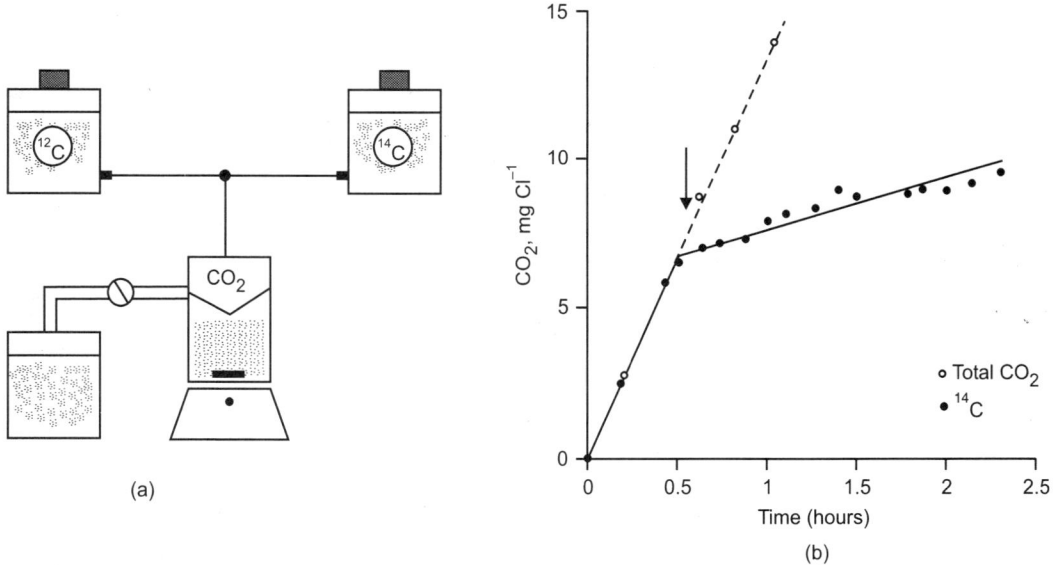

(a)

(b)

Fig. 2.9. Label substitution technique for determination of turnover rate of cell macromolecular constituents: (a) experimental setup including two medium reservoirs containing ^{14}C- and ^{12}C-glucose pumped into a cultivation vessel through a two-way valve; (b) example of $^{14}CO_2$ evolution dynamics before and after (arrow) switching of medium feed from ^{14}C to ^{12}C-glucose, glucose-limited culture of *Pseudomonas fluorescens* 1472, $D = 0.08$ hr^{-1}.

Maintenance Requirements and Wasteful Catabolism

The described concept of maintenance requirements was the subject of severe criticism. One of the strongest arguments against it was an apparent increase in Y^{max} observed in chemostat cultures limited by P, N, and other conserved substrates under conditions of energy excess. To preserve the constancy of the true yield, Pirt had to modify Eq. 2.29 in the following way:

$$q = \mu/Y^{max} + m + m'(1 - \mu/\mu_m) \qquad \qquad ...\,(2.32)$$

where, $m'(1 - \mu/\mu_m)$ is the second μ-dependent component of maintenance energy that operates under excess of energy substrate.

However, it is better to differentiate maintenance requirements *sensu stricto* as those more or less a minor component of the cell energy budget that is observed under energy-limitation and wasteful use of catabolic substrate under energy excess. In physiological terms, these two groups of nonproductive catabolic reactions are completely different. The first reactions are mainly responsible for compensation of turned-over macromolecules and therefore belong to the category of regular primary catabolism. The catabolic reactions of the second group include excretion into environment of partly oxidised substances (overflow metabolism), uncoupling of respiration from ATP generation by metabolic inhibitors, functioning of futile cycles, or substrate oxidation through alternative oxidases without ATP generation. These and related phenomena take place in chemostat culture limited by conserved substrates (opposite to limitation by energy source) as well as during lag phase of batch culture started from starving inoculum. We will discuss the mathematical formulation of these phenomena in the section devoted to growth kinetics.

Variation in Biomass Yield from Conserved Substrates

Yield on conserved substrates varies mainly as a result of alterations in biomass chemical composition expressed by parameter σ_s, the intracellular content of deficient element or cell quota (see Eq. 2.20). For most of known cases, the content σ_s increases parallel to growth acceleration (Fig. 2.10). As yield and cell quota are inversely related to each other (Eq. 2.20), then Y values decrease with growth rate. The physiological mechanisms of this variation are as follows. The intensive growth requires higher internal concentration of some conserved limiting substrates that preserve their chemical identity after uptake (K^+, Mg^{2+}, vitamins). Other conserved substrates (sources of P, N, S, etc.) are incorporated into macromolecular cell constituents (mainly nucleic acids and proteins) whose intracellular content also should be kept high at high growth rate. Both types of changes in cellular composition are manifested as σ increase, and both of them require additional maintenance .energy (to maintain concentration gradient or compensate turnover of macromolecules).

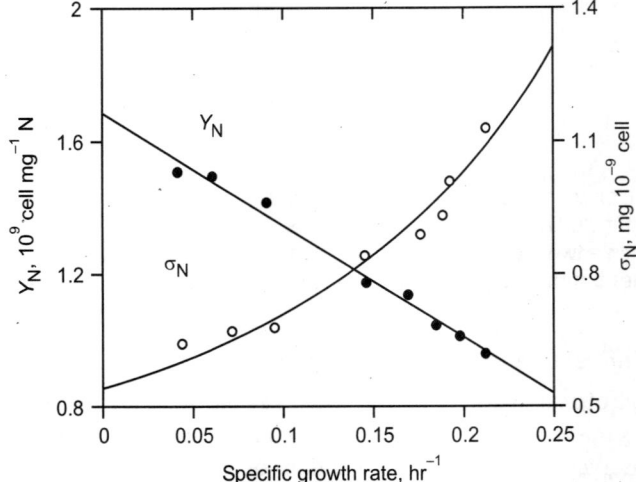

Fig. 2.10. Relationship between stoichiometric parameters Y and s and specific growth rates of *Chlorella vulgaris* grown in chemostat culture limited by nitrogen source. The curves are calculated using Eqs 2.34 and 2.35.

The observed μ-dependent variation in σ is, therefore, a compromise between biosynthetic requirements and energy conservation that is attained because of optimal metabolic control of cell performance. However, it would be erroneous to consider μ as truly independent variable setting up chemical composition of cells. In fact, both μ and σ are functions of one common independent variable, the limiting substrate concentration in the medium, s. For steady-state chemostat culture we have:

$$\mu = \frac{q}{\sigma} = \frac{1}{\sigma} \frac{Q\tilde{s}}{K_s + \tilde{s}}$$

$$\sigma = \sigma_0 + \frac{(\sigma_m - \sigma_0)\tilde{s}}{K_\sigma + \tilde{s}} \qquad \ldots (2.33)$$

where μ is specific growth rate, q is specific substrate uptake rates; σ_0 and σ_m are, respectively, lower and upper limits of σ variation; low limit $\sigma \to \sigma_0$ is attained when $\tilde{s} \to 0$ and upper limits $\sigma \to \sigma_m$ when $\tilde{s} \to \infty$. By excluding $\tilde{s}$ from both these equations we arrive at following relationship between σ and μ:

$$\mu = \mu_m \frac{\sigma_m(\sigma - \sigma_0)}{\sigma[\lambda(\sigma_m - \sigma_0) + \sigma - \sigma_0]}$$

$$\lambda = \frac{K_s}{K_\sigma} \qquad \ldots (2.34)$$

Under realistic assumption $\lambda \approx 1$ ($K_s \approx K_\sigma$) we have

$$\sigma = \frac{\sigma_0}{1 - (1 - \sigma_0/\sigma_m)\mu/\mu_m}$$

$$Y = Y_m - (Y_m - Y_0)\frac{\mu}{\mu_m} \qquad \ldots (2.35)$$

where, Y_m and Y_0 are, respectively, upper and lower limits of yield variation ($Y_m = 1/\sigma_0$, $Y_0 = 1/\sigma_m$). As we can see, the linear relationship between Y and μ is normally observed in chemostat culture (Fig. 2.10).

Microscopic Approach in Studies of Growth Stoichiometry

Equations 2.12 to 2.35 exemplify the macroscopic approach in studying of microbial growth stoichiometry. Its typical features are the use of gross formulas for biomass and metabolic products, evaluation of total mass balance for chemical elements (C, N, P) and formal description of microbial growth as a single-step conversion of substrate(s) into biomass. By contrast, the microscopic approach focuses on the much more complex real metabolic reactions and attempts to account for a limited but still quite large number of individual metabolic intermediates. The final aim of this approach is to organise the biochemical information into a consistent picture of microbial metabolism at the level of entire cell.

The microscopic approach has become possible by virtue of advancements in biochemistry, which has succeeded in establishing a sufficiently full picture of metabolic processes in certain micro-organisms. The pioneering work in this area was done by Bauchop and Elsden, who were able to sum up the balance of ATP for fermenting micro-organisms.

As a result, a relation was established between the biomass yield (a macroscopic quantity) and the number of generated ATP moles (a stoichiometric characteristic of real catabolic reactions):

$$Y_{ATP} = MY_E/n \qquad \text{... (2.36)}$$

where, n = mol of ATP made available to the organism by the metabolism of one mole of energy source, and M = molecular weight (g) of energy source. The following example illustrates the Y_{ATP} calculation: if biomass yield of some organisms aerobically grown on glucose is 0.52 g CDW/g, then Y_E is 1.49 g CDW per g of oxidised glucose (calculated from equation 6) or $Y_E = 1.49 \times 180 = 268$ g CDW/mol (180 is glucose molecular weight); assuming that P/O = 2 (that is, 2 mol of ATP produced per atom oxygen taken up) and that 2 ATP mol are produced via glycolysis (substrate phosphorylation) we arrived at $n = 2 + 12 \times 2 = 26$ and $Y_{ATP} = 268/26 = 10.3$ g CDW/mol ATP. Careful determination of n and Y_{ATP} is possible only for anaerobic growth of fermenting micro-organisms generating ATP via substrate phosphorylation. The mean value tends to be around 10.5 g CDW/mol ATP (Fig. 2.11). For aerobic growth, we need to make assumptions on the P/O ratio. As soon as the respiratory chain of bacteria differ widely for various organisms and growth conditions, this assumption can never be reliable. To avoid this obstacle, an interesting approach was proposed: microbial culture is grown in a chemostat limited by two carbon-containing energy sources, their ratio is varied while the total carbon feed rate is kept constant; yield measurements should allow one to determine both parameters (P/O and Y_{ATP}) independently by multiple linear regression.

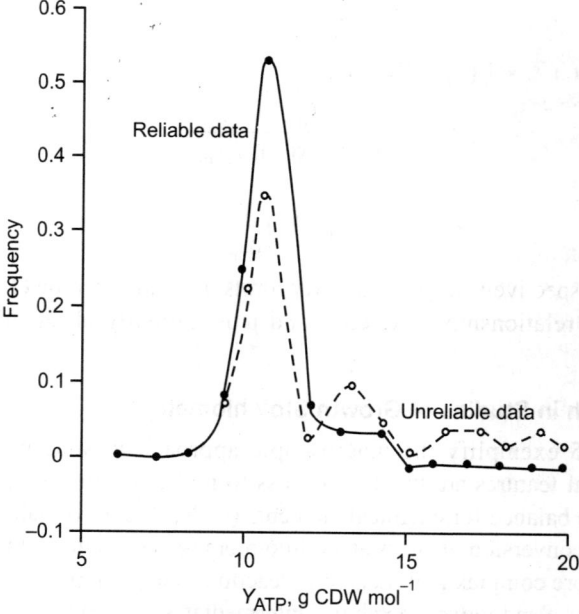

Fig. 2.11. Frequency distribution of experimentally measured values of Y_{ATP} at different degrees of creditability. The reliable data refer to studies of anaerobic growth with direct measurements of fermentation products. Note that these data are normally distributed with mean value 10.55, whereas all data display considerable skewness.

Today, microstoichiometry is quickly progressing as so-called metabolic balancing. Cell growth is viewed as a set of transport and intracellular metabolic reactions known for some particular organisms.

As a rule, the produced metabolic networks are composed of a combination of true stoichiometric equations for individual metabolites and empirical gross equations (Table 2.8). The amount of such equations vary in different models from 20 to 30 to more than 100. For example, van Gulik and Heijnen describe yeast growth by a set of more than 90 reactions including glycolysis and the citric acid cycle; PEP phosphotransferase; pentose phosphate pathway; glyoxylate shunt; oxidative phosphorylation; CO_2 interaction with THF; transport of inorganic P, NH_4^+, SO_4^{2-}, acetate, lactate, pyruvate, glucose, gluconate, succinate, and citrate (totally 10 transport reactions); amino acid synthesis and polymerisation; nucleotide synthesis; RNA synthesis; ATP consumption for maintenance; fatty acids synthesis; formation of glycogen and polysaccharides; and finally, the biomass formation from proteins, polysaccharides, RNA, fatty acids, and glycerol.

Table 2.8. Metabolic networks.

Reaction	Equation	Stoichiometric equation	Empirical gross equation
Glycolysis reaction	Glucose + ATP → glucose-6-P + ADP + H	x	–
	Glucose-6-P → fructose-6-P	x	–
	0.5 Fructose-6-P + 0.5 ATP → glyceraldehyde-3-P +0.5 ADP + 0.5 H	x	–
Oxidative phosphorylation	$NADH + 0.5O_2 + d_1ADP + d_2Pi + (1 + d_1) H →$ $(1 + d_1) H_2O + NAD + d_1ATD$	x	–
Biomass formation	a_1Proteins + $a_2$polysaccharides + a_3RNA + $a_4$lipids → biomass	–	x

For each compound, i, involved in a metabolic system, a mass balance can be defined:

$$\frac{dC_i}{dt} = r_{Ai} + \phi_i \qquad \dots (2.37)$$

where, C_i is concentration of ith compound, r_{Ai}, and ϕ_i denote the net rates of, respectively, i chemical conversion and transport over the boundaries of bioreactor (fluxes of CO_2, O_2, nutrients, cells, and products). Most metabolic balancing equations are applied to steady-state growth (which means that no intracellular accumulation of metabolites occurs). In such cases, the differential equations like Eq. 2.37 are reduced to linear algebraic ones. Besides, an extensive use of matrix calculus is customarily made to obtain a concise notation. The problem of experimental support of such model is especially important. The degree of freedom, df, of the resulting system of linear equations is equal to the total number of unknown rates (both intracellular and exchange reactions) minus the total number of linear equations. To resolve the system, df rates have to be measured, and then the system is fully determined. If the number of measured rates is greater than df, then the system is overdetermined, and the redundancy of the data can be used for statistical analysis and error minimisation. However, it is much more typical to have an underdetermined system when the sum of measured rates is less than df. In this case, the number of possible solutions is infinite unless additional constraints are applied (e.g. maximisation of biomass yield, minimisation of energy expenditure) to find the one and only one solution by the linear optimisation technique.

In most studies, flux estimates are obtained using measurements of substrate consumption and product formation. This approach has proved to be efficient in some particular biotechnological cases, such as when only specific pathways need to be considered or if the contribution of flux for cellular growth is weak, as with mammalian or hybridoma cells. The more complex microbial systems are turned out to be seriously underdetermined. In such cases, the application of metabolic balancing requires the use of one or another maneuvers: (i) to lump together several sets of reactions, and (ii) to utilise data from *in vitro* enzyme assays; to make assumptions on numeric values of some stoichiometric growth parameters, such as Y_{ATP}, P/O, and H^+/e ratios, which are the subject of controversial debates.

However, the best solution would be to get direct experimental data on *in vivo* flux and resolve the system. Isotopic tracers are one of the best candidates for such a purpose. This novel approach is based on the analytical power of ^{1}H-detected ^{13}C nuclear magnetic resonance. *Corynebacterium glutamicum* was grown in chemostat culture continuously fed with [1–^{13}C]-glucose; when steady-state was established, the cells were harvested and hydrolysed and the amino acids were separated by ion-exchange chromatography and analysed by NMR spectroscopy. NMR provides data on ^{13}C enrichment at each specified carbon position of amino acid. Because metabolic pathways for amino acid synthesis are exactly defined, then the entire central metabolism can be assessed for *in vivo* fluxes, including determination of the forward and back rates of bidirectional reactions. In *C. glutamicum*, the flux through the pentose phosphate pathway turned out to be 66.4 per cent (relative to glucose input flux 1.49 mmol g^{-1} CDW hr^{-1}); the entry into tricarboxylic acid cycle, 62.2 per cent; and the contribution of the succinylase pathway to lysine synthesis, 13.7 per cent. The total net flux of the anaplerotic reactions (carboxylation of PEP/pyruvate into oxaloacetatel/malate) was quantitated as 38 per cent, the true forward flux of C3 → C4 being 68.6 per cent (1.8 times of 38 per cent) and a back flux of C4 → C3 being 30.6 per cent (0.8 times of 38 per cent). The metabolic balancing proved to be very promising and useful to identify metabolic constraints for intensive synthesis (overproduction) of products such as amino acids. On the other hand, this approach still is restricted to steady-state and balanced growth and is not able to cope with complex dynamic behaviour of micro-organisms (transient growth, changes in biomass composition).

Chapter 3

Microbial Kinetics

INTRODUCTION

Kinetics, is a branch of natural science that deals with the rates and mechanisms of any processes—physical, chemical, or biological. Kinetic studies in microbiology cover all dynamic manifestations of microbial life: growth itself, survival and death, product formation, adaptations, mutations, cell cycles, environmental effects, and biological interactions. Kinetics provides a theoretical framework for optimal design in biotechnologies based on fermentation and enzyme catalysis, as well as on employment of outdoor activity of natural microbial populations (waste-water treatment, soil bioremediation, etc.).

Contrary to simple rates measurements, kinetic studies require the perception of the underlying basic mechanisms of studied processes. We will define mechanistic studies as those that interpret some complex process as an interplay of several simpler reactions, for example, cell growth can be explained through activity of enzymes and microbial community dynamics can be interpreted through behaviour of individual cells and populations. Ideally, mechanistic studies infer the coupling of experimental measurements with analysis of simulating mathematical models. The models formalise postulated mechanisms, so that the comparison of observations and the model's predictions allows one to discard an incorrect hypotheses.

The quantitative studies in microbiology often involve the assessment of growth stoichiometry. Stoichiometry is the quantitative relationship between reactants and products in a chemical reaction. In microbiology, stoichiometry stands for a quantitative relationship between substrates and products of microbial processes, including biomass formation (the consequence of complying with mass and energy conservation laws). In practical terms, kinetic and stoichiometry are tightly linked to each other, but stoichiometry mainly addresses problems of a static nature (how much? in what proportion?), whereas kinetics considers the dynamics questions (at what rate? by which mechanism?).

It is well known that micro-organisms fuel their lives by performing oxidation/reduction reactions that generate the energy and reducing power needed to construct and maintain themselves. Because redox reactions are nearly always very slow unless catalysed, micro-organisms produce enzyme catalysts that increase the kinetics of their essential reactions to rates fast enough for them to exploit the chemical resources available in their environment. Engineers want to take advantage of these microbially catalysed reactions, because the chemical resources of the micro-organisms usually are the pollutants that the engineers must control. For example, the biochemical oxygen demand (BOD) is an organic electron donor for heterotrophic bacteria, NH_4^+–N is an inorganic electron donor for nitrifying bacteria, NO_3^-–N is an electron acceptor for denitrifying bacteria, and PO_4^{3-} is a nutrient for all micro-organisms. In trying to employ micro-organisms for pollution control, engineers must recognise two interrelated principles: First, metabolically active micro-organisms catalyse the pollutant-removing reactions. The rate of pollutant removal depends on the concentration of the catalyst, or the active biomass. Second, the active biomass is grown and sustained through the utilisation of its energy- and electron-generating primary substrates, which are its electron donor and electron acceptor. The rate of production of active biomass is proportional to the utilisation rate of the primary substrates.

The connection between the active biomass (the catalyst) and the primary substrates is the most fundamental factor needed for understanding and exploiting microbial systems for pollution control. Because those connections must be made systematically and quantitatively for engineering design and operation, mass-balance modelling is an essential tool.

Quantitative description of cellular processes is an indispensable tool in the design of fermentation processes. The two most important quantitative design parameters, yield and productivity, are quantitative measures that specify how the cells convert the substrates to the product. The yield specifies the amount of product obtained from the substrate, and it is of particular importance when the raw material costs make up a large fraction of the total costs, as exemplified in the production of solvents, antibiotics, alcohol, and other primary metabolites. The productivity specifies the rate of product formation, and is particularly important when the capital investments play an important role, such as in a growing market where there is an increasing demand for producing the product by a given capacity (or factory). These two design parameters can easily be derived from experimental data but, what is more difficult to predict, is how they change with the operating conditions, e.g. if the medium composition changes or the temperature changes. To do this it is necessary to set up a mathematical model.

A model is a set of relationships between the variables in the system being studied. These relationships are normally expressed in the form of mathematical equations, but they may also be specified as logic expressions (or cause/effect relationships) which are used in the operation of a process. The variables include any property that are of importance for the process, such as the agitation rate, the feed rate, pH, temperature, concentrations of substrates, metabolic products and biomass and the state of the biomass — often represented by the concentration of a set of key intracellular compounds.

To set up a mathematical model it is necessary to specify a control volume wherein all the variables of interest are taken to be uniform. For fermentation processes the control volume is typically the whole bioreactor, but for large bioreactors the medium may be nonhomogeneous due to mixing problems and here it is necessary to divide the bioreactor into several control volumes. When the control volume is the whole bioreactor it may either be of constant volume or it may change with time depending on the operation of the bioprocess.

When the control volume has been defined, a set of balance equations can be specified for the variables of interest. These balance equations specify how material is flowing in and out of the control volume and how material is converted within the control volume. Rate equations (or kinetic expressions) specify the conversion of material within the control volume. They may be anything from a simple empirical correlation that specifies the product formation rate as a function of the medium composition to a complex model that accounts for all the major cellular reactions involved in the conversion of the substrates to the product.

Independent of the model structure, the process of defining a quantitative description of a fermentation process involves a number of steps, as shown in Fig. 3.1.

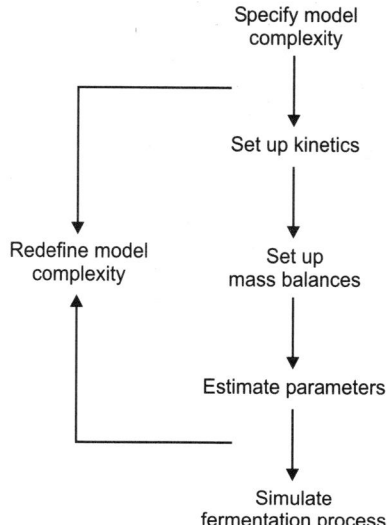

Specify model
complexity

Set up kinetics

Redefine model
complexity

Set up
mass balances

Estimate parameters

Simulate
fermentation process

Fig. 3.1. Different steps in quantitative description of fermentation processes.

A key aspect in setting up a model is to specify the model complexity. This depends on what the model is going to be used for. Specification of the model complexity involves defining the number of reactions to be considered in the model, and specification of the stoichiometry for these reactions. When the model complexity has been specified, rates of the cellular reactions considered in the model are described with mathematical expressions, i.e. the rates are specified as functions of the variables; namely the concentration of the substrates (and in some cases the metabolic products). These functions are normally referred to as kinetic expressions, since they specify the kinetics of the reactions considered in the model. This is an important step in the overall modelling cycle and in many cases, different kinetic expressions have to be examined before a satisfactory model is obtained.

The next step in the modelling process is to combine the kinetics of the cellular reactions with a model for the reactor in which the cellular process occurs. Such a model specifies how the concentrations of substrates, biomass, and metabolic products change with time, and what flows in and out of the bioreactor. These bioreactor models are normally represented in terms of simple mass balances over the whole reactor, but more detailed reactor models may also be applied, if inhomogeneity of the medium is likely to play a role. The combination of the kinetic and the reactor model makes up a complete mathematical description of the fermentation process and this model can be used to simulate the profile of the different variables of the process, e.g. the substrate and product concentrations. However, before this can be done it is necessary to assign values to the parameters of the model. Some of these parameters are operating parameters, which are dependent on how the process is operated, e.g. the volumetric flow in and out of the bioreactor, whereas others are kinetic parameters which are associated with the cellular system. To assign values to these parameters, it is necessary to compare model simulations with experimental data and hereby estimate a parameter set that gives the best fit of the model to the experimental data. This is referred to as parameter estimation. The evaluation of the fit of the model to the experimental data can be done by simple visual inspection of the fit, but generally it is preferential to use a more rational procedure, such as minimising the sum of squared errors between the model and the experimental data.

In the following, we will consider the two different elements needed for setting up a bioprocess model, namely kinetic modelling and mass balances. This will lead to a description of different types of bioreactor operation, and hereby simple design problems can be illustrated.

KINETIC MODELLING OF CELL GROWTH

All researchers in life sciences use models when results from individual experiments are interpreted and when results from several different experiments are compared with the aim of setting up a model that may explain the different observations. During the last 20 years there has been a revolution in experimental techniques applied in life sciences, and this has made possible far more detailed modelling of cellular processes. Furthermore, the availability of powerful computers has made it possible to solve complex numerical problems with a reasonable computational time; even complex mathematical models for biological processes can be handled and experimentally verified. However, often such detailed (or mechanistic) models are of little use in the design of a bioprocess, whereas they mainly serve a purpose in fundamental research of biological phenomena. In this presentation, we will focus on models which are useful for design of bioprocesses, but in order to give an overview of the different mathematical models applied to describe biological processes we start the presentation of kinetic models with a discussion of model complexity.

Model Structure and Model Complexity

Biological processes are *per se* extremely complex. Cell growth and metabolite formation are the result of a very large number of cellular reactions and events like gene expression, translation of mRNA into functional proteins, further processing of proteins into functional enzymes or structural proteins, and sequences of biochemical reactions leading to building blocks needed for synthesis of cellular components.

It is clear that a complete description of all these reactions and events cannot possibly be included in a mathematical model. In fermentation processes, where there is a large population of cells, non-homogeneity of the cells with respect to activity and function may add further to the complexity. In setting up fermentation models lumping of cellular reactions and events is, therefore, always done but the detail level considered in the model, i.e. the degree of lumping, depends on the aim of the modelling.

Fermentation models can roughly be divided into four groups depending on the detail level included in the model, (Fig. 3.2). The simplest description is the so-called unstructured models where the biomass is described by a single variable (often the total biomass concentration) and where no segregation in the cell population is considered.

These models can be combined with a segregated population model, where the individual cells in the population are described by a single variable, e.g. the cell mass or cell age, but often it is relevant to add further structure to the model when segregation in the cell population is considered. In the so-called structured models the biomass is described with more than one variable, i.e. structure in the biomass is considered. This structure may be anything from a few compartments to a detailed structuring into individual enzymes and macromolecular pools.

It is clear that a very important element in mathematical modelling of fermentation processes is defining the model structure (or specifying the complexity of the model), and for this, a general rule can be stated: As simple as possible but not simpler.

This rule implies that the basic mechanisms always should be included and that the model structure depends on the aim of the modelling exercise.

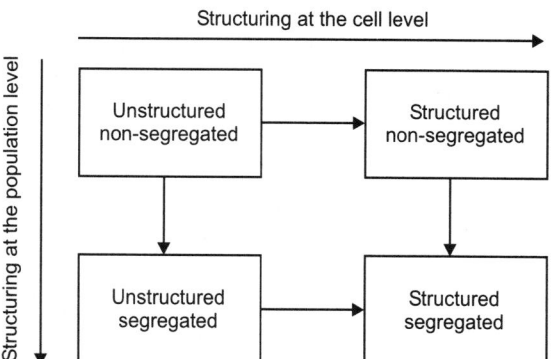

Fig. 3.2. Different types of model complexity, with increasing complexity going from the upper left corner to the lower right corner. When there is structuring at the cell level, specific intracellular events or reactions are considered in the model, and the biomass is structured into two or more variables. When there is structuring at the population level, segregation of the population is considered, i.e. it is accounted for that not all the cells in the population are identical.

Definitions of Rates and Yield Coefficients

Before we turn to describing different unstructured models, a few definitions are needed. Figure 3.3 is a representation of the overall conversion of substrates into metabolic products and biomass components (or total biomass). The rates of substrate consumption can be determined during a fermentation process by measuring the concentration of these substrates in the medium. Similarly, the rates of formation of metabolic products and biomass can be determined from measurements of the corresponding concentrations. It is, therefore, possible to determine what flows into the total pool of cells and what flows out of this pool.

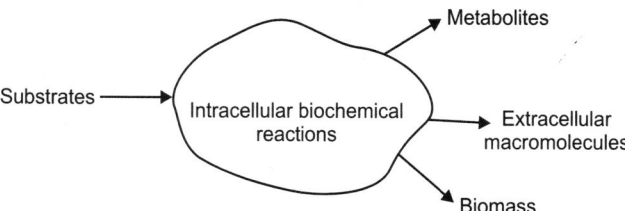

Fig. 3.3. General representation of cellular growth and product formation. Via a large number of intracellular biochemical reactions, substrates are converted into metabolic products, e.g. ethanol, acetate, lactate, or penicillin (and other secondary metabolites), extracellular macromolecules, e.g. a secreted enzyme, a heterologous protein, or a polysaccharide, and into biomass constituents, e.g. cellular protein, lipids, RNA, DNA, and carbohydrates.

The inflow of a substrate is normally referred to as the substrate uptake rate and the outflow of a metabolic product is normally referred to as the product formation rate. From the direct measurements of the concentrations, one obtains so-called volumetric rates. Often it is convenient to normalise the rates with respect to the amount of biomass present, since the rates hereby easily can be compared between fermentation experiments, even when the amount of biomass changes. Such normalised rates are referred to as specific rates, and these are often represented as r_i, where the subscript indicates whether it is a substrate (s) or a metabolic product (p). The specific growth rate of the total biomass is also a very important variable, and it is generally designated μ. The specific growth rate is related to the doubling time t_d (hr) of the biomass through:

$$t_d = \frac{\ln 2}{\mu} \qquad \text{... (3.1)}$$

The doubling time t_d is equal to the generation time for a cell, i.e. the length of a cell cycle for unicellular organisms, which is frequently used by life scientists to quantify the rate of cell growth.

The specific rates, or the flow in and out of the cell, are very important design parameters since they are related to the productivity of the cell. Thus, the specific productivity of a given metabolite directly indicates the capacity of the cells to synthesise this metabolite. Furthermore, if the specific rate is multiplied by the biomass concentration in the bioreactor one obtains the volumetric productivity, or the capacity of the biomass population per reactor volume. In simple kinetic models the specific rates are specified as functions of the variables in the system, e.g. the substrate concentrations. In more complex models where the rates of the intracellular reactions are specified as functions of the variables in the system, the substrate uptake rates and product formation rates are given as functions of the intracellular reaction rates. Another class of very important design parameters are the yield coefficients, which quantify the amount of substrate recovered in biomass and the metabolic products. The yield coefficients are given as ratios of the specific rates, e.g. for the yield of biomass on a substrate:

$$Y_{sx} = \frac{\mu}{r_s} \qquad \text{... (3.2)}$$

and similarly for the yield of a metabolic product on a substrate:

$$Y_{sp} = \frac{r_p}{r_s} \qquad \text{... (3.3)}$$

The yield coefficients are clearly determined by how the carbon in the substrate is distributed among the different cellular pathways towards the end products of the catabolic and anabolic routes. These parameters can be considered as an overall determination of metabolic fluxes, a key aspect in modern physiological studies where methods to quantify intracellular, metabolic fluxes have become an important tool in defining the activity of the different pathways within the complete metabolic network. In the production of low-value added products, e.g. ethanol, antibiotics, amino acids and baker's yeast, it is generally of utmost importance to optimise the yield of product on the substrate and the target is, therefore, to direct as much carbon as possible towards the product and minimise the carbon flow to by-products (including biomass in metabolite production processes). In this process the yield coefficient is the most important design parameter, both for characterising different mutants and for characterising different fermentation schemes.

For aerobic processes the yield of CO_2 from O_2 is often used to characterise the metabolism of the cells. This yield coefficient is referred to as the respiratory quotient (RQ). With complete respiration the RQ is close to 1 whereas if a metabolite is formed it deviates from 1.

The yield coefficients are always given with a double index that indicates the direction of the conversion, i.e. the yield for the conversion of substrate to biomass ($s \to x$) has the index sx. Thus, the yield coefficient Y_{xs} specifies the amount of substrate converted per unit biomass formed and, similarly, the yield coefficient, Y_{xp}, specifies the amount of product formed per unit biomass formed.

Black Box Models

The simplest mathematical presentation of cell growth is the so-called black box model, where all the cellular reactions are lumped into a single overall reaction. This implies that the yield of biomass on the substrate (as well as the yield of all other compounds consumed and produced by the cells) is constant. Consequently the specific substrate uptake rate can be specified as a function of the specific growth rate of the biomass, simply by rewriting Eq. (3.2):

$$r_s = Y_{xs}\mu \qquad \qquad ...(3.4)$$

Similarly, the specific uptake rate of other substrates, such as O_2, and the formation rate of metabolic products are proportional to the specific growth rate. In the black box model, the kinetics reduces to a description of the specific growth rate as a function of the variables in the system. In the most simple model description, it is assumed that there is only one limiting substrate, typically the carbon source, and the specific growth rate is, therefore, specified as a function of the concentration of this substrate only. A very general observation for cell growth on a single limiting substrate is that at low substrate concentrations (c_s) the specific growth rate, μ, is proportional with c_s, but for increasing concentrations there is an upper value for the specific growth rate. This verbal presentation can be described with many different mathematical models, but the most often applied is the Monod model, which states that:

$$\mu = \mu_{max} \frac{c_s}{c_s + K_s} \qquad \qquad ...(3.5)$$

K_s is the substrate concentration at which the specific growth rate is 0.5 μ_{max}, and is sometimes interpreted as the affinity of the cells towards the substrate s. Since the substrate uptake often is involved in the control of substrate metabolism, the value of K_s is also often in the range of the K_m values of the substrate uptake system of the cells.

However, K_s is an overall parameter for all the reactions involved in the conversion of the substrate to biomass, and it is, therefore, completely empirical and has no physical interpretation. The influence of the substrate concentration on the specific growth rate with the Monod model is illustrated in Fig. 3.4. Table 3.1 summarises the K_s value for different microbial systems.

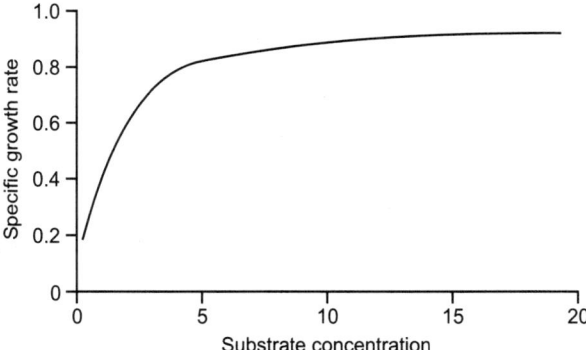

Fig. 3.4. The specific growth rate, μ, as function of the concentration of the limiting substrate, s, when the Monod model is applied.

The Monod model is not the only kinetic expression that has been proposed to describe the specific growth rate in the black box model. Many different kinetic expressions have been presented as shown in

Table 3.2. Except for the Moser model, all the kinetic expressions contain two adjustable parameters as in the Monod model. In the Contois kinetics, an influence of the biomass concentration, x, is included, i.e. at high biomass concentrations there is an inhibition of cell growth. It is unlikely that the biomass concentration as such inhibits cell growth but there may well be an indirect effect, e.g. the formation of an inhibitory compound by the biomass or high biomass concentrations may give a very viscous medium that results in mass transfer problems. Similarly, the Logistic law expresses a negative influence of the biomass concentration on the specific growth rate. These different expressions clearly demonstrate the empirical nature of these kinetic models, and it is, therefore, futile to discuss which model is to be preferred, since they are all simply data fitters, and one should simply choose the model that gives the best description of the system being studied.

Table 3.1. Compilation of K_s values for different microbial cells growing on different sugars.

Species	Substrate	K_s (mg^{-1})
Aspergillus oryzae	Glucose	5
Escherichia coli	Glucose	4
Klebsiella pneumoniae	Glucose	9
Aerobacter aerogenes	Glycerol	9
Klebsiella oxytoca	Glucose	10
	Arabinose	50
	Fructose	10
Penicillium chrysogenum	Glucose	4
Saccharomyces cerevisiae	Glucose	180

Table 3.2. Compilation of different unstructured, kinetic models.

Name	Kinetic expression
Tessier	$\mu = \mu_{max}(1 - e^{-c_s/K_s})$
Moser	$\mu = \mu_{max}\dfrac{c_s^n}{c_s^n + K_s}$
Contois	$\mu = \mu_{max}\dfrac{c_s}{c_s + K_s x}$
Blackman	$\mu = \begin{cases} \mu_{max}\dfrac{c_s}{2K_s}; & c_s \leq 2K_s \\ \mu_{max} & c_s \geq 2K_s \end{cases}$
Logistic law	$\mu = \mu_{max}\left(1 - \dfrac{x}{K_x}\right)$

All the kinetic expressions presented in Table 3.2 assume that there is only one limiting substrate, but often more than one substrate concentration influences the specific growth rate. In these situations, complex interactions can occur which are difficult to model with unstructured models unless many adjustable parameters are included. Several different multi-parameter, unstructured models for growth on multiple substrates have been proposed where it is often difficult to distinguish between whether a second substrate is growth enhancing or limiting growth. A general kinetic expression that accounts for both types of substrates is:

$$\mu = \left(1 + \sum_i \frac{c_{si,e}}{c_{si,e} + K_{e,i}}\right) \prod_j \frac{\mu_{max,j} c_{s,j}}{c_{s,j} + K_{s,j}} \qquad \ldots (3.6)$$

The presence of growth-enhancing substrates increases the specific growth rate whereas the essential substrates are necessary for growth to take place.

A special case of Eq. 3.6 is the growth in the presence of two essential substrates, $c_{s,1}$ and $c_{s,2}$:

$$\mu = \frac{\mu_{max,1} \, \mu_{max,2} \, c_{s,1} c_{s,2}}{(c_{s,1} + K_1)(c_{s,2} + K_s)} \qquad \ldots (3.7)$$

If both substrates are at concentrations where the specific growth rate for each substrate reaches 90 per cent of its maximum value, i.e. $c_{s,i} = 0.9 \, K_i$, then the total rate of growth is limited to 81 per cent of the maximum possible value. This is hardly practical and several alternatives to Eq. 3.7 have, therefore, been proposed, and one of these is:

$$\frac{\mu}{\mu_{max}} = \min\left(\frac{c_{s,1}}{c_{s,1} + K_1}, \frac{c_{s,2}}{c_{s,2} + K_2}\right) \qquad \ldots (3.8)$$

Growth on two or more substrates that may substitute each other, e.g. glucose and lactose, cannot be described by any of the unstructured models described above. Consider for example growth of *E. coli* on glucose and lactose. Glucose is the favoured substrate and will therefore be metabolised first. Only when this sugar is exhausted will the metabolism of lactose begin. The bacterium needs one of the sugars to grow but, in the presence of glucose, there is not a growth-enhancing effect of lactose. Application of Eq. 3.6 to this example of multiple substrates will clearly not be feasible. To describe this so-called diauxic growth it is necessary to apply a structured model and, in general, it is advisable always to consider only a single limiting substrate in black box models.

In some cases growth is inhibited either by high concentrations of the limiting substrate or by the presence of a metabolic product. In order to account for these aspects the Monod kinetics are often extended with additional terms. Thus, for inhibition by high concentrations of the limiting substrate:

$$\mu = \mu_{max} \frac{c_s}{c_s^2/K_i + c_s + K_s} \qquad \ldots (3.9)$$

and for inhibition by a metabolic product:

$$\mu = \mu_{max} \frac{c_s}{c_s + K_s 1 + p/K_i} \qquad \ldots (3.10)$$

Equations 3.9 and 3.10 may be a useful way of including product or substrate inhibition in a simple model. Extension of the Monod model with additional terms or factors should, however, be done with some restraint since the result may be a model with a large number of parameters but of little value outside the range in which the experiments were made.

Linear Rate Equations

In the black box model all the yield coefficients are taken to be constant. This implies that all the cellular reactions are lumped into a single, overall growth reaction where substrate is converted to biomass. A requirement for this assumption is that there is a constant distribution of fluxes through all the different cellular pathways under different growth conditions. In 1959, Denis Herbert clearly demonstrated this was not the case since he found that the yield of biomass on substrate was not constant. In order to describe his observations, he introduced the concept of endogenous metabolism and specified substrate consumption for this process in addition to that for biomass synthesis, i.e. substrate consumption takes place in two different reactions. In the same year Luedeking and Piret found that lactic acid bacteria produce lactic acid under non-growth conditions, which was consistent with an endogenous metabolism of the cells. Their results indicated a linear correlation between the specific lactic acid production rate and the specific growth rate:

$$r_p = \alpha r_x + \beta x \qquad \text{... (3.11)}$$

In 1965, John Pirt introduced a similar linear correlation between the specific substrate uptake rate and the specific growth rate. He suggested use of the term maintenance, which now is the most commonly used term for endogenous metabolism. The linear correlation of Pirt takes the form:

$$r_s = Y_{xs}^{true}\mu + m_s \qquad \text{... (3.12)}$$

The maintenance coefficients quantify the rate of substrate consumption for cellular maintenance, and it is normally given as a constant. In principle, this gives rise to a conflict since this may result in substrate consumption even when the substrate concentration is zero ($c_s = 0$), and in some cases it may, therefore, be necessary to specify m_s as a function of c_s.

With the introduction of the linear correlations the yield coefficients can obviously not be constants. Thus, for the biomass yield on the substrate:

$$Y_{sx} = \frac{\mu}{Y_{xs}^{true}\mu + m_s} \qquad \text{... (3.13)}$$

which shows that Y_{sx} decreases at low specific growth rates where an increasing fraction of the substrate is used to meet the maintenance requirements of the cell. For large specific growth rates the yield coefficient approaches the reciprocal of Y_{xs}^{true}, i.e. Y_{sx} becomes equal to Y_{xs}^{true}. This corresponds to the situation where the maintenance substrate consumption becomes negligible compared with the substrate consumption for biomass growth, and Eq. 3.12 can be approximated with Eq. 3.4. Despite its simple structure the linear rate Eq. 3.12 of Pirt is found to hold for many different species, and Table 3.3 compiles true yield coefficients and maintenance coefficients for various microbial species.

The empirically derived, linear correlations are very useful to correlate growth data, especially in steady state continuous cultures where linear correlations similar to Eq. 3.12 are found for most of the important specific rates.

The remarkable robustness and general validity of the linear correlations indicates that they have a fundamental basis and this basis is likely to be the continuous supply and consumption of ATP, since these two processes are tightly coupled in all cells. Thus, the role of the energy producing substrate is to provide ATP to drive both the biosynthetic and polymerisation reactions of the cell and the different maintenance processes according to the linear relationship:

$$r_{ATP} = Y_{xATP}\mu + m_{ATP} \qquad \text{... (3.14)}$$

which is a formal analogue to the linear correlation of Pirt, and states that the ATP being produced is balanced by its consumption for growth and for maintenance. If the ATP yield on the energy-producing substrate is constant, i.e. r_{ATP} is proportional to r_s, it is quite obvious that Eq. 3.14 can be used to derive the linear correlation Eq. 3.12. Y_{xATP} used in Eq. 3.14 is a true yield coefficient but it is normally specified without the superscript 'true'.

Table 3.3. True yield (g substrate needed to produce 1 g biomass) and maintenance coefficients (g substrate consumed for maintenance metabolism per g biomass per hour) for different microbial species and growth on glucose or glycerol.

Organism	Substrate	Y_{xs}^{true} $(g\ g^{-1})$	m_s $(g\ g^{-1} \cdot hr)$
Aspergillus awamori	Glucose	1.92	0.016
Aspergillus nidulans		1.67	0.020
Candida utilis		2.00	0.031
Escherichia coli		2.27	0.057
Klebsiella aerogenes		2.27	0.063
Penicillium chrysogenum		2.17	0.021
Saccharomyces cerevisiae		1.85	0.015
Aerobacter aerogenes		1.79	0.089
Bacillus megatarium		1.67	–
Klebsiella aerogenes	Glycerol	2.13	0.074

With the linear rate equations the cellular reactions can be structured into several individual reactions. This concept can, in principle, be extended to consider individual reactions for different cellular pathways, as illustrated in the Sonnleitner and Käppeli model for baker's yeast. During aerobic growth of baker's yeast (*Saccharomyces cerevisiae*) there may be a mixed metabolism with both respiration and fermentation being active. At high glucose uptake rates there is a limitation in the respiratory pathway which results in an overflow metabolism towards ethanol. The point at which the glucose uptake rate initiates fermentative metabolism is often referred to as the critical glucose uptake rate, and this is dependent on the oxygen concentration in the bioreactor. Thus, at low dissolved oxygen concentrations the critical glucose uptake rate is lower than at high dissolved oxygen concentrations (and clearly at anaerobic conditions there is only fermentative metabolism corresponding to the critical glucose uptake rate being zero).

Effect of Temperature and pH

The reaction temperature and the pH of the growth medium are other process conditions with a bearing on the growth kinetics. It is normally desired to keep both of these variables constant (and at their optimal values) throughout the cultivation process, hence they are often called culture parameters to distinguish them from other variables such as reactant concentrations, stirring rate, oxygen supply rate etc. which can change dramatically from the start to the end of a cultivation. The influence of temperature and pH on individual cell processes can be very different, and since the growth process is the result of many enzymatic processes the influence of both variables (or culture parameters) on the overall bioreaction is quite complex.

The influence of temperature on the maximum specific growth rate of a micro-organism is similar to that observed for the activity of an enzyme: an increase with increasing temperature up to a certain point where protein denaturation starts, and a rapid decrease beyond this temperature. For temperatures below the onset of protein denaturation the maximum specific growth rate increases in much the same way as for a normal chemical rate constant:

$$\mu_{max} = A \exp\left(-\frac{E_g}{RT}\right) \qquad \ldots (3.15)$$

Assuming that the proteins are temperature denatured by a reversible chemical reaction with free energy change ΔG_d and that denatured proteins are inactive one may propose an expression for μ_{max}:

$$\mu_{max} = \frac{A \exp(-E_g/RT)}{1 + B \exp(-\Delta G_d/RT)} \qquad \ldots (3.16)$$

Figure 3.5 is a typical Arrhenius plot (reciprocal of the absolute temperature on the abscissa and log μ on the ordinate) for *E. coli*. The linear portion of the curve between approximately 294 and 300.5 K is accurately represented by Eq. 3.27 while the sharp bend and rapid decrease of μ for T > 312 K (= 39°C) shows the influence of the denominator term in Eq. 3.16.

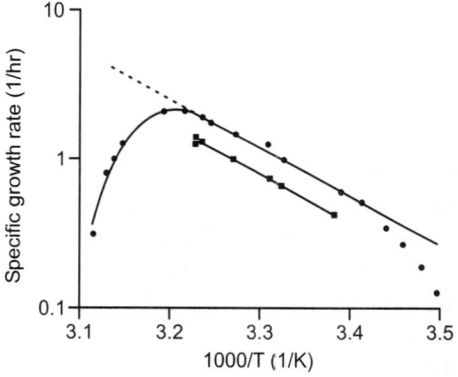

Fig. 3.5. The influence of temperature on the maximum specific growth rate of *Escherichia coli* B/r, (•) Growth on a glucose-rich medium; (■) growth on a glucose-minimal medium. The lines are calculated using the model in Eq. 3.28 with the parameters: E_g = 58 kj mole^{-1}, ΔG_d = 550 kj mole^{-1}, A = 10^{10} hr^{-1}, B = 3.0 10^{90}.

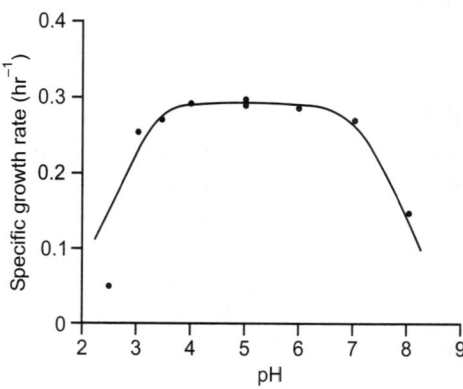

Fig. 3.6. The influence of pH on the maximum specific growth rate of the filamentous fungus *Aspergillus oryzae*. The line is simulated using Eq. 3.31 with K_1 = 4·10^{-3}, K_2 = 2·10^{-8}, and ke_{tot} = 0.3 hr^{-1}.

The influence of pH on the cellular activity is determined by the sensitivity of the individual enzymes to changes in the pH. Enzymes are normally only active within a certain pH range, and the total enzyme activity of the cell is, therefore, a complex function of the environmental pH. As an example, we shall consider the influence of pH on a single enzyme which is taken to represent the cell activity. The enzyme is assumed to exist in three forms:

$$e \leftrightarrow e^- + H^+ \leftrightarrow e^{2-} 2H^+ \qquad \qquad ...(3.17)$$

where, e^- is taken to be the active form of the enzyme while the two other forms are assumed to be completely inactive. With K_1 and K_2 being the dissociation constants for e and e^- respectively. The fraction of active enzyme e^- is calculated to be:

$$\frac{e^-}{e_{tot}} = \frac{1}{1 + [H^+]/K_1 + K_2/[H^+]} \qquad \qquad ...(3.18)$$

and the enzyme activity is taken to be $k = k_e e^-$. If the cell activity is determined by the activity of the enzyme considered above the maximum specific growth rate will be:

$$\mu_{max} = \frac{1}{1 + [H^+]/K_1 + K_2/[H^+]} \qquad \qquad ...(3.19)$$

Although the dependence of cell activity on pH cannot possibly be explained by this simple model it is, however, found that Eq. 3.19 gives an adequate fit for many micro-organisms, and Fig. 3.6 shows fit of the model for some data of the filamentous fungus *Aspergillus oryzae*.

MASS BALANCES FOR IDEAL BIOREACTORS

The last step in modelling of fermentation processes is to combine the kinetic model with a model for the bioreactor. A bioreactor model is normally represented by a set of dynamic mass balances for the substrates, the metabolic products and the biomass, which describes the change in time of the concentration of these state variables. The bioreactor may be any type of device ranging from a test tube or a shake flask to a well-instrumented bioreactor. Figure 3.7 is a general representation of a bioreactor. The feed is normally assumed to be sterile, i.e. the biomass concentration in the feed is zero.

The bioreactor may be operated in three different modes:

1. Batch, where $F = F_{out} = 0$, i.e. the volume is constant.
2. Continuous, where $F = F_{out} > 0$, i.e. the volume is constant.
3. Fed-batch (or semi-batch), where $F > 0$ and $F_{out} = 0$, i.e. the volume increases.

The mass balances for the different bioreactor modes can all be derived from a set of general mass balances, and we, therefore, start to consider these general balances.

General Mass Balance Equations

The basis for derivation of the general dynamic mass balances is the mass balance equation:

$$\text{Accumulated} = \text{Net formation rate} + \text{In} - \text{Out} \qquad \qquad ...(3.20)$$

The term accumulated specifies the rate of change of a compound in the bioreactor, such as the rate of increase in the biomass concentration during a batch fermentation. For substrates, the term Net formation rate is given by a substrate uptake rate (that is regarded as negative being the withdrawal of carbon from the system), whereas for metabolic products and biomass this term is given by the formation rate of these variables.

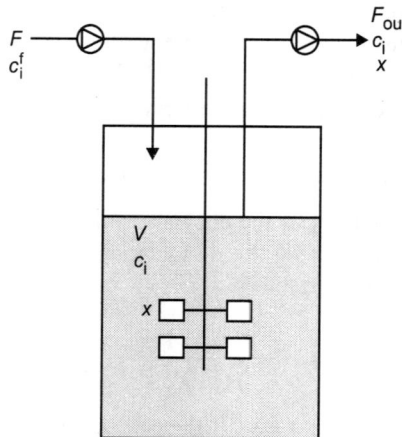

Fig. 3.7. General representation of a bioreactor with addition of fresh, sterile medium and removal of spent medium. c_i^f is the concentration of the i th compound (typically a substrate) in the feed and c_i is the concentration of the i th compound in the spent medium. The bioreactor is assumed to be very well mixed (or ideal), whereby the concentration of each compound in the spent medium becomes identical to its concentration in the bioreactor. In small volume bioreactors (<50 l) (including shake flasks) this can generally be achieved through aeration and agitation. In larger bioreactors there may, however, be significant concentration gradients throughout the bioreactor.

The term 'in' represents the flow of the compound into the bioreactor and the term 'out' the flow of the compound out from the bioreactor.

For the ith substrate, which is added to the bioreactor via the feed and is consumed by the cells present in the bioreactor, the mass balance is:

$$\frac{d(c_{s,i}V)}{dt} = -r_{s,i}xV + Fc_{s,i}^f - F_{out}c_{s,i} \qquad \text{... (3.21)}$$

The first term in Eq. 3.21 is the accumulation term, the second term accounts for substrate consumption (or net formation), the third term accounts for the inlet, and the last term accounts for the outlet. Rearrangement of Eq. 3.21 gives:

$$\frac{dc_{s,i}}{dt} = -r_{s,i}x + \frac{F}{V}c_{s,i}^f - \left(\frac{F_{out}}{V} + \frac{1}{V}\frac{dV}{dt}\right)c_{s,i} \qquad \text{... (3.22)}$$

Since for a fed-batch reactor:

$$F = \frac{dV}{dt} \qquad \text{... (3.23)}$$

and $F_{out} = 0$ the term within the parentheses becomes equal to the so-called dilution rate given by:

$$D = \frac{F}{V} \qquad \text{... (3.24)}$$

For both a continuous and a batch reactor, the volume is constant, i.e. $dV/dt = 0$, and $F = F_{out}$, and also for these bioreactor modes the term within the parentheses becomes equal to the dilution rate. Equation 3.24 therefore reduces to the mass balance (Eq. 3.25) for any type of operation.

$$\frac{dc_{s,i}}{dt} = -r_{s,i}x + D(c_{s,i}^f - c_{s,i}) \qquad \qquad \qquad ...(3.25)$$

The first term on the right hand side of Eq. 3.25 is the volumetric rate of substrate consumption, which is given as the product of the specific rate of substrate consumption and the biomass concentration. The second term accounts for the addition and removal of substrate from the bioreactor.

Dynamic mass balances for the metabolic products are derived in analogy with those for the substrates and takes the form:

$$\frac{dc_{p,i}}{dt} = -r_{s,i}x + D(c_{p,i}^f - c_{p,i}) \qquad \qquad \qquad ...(3.26)$$

where the first term on the right hand side is the volumetric formation rate of the ith metabolic product. Normally the metabolic products are not present in the sterile feed to the bioreactor and $c_{p,i}^f$ is, therefore, often zero.

With sterile feed the mass balance for the total biomass is:

$$\frac{d(xV)}{dt} = \mu x V - F_{out}x \qquad \qquad \qquad ...(3.27)$$

which in analogy with the substrate balance can be rewritten as:

$$\frac{dx}{dt} = (\mu - D)x \qquad \qquad \qquad ...(3.28)$$

Batch Reactor

This is the classical operation of the bioreactor that is used extensively. The disadvantage is that the experimental data produced are difficult to interpret since there are dynamic conditions throughout the experiment, i.e. the environmental conditions experienced by the cells vary with time. In well-instrumented laboratory bioreactors many variables, e.g. pH and dissolved oxygen tension, may be kept constant and this allows study of the effect of a single substrate on the biomass growth and product formation.

The dilution rate is zero for a batch reactor and the mass balances for the biomass and the limiting substrate (in a batch fermentation the limiting substrate is defined as the substrate that is first exhausted) therefore take the form:

$$\frac{dx}{dt} = \mu x; x(t = 0) = x_0 \qquad \qquad \qquad ...(3.29)$$

$$\frac{dc_s}{dt} = -r_s x; c_s(t = 0) = c_{s,0} \qquad \qquad \qquad ...(3.30)$$

According to these mass balances the biomass concentration will increase and the substrate concentration will decrease until its concentration reaches zero and growth stops. Assuming Monod kinetics, the mass balances for biomass and the limiting substrate can be rearranged into one first-order differential equation in the biomass concentration and an algebraic equation relating the substrate concentration to the biomass concentration. The algebraic equation is given by:

$$c_s = c_{s,0} - Y_{xs}(x - x_0) \qquad \qquad \qquad ...(3.31)$$

and the solution to the differential equation for the biomass concentration is given by:

$$\mu_{\max} t = \left(1 + \frac{K_s}{c_{s,0} + Y_{xs}x_0}\right) \ln\left(\frac{x}{x_0}\right) - \frac{K_s}{c_{s,0} + Y_{xs}x_0} \ln\left(1 + \frac{x_0 - x}{Y_{sx}c_{s,0}}\right) \qquad \text{... (3.32)}$$

Using these equations the profiles of the biomass and the glucose concentrations during a typical batch culture are easily derived, as shown in Fig. 3.8. Since the substrate concentration is zero at the end of the cultivation the overall yield of biomass on the substrate can be found from:

$$Y_{sx}^{\text{overall}} = \frac{x_{\text{final}} - x_0}{c_{s,0}} \qquad \text{... (3.33)}$$

Normally $x_0 \ll x_{\text{final}}$, and the overall yield coefficient can, therefore, be estimated from the final biomass concentration and the initial substrate concentration alone.

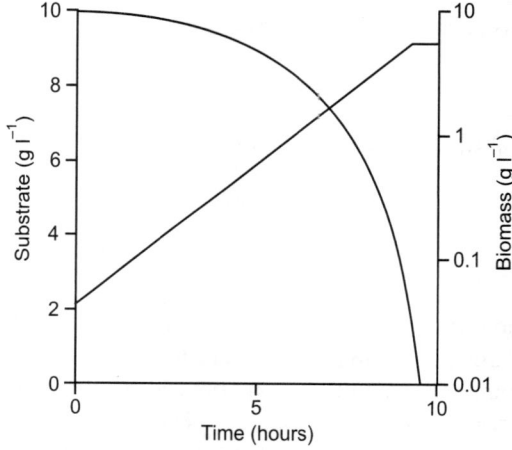

Fig. 3.8. Simulation of the biomass and glucose concentration during a batch culture. The simulation has been carried out using the Monod model with $\mu_{\max} = 0.5$ hr^{-1}; $K_s = 0.05$ g 1^{-1} and $Y_{sx} = 0.50$.

Notice that the yield coefficient determined from Eq. 3.33 is the overall yield coefficient and not Y_{sx} or Y_{sx}^{true}. The yield coefficient, Y_{sx}, may well be time dependent since it is the ratio between the specific growth rate and the substrate uptake rate (see Eq. 3.2). However, if there is little variation in these rates during the batch culture (e.g. if there is a long exponential growth phase and only a very short declining growth phase) the overall yield coefficient may be similar to the yield coefficient. If there is maintenance metabolism the true yield coefficient is difficult to determine from a batch cultivation since it requires information about the maintenance coefficients, which can hardly be determined from a batch experiment. However, in a batch cultivation the specific growth rate is close to its maximum throughout most of the growth phase and the substrate consumption due to maintenance is, therefore, negligible and, according to Eq. 3.14, the true yield coefficient is, therefore, close to the observed yield coefficient determined from the final biomass concentration.

Chemostat

A typical operation of the continuous bioreactor is the so-called chemostat, where the added medium is designed such that there is a single limiting substrate. This allows for controlled variation in the specific growth rate of the biomass. By varying the feed flow rate to the bioreactor, the environmental conditions can be varied and thereby valuable information concerning the influence of the environmental conditions on the cellular physiology can be obtained. For industrial applications, the continuous bioreactor is attractive since the productivity may be high. However, often the titre, i.e. the product concentration, is lower than what can be obtained in the fed-batch reactor. Furthermore, it is rarely used in industrial processes since it is sensitive to contamination, e.g. via the feed stream, and to the appearance of spontaneously formed mutants that may out-compete the production strain. Other examples of continuous operation besides the chemostat are the pH-stat, where the feed flow is adjusted to maintain the pH constant in the bioreactor, and the turbidostat, where the feed flow is adjusted to maintain the biomass concentration at a constant level.

From the biomass mass balance (Eq. 3.40), it is easily seen that in a steady state continuous reactor the specific growth rate equals the dilution rate:

$$\mu = D \qquad \qquad \text{... (3.34)}$$

Thus, by varying the dilution rate (or the feed flow rate) in a continuous culture different specific growth rates can be obtained. This allows detailed physiological studies of the cells when they are grown at a specified specific growth rate (corresponding to a certain environment experienced by the cells). At steady state the substrate mass balance (Eq. 3.25) gives:

$$0 = -r_s x + D(c_s^f - c_s) \qquad \qquad \text{... (3.35)}$$

which upon combination with Eq. 3.34 and the definition of the yield coefficient directly gives:

$$x = Y_{sx}(c_s^f - c_s) \qquad \qquad \text{... (3.36)}$$

Thus, the yield coefficient can be determined from measurement of the biomass and the substrate concentrations in the bioreactor. From measurements of the substrate concentration and the biomass concentration at steady state the specific glucose uptake rate can easily be calculated using Eq. 3.35, and similarly the specific rates of product formation can be determined from measurement of the product concentration and the biomass concentration.

If the Monod model applies the mass balance for the biomass gives:

$$D = \mu_{max} \frac{c_s}{c_s + K_s} \qquad \qquad \text{... (3.37)}$$

or

$$c_s = \frac{D K_s}{\mu_{max} - D} \qquad \qquad \text{... (3.38)}$$

Thus, the concentration of the limiting substrate increases with the dilution rate. When substrate concentration becomes equal to the substrate concentration in the feed the dilution rate attains its maximum value, which is often called the critical dilution rate:

$$D_{crit} = \mu_{max} \frac{c_s^f}{c_s^f + K_s} \qquad \qquad \text{... (3.39)}$$

When the dilution rate becomes equal to or larger than this value the biomass is washed out of the bioreactor. Equation 3.38 clearly shows that the steady state chemostat is well suited to study the influence of the substrate concentration on the cellular function, e.g. product formation, since by changing the dilution rate it is possible to change the substrate concentration as the only variable. Furthermore, it is possible to study the influence of different limiting substrates on the cellular physiology, e.g. glucose and ammonia.

Besides quantification of the Monod parameters the chemostat is well suited to determine the maintenance coefficient. Since the dilution rate equals the specific growth rate, combination of Eqs 3.13 and 3.36 gives:

$$x = \frac{D}{Y_{xs}^{true}D + m_s}(c_s^f - c_s) \qquad \qquad \dots (3.40)$$

which shows that the biomass concentration decreases at low specific growth rates, where the substrate consumption for maintenance is significant compared with that for growth. At high specific growth rates (high dilution rates) maintenance is negligible the yield coefficient becomes equal to the true yield coefficient, (see Fig. 3.10). Since $\mu = D$ at steady state, Eq. 3.12 expresses that there is a linear relation between the specific substrate uptake rate and the dilution rate. In this linear relationship the true yield coefficient and the maintenance coefficient can easily be estimated using linear regression.

For production of biomass, e.g. baker's yeast or single cell protein, and growth-related products the chemostat is very well suited since it is possible to maintain a high productivity over very long periods of operation. The productivity of biomass is given by:

$$P_x = Dx \qquad \qquad \dots (3.41)$$

and, in Fig. 3.9, the productivity is shown as a function of the dilution rate. By inserting the expression for the biomass concentration Eq. 3.40 in Eq. 3.41, with Eq. 3.38 inserted for the substrate concentration, it is possible to calculate the dilution rates which give the maximum productivity. If there is no maintenance, i.e. $m_s = 0$, the optimal dilution rate is given by:

$$D_{opt} = \mu_{max}\left(1 - \sqrt{\frac{K_s}{c_s^f + K_s}}\right) \qquad \qquad \dots (3.42)$$

It is important to emphasise that this optimum only holds for Monod kinetics without maintenance. When maintenance is included finding the optimum dilution rate will involve solving a third-degree polynomial. This polynomial will have one solution in the possible range of dilution rates. However, instead of solving the third-degree polynomial it is generally easier to find the solution numerically.

Fed-batch Reactor

This operation is probably the most common operation in industrial processes, since it allows for control of the environmental conditions, e.g. maintaining the glucose concentration at a certain level; it also enables formation of very high titres (up to several hundred grams per litre of some metabolites), which is of importance for subsequent downstream processing. There is striking similarity between the fed-batch reactor and the chemostat, and for the fed-batch reactor the mass balances for biomass and substrate are given by the general mass balance Eqs 3.25 and 3.28. Normally the feed concentration c_s^f is very high, i.e. the feed is a very concentrated solution, and the feed flow is low giving a low dilution rate. The dilution rate is given by:

$$D = \frac{1}{V}\frac{dV}{dt} \qquad \qquad \dots (3.43)$$

and if D is to be kept constant there needs to be an exponentially increasing feed flow to the bioreactor.

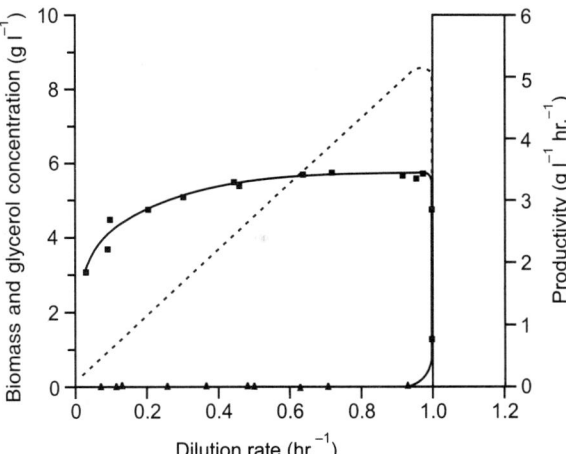

Fig. 3.9. Growth of *Klebsiella pneumaniae* (*Aerobacter aerogenes*) in a chemostat with glycerol as the limiting substrate. The biomass concentration (■) decreases at low dilution rates due to the maintenance metabolism, and when the dilution rate approaches the critical value the biomass concentration decreases rapidly. The glycerol concentration (▲) increases slowly at low dilution rates, but when the dilution rate approaches the critical value it increases rapidly. The lines are model simulations using the Monod model with maintenance, and with the parameter values: $c_s^f = 10$ g 1^{-1}; $\mu_{max} = 1.0$ hr^{-1}; $K_s = 0.01$ g 1^{-1}; $m_s = 0.08$ g g^{-1}·hr; $Y_{xs}^{true} = 1.70$ g g^{-1}. The broken line is the productivity according to Eq. 3.41.

If the yield coefficient is constant combination of the mass balances for the biomass and the substrate gives:

$$\frac{d(x + Y_{sx}c_s)}{dt}\left\{(\mu - D)x - Y_{sx}r_sx + Y_{sx}D(c_s^f - c_s)\right\} \qquad \dots (3.44)$$

or since $\mu = Y_{sx}r_s$

$$\frac{d\left(x - Y_{sx}(c_s^f - c_s)\right)}{dt} = -D\left(x - Y_{sx}(c_s^f - c_s)\right) \qquad \dots (3.45)$$

Through combination with Eq. 3.43 this differential equation can easily be solved with the solution given by:

$$\frac{Y_{sx}(c_s^f - c_{s,0}) - x_0}{Y_{sx}(c_s^f - c_s) - x} = \frac{V}{V_0} \qquad \dots (3.46)$$

where x_0, $c_{s,0}$ and V_0 define the biomass concentration, the substrate concentration and the reactor volume at the start of the fed-batch process. As mentioned above the substrate concentration in the feed c_s^f is normally very high and much higher than both the initial substrate concentration and the substrate concentration during the process (c_s). Furthermore, a very high c_s^f means that $Y_{sx}c_s^f$ is larger than the biomass concentration, both initially and during the process. Consequently the increase in volume can be kept low even when there is a very large increase in the biomass concentration.

If there is an exponential feed flow to the bioreactor there will be substantial biomass growth and, since the biomass concentration increases, this may lead to limitations in the O_2 supply. The feed flow is, therefore, typically increased until limitations in the O_2 supply set in and thereafter the feed flow is kept constant. This will give a decreasing specific growth rate. However, since the biomass concentration normally will increase, the volumetric uptake rate of substrates (including oxygen) may be kept approximately constant. From the above it is clear that there may be many different feeding strategies in a fed-batch process and optimisation of the operation is a complex problem that is difficult to solve empirically; and, even when a very good process model is available, calculation of the optimal feeding strategy is a complex optimisation problem. In an empirical search for the optimal feeding policy the two most obvious criteria are: (i) keep the concentration of the limiting substrate constant, and (ii) keep the volumetric growth rate of the biomass (or uptake of a given substrate) constant.

A constant volumetric growth rate (or uptake of a given substrate) is applied if there are limitations in the supply of oxygen or in heat removal. A constant concentration of the limiting substrate is often applied if the substrate inhibits product formation, and the chosen concentration, therefore, depends on the degree of inhibition and the desire to maintain a certain growth of the cells. The required feeding profile to maintain a constant substrate concentration $c_{s,0}$ corresponding to a constant specific growth rate μ_0 is quite simple to derive. From Eq. 3.27 with $F_{out} = 0$,

$$\frac{d(xV)}{dt} = \mu_0 xV \qquad \qquad \dots (3.47)$$

or

$$xV = x_0 V_0 e^{\mu_0 t} \qquad \qquad \dots (3.48)$$

Since the substrate concentration is constant the substrate balance gives:

$$-Y_{xs}\mu_0 x + D(c_s^f - c_s) = 0 \qquad \qquad \dots (3.49)$$

or

$$F(t) = \frac{Y_{xs}\mu_0}{c_s^f - c_s} xV = \frac{Y_{xs}\mu_0}{c_s^f - c_s} x_0 V_0 e^{\mu_0 t} \qquad \qquad \dots (3.50)$$

Finally, the biomass concentration $x(t)$ is obtained from Eq. 3.46 with $c_s = c_{s,0}$:

$$\frac{x(t)}{x_0} = \frac{e^{\mu_0 t}}{1 - ax_0 + ax_0 e^{\mu_0 t}} \qquad \qquad \dots (3.51)$$

where,

$$a = \frac{Y_{xs}}{c_s^f - c_s} \qquad \qquad \dots (3.52)$$

The bioreactor volume is given by:

$$\frac{V}{V_0} = 1 - ax_0 + ax_0 e^{\mu_0 t} \qquad \qquad \dots (3.53)$$

Figure 3.10 illustrates typical profiles for the biomass concentration, the bioreactor volume and the feed flow rate during a fed-batch process with constant substrate concentration.

Fed-batch processing is applied to processes where control of culture conditions is required, mainly to achieve high yields. Baker's yeast, secondary metabolites (where penicillins are the most prominent group of compounds), industrial enzymes and many other products are derived from fermentation processes.

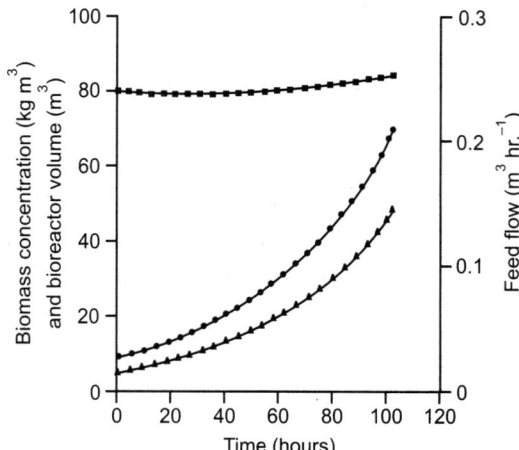

Fig. 3.10. The biomass concentration (•), the bioreactor volume (■), and the feed flow rate (▲) for a fed-batch reactor operated with a constant substrate concentration. The yield coefficient Y_{sx} is 0.5, the constant specific growth rate μ_0 is 0.02 hr^{-1}, and the substrate concentration in the feed c'_s is 400 kg m^{-3}. The substrate concentration is assumed to be much less than c'_s. The initial biomass concentration x_0 and the initial bioreactor volume are taken to be 10 kg m^{-3} and 80 m^3, respectively.

Nomenclature

a	constant
A	constant
B	Constant
c	concentration (g l^{-1} or moles l^{-1})
c_s	concentration of a substrate essential for growth (g l^{-1} or moles l^{-1})
$c_{s,0}$	initial concentration of the limiting substrate (g l^{-1} or moles l^{-1})
$c_{s,e}$	concentration of a growth enhancing substrate (g l^{-1} or moles l^{-1})
$c_{s,i}$	concentration (g l^{-1} or moles l^{-1})
D	dilution rate (hr^{-1})
D_{crit}	critical dilution rate (hr^{-1})
e^-	active form of the enzyme
e, e^{2-}	inactive forms of the enzyme
E_g	activation energy of the growth process (kJ mole^{-1})
F	flow rate (1 hr^{-1})
F_{out}	flow rate out of the bioreactor (1 hr^{-1})
ΔG_d	change in free energy (kJ mole^{-1})
K_I	inhibition constant (g g^{-1})
K_1	dissociation constant
K_2	dissociation constant
K_s	saturation coefficient (g l^{-1} or moles l^{-1})
m_s	maintenance coefficient (g g^{-1}·hr)
P_x	productivity (g l^{-1}·hr or moles l^{-1}hr)
r_i	specific rates (g g^{-1}·hr or moles g^{-1}·hr)

r_p	specific production rate (g g^{-1}·hr or moles g^{-1}·hr)
r_s	specific substrate uptake rate (g g^{-1}·hr or moles g^{-1}·hr)
T	temperature (K)
t	time (hr)
t_d	doubling time (hr)
V	volume (l)
x	biomass concentration (g l^{-1}).
Y_{ji}	yield coefficient specifying the amount of i produced per unit of j consumed (g$_j$ g$_i^{-1}$)
Y_{ij}	yield coefficient specifying the amount of j converted per unit of i produced (g$_i$ g$_j^{-1}$)
Y_{sx}	yield coefficient specifying the amount of biomass formed per unit substrate consumed (g g^{-1})
Y_{xp}	yield coefficient specifying the amount of product formed per unit biomass formed (g g^{-1})
Y_{xATP}	yield coefficient specifying the amount of ATP consumed per unit of biomass produced (g g^{-1})
Y_{xs}	yield coefficient specifying the amount of substrate used per unit biomass formed (g g^{-1})

Subscripts

e	growth enhancing compound
i	i-th substrate or product
j	essential growth compound
o	initial conditions
s	substrate
x	biomass
p	product

Superscripts

f	feed

Greek letters

α, β	coefficients in Eq. 3.11
ΔG_d	free energy change
μ	specific growth rate of the total biomass (g g^{-1}·hr or simply hr^{-1})
μ_{max}	maximum specific growth rate of the total biomass (g g^{-1}·hr or simply hr^{-1})

Chapter 4

Bioreactor Design

INTRODUCTION

In any fermentation process the bioreactor plays a central role in determining the process efficiency. Even with recombinant products where stringent quality control implies that downstream processing is the major cost component, it is the bioreactor performance which determines product yields.

Any vessel with facilities for aeration and agitation can be used as a bioreactor. Additionally, it must meet the requirements of aseptic operation and provide the cells with a controlled environment conducive to growth and product formation. Traditionally, the vessel of choice has been the stirred-tank bioreactor which consists of a vessel with a vertical rotating shaft with agitator blades (Fig. 4.1).

Since the vessel must be sterilised, it must meet the requirements of pressure vessel design (since steam is used under pressure to sterilise the bioreactor). Thus, the material of construction is usually 4–5 mm thick stainless steel, which is also resistant to the acids that are typically produced during fermentation. The height to diameter ratio (H/D) varies from 1 (for small reactors) to 3 (for larger vessels). A high H/D ratio provides for a smaller footprint (space saving), ease of construction and better mixing since the agitator blades need to be proportionally larger as the vessel diameter increases. However, tall tabular reactor with a high H/D ratio often leads to oxygen starvation in the gas phase which affects oxygen transfer rates. The other factor which is critical for large reactors is heat transfer since the metabolic heat generated during growth has to be removed. Cooling coils are used to carry cold water or a mixture of glycerol and water if the temperature of the coolant has to be less than 0°C.

The design of the agitator blade plays a crucial role in oxygen transfer and mixing. Traditionally, the flat blade impeller, the so-called Rushton stirrer (Fig. 4.2) was used. This stirrer provides good radial mixing and does not get 'flooded' with air bubbles even with high air-flow rates. However, it provides poor bulk mixing and this becomes a problem for fungal fermentations. This is because fungal broths shows non-Newtonian behaviour where the viscosity changes with the shear force. Thus the air bubbles get channelled through the centre of the fermenter where the viscosity is low (due to high mixing) effectively starving the media which are close to the walls of oxygen. To prevent this, agitators with better bulk mixing characteristics have been designed, such as the Scaba agitator and the Prochem Maxflow agitator (Fig. 4.2). When cells are shear sensitive the agitator is designed like a marine propeller which gives good axial mixing.

Often the problems of heat and oxygen transfer cannot be addressed with the conventional stirred-tank design. Airlift reactors are then used to provide better oxygen transfer. These reactors are modifications of bubble column reactors which have been used in beer production.

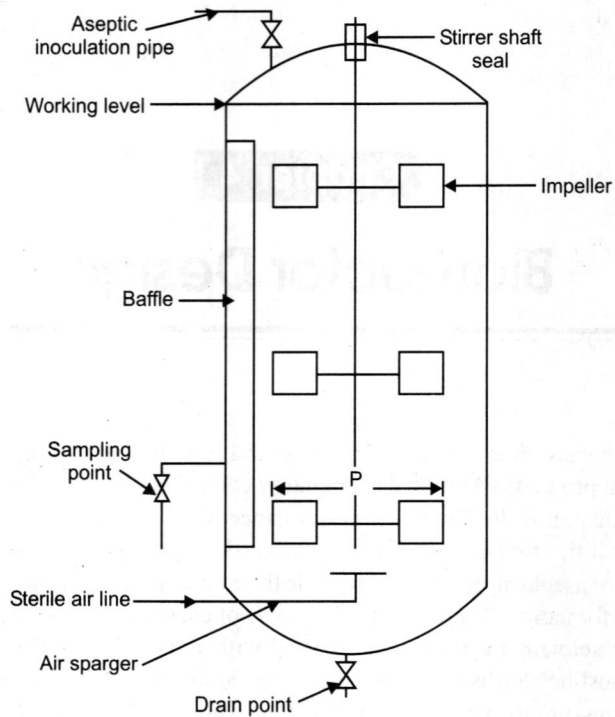

Fig. 4.1. Schematic of a stirred-tank bioreactor.

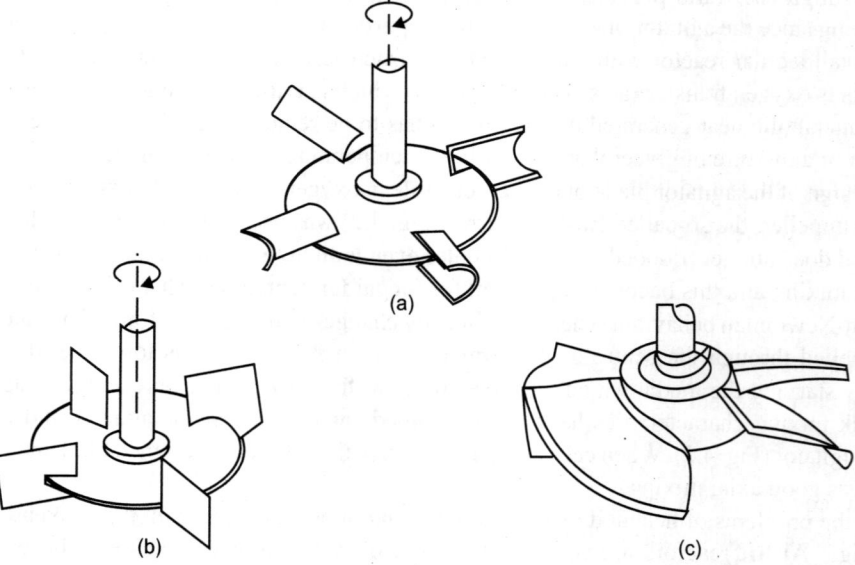

Fig. 4.2. Design of various agitators: (a) Scaba agitator, (b) Rushtor stirrer, and (c) Prochem Maxflow agitator.

In bubble columns the mixing is provided by the stream of bubbles entering the reactor at the bottom which helps to reduce construction and operating costs. In airlift reactors the liquid also rises with the bubbles through the 'riser', disengages with the gas phase and comes down through the downcomer. This 'downcomer' may be internal or external to the reactor. The circulation loop set up helps in improving heat and mass transfer rates. Other specialised bioreactors are required for specific needs. Thus, photobioreactors need to have a large specific surface area (i.e. surface area per unit volume) since the growth of cells is dependent on the incident sunlight. Thus, instead of a large tank, the cells are grown in tube banks (i.e. tubes arranged parallel to each other) and the material of construction is Plexiglas which is transparent to sunlight. The media (usually seawater) enters with a small inoculum, flows through the tubes like in a plug glow reactor and provides a high cell density at the outlet. Often a small fraction of the outlet cells is recycled to provide a continuous inoculum. Many novel bioreactors have been designed, like the pulsed column bioreactor which combines a pneumatic or mechanical pulsing of the reactor medium with a bubble column design. This helps in bubble break up thereby increasing the surface area and oxygen transfer rates. Since the shear forces are low, this set-up can be used for highly aerobic but shear sensitive organisms. However, most of the designs remain at the laboratory bench as they have not been taken up by industry which still prefers conventional and time-tested designs for large-scale operation.

CLASSIFICATION OF BIOCHEMICAL REACTOR

The biochemical reactor designs can be broadly classified into:

1. Submerged reactor—micro-organism remains submerged all the time inside the liquid. Gas-to-liquid mass transfer is achieved by dispersing the gas in the liquid through continuous input of energy
2. Surface reactor—the culture adheres to solid surface and oxygen is supplied from the gas phase to the continuously wetted solid surface.

Submerged reactors are further classified depending upon the nature of the energy input, namely:

1. Mechanically stirred systems with agitators.
2. Forced convection of the liquid using recirculating pumps.
3. Operation by pumping compressed air.

Mechanically Stirred Tank Reactor

In a mechanically stirred tank reactor, air is introduced from the bottom through a sparging arrangement and the contents are agitated with mechanical stirrers. Different types of stirrer designs are available for creating a good mixing between the gas and liquid and for breaking the large gas bubbles into finer bubbles. An agitator has to create not only axial movement but also radial movement. As the shear near the tip of the agitator blades are high, shear sensitive micro-organisms break easily. Long thin organisms can break as they get entangled in the rotating shaft. Baffles are provided to prevent vortex formation and improve mixing. The reactor is provided with a jacket or coils for heating and cooling the liquid contents. Power consumption in large designs is an issue in this type of reactor. Gas sparging decreases the power requirement for the agitator motor.

When the gas is sparged in the eye of the impeller the blades break up the large bubbles into smaller ones. The larger bubbles rise in the fluid phase faster than smaller bubbles. In highly viscosity fluids the rise of the bubbles is very slow. If the impeller speed is high enough the gas bubbles, having diameters too small to escape from the liquid phase, will be continuously recirculated with the incoming fresh gas phase. As a result one can assume a complete mixing of the gas phase under well-agitated conditions. If the mixing mechanism is the same as the liquid phase, the mixing time for gaseous phase also can be approximated by the liquid phase mixing time. The mixing pattern in a stirred vessel in the presence of air is different than that in the absence of it. At a higher impeller speed and low aeration rate, the pattern is more or less as that in an unaerated vessel. On increasing air flow rate, the flow pattern gets increasingly dominated by air flow. At a very high air flow rate, the air is not dispersed at all with a reversal of circulation flow at the centre. In this condition, the impeller is said to be flooded where energy dissipation by air is higher than the energy dissipation by the impeller.

Multicompartment Reactor or Cascade Reactor

A multicompartment reactor or a cascade reactor consists of a tall column, separated into several compartments and a single stirrer assembly with multiple blades agitates each of these compartments independently. Mixing and dispersion of gas into the liquid takes place in each chamber. Liquid flows down from the top compartment while gas rises upwards. The circulation pattern set up by multiple impellers depends on the type of the impellers, the speed of the agitator, geometry of the vessel and distance between impellers. For impellers spacing higher than the diameter of the vessel, the flow patterns creatred by each impeller are quite independent of each other. For spacing equal to the impeller diameter the flow patterns can either merge with each other or work against each other.

Typical reactors used in environmental applications are illustrated in Fig. 4.3. Table 4.1 contains a summary of typical applications for each type. The three basic reactors may find application as either suspended growth or biofilm reactors.

Table 4.1. Reactor types and their typical uses.

Reactor type	Typical uses
Basic reactors	
Batch	BOD test, high removal efficiency of individual waste-water constituents
Continuous-flow stirred-tank (CSTR)	Anaerobic digestion of sludges and concentrated wastes, aerated lagoon treatment of industrial wastes, stabilisation ponds for municipal and industrial wastes, part of activated sludge treatment of municipal and industrial waste-waters
Plug-flow (PFR)	Activated sludge treatment of municipal and industrial wastes, aerated lagoon treatment of industrial wastes, stabilisation ponds for municipal and industrial wastes, nitrification, high-efficiency removal of individual waste-water constituents
Biofilm reactors	
Packed bed	Aerobic and anaerobic treatment of municipal and industrial waste-waters, organic removal, nitrification, denitrification
Fluidised bed	Aerobic treatment of low BOD concentration waste-waters, toxic organic biodegradation, anaerobic treatment, denitrification
Rotating biological contactor (RBC)	Aerobic treatment of municipal and industrial waste-waters, organic removal, nitrification
Reactor arrangements	
Recycle	General aerobic and anaerobic treatment of municipal and industrial waste-waters, especially medium to low concentration BOD, organic removal, nitrification, denitrification

(Contd ...)

Reactor type	Typical uses
Series	BOD removal combined with nitrification or with nitrification and denitrification or combined with biological phosphorus removal, anaerobic staged treatment, stabilisation pond treatment, sequential anaerobic and aerobic treatment of waste-waters such as for removal of specific toxic organic chemicals
Parallel	Generally used for redundancy and reliability in plant operation, especially with high overall waste-water flow rates
Hybrid	Used for combined forms of treatment such as organic removal and nitrification, or organic removal, nitrification, and denitrification, or organic, nitrogen, and phosphorus removal; anaerobic treatment of industrial waste-waters
Sequencing batch	Useful for high-efficiency removal of individual constituents such as biodegradable but hazardous organics, combined removals of organics, nitrogen, and phosphorus; combination of aerobic and anaerobic processes with same micro-organisms

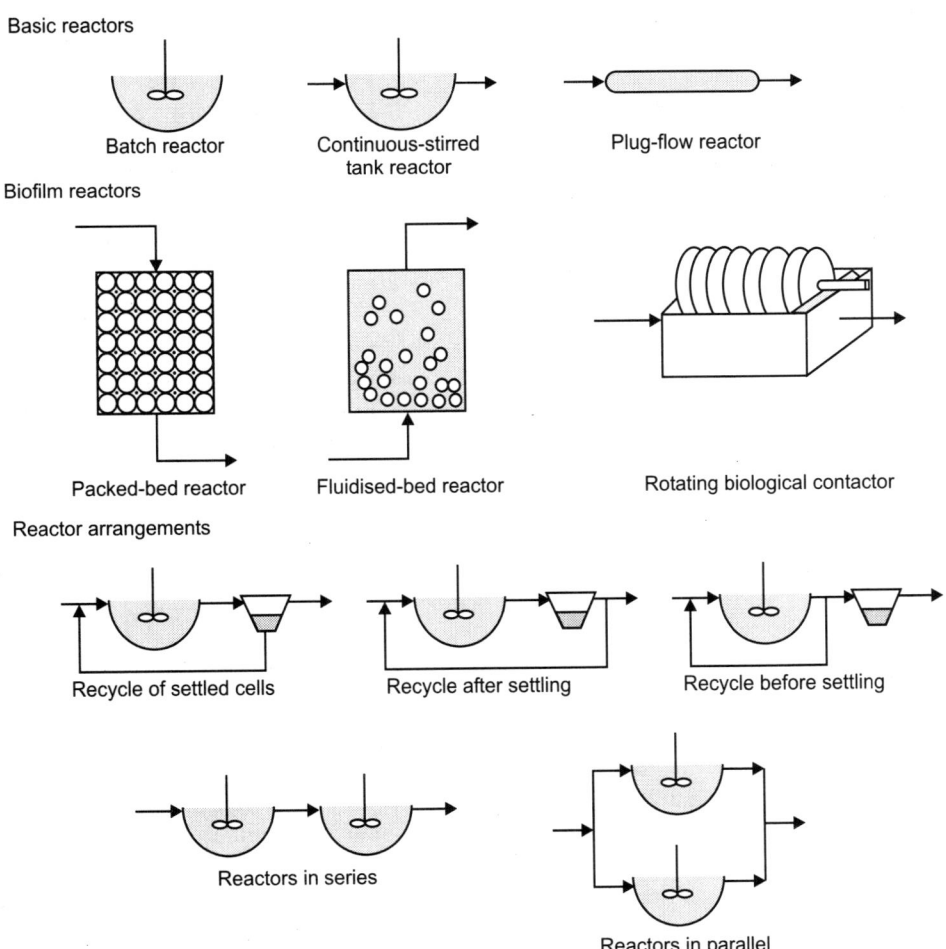

Fig. 4.3. Various reactor types and arrangements.

Bubble Columns

A bubble column bioreactor is shown in Fig. 4.4. Usually, the column is cylindrical with an aspect ratio of 4–6 (height-to-diameter). Gas is sparged at the base of the column through perforated pipes, perforated plates, or sintered glass or metal micro-porous spargers. O_2 transfer, mixing and other performance factors are influenced mainly by the gas flow rate and the rheological properties of the fluid. Internal devices such as horizontal perforated plates, vertical baffles and corrugated sheet packings may be placed in the vessel to improve mass transfer and modify the basic design. The column diameter does not affect its behaviour so long as the diameter exceeds 0.1 metre. One exception is the axial mixing performance. For a given gas flow rate, the mixing improves with increasing vessel diameter.

Mass and heat transfer and the prevailing shear rate increase as gas flow rate is increased. In bubble columns the maximum aeration velocity does not usually exceed 0.1 ms⁻¹. The liquid flow rate does not influence the gas-liquid mass transfer coefficient so long as the superficial liquid velocity remains below 0.1 ms⁻¹.

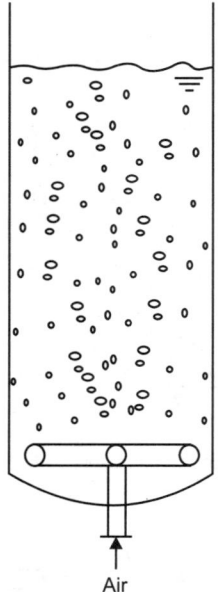

Air

Fig. 4.4. A bubble column.

Airlift Bioreactor Systems

An airlift bioreactor also known as a tower reactor can be described as a bubble column containing a draught tube. Many types of airlift bioreactors are currently in use today. The simple design of a concentric draught tube bioreactor with annular liquid downflow is shown in Fig. 4.5.

The gas supply is given by means of a sparger at the bottom into the inner cylinder and moves into the annular space creating a swarm of bubbles that induce significant aeration.

Air is fed through the sparger ring into the bottom of a central draught tube that controls the circulation of air and the medium. Air flows up the tube, forming bubbles, and exhaust gas disengages at the top of the column. The degassed liquid then flows downwards and the product is drained from the tank. The tube can be designed to serve as an internal heat exchanger, or a heat exchanger can be added to an internal circulation loop. Airlift systems provide some advantages against more conventional bioreactors as fermenters:

1. Simple design with no moving parts or agitator shaft seals for less maintenance, less risk of defects and easier sterilisation.
2. Lower shear rate, for greater flexibility—the system can be used for growing both plant and animal cells.
3. Efficient gas phase disengagement.
4. Large, specific interfacial contact area with low energy input.
5. Well-controlled flow and efficient mixing.
6. Well-defined residence time for all phases.
7. Increased mass transfer due to enhanced oxygen solubility achieved in large tanks with greater pressure.
8. Large volume tanks possible, increasing the output.
9. Greater heat removal vs conventional stirred tanks.

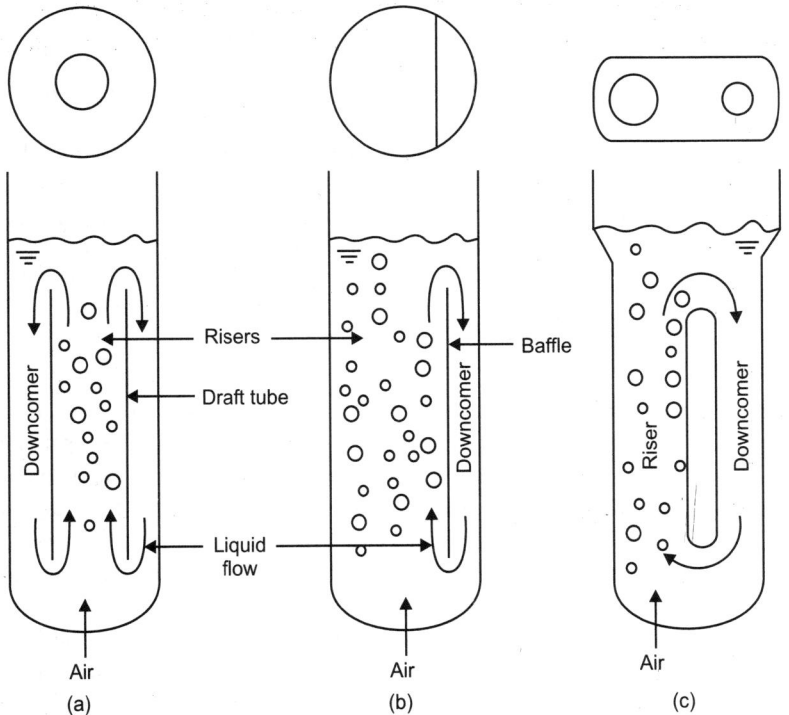

Fig. 4.5. Airlift bioreactor: (a) draft-tube internal loop configuration, (b) a split cylinder device, and (c) an external loop system.

The main disadvantages are as follows:

1. Higher initial capital investment due to large-scale processes.
2. Greater air throughput and higher pressures needed, particularly for large-scale operations.
3. Low friction with an optimal hydraulic diameter for the riser and the downcomer.
4. Lower efficiency of gas compression.

5. Inherently impossible to maintain consistent levels of substrate, nutrients in oxygen with organisms circulating through the bioreactor and conditions changing.
6. Inefficient gas/liquid separation and foaming occurs.

Fluidised Beds

Fluidised bed bioreactors are suited to reactions involving a fluid-suspended particulate biocatalyst such as the immobilised enzyme and cell particles or microbial flocs. An up-flowing stream of liquid is used to suspend or 'fluidise' the solids. Geometrically, the reactor is similar to a bubble column except that the top section is expanded to reduce the superficial velocity of the fluidising liquid to a level below that needed to keep the solids in suspension. Consequently, the solids sediment in the expanded zone and drop back into the narrower reactor column below; hence, the solids are retained in the reactor whereas liquid flows out.

A liquid fluidised bed may be sparged with air or some other gas to produce a gas-liquid-solid fluid bed. If the solid particles are too light, they may have to be artificially weighted, for example by embedding stainless steel balls in an otherwise light solid matrix. A high density of solids improves solid-liquid mass transfer by increasing the relative velocity between the phases. Denser solids are also easier to sediment but the density should not be too high relative to that of the liquid, or fluidisation will be difficult. Liquid fluidised beds tend to be fairly quiescent but introduction of a gas substantially enhances turbulence and agitation. Even with relatively light particles, the superficial liquid velocity needed to suspend the solids may be so high that the liquid leaves the reactor much too quickly, i.e. the solid-liquid contact time is insufficient for the reaction. In this case, the liquid may have to be recycled to ensure a sufficiently long cumulative contact time with the biocatalyst. The minimum fluidisation velocity, i.e. the superficial liquid velocity needed to just suspend the solids from a settled state — depends on several factors, including the density difference between the phases, the diameter of the particles, and the viscosity of the liquid.

Packed Bed Columns

A bed of solid particles, usually with confining walls, constitutes a packed bed. The biocatalyst is supported on, or within, the matrix of solids that may be porous or a homogeneous nonporous gel. The solids may be particles of compressible polymeric or more rigid material. A fluid containing nutrients flows continuously through the bed to provide the needs of the immobilised biocatalyst. Metabolites and products are released into the fluid and removed in the outflow. The flow may be upward or downward, but downflow under gravity is the norm. If the fluid flows up the bed, the maximum flow velocity is limited because the velocity cannot exceed the minimum fluidisation velocity or the bed will fluidise.

The depth of the bed is limited by several factors, including the density and the compressibility of the solids, the need to maintain a certain minimal level of a critical nutrient, such as O_2, through the entire depth, and the flow rate that is needed for a given pressure drop. For a given void volume (i.e. solids-free volume fraction of the bed) the gravity-driven flow rate through the bed declines as the depth of the bed increases. Nutrients and substrates are depleted as the fluid moves down the bed. Conversely, concentrations of metabolites and products increases. Thus, the environment of a packed bed is non-homogeneous but concentration variations along the depth can be decreased by increasing the flow rate. Gradients of pH may occur if the reaction consumes or produces H^+ or OH^-. Because of poor mixing, pH control by addition of acid and alkali is nearly impossible. Beds with greater void volume permit greater flow velocities through them but the concentration of the biocatalyst in a given bed volume declines as the voidage (void volume) is increased. If the packing, i.e. the biocatalyst-supporting solids, is compressible, its weight may compress the bed unless the packing height is kept low. Flow is difficult through a compressed bed because of a reduced voidage. Packed beds are used extensively as immobilised enzyme reactors. Such reactors are particularly attractive for product inhibited reactions: the product concentration varies from a low value at the inlet of the bed to a high value at the exit; thus, only a part of the biocatalyst is exposed to high inhibitory levels of the product.

BIOREACTOR DESIGN FEATURES

Irrespective of the specific bioreactor configuration used, the vessel must be provided with certain common features. Some of the principal features are illustrated in Fig. 4.6. The reactor vessel is provided with a vertical sight glass and side ports for pH, temperature, and dissolved O_2 sensors as minimum requirements. Retractable sensors that can be replaced during operation are increasingly used. Connections for acid and alkali (for pH control), antifoam agents, and inoculum are located above the liquid level in the reactor vessel. Air (or other gases, such as CO_2 or ammonia for pH control) is introduced through a sparger situated near the bottom of the vessel. The agitator shaft is provided with steam-sterilisable single or double mechanical seals. Double seals are preferred but they require lubrication with cooled, clean steam condensate. Alternatively, when torque limitations allow, magnetically coupled agitators may be used thereby eliminating the mechanical seals.

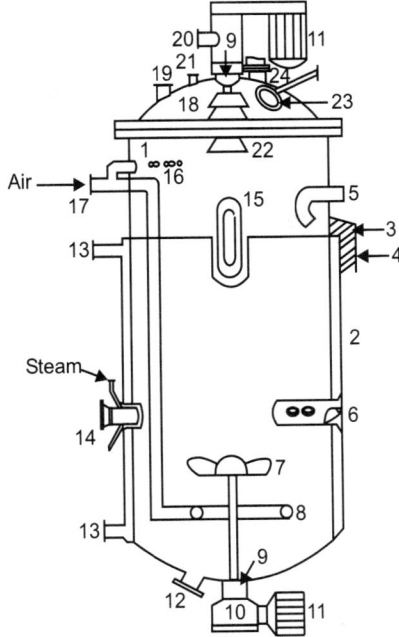

Fig. 4.6. A typical bioreactor: (1) reactor vessel, (2) jacket, (3) insulation, (4) shroud, (5) inoculum connection, (6) ports for pH, temperature and dissolved oxygen sensors, (7) agitator, (8) gas sparger, (9) mechanical seals, (10) reducing gearbox, (11) motor, (12) harvest nozzle, (13) jacket connections, (14) sample valve with steam connection, (15) sight glass, (16) connections for acid, alkali and antifoam chemicals, (17) air inlet, (18) removable top, (19) medium or feed nozzle, (20) air exhaust nozzle, (21) instrument ports (several), (22) foam breaker, (23) sight glass with light (not shown) and steam connection, and (24) rupture disc nozzle.

Aeration and agitation will inevitably produce foam that is controlled with a combination of chemical antifoam agents and mechanical foam breakers. Foam breakers are used exclusively when the presence of antifoam in the product is not acceptable or if the antifoam interferes with downstream processing operations such as membrane based separations or chromatography. The shaft of the high-speed mechanical foam breaker must also be sealed using double mechanical seals.

In most instances, the bioreactor is designed for a maximum allowable working pressure of 377–412 kPa (absolute). Although the sterilisation temperature generally does not exceed 121°C, the vessel is designed for a higher temperature, typically 150°–180°C. The vessel is designed to withstand full vacuum, or it could collapse while cooling after sterilisation. The reactor can be sterilised in place using saturated clean steam at a minimum absolute pressure of 212 kPa. Over-pressure protection is provided by a rupture disc located on top of the bioreactor. Usually this is a graphite burst disc because it does not crack or develop pinholes without failing completely. The rupture disc is piped to a contained drain. Other items located on the head plate of the vessel are nozzles for media or feed addition and for sensors (e.g. the foam electrode), and instruments (e.g. the pressure gauge).

The vessel should have as few internals as practically possible and the design should take into account the needs of clean-in-place and sterilisation-in-place procedures. The vessel should be free of crevices and stagnant areas where pockets of liquids and solids may accumulate. Attention to design of such apparently minor items as the gasket grooves is important. Easy-to-clean channels with rounded edges are preferred. As far as possible, welded joints should be used in preference to couplings. Steam connections should allow for complete displacement of all air pockets in the vessel and associated pipework. Even the exterior of a bioprocess plant should be cleanly designed with smooth contours and minimum bare threads. The reactor vessel is invariably jacketed. In the absence of especial requirements, the jacket is designed to the same specifications as the vessel. The jacket is covered with chloride-free fibreglass insulation that is fully enclosed in a protective shroud as shown in Fig. 4.6. The jacket is provided with over-pressure protection through a relief valve located on the jacket or its associated piping. For a great majority of applications, austenitic stainless steels are the preferred material of construction for bioreactors. The bioreactor vessel is usually made in Type 316L stainless steel, while the less expensive Type 304 (or 304L) is used for the jacket, the insulation shroud and other surfaces not coming into direct contact with the fermentation broth. The L grades of stainless steel contain less than 0.03 per cent carbon, which reduces chromium carbide formation during welding and lowers the potential for later intergranular corrosion at the welds. The welds on internal parts should be ground flush with the internal surface and polished.

DESIGN FOR STERILE OPERATION

Most commercial fermentation processes are mono-cultures. To establish and maintain aseptic conditions are vital for the success of these processes. Hence, a bioreactor must be sterilised prior to inoculation and contamination during operation must be prevented. Contamination during culture is a common cause of process failure.

Sterilisation-in-place

A bioreactor intended for *in situ* sterilisation requires a complex arrangement of pipe work, valves, and filters to enable initial sterilisation and maintenance of sterility. A typical arrangement for *in situ* sterilisation is shown in Fig. 4.7. Because almost all biopharmaceutical production processes involve aeration, the figure includes aeration and exhaust groups that must also be sterilised. The air inlet and exhaust lines have *in situ* steam-sterilisable gas filtres. Typically, hydrophobic membrane cartridge filters are used. These filters are rated for removing particles down to 0.45 μm or even 0.1 μm. Often the gas streams have two filter cartridges in series; with the first serving to protect the final filter.

A good system is designed so that the different sections can be sterilised independently of any of the others, thus sterilisation of any section during fermentation can be carried out if, and when, required. Saturated clean steam (1.1–1.4 bar gauge) is used for sterilisation. The air inlet and exhaust groups are sterilised first, and then, in a second step, the bioreactor. The system is designed so that the filters, valves and the associated pipe-work reach sterilisation temperature (~121°C) very quickly (~1 minute), and are held at the temperature for the required time (25–30 minutes).

Apart from the harvest valve, all other valves shown in Fig. 4.7 should either be diaphragm or pinch valves. The harvest valve is usually a piston valve with a metal bellows sealed stem. The valve closes flush with the internal surface of the bioreactor and there is an unobstructed flow path through the valve body. The valves may be operated manually, but pneumatic operation under automatic control is more efficient and reproducible. The bioreactor is sterilised either filled with the medium or without. Empty sterilisation is the norm in cell culture applications where the media are invariably heat sensitive. In this case, filter sterilisation is used to sterilise the medium.

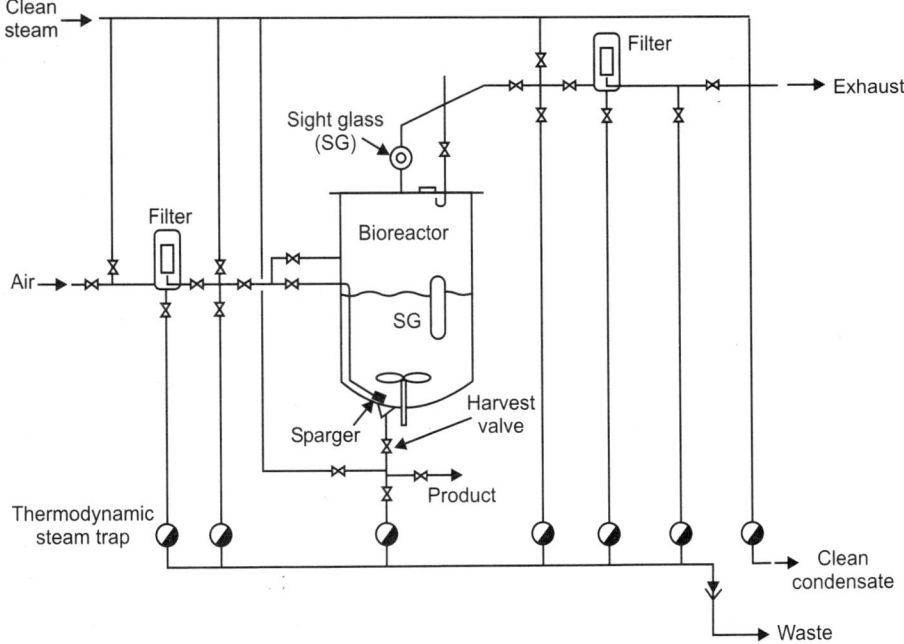

Fig. 4.7. A bioreactor with air inlet and exhaust groups arranged for in-place sterilisation with steam.

Proper closing and opening sequence of the various valves is important for attaining sterility and preventing recontamination from the adjacent non-sterile areas. Once the sterilising steam supply is shut off, the bioreactor is immediately pressurised with sterile air through the air inlet filter so that any leakage from the outside to the sterile vessel is prevented. In bioreactors with stirrer or foam breaker shaft penetrations, the shaft seals require suitable piping and valves for steam sterilisation and maintenance of a sterile barrier fluid between the contents of the fermenter and the outside.

Clean-in-place Considerations

Industrial bioreactors and much of the other processing equipment are cleaned in-place using automated methods. Automation ensures consistency of cleaning and reduces down-time (i.e. unproductive time of a machine). Attaining an acceptable state of cleanliness is essential to prevent contamination and cross-contamination of biopharmaceuticals and food products. An effective and trouble-free cleaning capability requires attention to design of the bioreactors and the clean-in-place (CIP) systems. At any given time a plant may have several bioreactors at different stages of processing and some empty reactors which need to cleaned along with any associated transfer piping. The CIP devices and procedures must be matched to the specific configuration of the bioreactor and to the fermentation process to ensure satisfactory cleaning. Generally, a bioreactor which has processed hybridoma or other animal cell culture broth is far easier to clean than one which has processed broths of *Streptomyces* or mycelial fungi such as *Penicillium*.

Design aspects

To ensure removal of solid particles and avoid sedimentation, the minimum flow velocity through piping should be 1.5 ms^{-1}, but a higher value of 2.0 ms^{-1} is preferred. In addition, the piping should be free of dead spaces as much as possible; if unavoidable, the depth of the dead zone must be less than two pipe diameters to ensure adequate cleaning using CIP techniques. Only valves with a metal-bellows-sealed stem, or diaphragm and pinch valves are recommended as all other valves carry a significant risk of contaminating reactors with accumulated debris during the final rinse cycle. For adequate cleaning, the CIP solutions are sprayed into the reactor through one or more removable, static or dynamic spray balls, or dynamic spray nozzles (Fig. 4.8). In addition, the piping for air exhaust, which is upstream of the exhaust gas filter, and the air inlet piping, should also receive the cleaning solutions. For cleaning with jet spray, pressures of 308 to 377 kPa (absolute) are optimal. Permanently installed spray heads are not recommended for bioreactors because of potential difficulties with sterilisation. These devices must be inserted into the reactor through one of the ports on the head plate. Often, the spray heads are designed to spray the upper one-third of the tank and the falling liquid film irrigates the remaining surface.

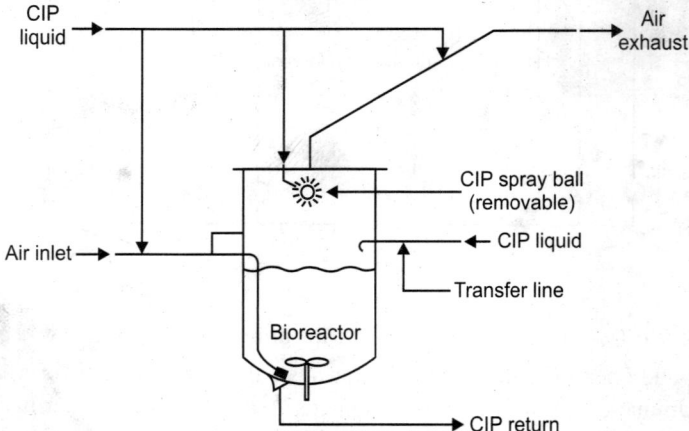

Fig. 4.8. Delivery of the clean-in-place (CIP) liquids to the bioreactor. The flow of CIP solutions is sequenced through the transfer line, the air inlet and exhaust groups and the spray ball of the bioreactor.

For bioreactors for parenteral (injectable) products and other biopharmaceuticals, potable quality deionised water is recommended for all pre-rinsing and detergent formulations. Pre-rinse should be on a once-through basis without recirculation. A five minute pre-rinse is usually sufficient for bacterial, yeast and animal cell culture reactors. Following pre-rinse, 1 per cent (w/v) NaOH at 75°–80°C should be circulated through the equipment so that all product contact surfaces are exposed to this solution for 15–20 minutes. The alkali should be discarded afterwards. Dilution, contamination with soil and microbial spores that can survive for long periods and loss of quality definition of the starting material for the next cleaning, are some of the arguments against reuse of cleaning chemicals. A deionised or reverse osmosis water rinse at 25°–35°C is used to remove all alkali from the system. Process equipment for products that are injected into the body must undergo a final wash with hot water-for-injection grade water. This ensures that all residual water complies with the requisite quality standards.

In mechanically agitated bioreactors, the spray of cleaning solutions may be unable to achieve proper cleaning of the agitators, magnetic couplings, mechanical seals and the lower portions of baffles. Therefore, filling of the vessel to at least above the level of the lower most impeller and agitation at impeller Reynolds numbers of 10^8–$10^{8.5}$ is recommended during pre-rinse, alkali recirculation and the final rinse. Agitation for 2–3 minutes is sufficient to dislodge adhering dirt or soil. These recommendations assume that reactors are being cleaned in-place soon after use and caking of dirt has not occurred.

PHOTOBIOREACTORS

Certain micro-algae and cyanobacteria provide important chemicals, such as astaxanthin and β-carotene, in addition to being used as aquaculture feed for bivalves and fish hatchlings. Cyanobacteria, such as *Spirulina*, are also grown as human health-foods. Photosynthetic cultures require sunlight or artificial illumination. Although some algae may be grown heterotrophically, i.e. without sunlight, this type of growth requires an alternative organic energy source, usually glucose. Heterotrophically grown cultures often lack photosynthetic pigments and may not yield the same products as a photosynthesising population. However, much progress is being made in developing heterotrophic strains for production of commercially valuable products.

Artificial illumination is impractically expensive; only outdoor photobioreactors appear to be promising for large-scale production. Open ponds and 'raceways' are often used to culture micro-algae, but mono-septic culture requires fully closed photobioreactors. Because it needs light, photosynthesis can occur only at relatively shallow depths. Algal ponds are typically no deeper than 0.15 m. However, too much light causes photoinhibition; a situation in which slightly reducing the light intensity will actually improve the rate of photosynthesis. With increasing cell population, the self-shading effect of cells further limits light penetration. In addition to light, photosynthesising algal cells need a source of carbon, usually carbon dioxide. Part of the carbon may be derived from dissolved bicarbonate species. Cells convert CO_2 to carbohydrate and other cellular components. Too high a concentration of CO_2 can reduce photosynthetic productivity.

Closed photobioreactors for monoculture consist of arrays of transparent tubes that may be made of glass, or more commonly, a clear plastic. The tubes may be laid horizontally, or arranged as long rungs on an upright ladder (Fig. 4.9). A continuous single run tubular loop configuration is also used, or the tube may be wound helically around a vertical cylindrical support. In addition to the tubes, flat or inclined thin panels may be employed in relatively small-scale operations. An array of tubes or a flat panel constitutes a 'solar receiver'. The culture is circulated through the solar receiver by a variety of methods, including centrifugal pumps, positive displacement mono pumps. Archimedean screws and airlift devices. Airlift pumps perform well, have no mechanical parts, are easy to operate aseptically and are suited to shear sensitive applications.

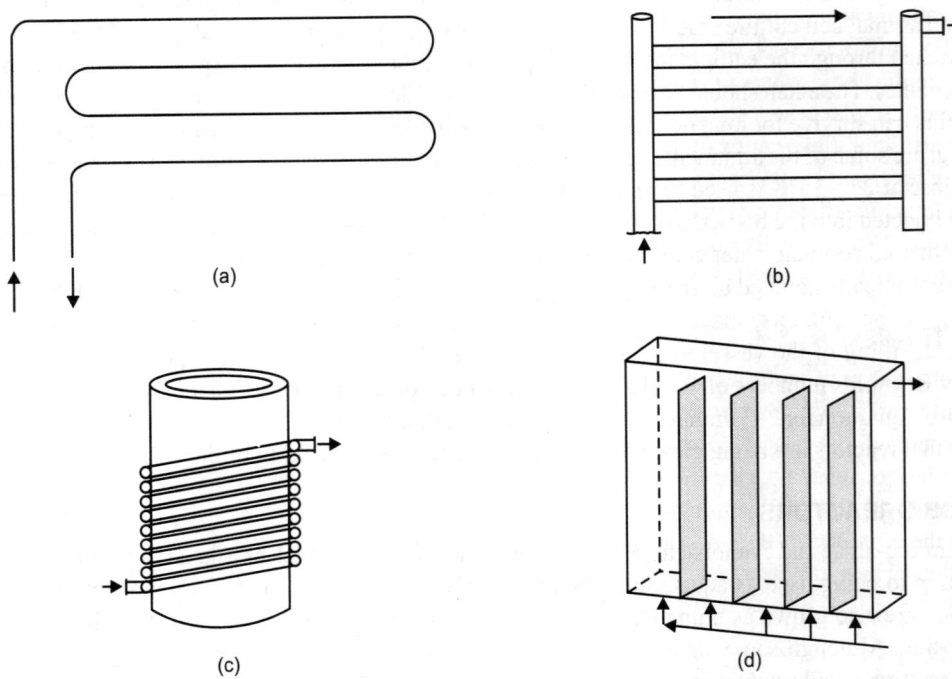

Fig. 4.9. Photobioreactors for monoculture: (a) continuous run tubular loop, (b) a solar receiver made of multiple parallel tubes, (c) helical wound tubular loop, (d) flat panel configuration. Configurations (a) and (b) may be mounted vertically, or parallel to the ground.

The flow in a solar receiver tube or panel should be turbulent enough to aid periodic movement of cells from the deeper poorly lit interior to the regions nearer the walls. Generally, a minimum Reynolds number value of 10^4 is recommended. While turbulence is needed to improve radial mixing, too much turbulence can be harmful. The velocity everywhere should be sufficient to prevent sedimentation of cells. Typical linear velocities through receiver tubes tend to be 0.3–0.5 ms^{-1}.

Because of the need to maintain adequate sunlight penetration, a tubular solar receiver cannot be scaled up by simply increasing the tube diameter. The diameter should not exceed 6 cm, although this constraint may be relaxed somewhat by deploying specially designed static mixers that improve radial mixing inside the tube. Without the mixers, reducing the tube diameter from 6 cm to 5 cm and further to 2 cm noticeably improves culture performance. Light penetration depends on biomass density, cellular morphology and pigmentation, and absorption characteristics of the cell-free culture medium.

Photobioreactors are normally operated in continuous mode. Micro-algae grow slowly; the doubling time of *Chlorella pyrenoidosa* is approximately 9 hours. Consequently, the dilution rate is kept low; about one culture volume per day, confined to daylight hours. Although the biomass grows only during daylight, certain products are produced predominantly during the dark hours. Biomass productivity of outdoor cultures is generally less than 2 g l^{-1} day, often no more than 1.5 g l^{-1} day. Culture is generally carried out at 22°–37°C. During daylight hours, the solar receiver tubes need to be cooled to prevent temperature rise to damaging levels.

A solar receiver is more amenable to scale-up by increasing the length of a continuous run tube; however, the maximum permissible length should not exceed 50–100 metre because the photosynthetically generated O_2 builds up along the tube and high oxygen concentrations inhibit photosynthetic productivity. An alternative to a long continuous run tube is an array of multiple parallel tubes. For minimal costs, each tube of the multi-tube arrangement should be as long as possible but within the threshold where O_2 levels become inhibitory. The rate of photosynthesis and, consequently, the rate of O_2 generation depend on the amount of sunlight available. With *Spirulina platensis* under intense artificial illumination O_2 production rates have been estimated at 0.35–0.5 g l^{-1} hr. for radiation intensity levels of 1500–2600 μE $m^{-2}s$.

In a long tube, the rate of photosynthesis varies along the tube because of several factors: (i) the light intensity declines because of increasing cell concentration, (ii) the CO_2 is depleted, and (iii) O_2 concentration may increase to inhibitory levels.

HEAT TRANSFER

The metabolic heat generated by the cells needs to be removed because it is important to maintain a constant temperature in the reactor. The overall heat balance on a reactor would include: the metabolic heat generated, the heat generated due to stirring and agitation, the heat lost due to evaporation, the sensible heat content of the input and output flows and the heat exchanged with the surroundings. In a large reactor only the first two terms are important, with the metabolic heat often contributing more than 80 per cent of the heat load on the system. It is fairly easy to calculate this load if we know the rates of biomass formation (which are determined by growth kinetics) and the enthalpy efficiency of the process (η_H):

$$Q_{met} = F_x \Delta H_x (1 - \eta_H)/\eta_H$$

Since η_H represents the fraction of substrate energy going for biomass formation and $(1 - \eta_H)$ is the fraction which is lost as metabolic heat. We need to look into the basic principles of heat transfer, to be able to design the heat transfer equipment (cooling coils, etc.) to take care of this heat load.

Heat transfer rate is determined by Newton's law of cooling:

$$q = kA \, dT/dX$$

where q is the heat transfer rate (J s^{-1}), k is the conductivity [J s^{-1} (°Cm)], A is the area of heat transfer (m^2) and dT/dX is the temperature gradient (°C/m). Therefore, $q = kA(T_1 - T_2)/\Delta x$ (Fig. 4.10).

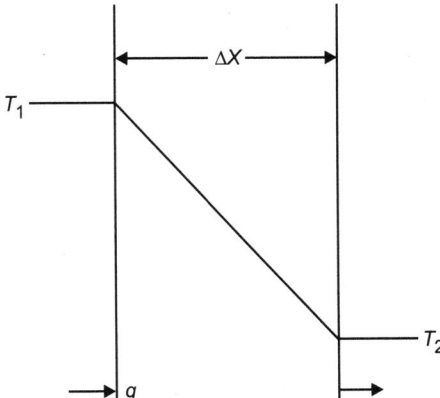

Fig. 4.10. Temperature gradient for steady-state heat flow through one slab.

The heat flow at steady-state is proportional to the temperature gradient and conductivity. As such the analogy with Ohm's law for the flow of electricity is obvious:

$$i = kV$$

where i is the current, V the voltage and k the conductivity. This is true for many transport processes at steady state and the general equation can be written as:

Flux = Driving force/Resistance

where resistance is the inverse of conductivity. We can, thus, use the principle of resistance in series $(R = R_1 + R_2 + R_3 + ...)$ as given by Ohm's law to calculate heat fluxes and temperature changes when more than one resistance to heat flow is involved. We have to substitute the voltage by temperature difference (driving force), current by heat flux and resistance by the thickness of the slab divided by its conductivity.

Figure 4.11 shows steady-state heat transfer through two slabs of thickness Δx_1 and Δx_2 with conductivities K_1 and K_2. Now we determine the heat flux and the interfacial temperature. We have $R_1 = \Delta X_1/K_1$ and $R_2 = \Delta X_2/K_2$. Therefore,

$$R = \Delta X_1/K_1 + \Delta X_2/K_2$$
$$(T_1 - T_2) = (q/A)(\Delta X_1/K_1 + \Delta X_2/K_2)$$

which is similar to $V = iR$

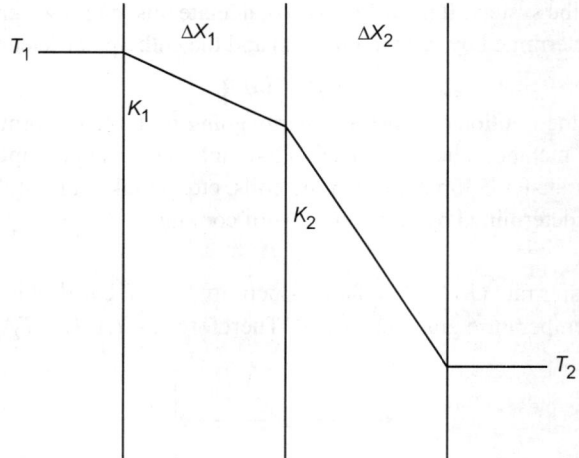

Fig. 4.11. Temperature gradient for steady-state heat flow through two slabs.

The numerical values can be substituted to determine q/A. Similarly, since voltage drop is proportional to resistance, we have:

$$T_1 - T_{\text{interface}}/(T_1 - T_2) = (\Delta X_1/K_1)/(\Delta X_1/K_1 + \Delta X_2/K_2)$$

which can be solved to determine $T_{\text{interface}}$.

Let us now look at the various resistances to heat flow when a cooling coil is used to remove heat. Figure 4.12 shows an expanded view of the wall of a cooling coil, whose outside surface is in contact with the fermenter medium (of temperature T_b) and inside has cooling liquid (usually water) flowing at temperature T_c. Note that the temperature of the outside wall surface is T_{wo} which is less than T_b and similarly the temperature of the inside surface of the wall is T_{wi} which is greater than T_c. This is because heat flows from the outside to the inside and there is a resistance to heat flow which shows up in this temperature gradient. We can postulate the existence of a thin film of liquid of thickness δ across which the temperature drop takes place (from the wall to the bulk liquid) and thus have

$$q = k_o A (T_b - T_{wo})/\delta_o$$
$$q = k_i A (T_{wi} - T_c)\delta_i$$

where, k_o and k_i are the conductivities of these films (of liquid) and δ_o and δ_i are the thicknesses. Since it is impossible to experimentally measure this film thickness we can couple this with the conductivity of the film and define a film heat transfer coefficient h given by:

$$h_o = k_o/\delta_o \text{ and } h_i = k_i/\delta_i$$

there by getting

$$q = h_o A (T_b - T_{wo})$$
$$q = h_i A (T_{wi} - T_c)$$
$$q = k A (T_{wo} - T_{wi})/\Delta X$$

where k is the conductivity of the wall (typically stainless steel which is the material of construction of the cooling tube) and ΔX is the thickness of the cooling tube. Adding up the resistances we have:

$$1/U = 1/h_o + \delta X/k + h_i$$

where U is defined as the overall conductivity and h_o and h_i are the external and internal 'film heat transfer coefficients,' respectively. We can now write the heat balance as:

$$q = UA \, \Delta T = UA(T_b - T_c)$$

where q is the heat removed by the cooling coil, A is the surface area of the coil and ΔT is the temperature difference between the fermenter culture medium and the cooling liquid. The student can try and derive the above expression using basic algebraic techniques which involve using the three equations given earlier to get rid of the two unknowns, namely, T_{wo} and T_{wi}.

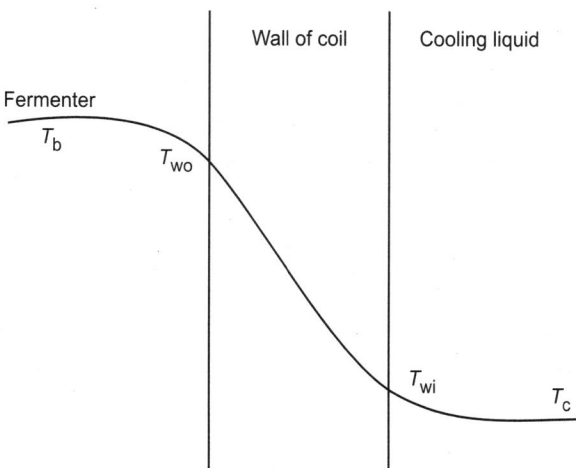

Fig. 4.12. Temperature gradient for steady-state heat flow between fermenter and cooling liquid.

However, this temperature difference ($T_b - T_c = \Delta T$) is not a constant since the temperature of the cooling liquid rises as it flows inside the fermenter (here it picks up the heat generated by the growing culture). This change in the cooling coil temperature (ΔT_c) changes ΔT between the coil and fermenter medium (Fig. 4.13). Thus, an average value of ΔT needs to be used while using the above equation.

This average ΔT can be determined if we know the ΔT at the inlet and the outlet of the cooling coil. We have:

$$q = mC_p \, \Delta T_c$$

where m is the mass flow rate of the cooling liquid and C_p is its heat capacity.

If we consider the heat exchange in the small shaded portion in the Fig. 4.9, we have

$$dq = UdA\Delta T$$

where, dA is the area of the shaded part. Also from the temperature increase of the cooling liquid we have

$$dq = mC_p \, d(\Delta T)$$

since the change in ΔT is because of the rise in temperature of the cooling liquid. Thus

$$mC_p \, d(\Delta T) = U \, dA \, \Delta T$$

Rearranging and integrating across the whole length of the coil, we get

$$mC_p \int d(\Delta T) / \Delta T = U \int dA$$
$$\Rightarrow mC_p \cdot \ln(\Delta T_1 / \Delta T_2) = UA$$

where, ΔT_1 and ΔT_2 are the temperature differences at the inlet and the outlet of the cooling coil. We also have

$$\Delta T_C = \Delta T_1 - \Delta T_2$$

therefore,

$$q = mC_p(\Delta T_1 - \Delta T_2)$$

Substituting for mC_p in the above equation we get:

$$q = UA[(\Delta T_1 - \Delta T_2)/\ln \Delta T_1/\Delta T_2]$$

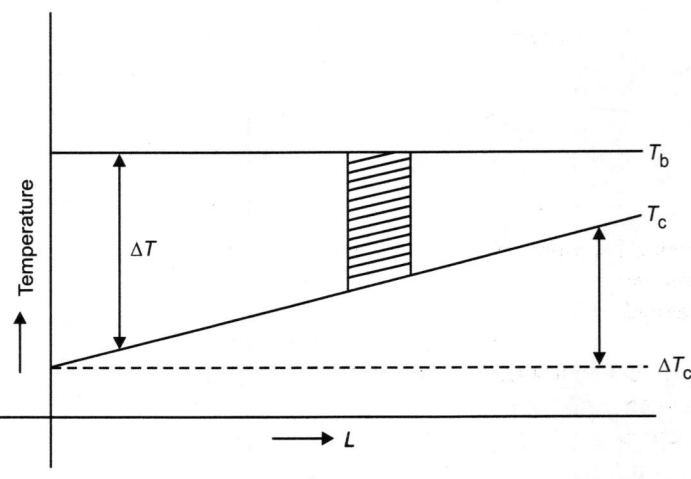

Fig. 4.13. Temperature gradient showing rise in temperature of cooling water and hence change in ΔT.

The term within brackets is referred to as the log mean temperature difference (LMTD) and the use of this logarithmic mean instead of the arithmetic mean of the temperature differences (ΔT_{avg}) gives a more accurate estimate of the heat transfer rate. Thus

$$q = UALMTD$$

DIMENSIONAL ANALYSIS

While data for typical ranges of values of overall heat transfer coefficients (U) are available, often precise design calculations require estimating values of the individual film heat transfer coefficients (h_0 and h_i) and then calculating U from the equation given earlier.

The values of the film heat transfer coefficients are dependent on a large number of parameters. Thus 'h_i' is a function of the conductivity of the cooling liquid k, the pipe diameter (D), the liquid viscosity (μ), the heat capacity (C_p), the liquid velocity (v) and the density (ρ), that is:

$$h = f(K, D, \mu, C_p, v, \rho)$$

These functional relationships need to be determined empirically. However, since there is a physical basis to these relationships we postulate that the form of these relationships require that they be dimensionally homogenous. This means that the LHS and RHS of this equation have the same units in terms of the four fundamental units, viz. mass (M), length (L), time (t) and temperature (T). The requirement of dimensional homogeneity imposes constraints on the nature of the equation that can be formulated and thus reduces the number of constants that need empirical determination. The strategy outlined below is called the Buckingham Pi method and though we are applying it now to determine the relationship between h and other variables, it has applicability in a wide range of other cases. We define a power law relationship:

$$h = C k^a D^b \mu^c C_p^d v^e \rho^f$$

where, C is a dimensionless constant and a,b,c, . . . are the exponents. Note that if there were no constraints on this equation we would need to empirically determine the value of the seven constants. The dimensional units of the variables are:

$$h = [Mt^{-3} T^{-1}]; k = [MLt^{-3} T^{-1}]; D = [L]$$
$$\mu = [ML^{-1} t^{-1}]; C_p = [L^2 t^{-2} T^{-1}]; v = [Lt^{-1}]$$
$$\rho = [ML^{-3}]$$

The equation in terms of the dimensional units is (C being a constant has no units)

$$[Mt^{-3} T^{-1}] = [MLt^{-3} T^{-1}]^a [L]^b [ML^{-1} t^{-1}]^c [L^2 t^{-2} T^{-1}]^d [Lt^{-1}]^e [ML^{-3}]^f.$$

Equating the units of LHS and RHS, we get

$$\text{for M:} \quad 1 = a + c + f \qquad\qquad\qquad \dots (4.1)$$
$$\text{for L:} \quad 0 = a + b - c + 2d + e - 3f \qquad \dots (4.2)$$
$$\text{for t:} \quad -3 = -3a - c - 2d - e \qquad\qquad \dots (4.3)$$
$$\text{for T:} \quad -1 = -a - d \qquad\qquad\qquad\quad \dots (4.4)$$

We have four equations but six unknowns and thus we can express four of the above exponents in terms of the other two. Retaining the variables 'd' and 'f' (this makes the job easier), we get

from Eq. 4.8 $\qquad a = (1 - d)$

from Eq. 4.5 $\qquad c = (1 - a - f) = (d - f)$

from Eq. 4.7 $\qquad e = f$

from Eq. 4.6 $\qquad b = -1 + f$

Substituting we can write in terms of d and f only:

$$h = Ck^{(1-d)} D^{(-1+f)} \mu^{(d-f)} C_p^d v^f \rho^f$$

Rearranging the terms we get

$$(hD/k) = C(C_p\mu/k)^d (\rho vD/\mu)^f$$

Note that this equation is dimensionally homogenous whatever values we choose for d and f. This is possible because each of the groups within brackets represents a combination of variables which taken together have no units. They are, thus, referred to as dimensionless numbers. Thus (hD/k) is called the Nusselt number (Nu), $(C_p\mu/k)$ is the Prandtl number (Pr) and $(\rho vD/\mu)$ is the Reynolds number (Re). The Buckingham Pi method, thus, becomes a technique for generating these dimensionless numbers. Here we have:

$$Nu = C(Pr)^\alpha(Re)^\beta$$

where the constant C and the values of α and β need to be determined empirically. We have, thus, reduced the number of constants that need empirical determination from seven to three. Typical values of C, α and β are available in literature helping us to correlate the above dimensional numbers. Thus, the Dittus Boelter equation for liquid flowing inside pipes is:

$$(Nu) = 0.0265(Re)^{0.8}(Pr)^{0.3}$$

for $(Re) > 10000$ and $0.7 < (Pr) < 170$.

A lot of literature is available on such correlations linking up different dimensionless numbers which are applicable within a range of operating conditions. These correlations can be used to determine the values of different parameters like film heat transfer coefficients.

MASS TRANSFER

Mass transfer deals with the problem of diffusive transfer. Diffusion is controlled by concentration gradients and given by Fick's first law:

$$N_A = D(dC_A/dx)$$

where N_A is the flux of component A per unit area, D is the diffusivity and (dCA/dx) is the concentration gradient. This is similar in form to the equation governing heat transfer. We are concerned with mass transfer primarily because cells growing inside a fermenter need oxygen which has to be supplied by bubbling air/oxygen into the fermenter.

For the transfer of oxygen to the cells, oxygen has to first diffuse through the bubbles into the fermenter medium and then into the cells from the liquid medium. The equilibrium relationship governing gas solubilities in a liquid is governed by Henry's law:

$$p_A = Hc_A$$

where, p_A is the partial pressure in the gas phase, c_A is the solubility (referred to as the dissolved oxygen concentration) in the liquid phase and H is Henry's constant. The value of H is a function of pH, temperature, ionic strength and presence of dissolved solutes and hence varies from medium to medium. When air is bubbled inside liquid (either water or fermenter medium) so that equilibrium is reached, the dissolved oxygen concentration reaches its saturation value $c*$ given by $p_A = Hc_A*$ which is typically in the range of 1.0 ± 0.2 m moles l^{-1}.

Let us now consider the situation where oxygen is transferred from bubbles to medium containing growing cells and simultaneously taken up from the medium by these cells for respiration. A material balance on the liquid phase for oxygen gives

$$V(dc_L/dt) = OTR - OUR$$

where, $V(dc_L/dt)$ represents the rate of accumulation of oxygen in the liquid, OTR is the oxygen transfer rate from the bubbles to the liquid and OUR is the oxygen uptake rate by the growing cells given by:

$$OUR = \mu x/Y_{X/O}$$

At steady state $dc_L/dt = 0$ and we have OTR = OUR

Note that the dissolved oxygen concentration at steady state given by c_L is lower than c^* (the saturation value), thus allowing continuous oxygen transfer from the gas to the liquid phase.

To determine OTR we consider the resistance to diffusive flow of oxygen due to two films, one on the gas side causing the partial pressure of oxygen (which is the driving force) to drop from p_b (the bulk gas phase oxygen partial pressure) to p_i (the partial pressure at the interface) (Fig. 4.14).

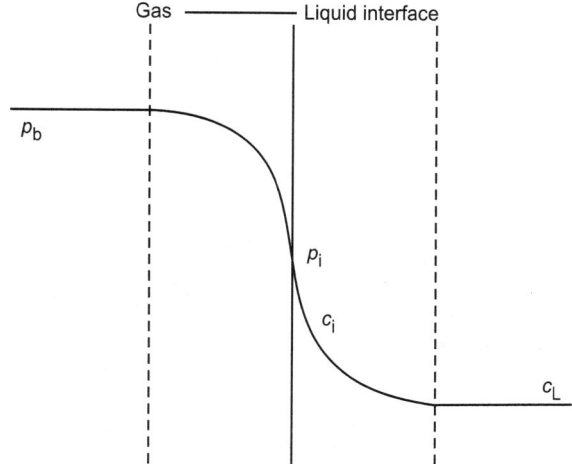

Fig. 4.14. Oxygen gradient due to diffusion of oxygen from bubbles to culture medium containing growing cells.

Similarly the film on the liquid side causes the dissolved oxygen concentration to fall from c_i and c_L, where c_i and c_L are the dissolved oxygen concentrations at the interface and bulk liquid, respectively. (This formulation is similar to the formulation for heat transfer.) We can now write the equations for mass transfer as

$$N = K_G A(p_b - p_i)$$

where, N is the flux of oxygen, K_G is the gas side film mass transfer coefficient, A is the surface area of the bubbles. Also

$$N = K_L A(c_i - c_L)$$

where, K_L is the liquid-side mass transfer coefficient.

Since the interface has zero thickness it cannot provide any resistance to flow. We consider that p_i and c_i are in equilibrium with each other and hence governed by Henry's law, that is

$$p_i = Hc_i$$

Solving these three equations to get rid of p_i and c_i, we have $N = K_L A(p_b/H - c_L)$, where $1/K_L = 1/K_L + 1/K_GH$. K_L is the overall mass transfer coefficient incorporating both the gas-side and liquid-side mass transfer coefficients.

We can substitute c^* for p_b/H where c^* is the saturated dissolved oxygen concentration in the liquid phase, in equilibrium with oxygen in the gas phase. We need to assume that the bulk gas-phase concentration does not change significantly between entry and exit (even though some oxygen gets transferred to the liquid phase). This assumption is not valid for tall tubular reactors where air enters at the bottom and leaves at the top.

Also since the oxygen flux is measured per litre of reactor volume we define a specific surface area of the gas bubbles as $a = A/V$ where A is the total surface area of the bubbles and V is the reactor volume. We have:

$$N/V = K_L a(c^* - c_L)$$

The specific surface area (a) can be estimated if we know the volume of gas held up in the reactor (V_g) and the radius of the bubbles (r). We therefore have:

$$\varepsilon = V_g/V_T$$

where ε is called the gas hold up ratio. Also the specific surface area of a bubble is given by its area per unit volume, that is:

$$a = (4\pi r^2)/(4\pi r^3/3) = 3/r$$

Thus, the specific surface area per unit reactor volume is given by $V_g \times a/V_T = 3\varepsilon/r$.

[Since we have a bubble size distribution we need to use r_{avg}, a mean radius of the bubbles where the concept of 'Sauter mean radius', r_{sm}, is used ($r_{sm} = \Sigma r_i^3/\Sigma r_i^2$). The student can check that the Sauter mean radius gives an accurate measure of the specific surface area.]

Correlations are available for K_L in terms of the diffusivity D and other variables in the form of dimensionless numbers. Similarly correlations for a are also available in literature. However, for practical purposes since both K_L and a affect the OTR, we use correlations which estimate $K_L a$ as a single parameter. A typical correlation is

$$K_L a = C (P/V)^\alpha (v_s)^\beta$$

where, C is a constant, P is the power consumed due to agitation, V is the reactor volume and v_s is the superficial gas velocity (given by the gas flow rate divided by the cross-sectional area of the reactor).

The power consumption for agitation can be related in turn to other variables using dimensionless numbers. Thus,

$$P = f(N, D, \rho, g, \mu)$$

where, N is the rpm of the agitator, D the diameter of the agitator, ρ the liquid density, g is gravity and μ is the viscosity of the liquid. The dimensionless numbers relating the above variables are (the students can derive this from the Buckingham P_i method described earlier).

$$(P/N^3 D^5 \rho) = c(\rho ND^2/\mu)^\alpha N^2 D/g)^\beta$$

The LHS of the equation is the Power number (P_0), the term ($\rho ND^2/\mu$) is the modified Reynolds number for agitated liquids (Re) and ($N^2 D/g$) is the Froude number.

Typically 'baffles' are used in reactors to break up vortex formation. These are thin strips of metal stuck to the inside wall of the reactor (in the perpendicular direction), which break up the circular motion of the liquid and thus cause turbulence. Under these circumstances the Froude number has little effect on the power consumption. A plot of Power number vs. Reynolds number is given in Fig. 4.15, where three zones can be identified during agitation. These are:

1. Laminar zone: It is the zone where P_0 declines with increasing R_e.
2. Transient zone: It is the zone where a complex relationship exist between P_0 and R_e.
3. Turbulent zone: It is the zone where P_0 is a constant (and hence independent of Re).

Most fermenters are run in the turbulent zone and, therefore, the Power number is a constant which is independent of the Reynolds number. We thus have:

$$P = P_0(N^3D^5\rho)$$

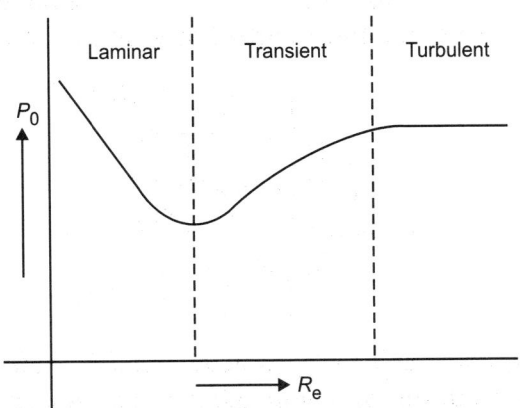

Fig. 4.15. Plot of Power number vs. Reynolds number.

This relationship can also be derived from basic principles if we note that the power consumption is proportional to the kinetic energy (KE) it imparts to the liquid while mixing. Thus, the mass of liquid an agitator blade displaces while rotating is proportional to 'ρND^3' (where D^3 is proportional to the volume displaced by the agitator blades, so ND^3 is the volume displaced per unit time) and the velocity it imparts to this liquid is 'ND' (which is the tip velocity of the agitator blade). Thus, the KE imparted is

$$\tfrac{1}{2}mv^2 \propto \rho ND^3 \times (ND)^2 = \rho N^3D^5$$

Therefore, $P \propto \rho N^3D^5$ and the proportionality constant is the Power number.

The Power number depends on the number and shape of the agitator blades and whether the system is aerated or not (since the effective density of the liquid culture would fall with aeration and gas hold up). The above correlations allow us to identify the effect of operating variables like agitator rpm on the power consumption and OTR.

Scale-up: In the earlier sections, we have developed stoichiometric and kinetic relationships which were scale independent and could thus be applied to large-scale systems after they had been determined in the small scale. In a similar fashion, parameters like K_La (which determine the OTR), power consumption per unit volume (P/V) and maximum shear rate (given by the tip velocity of the impeller blades, ND) need to be determined upon scale-up. Since it is not possible to keep all the above operational variables constant as scale-up is done, only the critical parameters are considered and kept constant. Thus, if oxygen supply is the critical parameter then K_La would be kept constant but if the cells are shear sensitive then shear has to be kept constant. Note that geometric similarity is maintained during scale-up and thus parameters which are length dependent increase as L, those which are area dependent increase as L^2 and those which are volume dependent increase as L^3.

SHEAR EFFECTS IN CULTURE

Shear rate is a measure of spatial variation in local velocities in a fluid. Cell damage in a moving fluid is sometimes associated with the magnitude of the prevailing shear rate. But the shear rate in the relatively turbulent environment of most bioreactors is neither easily defined nor easily measured. Moreover, the shear rate varies with location within the vessel. Attempts have been made to characterise an average shear rate or a maximum shear rate in various types of bioreactors. In bubble columns an average shear rate has been defined as a function of the superficial gas velocity as follows:

$$\gamma = kU_G^a \qquad \ldots (4.5)$$

where the parameter a equals 1.0 in most cases, but the k value has been reported variously as 1000, 2800, 5000 m^{-1}, etc. Equation 4.5 has been applied also to airlift bioreactors using the superficial gas velocity in the riser zone as a correlating parameter; however, that usage is incorrect. A more suitable form of the equation for airlift reactors is:

$$\gamma = \frac{kU_{Gr}}{1 + \dfrac{A_d}{A_r}} \qquad \ldots (4.6)$$

Depending on the value of k equations such as (4.5) and (4.6) produce wildly different values of the supposed shear rate. In addition the equations fail to take into account the momentum transfer capability, i.e. the density and the viscosity of the fluid. Both of these will influence the shear rate.

An average shear rate in stirred fermenters is given by the equation:

$$\gamma = k_i \left(\frac{4n}{3n+1} \right)^{n/(n-1)} N \qquad \ldots (4.7)$$

where, n the flow index of a fluid, equals 1.0 for a Newtonian liquid such as water and thick glucose syrup. Some typical k_i values are: 11–13 for 6-bladed disc turbines, 10–13 for paddle impellers, ~10 for propellers, and ~30 for helical ribbon impellers. The maximum shear rate on a Rushton disc turbine in Newtonian fluids has been expressed as:

$$\gamma_{max} = 3.3N^{1.5}d_i \left(\frac{\rho_L}{\mu_L} \right)^{1/2} \qquad \ldots (4.8)$$

Equation 4.8 applies when $100 \leq (Nd_i^2\rho_L/\mu_L) \leq 29,000$. It also applies to non-Newtonian fluids if μ_L is taken as the zero shear viscosity. The shear rate can be converted to a parameter known as shear stress τ, where

$$\tau = \gamma\mu_L \qquad \ldots (4.9)$$

The susceptibility of some animal cells to shear stress levels has been characterised in well-defined laminar flow environments.

Another method of deciding whether the turbulence in a fluid could potentially damage a suspended biocatalyst is based on comparing the dimensions of the cell or the biocatalyst floc with the length scale of the fluid eddies.

The mean length, ℓ, of the fluid eddy depends on the energy dissipation rate per unit mass of the fluid in the bioreactor; thus,

$$\ell = \left(\frac{\mu_L}{\rho_L}\right)^{3/4} E^{-1/4} \qquad \qquad ...(4.10)$$

In most cases, all the energy input to the fluid is dissipated in fluid eddies and E equals the rate of energy input. Equation 4.10 applies to isotropically turbulent fluid, i.e. one in which the size of the primary eddies generated by the turbulence producing mechanism is a thousand-fold or more compared to the size of the energy dissipating micro-eddies. The size of the micro-eddies is calculated with Eq. 4.10. The length scale of the primary eddies is often approximated as the width of the impeller blade or the diameter of the impeller in a stirred tank. In bubble columns and airlift bioreactors, the length scale of primary eddies is approximated as the diameter of the column (or the riser tube) or the diameter of the bubble issuing from the gas sparger. Generally, if the dimensions of the biocatalyst particle are much smaller than the calculated length, ℓ, of the micro-eddies, the particle is simply carried around by the fluid eddy; the particle does not experience any disruptive force.

On the other hand, a particle that is larger than the length scale of the eddy will experience pressure differentials on its surface and if the particle is not strong enough it could be broken by the resulting forces.

In addition to turbulence within the fluid, other damage-causing phenomena in a bioreactor include inter-particle collisions; collisions with walls, other stationary surfaces, and the impeller; shear forces associated with bubble rupture at the surface of the fluid; phenomena linked with bubble coalescence and break-up; and bubble formation at the gas sparger.

Effects of interfacial shear rate around rising bubbles and those due to bubble rupture at the surface can be minimised by adding non-ionic surfactants to the culture medium. These surfactants reduce adherence of animal cells to bubbles; hence, fewer cells experience interfacial shear and rupture events at the surface of the liquid.

In micro-carrier culture of animal cells where spherical carriers as small as 200 µm in diameter are suspended in the culture fluid to support adherent cells on the surface of the carrier, inter-particle collisions are generally infrequent under the conditions that are typically employed. However, the size of the fluid eddies in micro-carrier culture systems may be similar to or smaller than the dimensions of the carriers; hence, the adhering cells may experience turbulence-related damage. Freely suspended animal cells are generally too small to be damaged by fluid turbulence levels that are typically employed in cell culture bioreactors.

In micro-carrier culture, shear stress levels as low as 0.25 Nm^{-2} may interfere with the initial attachment of cells on micro-carriers.

Chapter 5

Microbes and Metabolism

INTRODUCTION

Microbes are referred to as such, simply because they cannot be seen by the naked eye. Microbial metabolism is the means by which a microbe obtains the energy and nutrients (e.g. carbon) it needs to live and reproduce. Microbes use many different types of metabolic strategies and species can often be differentiated from each other based on metabolic characteristics. The specific metabolic properties of a microbe are the major factors in determining that microbe's ecological niche, and often allow for that microbe to be useful in industrial processes or responsible for biogeochemical cycles.

HETEROTROPHIC MICROBIAL METABOLISM

Most microbes are heterotrophic (more precisely chemoorganoheterotrophic), using organic compounds as both carbon and energy sources. Heterotrophic microbes live off of nutrients that they scavenge from living hosts (as commensals or parasites) or find in dead organic matter of all kind (saprophages). Microbial metabolism is the main contribution for the bodily decay of all organisms after death. Many eukaryotic micro-organisms are heterotrophic by predation or parasitism, properties also found in some bacteria such as *Bdellovibrio* (an intracellular parasite of other bacteria, causing death of its victims) and *Myxobacteria* such as *Myxococcus* (predators of other bacteria which are killed and lysed by cooperating swarms of many single cells of *Myxobacteria*). Most pathogenic bacteria can be viewed as heterotrophic parasites of humans or whatever other eukaryotic species they affect. Heterotrophic microbes are extremely abundant in nature and are responsible for the breakdown of large organic polymers such as cellulose, chitin or lignin which are generally indigestible to larger animals. Generally, the breakdown of large polymers to carbon dioxide (mineralisation) requires several different organisms, with one breaking down the polymer into its constituent monomers, one able to use the monomers and excreting simpler waste compounds as by-products and one able to use the excreted wastes. There are many variations on this theme, as different organisms are able to degrade different polymers and secrete different waste products. Some organisms are even able to degrade more recalcitrant compounds such as petroleum compounds or pesticides, making them useful in bioremediation.

Metabolic pathways are interlinked to produce what can develop into an extraordinarily complicated network, involving several levels of control. However, they are fundamentally about the interaction of natural cycles and represent the biological element of the natural geobiological cycles. These impinge on all aspects of the environment, both living and nonliving. Using the carbon cycle as an example, carbon dioxide in the atmosphere is returned by dissolution in rainwater, and also by the process of photosynthesis to produce sugars, which are eventually metabolised to liberate the carbon once more. In addition to constant recycling through metabolic pathways, carbon is also sequestered in living and nonliving components such as in trees in the relatively short term, and deep ocean, systems or ancient deposits, such as carbonaceous rocks, in the long term. Cycles which involve similar principles of incorporation into biological molecules and subsequent re-release into the environment operate for nitrogen, phosphorus and sulphur. All of these overlap in some way, to produce the metabolic pathways responsible for the synthesis and degradation of biomolecules. Superimposed, is an energy cycle, ultimately driven by the sun, and involving constant consumption and release of metabolic energy,

To appreciate the biochemical basis and underlying genetics of environmental biotechnology, at least an elementary grasp of molecular biology is required.

IMMOBILISATION, DEGRADATION OR MONITORING OF POLLUTANTS FROM A BIOLOGICAL ORIGIN

Removal of a material from an environment takes one of two routes: it is either degraded or immobilised by a process which renders it biologically unavailable for degradation and so is effectively removed.

Immobilisation can be achieved by chemicals in the excreted by an organism or by chemicals in the neighbouring environment which trap or chelate a molecule thus making it insoluble. Since virtually all biological processes require the substrate to be dissolved in water, chelation renders the substance unavailable. In some instances this is a desirable end result and may be viewed as a form of remediation, since it stabilises the contaminant. In other cases it is a nuisance, as digestion would be the preferable option. Such 'unwanted' immobilisation can be a major problem in remediation, and is common state of affairs with aged contamination. Much research effort is being applied to find methods to reverse the process.

Degradation is achieved by metabolic pathways operating within an organism or combination of organisms, sometimes described as consortia. These processes are the crux of environmental biotechnology and thus form the major part of this chapter. Such activity operates through metabolic pathways functioning within the cell, or by enzymes either excreted by the cell or, isolated and applied in a purified form.

Biological monitoring utilises proteins, of which enzymes are a subset, produced by cells, usually to identify, or quantify contaminants. This has recently developed into an expanding field of biosensor production.

The biological players in these processes, their attributes which are so essential to this science and types of biological material are discussed in this chapter.

THE PLAYERS

Traditionally, life was placed into two categories—those having a true nucleus (eukaryotes) and those that do not (prokaryotes). This view was dramatically disturbed when Carl Woese proposed a third domain, the archaebacteria, now described as archaea, arguing that although apparently prokaryote at first glance they contain sufficient similarities with eukaryotes, in addition to unique features of their own, to merit their own classification.

It is primarily to the archaea, which typically inhabit extreme niches with respect to temperature, pressure, salt concentration or osmotic pressure, that a great debt of gratitude is owed for providing this planet with the metabolic capability to carry out processes under some very odd conditions indeed.

An appreciation of the existence of these classifications is important, as they differ from each other in the detail of their cell organisation and cellular processes making it unlikely that their genes are directly interchangeable. However, it is interesting to examine the potentially prokaryotic origins of the eukaryotic cell. There are many theories but the one which appears to have the most adherents is the endosymbiotic theory. It suggests that the 'proto' eukaryotic cell lost its cell wall, leaving only a membrane, and phagocytosed or subsumed various other bacteria with which it developed a symbiotic relationship. These included an aerobic bacterium, which became a mitochondrion, endowing the cell with the ability to carry out oxidative phosphorylation, a method of producing chemical energy able to be transferred to the location in the cell where it is required. Similarly, the chloroplast, the site of photosynthesis in higher plants, is thought to have been derived from cyanobacteria, the so-called blue–green algae. Chloroplasts are a type of plastid. These are membrane-bound structures found in vascular plants. Far from being isolated cellular organelles, the plastids communicate with each other through interconnecting tubules. Various other cellular appendages are also thought to have prokaryotic origins such as cilia or the flagellum on a motile eukaryotic cell which may have formed from the fusion of a spirochete bacterium to this 'proto' eukaryote. Nuclei may well have similar origins but the evidence is still awaited.

No form of life should be overlooked as having a potential part to play in environmental biotechnology. However, the organisms most commonly discussed in this context are microbes and certain plants. They are implicated either because they are present by virtue of being in their natural environment or by deliberate introduction.

Microbes

Microbes are referred to as such, simply because they cannot be seen by the naked eye. Many are bacteria or archaea, all of which are prokaryotes, but the term 'microbe' also encompasses some eukaryotes, including yeasts, which are unicellular fungi, as well as protozoa and unicellular plants. In addition, there are some microscopic multicellular organisms, such as rotifers, which have an essential role to play in the microsystem ecology of places such as sewage treatment plants. An individual cell of a eukaryotic multicellular organism like a higher plant or animal, is approximately 20 microns in diameter, while a yeast cell, also eukaryotic but unicellular, is about five microns in diameter. Although bacterial cells occur in a variety of shapes and sizes, depending on the species, typically a bacterial cell is rod shaped, measuring approximately one micron in width and two microns in length. At its simplest visualisation, a cell, be it a unicellular organism, or one cell in a multicellular organism, is a bag, bounded by a membrane, containing an aqueous solution in which are all the molecules and structures required to enable its continued survival. In fact, this 'bag' represents a complicated infrastructure differing distinctly between prokaryotes and eukaryotes, but a discussion of this is beyond the scope of this chapter.

Depending on the microbe, a variety of other structures may be present, for instance, a cell wall providing additional protection or support, or a flagellum a flexible tail, giving mobility through the surrounding environment. Survival requires cell growth, replication of the DNA and then division, usually sharing the contents into two equal daughter cells. Under ideal conditions of environment and food supply, division of some bacteria may occur every 20 minutes, however, most take rather longer. However, the result of many rounds of the binary division just described, is a colony of identical cells. This may be several millimetres across and can be seen clearly as a contamination on a solid surface, or if in a liquid, it will give the solution a cloudy appearance. Other forms of replication include budding off, as in some forms of yeast, or the formation of spores as in other forms of yeast and some bacteria. This is a type of DNA storage particularly resistant to environmental excesses of heat and pH, for example. When the environment becomes more hospitable, the spore can develop into a bacterium or yeast, the formation of spores as in other forms of yeast and some bacteria. This is a type of DNA storage particularly resistant to environmental excesses of heat and pH, for example. When the environment becomes more hospitable, the spore can develop into a bacterium or yeast, according to its origins, and the life cycle continues.

Micro-organisms may live as free individuals or as communities, either as a clone of one organism, or as a mixed group. Biofilms are examples of microbial communities, the components of which may number several hundred species. This is a fairly loose term used to describe any aggregation of microbes which coats a surface, consequently, biofilms are ubiquitous. They are of particular interest in environmental biotechnology since they represent the structure of microbial activity in many relevant technologies such as trickling filters. Their structure, and interaction between their members, is of sufficient interest to warrant at least one major symposium. Commonly, biofilms occur at a solid/liquid interphase. Here, a mixed population of microbes live in close proximity which may be mutually beneficial. Such consortia can increase the habitat range, the overall tolerance to stress and metabolic diversity of individual members of the group. It is often thanks to such communities, rather than isolated bacterial species, that recalcitrant pollutants are eventually degraded due to combined contributions of several of its members. Another consequence of this close proximity is the increased likelihood of bacterial transformation. This is a procedure whereby a bacterium may absorb free deoxyribonuclenic acid (DNA), the macromolecule which stores genetic material, from its surroundings released by other organisms, as a result of cell death, for example. The process is dependent on the ability, or competence, of a cell to take up DNA, and upon the concentration of DNA in the surrounding environment. This is commonly referred to as horizontal transfer as opposed to vertical transfer which refers to inherited genetic material, either by sexual or asexual reproduction. Some bacteria are naturally competent, others exude competence factors and recently, there is laboratory evidence that lighting can impart competence to some bacteria. It is conceivable that conditions allowing transformation prevail in biofilms considering the very high local concentration of microbes. Indeed there is evidence that such horizontal transfer of DNA occurs between organisms in these communities. In addition to transformation, genes are readily transferred on plasmids as described later in this section. It is now well established that, by one method or another, there is so much exchange of genetic material between bacteria in soil or in aquatic environments, that rather than discrete units, they represent a massive gene pool.

The sliminess often associated with biofilms is usually attubuted to excreted molecules often protein and carbohydrate in nature, which may coat and protect the film. Once established, the biofilm may proliferate at a rate to cause areas of anoxia at the furthest point from the source of oxygen, thus encouraging the growth of anaerobes. Consequently, the composition of the biofilm community is likely to change with time. To omplete the picture of microbial communities, it must be appreciated that they can include the other micro-organisms listed above, namely, yeasts, protozoa, unicellular plants and some microscopic multicellular organisms such as rotifers.

Plants

In contrast with microbes, the role of plants in environmental biotechnology is generally a structural one, exerting their effect by oxygenation of a microbe-rich environment, filtration solid-to-gas conversion, or extraction of the contaminant.

METABOLISM

The energy required to carry out all cellular processes is obtained from ingested food in the case of chemotrophic cells, additionally from light in the case of phototrophs and from inorganic chemicals in lithotrophic organisms. Since all biological macromolecules contain the element carbon, a dietary source of carbon is a requirement. Ingested food is therefore, at the very least, a source of energy and carbon, the chemical form of which is rearranged by passage through various routes called metabolic pathways. One purpose of this reshuffling is to produce, after addition or removal of other elements such as hydrogen, oxygen, nitrogen, phosphorus and sulphur, all the chemicals necessary for growth. The other is to produce chemical energy in the form of adenosine triphosphate (ATP), also one of the 'building blocks' of nucleic acids. Where an organism is unable to synthesise all its dietary requirements, it must ingest them, as they are by definition essential nutrients. The profile of these can be diagnostic for that organism and may be used in its identification in the laboratory. An understanding of nutritional requirements of any given microbe, can prove essential for successful remediation by bioenhancement.

At the core of metabolism are the central metabolic pathways of glycolysis and the tricarboxylic acid (TCA) cycle on which a vast array of metabolic pathways eventually converge or from which they diverge. Glycolysis is the conversion of the six-carbon phosphorylated sugar, glucose 6-phosphate, to the three-carbon organic acid, pyruvic acid, and can be viewed as pivotal in central metabolism since from this point pyruvate may enter various pathways determined by the energy and synthetic needs of the cell at that time. A related pathway, sharing some but not all of the reactions of glycolysis, and which operates in the opposite direction is called gluconeogenesis. Pyruvate can continue into the TCA cycle whose main function is to produce and receive metabolic intermediates and to produce energy, or into one of the many fermentation routes. The principles of glycolysis are universal to all organisms known to date, although the detail differs between species. An outline of glycolysis, the TCA, and its close relative the glycolysis, cycles is given in Fig. 5.1, together with an indication of the key points at which the products of macromolecule catabolism, or breakdown, enter these central metabolic pathways. The focus is on degradation rather than metabolism in general, since this is the crux of bioremediation. A description of the biological macromolecules which are lipids, carbohydrates, nucleic acids and proteins are given in the appropriate figures (Figs 5.2 to 5.5).

Not all possible metabolic routes are present in the genome of anyone organism. Those present are the result of evolution, principally of the enzymes which catalyse the various steps, and the elements which control their expression. However, an organism may have the DNA sequences, and so have the genetic capability for a metabolic route even though it is not 'switched on'. This is the basis for the description of 'latent pathways' which suggests the availability of a route able to be activated when the need arises, such as challenge from a novel chemical in the environment. Additionally, there is enormous, potential for uptake and exchange of genetic information as discussed earlier in this chapter. It is the enormous range of metabolic capability which is harnessed in environmental biotechnology.

The basis of this discipline is about ensuring that suitable organisms are present which have the capability to perform the task required of them. This demands the provision of optimal conditions for growth, thus maximising degradation of removal of the contaminant. Linked to many of the catalytic steps in the metabolic pathway are reactions which release sufficient energy to allow the synthesis of ATP. This is the energy 'currency' of a cell which permits the transfer of energy produced during degradation of a food to a process which may be occurring in a distant location and which requires energy.

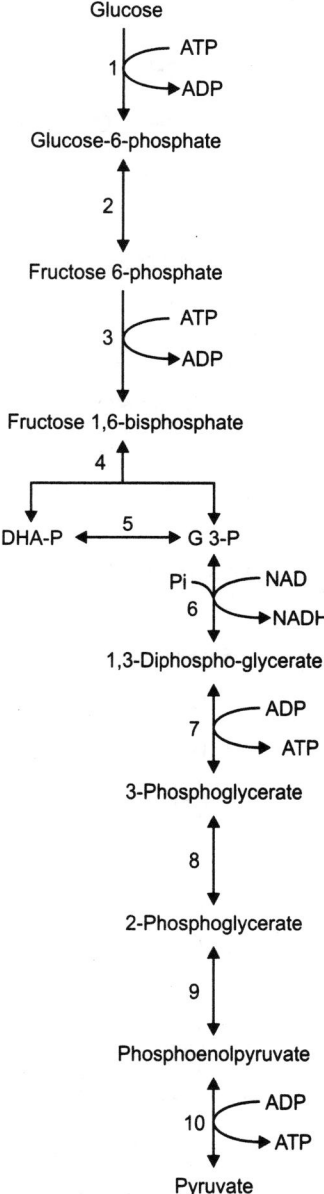

Fig. 5.1. Glycolysis, the TCA and glyoxalate cycle.

For brevity, the discussions in this chapter consider the metabolic processes of prokaryotes and unicellular eukaryotes as equivalent to a single cell of a multicellular organism such as an animal or plant.

This is a hideous oversimplification but justified when the points being made are general to all forms of life. Major differences are noted.

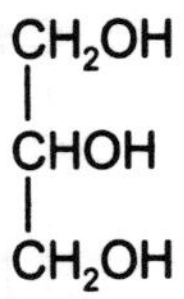

Glycerol

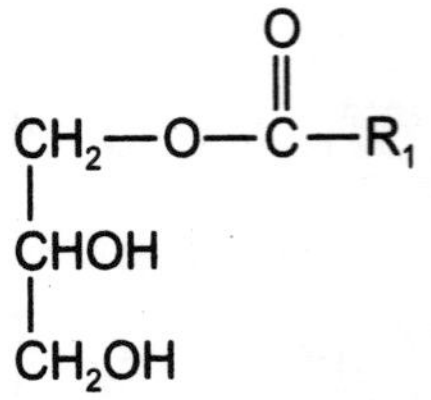

1-Monoacyl glycerol

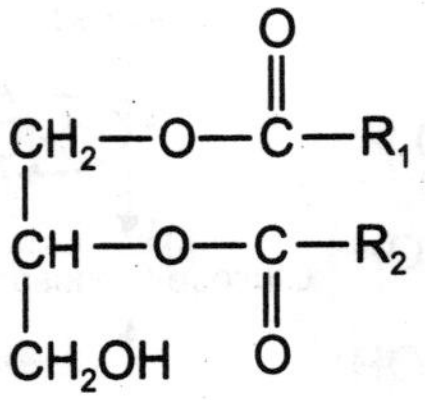

1,2-Diacyl glycerol

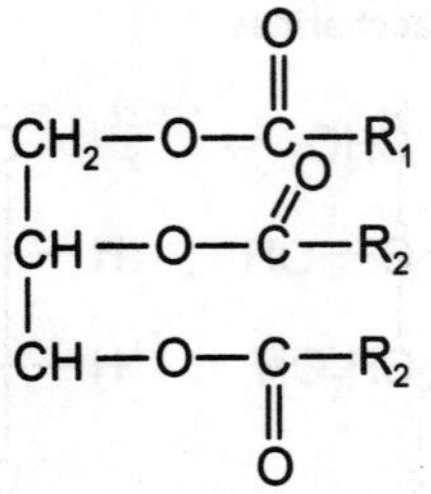

1,2,3-Triacyl glycerol

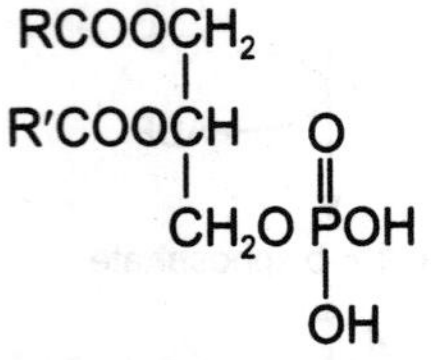

L-α-Phosphatidic acid

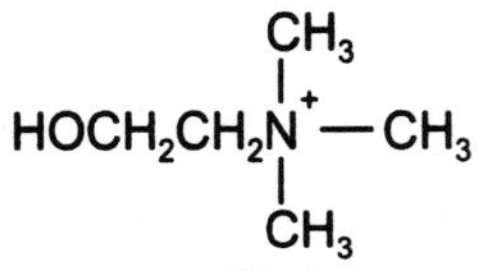

Choline

$HOCH_2CH_2NH_2$

Ethanolamine

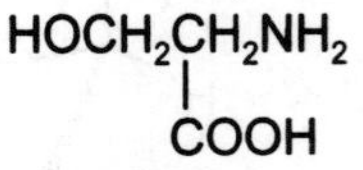

L-Serine

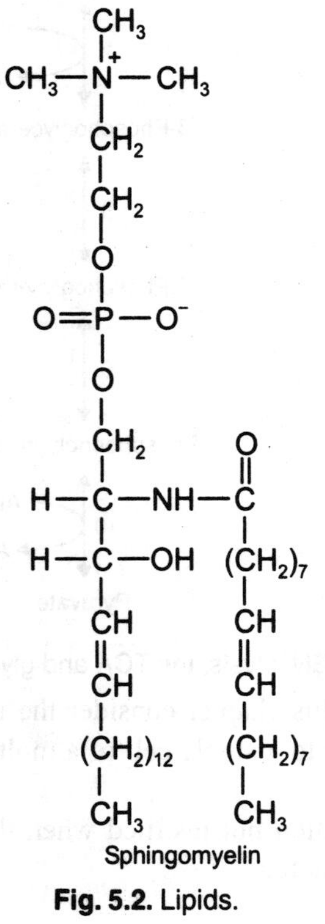

Sphingomyelin

Fig. 5.2. Lipids.

Polysaccharides

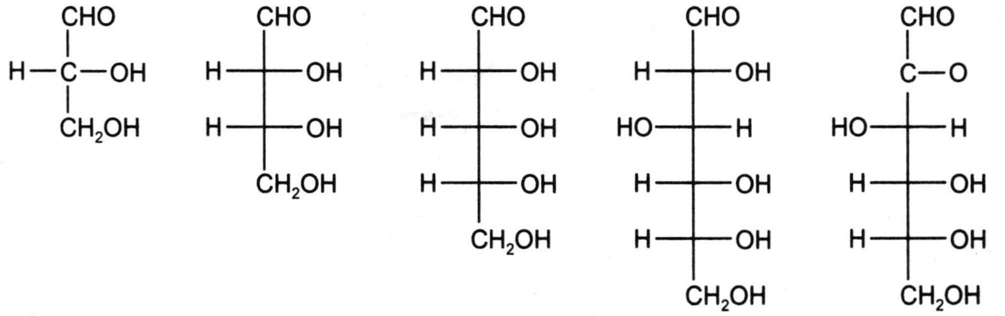

Glyceraldehyde	Erythrose	Ribose	Glucose	Fructose

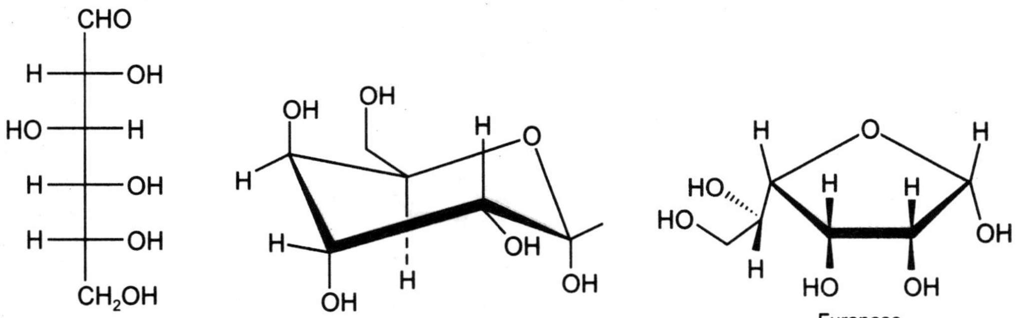

Linear form   Pyranose form   Furanose

Disaccharides

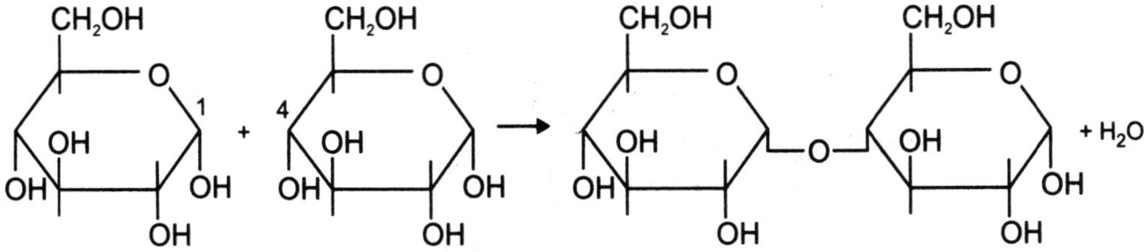

α-D-Glucose   α-D-Maltose

Monosaccharides

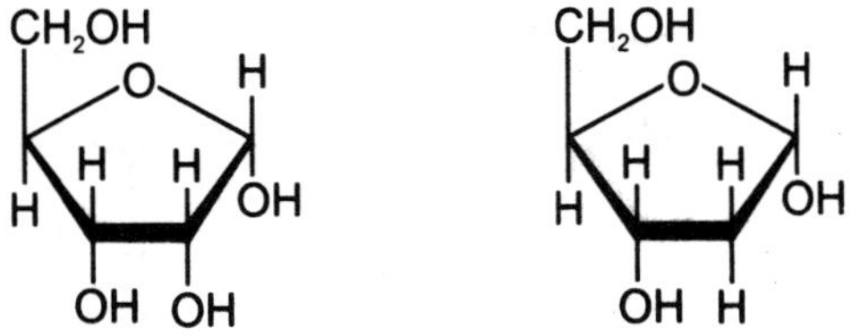

Ribose (RNA)   Deoxyribose (DNA)

Fig. 5.3. Carbohydrates.

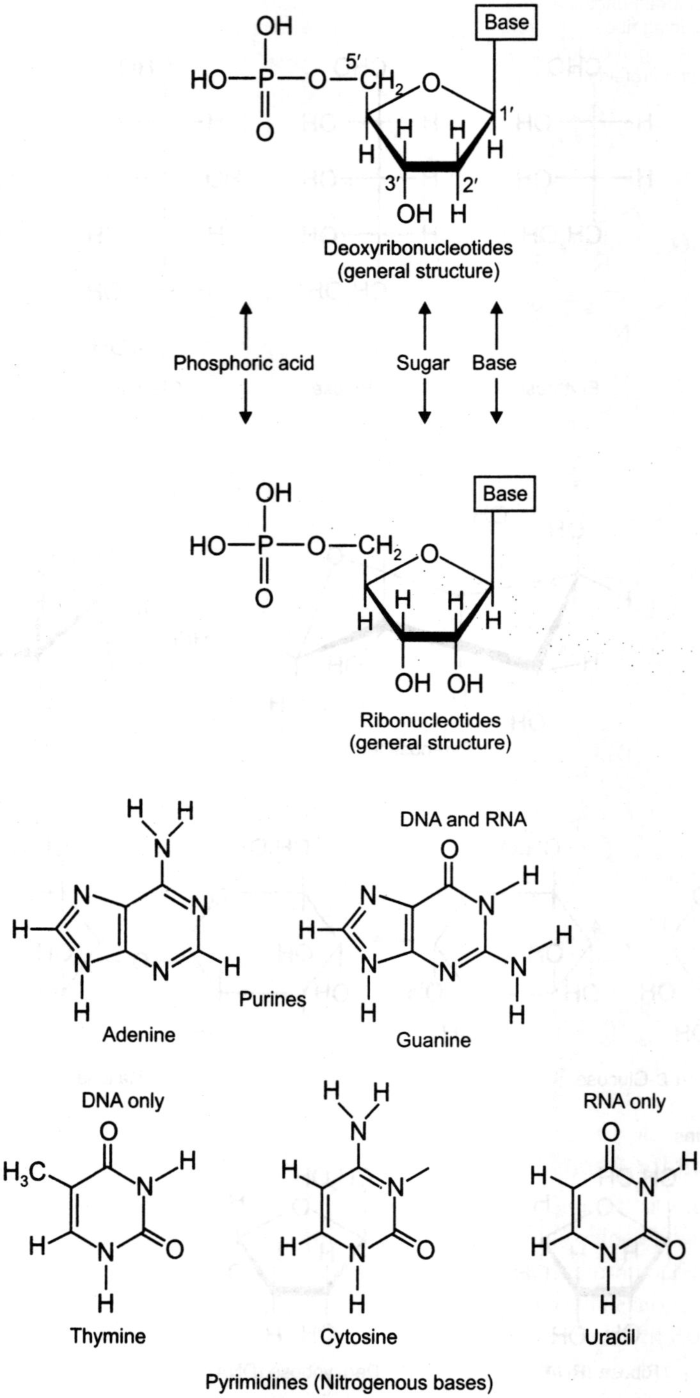
OH
HO—P—O—CH2
O
Base
5′
1′
3′
2′
OH H
Deoxyribonucleotides
(general structure)
Phosphoric acid
Sugar
Base
Ribonucleotides
(general structure)
OH OH
Adenine
Purines
DNA and RNA
Guanine
DNA only
Thymine
Cytosine
RNA only
Uracil
H3C
Pyrimidines (Nitrogenous bases)

Fig. 5.4. Nucleic acids.

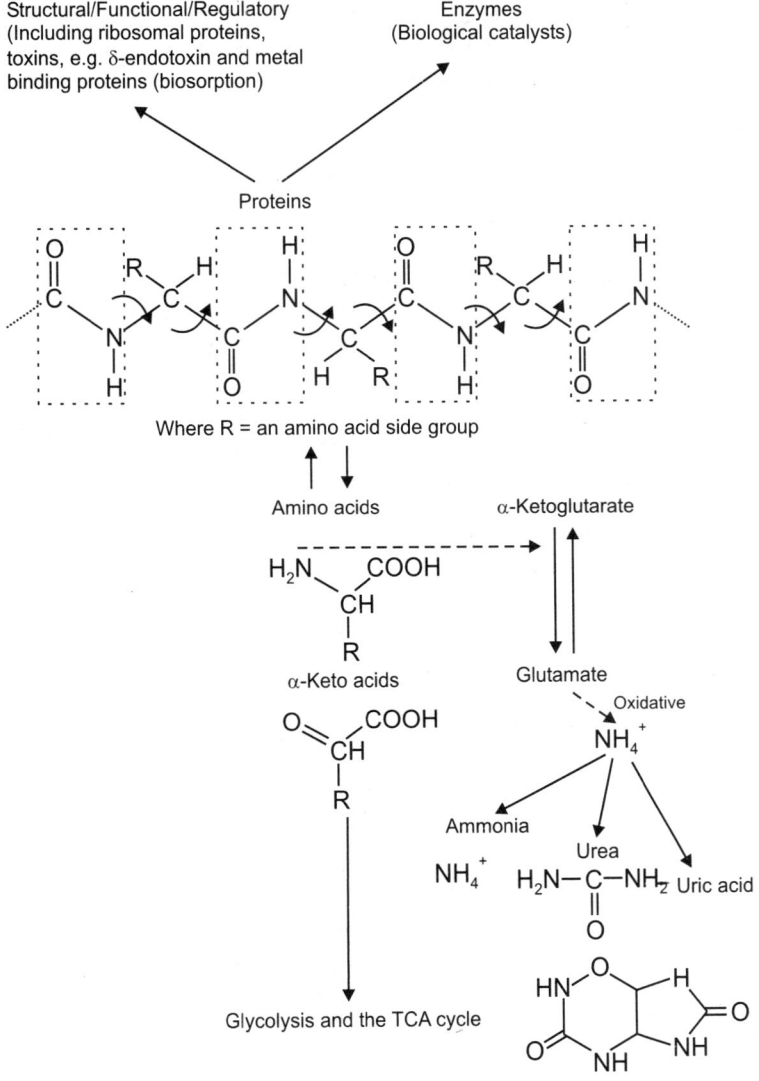

Fig. 5.5. Proteins.

Genetic Blueprint for Metabolic Capability

Metabolic capability is the ability of an organism or food. Obviously, the first requirement is that the food cell to digest available should be able to enter the cell which sometimes requires specific carrier proteins to allow penetration across the cell membrane. Once entered, the enzymes must be present to catalyse all the reactions in the pathway responsible for degradation, or catabolism. The information for this metabolic capability, is encoded in the DNA. The full genetic information is described as the genome and can be a single circular piece of DNA as in bacteria, or may be linear and fragmented into chromosomes as in higher animals and plants.

Additionally, many bacteria carry plasmids, which are much smaller pieces of DNA, also circular and self-replicating. These are vitally important in the context of environmental biotechnology in that they frequently carry the genes for degradative pathways. Many of these plasmids may move between different bacteria where they replicate, thus making the metabolic capability they carry, transferable. Bacteria show great promiscuity with respect to sharing their DNA. Often, bacteria living in a contaminated environment, themselves develop additional degradative capabilities. The source of that genetic information new to the organism, whether it is from modification of DNA within the organism or transfer from other microbes, or DNA free in the environment, is a source of hot debate between microbiologists. DNA not only codes for RNA which is translated into proteins but also for RNAs which are involved in protein synthesis, namely transfer RNA (tRNA) and ribosomal RNA (rRNA), also, small RNAs which are involved in the processing of rRNA. These are illustrated in Fig. 5.6.

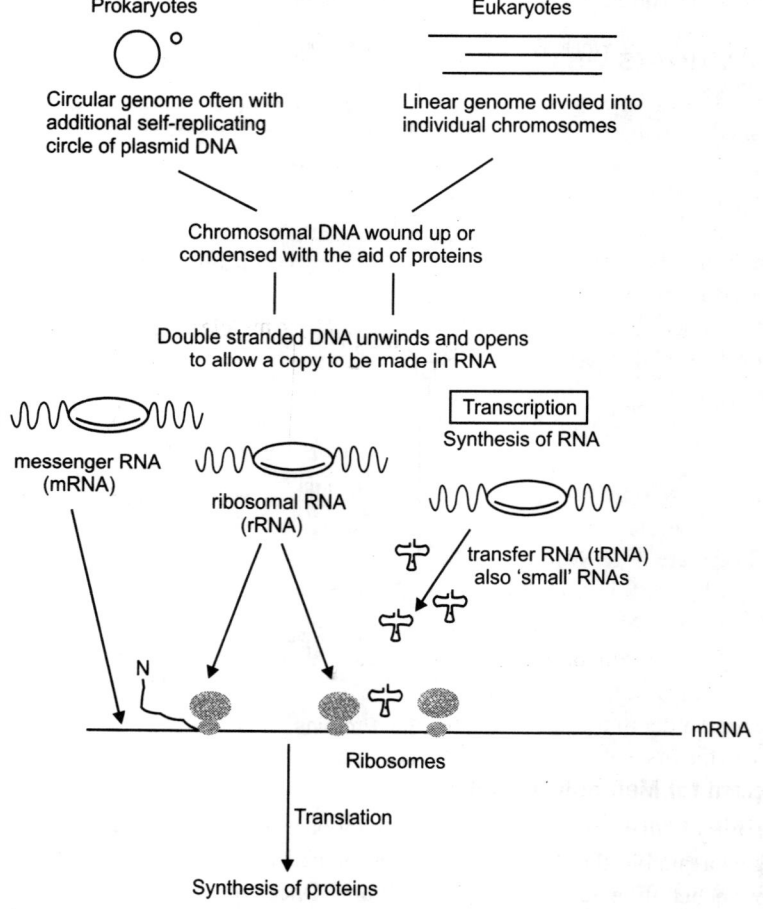

Fig. 5.6. Storage and expression of genetic information.

There have been many systems used to describe the degree of relatedness between organisms, but the most generally accepted is based on the sequence of the DNA coding for ribosomal RNA, the DNA. For completeness, it is important to mention the retroviruses which are a group of eukaryotic viruses with RNA rather than DNA as their genome. They carry the potential for integration into inheritable DNA due to the way in which they replicate their genomic RNA by way of a DNA intermediate.

MICROBIAL DIVERSITY

Microbes have been discovered in extraordinarily hostile environments where their continued survival has made demands on their structure and metabolic capability. These organisms, frequently members of the archaea, are those which have the capacity to degrade some of the most hazardous and recalcitrant chemicals in our environment and thus provide a rich source of metabolic capacity to deal with some very unpleasant contaminants. This situation will remain as long as the environments which harbour these invaluable microbes are recognised as such and are not destroyed. Microbial life on this planet, taken as a whole, has an immense capability to degrade noxious contaminants; it is essential to maintain the diversely and to maximise the opportunity for microbes to metabolise the offending carbon source.

METABOLIC PATHWAYS WHICH ARE PARTICULAR RELEVANCE TO ENVIRONMENTAL BIOTECHNOLOGY

Having established that the overall strategy of environmental biotechnology is to make use of the metabolic pathways in micro-organisms to break down or metabolise organic material, this chapter now examines those pathways in some detail. Metabolic pathways operating in the overall direction of synthesis are termed anabolic while those operating in the direction of breakdown or degradation are described as catabolic: the terms catabolism and anabolism being applied to describe the degradative or synthetic processes respectively.

It has been mentioned already in this chapter and it will become clear from the forthcoming discussion, that the eventual fate of the carbon skeletons of biological macromolecules is entry into the central metabolic pathways.

GLYCOLYSIS

As the name implies, glycolysis is a process describing the splitting of a phosphate derivative of glucose, a sugar containing six carbon atoms, eventually to produce two pyruvate molecules, each having three carbon atoms. There are at least four pathways involved in the catabolism of glucose. These are the Embden–Meyerthof (Fig. 5.1), which is the one most typically associated with glycolysis, the Entner–Doudoroff and the phosphoketolase pathways and the pentose phosphate cycle, which allows rearrangement into sugars containing 3, 4, 5, 6 or 7 carbon atoms. The pathways differ from each other in some of the reactions in the first half up to the point of lysis to two three-carbon molecules, after which point the remainder of the pathways are identical. These routes are characterised by the particular enzymes present in the first half of these pathways catalysing the steps between glucose and the production of dihydroxyacetone phosphate in equilibrium with glyceraldehyde 3-phosphate. All these pathways have the capacity to produce ATP and so function in the production of cellular energy. The need for four different routes for glucose catabolism, therefore, lies in the necessity for the supply of different carbon skeletons for anabolic processes and also for the provision of points of entry to glycolysis for catabolites from the vast array of functioning catabolic pathways. Not all of these pathways operate in all organisms. Even when several are encoded in the DNA, exactly which of these are active in an organism at any time, depends on its current metabolic demands and the prevailing conditions in which the microbe is living.

The point of convergence of all four pathways is at the triose phosphates which is the point where glycerol as glycerol phosphate enters glycolysis and so marks the link between catabolism of simple lipids and the central metabolic pathways. The addition of glycerol to the pool of trioses is compensated for by the action of triose phosphate isomerase maintaining the equilibrium between glyceraldehyde 3-phosphate and dihydroxyacetone phosphate which normally lies far in favour of the latter. This is perhaps surprising since it is glyceraldehyde 3-phosphate which is the precursor for the subsequent step. The next stage is the introduction of a second phosphate group to glyceraldehyde 3-phosphate with an accompanying oxidation, to produce glyceraldehyde 1,3-diphosphate. The oxidation involves the transfer of hydrogen to the coenzyme, NAD, to produce its reduced form, NADH. In order for glycolysis to continue operating, it is essential for the cell or organism to regenerate the NAD^+ which is achieved either by transfer of the hydrogens to the cytochromes of an electron transport chain whose operation is associated with the synthesis of ATP, or to an organic molecule such as pyruvate in which case the opportunity to synthesise ATP is lost.

This latter method is the first step of many different fermentation routes. These occur when operation of electron transport chains is not possible and so become the only route for the essential regeneration of NAD^+. Looking at the Embden–Meyerhof pathway, this is also the third stage at which a phosphorylation has occurred. In this case, the phosphate was derived from an inorganic source, in a reaction which conserves the energy of oxidation.

The next step in glycolysis is to transfer the new phosphate group to ADP, thus producing ATP and 3-phosphoglycerate, which is therefore the first substrate level site of ATP synthesis. After rearrangement to 2-phosphoglycerate and dehydration to phosphoenolpyruvic acid, the second phosphate is removed to produce pyruvic acid and ATP, and so is the second site of substrate level ATP synthesis. As mentioned above, depending on the activity of the electron transport chains and the energy requirements of the cell balanced against the need for certain metabolic intermediates, pyruvate, or its derivatives may now be reduced by accepting the hydrogen from NADH and so continue on a fermentation route or it may be decarboxylated to an acetyl group and enter the TCA cycle.

The overall energy balance of glycolysis is discussed later when considering chemical cellular energy production in more detail.

TCA CYCLE

Pyruvate decarboxylation produces the acetyl group bound to coenzyme A, ready to enter the TCA cycle otherwise named Kreb's citric acid cycle in tribute to the scientist who discovered it. Not only is this cycle a source of reduced cofactors which 'fuel' electron transport and thus, the synthesis of ATP, but it is also a great meeting point of metabolic pathways.

Cycle intermediates are constantly being removed or replenished. During anaerobic fermentation, many of the reactions seen in the TCA cycle are in operation even though they are not linked to electron transport.

GLYOXALATE CYCLE

This is principally the TCA cycle, with two additional steps forming a 'short circuit', involving the formation of glyoxalate from isocitrate. The second reaction requires the addition of acetyl CoA to glyoxalate to produce malic acid and thus rejoin the TCA cycle. The purpose of this shunt is to permit the organism to use acetyl CoA, which is the major breakdown product of fatty acids, as its sole carbon source.

MACROMOLECULES—DESCRIPTION AND DEGRADATION

Lipids

This class of macromolecules (Fig. 5.2) includes the neutral lipids which are triacylglycerols commonly referred to as fats and oils. Triacylglycerols are found in reservoirs in micro-organisms as fat droplets, enclosed within a 'bag', called a vesicle, while in higher animals, there is dedicated adipose tissue, comprising mainly cells full of fat. These various fat stores are plundered when energy is required by the organism as the degradation of triacylglycerols is a highly exergonic reaction and therefore a ready source of cellular energy. Gram for gram, the catabolism of these fats releases much more energy than the catabolism of sugar which explains in part why energy stores are fat rather than sugar. If this were not the case the equivalent space taken up by a sugar to store the same amount of energy would be much greater. In addition, sugar is osmotically active which could present a problem for water relations within a cell, should sugar be the major energy store.

Triacylglycerois comprise a glycerol backbone onto which fatty acids are esterified to each of the three available positions. They are insoluble in an aqueous environment due to the nonpolar nature of the fatty acids forming 'tails' on the triacylglycerol. However, diacylglycerols and monoacylglycerols which are esterified at only two or one position respectively, may form themselves into micelles due to their polar head, and so may exhibit apparent solubility by forming an emulsion. The tri-, di- and monoacylglycerols have in the past been described as tri-, di- or monoglycerides. Although these are inaccurate descriptions of the chemistry of these compounds the terms tri-, di- and monoglycerides are still in common usage. Chemically, fats and oils are identical. If the compound in question is a liquid at room temperature, frequently it is termed an oil, if solid it is described as a fat. The melting point of these compounds is determined to a large extent by the fatty acid content, where in general, saturated fatty acids, due to their ability to pack together in an orderly manner, confer a higher melting point than unsaturated fatty acids.

Their catabolism is by hydrolysis of the fatty acids from the glycerol backbone, followed by oxidation of the fatty acids by β-oxidation. This process releases glycerol which may then be further degraded by feeding into the central pathways of glycolysis, and several units of the acetyl group attached to the carrier coenzyme A (Fig. 5.2), which may feed into the central metabolic pathways just prior to entry into the TCA cycle (Fig. 5.1).

Compound lipids include the phosphoglycerides which are a major component of cell membranes. These can have very bulky polar head groups and nonpolar tails which allow them to act as surfactants and in this specific context, biosurfactants.

The most common surfactants are glycolipids (Fig. 5.7), which do not have a glycerol backbone, but have sugar molecules forming a polar head and fatty acids forming nonpolar tails, in an overall structure similar to that shown for phospholipids in Fig. 5.2. Derived lipids include fat soluble vitamins, natural rubber, cholesterol and steroid hormones. It is interesting to note here that bacteria do not synthesise steroids, and yet some, for example, *Comamonas testosteroni*, are able to degrade specific members of the group; testosterone in the case given.

However, oestrogen and its synthetic analogues used in the contraceptive pill, are virtually recalcitrant to decomposition by bacteria. This is proving a problem in waterways especially in Canada where the level of such endocrine disrupters has become so high in some lakes that the feminisation of fish is becoming a concern.

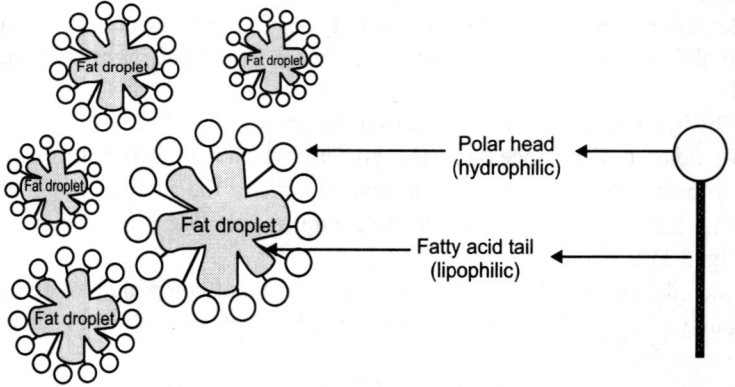

Rhamnolipid from *Pseudomonas* (glycolipid)

Micelle structure allowing dispersion of fats and oils is an aqueous medium

Fig. 5.7. Biosurfactants.

Proteins

The first catabolic step in protein degradation (Fig. 5.5) is enzymatic hydrolysis of the peptide bond formed during protein synthesis resulting in the release of short pieces, or peptides, and eventually after further degradation, amino acids. The primary step in amino acid catabolism is to remove the amino group thus producing an α-keto acid. This is usually achieved by transfer of the amino group to the TCA cycle intermediate, α-ketoglutarate, resulting in the amino acid, glutamate. Amino groups are highly conserved in all organisms due to the small number of organisms able to fix atmospheric nitrogen and so the source of an amino group is usually by transfer from another molecule. However, eventually, nitrogen is removed by oxidative deamination and is excreted in a form which depends upon the organism. Ammonia is toxic to most cells, but if an organism lives in an aqueous habitat, it may release ammonia directly into its surroundings where it is diluted and so made harmless. However, even in such an environment, if dilution should prove insufficient, ammonia concentration will increase, likewise the pH, consequently, the well-being of the organism will be compomised. Organisms which cannot make use of dilution, rid themselves of ammonia by converting it first into a less toxic form such as urea in the case of mammals and the fairly insoluble uric acid in the case of birds and most reptiles. Bacteria may then convert the excreted ammonia, urea or uric acid into nitrite and then oxidise it to nitrate which may then be taken up by plants. From there it is included in anabolic processes such as amino acid synthesis to produce material ingested by higher animals and the whole procedure of amino group transfer repeats itself. This is the basis of the nitrogen cycle which forms a central part of much of the sewage and effluent treatment.

The α-keto acid resulting from deamination of the amino acid is degraded by a series of reactions, the end product being dependent on the original amino acid, but all will finally result as a glycolysis or TCA cycle intermediate. A fascinating story of catabolism showing collaboration between mammals and bacteria resident in the gut, is the degradation of haemoglobin, the component of blood which carries oxygen and carbon dioxide. Haemoglobin comprises the protein, globin, into which was inserted during synthesis, the haeme ring system where the exchange between binding of oxygen or carbon dioxide takes place in circulating blood. The first step of haemoglobin degradation, performed in the mammalian system, is removal of the haeme ring structure releasing globin which is subject to normal protein degradation. Haeme has its origins in the amino acids in that the starting point for the ring structure is the amino acid, glycine. The degradation pathways starts with removal of iron and release of carbon monoxide to produce the linear structure, bilirubin. This is eventually excreted into the gut where enteric (gut) bacteria degrade the bilirubin to urobilinogens which are degraded further, some being excreted in the urine and others, such as stercobilin, are excreted in the faeces. All these products are further metabolised by microbes, for example, in the sewage treatment plant.

Nucleic Acids

Degradation of nucleic acids (Fig. 5.4) is also a source of ammonium ion. The purines are broken down to release CO_2 and uric acid which is reduced to allantoin. This is then hydrolysed to produce urea and glyoxylate which can enter the TCA cycle by the glyoxylate pathway present in plants and bacteria but not mammals. The urea thus produced may be further hydrolysed to ammonium ion or ammonia with the release of carbon dioxide. The form in which the nitrogen derived from the purines is excreted, again depends upon the organism.

Pyrimidines are hydrolysed to produce ammonia which enters the nitrogen cycle, carbon dioxide and β-alanine or β-aminoisobutyric acid both of which are finally degraded to succiuyl CoA which enters the TCA cycle.

Carbohydrates

The carbohydrates (Fig. 5.3) form a ready source of energy for most organisms as they lead, by a very short route, into the central metabolic pathways from which energy to fuel metabolic processes is derived. When several sugar units, such as glucose, are joined together to form macromolecules, they are called polysaccharides. Examples of these are glycogen in animals, and cellulose in plants. In nature, the sugars usually occur as ring structures and many have the general formula, $C(H_2O)_n$, where carbon and water are present in equal proportion. Catabolism of glucose has been described earlier in this chapter. As stated earlier, the resulting metabolite from a given carbon source, or the presence of specific enzymes, can be diagnostic of an organism. Whether or not the enzymes of a particular route are present can help to identify a microbe, and carbohydrate metabolism is frequently the basis of micro-organism identification in a Public Health laboratory. Glucose enters the glycolytic pathway to pyruvate, the remainder of which is determined in part by the energy requirements of the cell and in part by the availability of oxygen. If the organism or cell normally exists in an aerobic environment, there is oxygen available and the pyruvate is not required as a starting point for the synthesis of another molecule, then it is likely to enter the TCA cycle. If no oxygen is available, fermentation, defined later in this chapter, is the likely route. The function of fermentation is to balance the chemical reductions and oxidations performed in the initial stages of glycolysis.

PRODUCTION OF CELLULAR ENERGY

Cellular energy is present mainly in the form of ATP and to a lesser extent, GTP (Fig. 5.4) which are high energy molecules, so called because a large amount of chemical energy is released on hydrolysis of the phosphate groups. The energy to make these molecules is derived from the catabolism of a food, or from photosynthesis. A food source is commonly carbohydrate, lipid or to a lesser extent, protein but if a compound considered to be a contaminant can enter a catabolic pathway, then it can become a 'food' for the organism. This is the basis of bioremediation. The way in which energy is transferred from the 'food' molecule to ATP may take two substantially different routes. One is cytoplasmic synthesis of ATP which is the direct transfer of a phosphate group to ADP, storing the energy of that reaction in chemical bonds. The other involves a fairly complicated system involving transfer of electrons and protons, or hydrogen ions, which originated from the oxidation of the 'food' at some stage during its passage through the catabolic pathways. The final sink for the electrons and hydrogen ions is oxygen, in the case of oxidative phosphorylation, to produce water. This explains the need for good aeration in many of the processes of environmental biotechnology, where organisms are using oxidative phosphorylation as their main method for synthesising ATP. An example of this is the activated sludge process in sewage treatment. However, many microbes are anaerobes, an example being a class of archaea, the methanogens, which are obligate anaerobes in that they will die if presented with an oxygenated atmosphere. This being the case, they are unable to utilise the oxidative phosphorylation pathways and so instead, operate an electron transport chain similar in principle, although not in detail. It has as the ultimate electron and hydrogen sink, a variety of simple organic compounds including acetic acid, methanol and carbon dioxide. In this case, the end product is methane in addition to carbon dioxide or water depending on the identity of the electron sink. These are the processes responsible for the production of methane in an anaerobic digester which explains the necessity to exclude air from the process.

FERMENTATION AND RESPIRATION

The electrons derived from the catabolism of the carbon source are eventually either donated to an organic molecule in which case the process is described as fermentation, or donated to an inorganic acceptor by transfer along an electron chain. This latter process is respiration and may be aerobic where the terminal electron acceptor is oxygen, or anaerobic where the terminal electron acceptor is other than oxygen such as nitrate, sulphate, carbon dioxide, sulphur or ferric ion. Unfortunately, respiration is a term which has more than one definition. It may also be used to describe a subset of the respiration processes mentioned above to include only oxidation of organic material and where the ultimate electron acceptor is molecular oxygen. This latter definition is the basis of biological oxygen demand (BOD), which is often used to characterise potential environmental pollutants, especially effluents, being a measure of the biodegradable material available for oxidation by microbes.

Fermentations

In modern parlance, there are many definitions of the term 'fermentation'. They range from the broadest and somewhat archaic to mean any large-scale culture of micro-organisms, to the very specific, meaning growth on an organic substance and which is wholly dependent on substrate-level phosphorylation. This is the synthesis of ATP by transfer of a phosphate group directly from a high energy compound and not involving an electron transport chain. Additionally, and a source of great confusion, is that fermentation may refer simply to any microbial growth in the absence of oxygen but equally may be used generally to mean microbial growth such as food spoilage where the presence or absence of oxygen is unspecified. The definition used throughout, except with reference to eutrophic fermentation is that of growth dependent on substrate-level phosphorylation.

There are very many fermentation routes but all share two requirements, the first being the regeneration of NAD^+ from NADH produced during glycolysis which is essential to maintain the overall reduction: oxidation equilibrium, and the second being that pyruvate, or a derivative thereof, is the electron acceptor during the reoxidation of NADH. What this means is that all fermentation routes start with pyruvate, the end-point of glycolysis, and proceed along a variety of pathways to an end product indicative, if not diagnostic, of the organism. Fermentation is therefore an option under conditions where there is an active electron transport chain as discussed in the following section, but becomes essential when fermentation is the only method for regenerating NAD^+.

As noted above, the end product of fermentation for any given carbon source may be diagnostic of the identity of a specific organism. This is more relevant for bacteria than for yeast or other eukaryotic cells and arises from the predisposition of that organism, to use a particular fermentation pathway. These are summarised in Fig. 5.8.

Electron Transport Chains: Oxidative Phosphorylation and Methanogenesis

As described in the previous section, NADH and other reduced cofactors may be reoxidised by the reduction of organic receptors such as pyruvate. This is the fermentation route.

Alternatively, the reducing agent (or reductant) can transfer the electrons to an electron transport chain which ultimately donates them to an inorganic receptor (the oxidising agent or oxidant). In aerobic respiration, this receptor is oxygen. However, some bacteria have electron transport chains which use other electron sinks such as nitrate, sulphate, carbon dioxide and some metals, with respiration being described as anaerobic in these cases. The use of nitrate in this role leads to the process of denitrification, which plays an important part in many aspects of the applications of environmental biotechnology.

A number of events occur during the flow of electrons along the chain which have been observed and clearly described for a number of organisms and organelles, most especially the mitochondria of eukaryotic cells.

These are fully discussed in many biochemistry textbooks, an excellent example being Lehninger, the gist of which is outlined in this section. The details of exactly how these phenomena combine to drive the synthesis of ATP is still unclear but various models have been proposed.

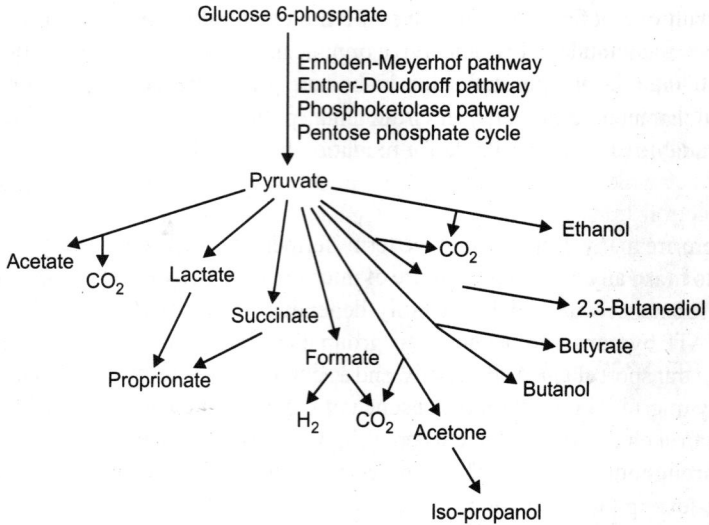

Glucose 6-phosphate

Embden-Meyerhof pathway
Entner-Doudoroff pathway
Phosphoketolase patway
Pentose phosphate cycle

Example of end products of pyruvate fermentation typically shown by the organisms listed:

Acetate	Enterobacteria, Clostridia
Acetoin	Yeast
Acetone	Clostridia
2,3-Butanediol	Yeast, aerobacter
Butanol	Clostridia
Butyrate	Clostridia
Ethanol	Yeast, acetobacter, enterobacteria
Formate	Enterobacteria
Iso-propanol	Clostridia
Lactate	Lactic acid bacteria (*Streptococcus*, *Lactobacillus*)
Proprionate	*Clostridium proprionicum*

Fig. 5.8. Fermentations.

The chemiosmotic model, proposed by Peter Mitchell, states that the proton, or hydrogen ion, gradient which develops across an intact membrane during biological oxidations is the energy store for the subsequent synthesis of ATP. This model somewhat revolutionised the then current thinking on the energy source for many cellular processes, as the principles of energy storage and availability according to the chemiosmotic theory were applicable to many energy-demanding cellular phenomena including photosynthetic phosphorylation and some cross-membrane transport systems. It could even account for the movement of flagellate which propel those bacteria possessing them, through a liquid medium. The chemiosmotic theory accounts for the coupling of the transmembrane proton gradient to ATP synthesis. It implies that during oxidation, the electrons flow down from high to low energy using that energy to drive protons across a membrane against a high concentration, thus developing the proton gradient. When the electron flow stops, the protons migrate down the concentration gradient, simultaneously releasing energy to drive the synthesis of ATP through membrane-associated proteins. The model system described first is that of mitochondria and, later in this chapter, comparisons with bacterial systems associated with oxidative phosphorylation and those systems associated with methanogenesis will be made.

Electron transport chains comprise cytochrome molecules which trap electrons, and enzymes which transfer electrons from a cytochrome to its neighbour. The quantity of energy released during this transfer is sufficient to drive the synthesis of approximately one ATP molecule by the enzyme ATP synthetase. The whole system is located in a membrane which is an essential requirement of any electron transport chain because of the need to organise it topographically, and to allow the establishment of a pH gradient. Also there is evidence that during active electron transport, the morphology of the membrane changes and is believed to store energy in some way yet to be elucidated. Consequently, an intact membrane is essential. Any toxic substance which damages the integrity of a membrane has the potential to interrupt the functioning of the electron transport chain thereby reducing the facility for ATP synthesis and potentially killing the organism. The chain may also be disrupted by interference with the electron carriers. Such a chemical is cyanide, which complexes with cytochrome oxidase, and for which research into a biological remediation route is underway.

Mitochondrial electron transport system and oxidative phosphorylation

The electron transport system in eukaryotes is located in the inner membrane of mitochondria. A representation of the system is given in Fig. 5.9. The chain is a series of complexes comprising cytochromes, and enzymes involved in oxidation reduction reactions whose function is to transfer electrons from one complex to the next. The ratios of the complexes one to another varies from cell type to cell type.

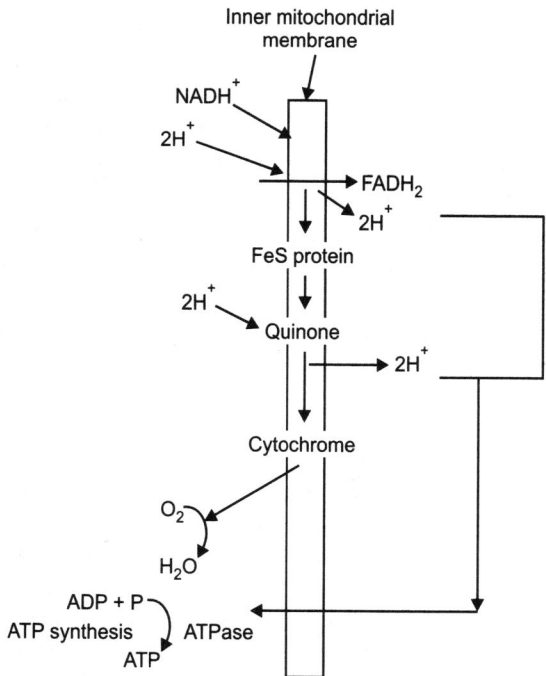

Fig. 5.9. Mitochondrial electron transport chain.

However, the concentration of the cytochrome a complex per unit area of inner membrane stays fairly constant. What changes from cell type to cell type is the degree of infolding of the inner membrane, such that cells requiring a large amount of energy have mitochondria which have a very large surface area of inner membrane, which is highly convoluted thus providing a high capacity for electron transport.

The process which couples ATP synthesis to electron transport in mitochondria and which still evades a complete description, is oxidative phosphorylation or more accurately, respiratory-chain phosphorylation. There are three sites within the mitochondrial chain which span the interaction between two neighbouring complexes, which on the basis of energy calculations are thought to witness a release of energy sufficient to synthesise almost one molecule of ATP from ADP and phosphate, as a result of electron transfer from one complex to its neighbour. These are designated site I between NADH and coenzyme Q, site II between cytochromes b and c, and site III between cytochrome a and free oxygen. Site III occurs within complex IV, the final complex which may also be referred to as cytochrome oxidase. Its overall function is to transfer electrons from cytochrome c to cytochrome a, then to a_3 and finally to molecular oxygen. It is this final stage which is blocked by the action of cyanide and by carbon monoxide. Associated with the electron flow, is the ejection of hydrogen ions from inside the mitochondrion, across the membrane, and in complex IV, the reduction of the oxygen molecule with two hydrogen ions originating from inside the mitochondrion. If all three sites were involved, the amount of energy released is sufficient to drive the synthesis of two and a half molecules of ATP for each pair of electrons transported. If the first site was omitted, the number falls to one and a half. In neither case is it a complete integer because there is not, a direct mole for mole relationship between electron transport and ATP synthesis but as described earlier, it is part of a much more complicated process described above as the chemiosmotic theory.

Bacterial electron transport systems and oxidative phosphorylation

Bacterial electron transport chains have fundamentally the same function as that described for mitochondrial electron transport chains but with several notable differences in their structure. For example, the cytochrome oxidase which is the final complex nearest the oxygen in mitochondria, is not present in all bacteria. The presence or absence of this complex is the basis of the 'oxidase' test for the identification of bacteria. In these organisms, cytochrome oxidase is replaced by a different set of cytochromes. An interesting example is *Escherichia coli*, an enteric bacterium and coliform, which is commonly found in sewage. It has replaced the electron carriers of cytochrome oxidase with a different set including cytochromes b_{558}, b_{595}, b_{562}, d and o, which are organised in response to the level of oxygen in the local environment. Unlike the mitochondrial chain, the bacterial systems may be highly branched and may have many more points for the entry of electrons into the chain and exit of electrons to the final electron acceptor.

Bacterial electron transport systems, denitrification and methanogenesis

As previously mentioned, the term respiration is applied to many processes. Without further specification it is usually used to mean the consumption of molecular oxygen, by reduction to water in the case of the electron transport discussed above, or by oxidation of an organic molecule to produce carbon dioxide and serine in the case of photorespiration, discussed later in this chapter. Thus the term anaerobic respiration seems a contradiction. It does, however, describe fundamentally the same process of electron transfer to a final acceptor which although inorganic, in this case is not oxygen. An example of such an electron acceptor is nitrate which is converted to nitrite. This is a toxic substance, and so many bacteria have the facility to convert nitrite to nitrogen gas. This overall series of reactions is described as denitrification and is the basis of the process by which denitrifying bacteria such as members of the *Pseudomonas* and *Bacillus* genera are able to reduce nitrate and nitrite levels down to consent values during sewage treatment. Such bacteria have different components in their electron transport chain in comparison with mitochondria, which have the necessary enzymatic activities to carry out these processes.

Like mitochondrial electron transport, denitrification can be associated with synthesis of ATP although with much reduced efficiency.

Other examples of terminal electron acceptors are firstly sulphate, in which case one of the final products is elemental sulphur. This process is carried our by the obligate anaerobe, *Desulfovibrio* and members of the archaean genus *Archaeglobus*. Another anaerobe, *Alkaliphilus transvaaleasis*, an extreme alkaliphile, growing at a pH of 8.5 to 12.5, isolated from an ultra-deep gold mine in South Africa, can use elemental sulphur, thiosulphate or fumarate as an additional electron acceptor. Secondly, carbon dioxide may be the final electron acceptor in which case one of the final products is methane. This process is also carried out by obligate anaerobes, in this case, the methanogens, all of which are archaeans and are responsible for methane production in anaerobic digesters and landfill sites. Again, it functions on much the same principles as the other chains mentioned above but has a different set of cofactors which are most unusual. For both of the above obligate anaerobes, anaerobic respiration is an important mechanism of ATP synthesis. It is less efficient than aerobic respiration due to the smaller drop in electropotential between sulphate or carbon dioxide and NADH compared with the difference between NADH and oxygen, and so less energy is available to be released during electron transport and consequently less ATP is synthesised per mole of NADH entering the pathway. Anaerobic respiration is, however, more efficient than fermentation and so is the route of choice for ATP synthesis for an anaerobe.

Energy balance sheet between substrate level and electron transport linked ATP synthesis

An approximate comparison may be made between the efficiency with respect to energy production, of ATP synthesis by substrate-level phosphorylation and by association with electron transport. For one mole of glucose passing through glycolysis by the Embden-Meyerhof pathway to produce two moles of pyruvate, there is net production of two moles of ATP. For most fermentation pathways, no further ATP is synthesised.

There are exceptions, of course, such as the conversion of an acyl CoA derivative such as acetyl CoA or butyrl CoA to the free acid which in these cases are acetate and butyrate respectiviely. Each of these reactions releases sufficient energy to drive the phosphorylation of one mole of ADP.

Conversely, if the electron transport chain is functioning. NADH may be oxidised by relinquishing electrons to the cytochromes in the chain thus regenerating the oxidised cofactor. In this scenario, pyruvate may enter the TCA cycle rather than a fermentation route, thus a further mole of ATP is produced at substrate level during conversion of succinyl CoA to succinate via GTP, which then transfers the terminal phosphate to ATP. In addition, NADH and $FADH_2$ are produced during the TCA cycle thus generating up to 15 moles of ATP per mole of pyruvate. An overall comparison may be made between glycolysis followed by reoxidation of NADH by fermentation or, alternatively, glycolysis followed by entry into the TCA cycle and reoxidation of cofactors via the electron transport chain. Remembering that one mole of glucose generates two moles of pyruvate during glycolysis, and that the two moles of NADH produced during glycolysis may also be reoxidised by transfer to the electron transport chain and not through fermentation, the net result is that glucose catabolised by the glycolysis-fermentation route results in the production of two moles of ATP whereas catabolism by the glycolysis-TCA cycle-electron transport/oxidative phosphorylation route produces up to 32 moles of ATP.

Anaerobic respiration is less efficient than aerobic respiration. Oxidation of the same amount of cofactor by methanogenesis rather than oxidative phosphorylation would produce fewer moles of ATP.

Consequently, for a given amount of ATP production, the flux of glucose through glycolysis followed by fermentation would have to be approximately 16 times greater than through glycolysis followed by oxidative phosphorylation, and the flux through methanogenesis is somewhat intermediate. It is the metabolic capability of the organism and the presence or absence of the appropriate inorganic electron acceptor which determines the fate of pyruvate on the grounds of energy considerations. On a practical basis this may explain why anaerobic processes, such as the anaerobic digestion of sewage sludge and municipal solid waste, are considerably less exothermic than their aerobic counterparts. For a given quantity of carbon source, an aerobic process will be able to extract in the order of 10 times the amount of energy than that generated by an anaerobic process.

Regeneration of NAD⁺ in plants

In addition to the processes discussed above for the production of NADH, plant mitochondria operate an additional system whereby the required protons are derived from two molecules of the amino acid glycine. During this mitochondrial process, one molecule of molecular oxygen is consumed in the production of carbon dioxide and the amine acid, serine. The superfluous amino group from the second glycine molecule is released as ammonia. The glycine molecules were derived from phosphoglycolate, the metabolically useless product of photorespiration. This subject is very important with regard to plant breeding and development and so is discussed in some detail alongside the related subject of photosynthesis.

PHOTOSYNTHESIS AND THE BASIS OF PHYTOTECHNOLOGY

The sun is the biosphere's ultimate source of energy and photosynthesis is the only means there is on this planet to trap incident sunlight and convert it into chemical energy available to biological processes. Thus, with very rare exceptions, organisms which do not photosynthesise, which is the majority, are totally dependent on those which do. With this introduction it is hardly surprising to find a description of this process in a book which specifically addresses the capabilities of biological organisms and their interplay. Leafy plants obviously feature in this section but so too do photosynthetic eukaryotic microorganisms and bacteria. A knowledge of this vital process is essential to appreciating the role which photosynthesising organisms play in the environment, their limitations and the strengths upon which biotechnology can capitalise.

The energy from this process is used to drive all the biochemical synthesis and degradation reactions occurring in the cell in addition to various other energy-requiring processes such as the movement and transport of molecules across membranes. Energy is finally dissipated as heat, and entropy rises in accordance with the laws of thermodynamics. Any interference with the flow from the sun either by reducing the ability of the energy to penetrate the atmosphere, or by reducing the total photosynthetic capacity of the planet, has dramatic consequences to all forms of life. Conversely, too intense a radiation from the sun resulting from thinning of the ozone layer runs the risk of damaging the photosynthetic machinery. This can be compensated for by the organism acquiring pigments to absorb harmful radiation, but this requires time for such an evolutionary adjustment to take place.

It is noteworthy that the bulk of photosynthesis is performed by unicellular organisms, such as photosynthetic algae, rather than the macrophytes as might reasonably be supposed. Photosynthesis occurs in two parts; the first is the trapping of light with associated reduction of NADP⁺ and ATP synthesis, and the second is the fixing of carbon dioxide by its incorporation into a carbohydrate molecule. This is most commonly a hexose sugar, and typically glucose, the synthesis of which utilises the NADPH and ATP produced in the light-dependent part 1. The processes of carbohydrate synthesis occurring in the second part are described as the dark reactions, so called because they may proceed in the dark after a period of illumination to activate part 1. The sugar produced during these dark reactions will then be utilised by the cell, transferred to another cell or ingested by a larger organism and eventually catabolised to carbon dioxide and water, releasing the energy consumed originally to synthesise the molecule. Here is another example of a natural cycle, where carbon is introduced, as carbon dioxide, into the synthesis of a sugar which is then interconverted through the various metabolic pathways until finally it is released as carbon dioxide thus completing the cycle. Eukaryotes capable of carrying out photosynthesis include higher green plants, multicellular green, brown and red algae and various unicellular organisms such as the euglenoids and dinoflagellates both of which are commonly found in fresh water environments, and diatoms which are also found in salt water. The diatoms which are unicellular algae, are particularly noteworthy given the current estimates that they are responsible for fixing 20 to 25 per cent of the world's carbon through photosynthesis. Prokaryotes capable of photosynthesis include blue-green algae, and both the sulphur and nonsulphur purple and green bacteria. The blue-green algae which are oxygenic bacteria and are alternatively named cyanobacteria, operate light reactions very similar to those of eukaryotes. Conversely, the green and the purple nonsulphur bacteria which are both facultative aerobes and the strictly anaerobic green and the purple sulphur bacteria utilise a rather different set of light reactions as a consequence of their possessing a 'simpler' photosystem. Eukaryotic and bacterial systems are both described in the following sections.

LIGHT REACTIONS

Visible light is the outcome of the nuclear fusion of hydrogen atoms, resulting in the production of helium atoms, gamma radiation and two electrons. This fusion occurs in the sun at a temperature of approximately 2,00,00,000 K. The gamma radiation and electrons combine to produce quanta of visible light. The entrapment of light is performed in photosynthetic cells by pigments; the most important of which are the chlorophylls. These are flat ring structures, with regions of conjugated double and single bonds, and a long hydrophobic tail well designed for anchoring the pigments into membrane. Only red and blue light is absorbed by the chlorophylls in most organisms. Consequently, when white light from the sun shines upon them, they reflect green light. Thus making these organisms appear green. Variation in the types of chlorophylls and the presence of additional accessory pigments all contribute to the observed colour of the organism and are the result of evolution which has developed the 'best fit' of light-trapping molecules to suit the ecological niche of the organism. It is worth pointing out that wholesale transport of the plant or bacterium for biotechnology purposes has to take this factor into account. It is important to test the growth and performance characteristics of any translocated plant or bacterium to ensure that the new environment does not produce disappointing results. The purpose of the accessory pigments referred to above, which include the carotenoids and phycobiliproteins, the latter found in red algae and cyanobacteria, is to extend the range of absorbed wavelengths thus maximising the amount of energy trapped from light and protecting the photosynthetic system from potential damage by oxidation. A rather unusual pigment which functions as a primary pigment, is bacteriorhodopsin which causes the archaea which express it, to appear purple. Returning to the principally eukaryotic process, the chlorophylls described above which receive the incident light are clustered in highly organised structures called antennae located on the cell surface. The incident light excites the energy state of the recipient chlorophyll to a higher energy state. When the chlorophyll returns to its normal level it releases electrons which are transferred to a neighbouring chlorophyll. The transfer is repeated until the electrons arrive at a photosystem, from which point they enter an electron transport chain linked to the reduction of NAD^+ and the synthesis of ATP. There are many similarities between electron transport in respiration and in photosynthesis in that they are both membrane bound and may be coupled to phosphorylation and thus synthesis of ATP, according to Mitchell's chemiosmotic theory, by employing a similar strategy of a proton gradient described earlier for respiration. In eukaryotic higher organisms, photosynthesis occurs in the chloroplast while in bacteria it occurs in the cytoplasmic membrane. The precise location in bacteria is sometimes described as being the mesosome. This has been reported as an infolding of the bacterial cellular membrane which sometimes appears to be in association with the bacterial DNA and often is found near nascent cell walls. Although considerable effort has been invested in determining its function, there is still disagreement as to whether or not the mesosome is indeed a bacterial cell structure or is simply an artefact occurring during preparation of samples for microscopy. Thus the site of bacterial photosynthesis remains uncertain beyond it being bound in the cytoplasmic membrane.

Photosystems in Eukaryotes and Cyanobacteria

There are two types of photosystem which may occur in photosynthetic organisms indicated in Fig. 5.10: photosystemt which receives electrons from photosystem 2 but may also operate independently by cyclic electron transport, and photosystem 2 which is not present in all such organisms. The pathway for electron transport has two principal routes. One involves only photosystem 1. In this, electrons transferred from the antennae to photosystem 1 cause excitation of the chlorophyll in this system. When the chlorophyll returns to its lower energy state, the electrons are transferred to ferredoxin, which is one of the iron-containing proteins in the chain of electron carriers. From this point there is a choice of routes; either the cyclic path by way of a chain of cytochrome molecules starting with cytochrome b_{563} and finally returning to chlorophyll a, or by the noncyclic route which is the transfer of electrons to $NADP^+$.

The source of the hydrogen atom required to reduce the $NADP^+$ to NADPH in this system is the water molecule which donates its electrons to photosystem 2 to replace those lost to $NADP^+$. It is the origin of the oxygen released during photosynthesis, hence the term oxygenic. Thus the overall flow of electrons in the noncyclic pathway is from the water molecule, through photosystem 2, along a series of cytochromes to photosystem 1 and thence to ferredoxin and finally $NADP^+$, which also collects a hydrogen atom to complete the reduction to NADPH. Both the cyclic and the noncyclic pathways produce a proton gradient which drives the synthesis of ATP, but only the cyclic route has the facility of producing NADPH. A combination of cyclic and noncyclic pathways are used by the organism to produce the required amounts of NADPH and ATP used in the dark reactions for the synthesis of carbohydrate. So far the description has been of photosynthesis in eukaryotes and cyanobacteria.

Photosystems in Purple and Green Bacteria

Looking at the general equation for the chemical reactions in photosynthesis shown in Fig. 5.11, it may be seen that water is the electron donor during oxygenic photosynthesis while several molecules may play the same role in anoxygenic systems. Suitable molecules are listed in the figure, from which several interesting observations may be made.

If the electron donor is hydrogen sulphide, which is the principal gas responsible for the foul smell, reminiscent of rotten eggs, typically found in wet and untilled soil, for example in the bottom of ponds, the product is sulphate or elemental sulphur. Examination of bacterial photosystems explains how this occurs.

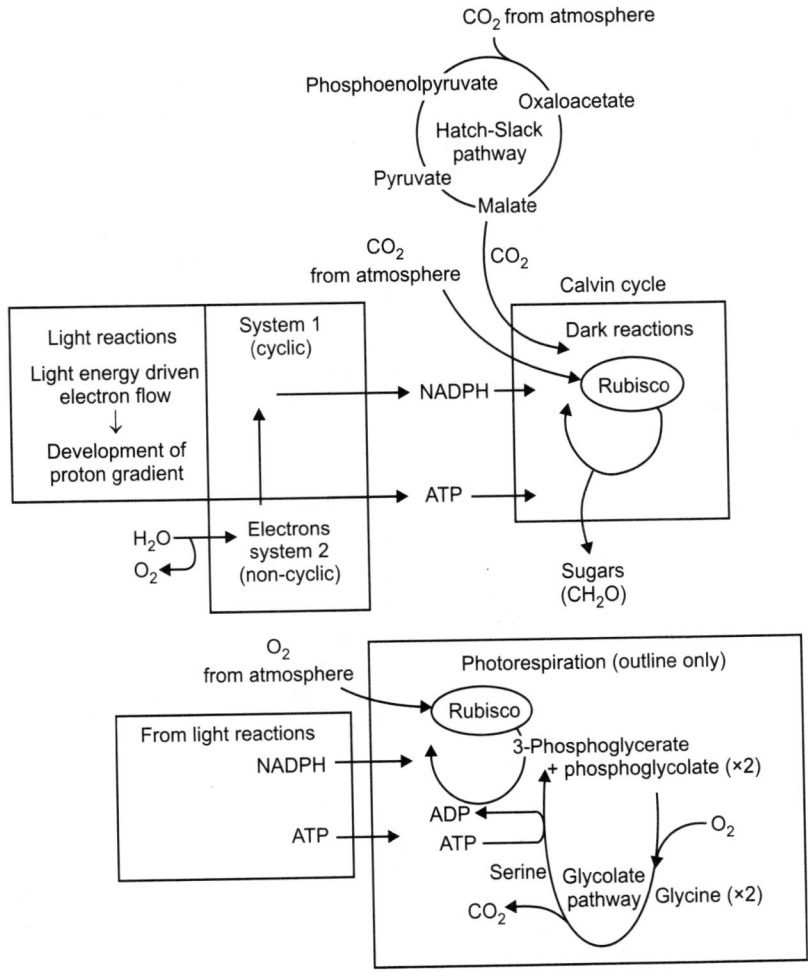

Fig. 5.10. Oxygenic photosynthesis, photorespiration and the Hatch-Slack pathway.

Green and purple bacteria possess only one photosystem which is a fairly basic equivalent to photosystem 1 of eukaryotes and cyanobacteria, but employing a different set of electron carriers. In purple nonsulphur bacteria, this is only capable of cyclic electron flow which produces a proton gradient and thus allows ATP photosynthesis, but this process does not lead to NADPH production. A similar system exists in green nonsulphur bacteria.

The lack of a photosystem equivalent to photosystem 2 in eukaryotes, requires these bacteria to provide a different route for the regeneration of NADH which serves much the same function as NADPH in carbohydrate synthesis.

Their solution to this problem is to use as electron donors, molecules which have a more negative reduction potential than water and so are easier to oxidise. These include hydrogen, hydrogen sulphide, elemental sulphur and a variety of organic compounds including sugars, and various organic acids such as amino acids, and succinate.

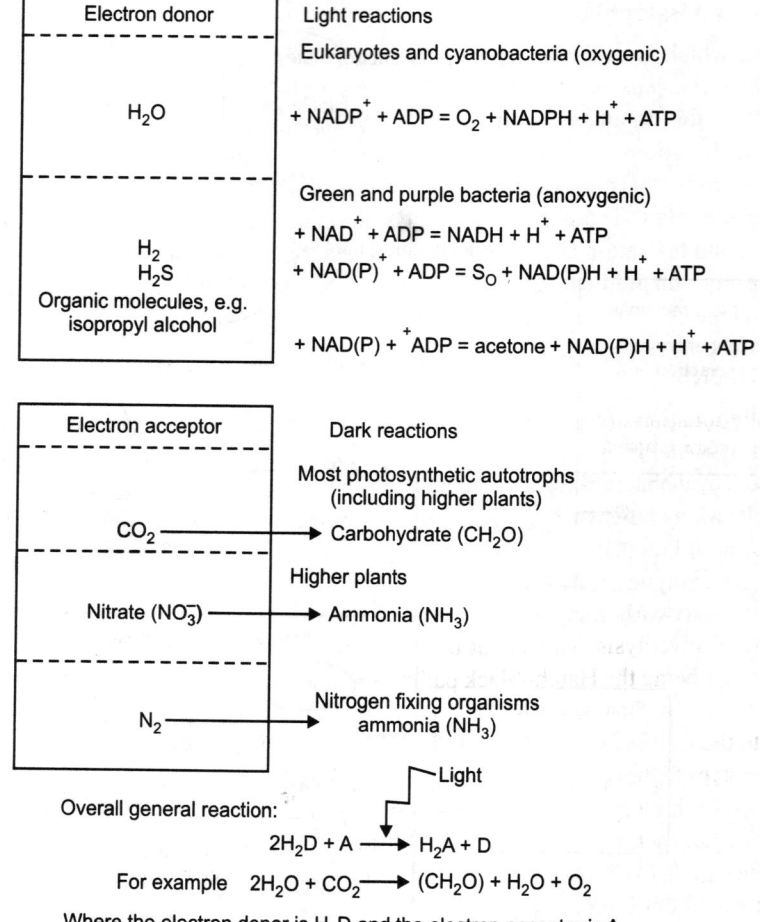

Fig. 5.11. Reactions of photosynthesis.

There are many ways in which green and purple nonsulphur bacteria may produce NADH. For example, direct reduction is possible if they are growing in the presence of dissolved hydrogen gas due to the fact that hydrogen has a more negative reduction potential than NAD^+. In addition, purple nonsulphur photosynthetic bacteria may use ATP or the proton gradient established during photosynthesis to reverse the electron flow such that the direction is from one of the electron donors noted above to NAD^+.

Green and purple sulphur bacteria are rather different in that in addition to having a cyclic system broadly similar to that of purple bacteria, they have an additional enzyme activity which allows the nonlinear transfer of electrons to ferredoxin linked to NAD^+ resulting in the production of NADH. One of the sources of electrons to replace those used in this reduction is the oxidation of hydrogen sulphide to sulphate or elemental sulphur, in a process comparable to the oxidation of water in oxygenic organisms. Other electron donors which may be used in this way are hydrogen and elemental sulphur. Both of these nonsulphur bacteria are strict anaerobes.

Photosystem in a Halophile

A photosystem which is different again from those described so far is that found in the halophile *Halobacterium salinarium* which has previously been classified as *Halobacteriun halobium*. Under normal conditions this organism obtains its energy by respiration, but in order to survive conditions of low oxygen concentrations, it can photosynthesise provided there is sufficient light. The pigment which has been developed for this purpose is bacteriorhodopsin, which is very similar to the rhodopsin pigment found in vertebrate eyes. The part of the molecule which absorbs light is retinal. When this occurs, changes in the bond formation of this chromophore result in expulsion of protons across the membrane thus producing a proton gradient. As described for other systems, this proton gradient may then be used to drive ATP synthesis.

DARK REACTIONS

The result of illumination of a photosynthetic organism is to stimulate electron transport which leads to the production of NADPH or NADH, and synthesis of ATP. Both are required for the next stage which in eukaryotes and cyanobacteria (blue-green algae) is the synthesis of sugar from carbon dioxide involving the Calvin cycle. Many biochemistry textbooks give excellent descriptions of this process and so only a summary is given in Fig. 5.10.

In brief, ribulose diphosphate is carboxylated with carbon dioxide catalysed by the enzyme rubisco to form an unstable six-carbon sugar which is then cleaved to form two molecules of 3-phosphoglycerate, an intermediate of glycolysis. This is not the only route of entry of carbon dioxide into carbohydrate synthesis, the other being the Hatch–Slack pathway. This subject is discussed in more detail later in this chapter.

Returning to the Calvin cycle, rearrangements of 3-phosphoglycerate produced by rubisco then take place by similar steps to the reversible steps of glycolysis and reactions of the pentose phosphate pathway. After completion of three cycles, the net result is the fixation of three molecules of carbon dioxide into a three-carbon sugar, each cycle regenerating a ribulose phosphate molecule. After phosphorylation of the trioses at the expense of ATP, they may enter into glycolysis and be converted into glucose and then to starch to be stored until required. The Calvin cycle is so familiar that it is easy to overlook the fact that not all reducing equivalents are channelled through rubisco to this cycle and carbohydrate synthesis.

Some organisms may use additional pathways involving other electron acceptors such as nitrate, nitrogen and hydrogen atoms, the reduction of which obviously does not produce carbohydrate but different essential nutrients which may then also be available to other organisms. These products are summarised in Fig. 5.11. For example, when nitrogen or nitrate is the electron donor, the product is ammonia which becomes incorporated by amino transfer into amino acids and thus forms part of the nitrogen cycle. Nitrogen is a particularly noteworthy case in the context of this chapter as it is the process of nitrogen fixation. This is performed by a number of nitrogen fixing bacteria some of which are free living in the soil and some form symbiotic relationships with certain leguminous plants, forming root nodules. Nitrogen fixation is, by necessity, an anaerobic process, and so one essential role for the plant is to provide a suitable oxygen-free environment for these bacteria, the other, to provide energy. It is relevant to point out here that the suggestion is often mooted of introducing the genes responsible for allowing nitrogen fixation to be transferred from the relevant bacteria into suitable plants. The symbiotic relationship between plant and bacteria is very difficult to create artificially and has been a stumbling block in the drive to increase the number of plant species able to host nitrogen fixation. The complicated interaction between plant and bacterium involves intricacies of plant physiology as well as genetic capability provided by the bacterium and so it is unlikely that a simple transfer of nitrogen fixation genes from bacterium to plant will be successful. This, however, remains a research area of major importance.

The issue of nitrogenous material, particularly in respect of sewage and associated effluents, is of considerable relevance to the environmental application of biotechnology. In addition, there is great potential for phytotechnological intervention to control nitrogen migration, most especially in the light of the burgeoning expansion of nitrate-sensitive areas within the context of agricultural fertiliser usage. Hence, bioengineering of the nitrogen cycle, at least at the local level, provides an important avenue for the control of pollution and the mitigation of possible eutrophication of aquatic environments. The cycle itself, and some of the implications arising, are discussed later in this chapter.

C_3 and C_4 Plants

Plants for which the reaction catalysed by rubisco is the first point of entry of atmospheric carbon dioxide into carbohydrate metabolism are termed C_3 plants due to the product of rubisco being two molecules of 3-phosphoglycerate which contains three carbons. This is the typical route for temperate organisms. An alternative to direct carboxylation for introducing carbon dioxide into the Calvin cycle used by some tropical plants, is the Hatch-Slack pathway illustrated in Fig. 5.10. In this case the first step of entry for atmospheric carbon dioxide is by carboxylation of phosphoenolpyruvate by phosphoenolpyruvate carboxylase to produce the four-carbon molecule, oxaloacetate. Hence, plants able to use this pathway are termed C_4 plants. The oxaloacetate is part of a cycle which carries the carbon dioxide into the bundle-sheath cells and so away from the surface of the plant, to where the oxygen concentration is lower. Here the carbon dioxide, now being carried as part of malate is transferred to rubisco thus releasing pyruvate which returns to the mesophyll cells at the surface of the plant where it is phosphorylated at the expense of ATP to phosphoenolpyruvate ready to receive the next incoming carbon dioxide molecule from the atmosphere.

The overall effect is to fix atmospheric carbon dioxide, transfer it to a site of lower oxygen concentration compared with the surface of the plant, concentrate it in the form of malate and then transfer the same molecule to rubisco where it enters the Calvin cycle. Although the Hatch-Slack pathway uses energy, and therefore may seem wasteful, it is of great benefit to plants growing in the warmer regions of the globe The reason for this is that the enzyme involved in carbon dioxide fixation in C_4 plants namely phosphoenolpyruvate carboxylase has a very high affinity for carbon dioxide and does not use oxygen as a substrate, contrasting with rubisco. The result of this competition between oxygen and carbon dioxide for binding to rubisco is the futile process of photorespiration, described in the next section. The affinity of carbon dioxide for rubisco falls off with increasing temperature and so in a tropical environment the efficiency of rubisco to fix carbon dioxide is low. In this situation, the disadvantage in using energy to operate the Hatch–Slack pathway is more than compensated for by the advantage of being able to fix carbon dioxide efficiently at elevated temperatures. So advantageous is this that much research is being directed to transferring the capability to operate the Hatch–Slack pathway into selected C_3 plants.

In the broadest sense of environmental biotechnology, the potential maximisation of solar energy usage, either as a means to the remediation of contamination or to reduce potential pollution by, for example, excessive fertiliser demand, could be of considerable advantage. Hence, appropriately engineered C_3 plants in either role offer major advantages in solar efficiency, which, in temperate climes, could provide significant environmental benefits.

Photorespiration

Returning to synthesis of carbohydrate by the Calvin cycle, as mentioned above, the first step is the carboxylation of the five-carbon sugar, ribulose diphosphate catalysed by rubisco. As mentioned in the preceding section, this enzyme may also function as an oxidase indicated by its full name ribulose diphosphate carboxylase oxidase. When this occurs and oxygen replaces carbon dioxide, the ensuing reaction produces phosphoglycolate in addition to 3-phosphoglycerate. Since, as a result of illumination, oxygen is consumed and carbon dioxide is released during the reactions of the glycolate pathway, this process is termed photorespiration and occurs alongside photosynthesis.

The higher the ambient temperature in which the organism is growing, and the higher the oxygen concentration relative to carbon dioxide, the more pronounced the oxidase activity becomes and consequently the less efficient rubisco is at introducing carbon dioxide into carbohydrate synthesis. The phosphoglycolate formed as a result of oxygen acting as substrate for rubisco, is then dephosphorylated to form glycolic acid. There follows a series of reactions forming a salvage pathway for the carbons of glycolic acid involving transfer of the carbon skeleton to the peroxisomes, then to the mitochondria, back to the peroxisomes and finally back to the chloroplast in the form of glycerate which is then phosphorylated at the expense of ATP to re-enter the Calvin cycle as 3-phosphoglycerate. The result of this detour, thanks to the oxidase activity of rubisco is to lose a high energy bond in phosphoglycolate, to consume ATP during phosphorylation to produce 3-phosphoglycerate, consumption of oxygen and release of carbon dioxide. This pathway resulting from the oxidase activity of rubisco, shown in Fig. 5.10 is wasteful because it consumes energy obtained by the light reactions with no concomitant fixation of carbon dioxide into carbohydrate.

The C_3 plants are therefore operating photosynthesis under suboptimal conditions especially when the oxygen tension is high and carbon dioxide tension is low. Why rubisco has not evolved to lose the oxidase activity is unclear: presumably evolutionary pressures of competition have been insufficient to date. For the reasons indicated in the preceding section, C_4 plants show little or no photorespiration due to their ability to channel carbon dioxide to rubisco by a method independent of oxygen tension. Therefore they are considerably more efficient than their C_3 counterparts and may operate photosynthesis at much lower concentrations of carbon dioxide and higher concentrations of oxygen. It is interesting to contemplate the competitive effects of introducing C_4 style efficiency into C_3 plants, but at the moment this is just speculation.

Balancing the Light and the Dark Reactions in Eukaryotes and Cyanobacteria

Using the six-carbon sugar, glucose, as an example, synthesis of one molecule requires six carbon dioxide molecules, 12 molecules of water, 12 protons, 18 molecules of ATP and 12 molecules of NADPH. Since photophosphorylation is driven by a proton gradient established during electron flow after illumination, there is not a stoichiometric relationship between the number of photons exciting the systems and the amount of ATP produced.

However, it is now established that for every eight photons incident on the two photosystems, four for each system, one molecule of oxygen is released, two molecules of $NADP^+$ are reduced to NADPH and approximately three molecules of ATP are synthesised.

Since this may leave the dark reactions slightly short of ATP for carbohydrate synthesis, it is postulated that photosystem 2 passes through one extra cycle thus producing additional ATP molecules with no additional NADPH.

NITROGEN CYCLE

Nitrogen is constantly taken, or fixed, from the atmosphere, oxidised to a form able to be utilised by plants and some bacteria, to be subsumed into metabolic pathways, and through the various routes described above is then excreted into the environment as reduced nitrogen where it may be reoxidised by bacteria or released back into the atmosphere as nitrogen gas. These combined processes are known collectively as the nitrogen cycle. The previous discussions have referred to the release of nitrogen during degradation of proteins and nucleic acid bases, either in the form of ammonia, the ammonium ion, urea or uric acid. The fate of all these nitrogen species is to be oxidised to nitrite ion by *Nitrosomas*, a family of nitrifying bacteria. The nitrite ion may be reduced and released as atmospheric nitrogen, or further oxidised to nitrate by a different group of nitrifying bacteria, *Nitrobacter*. The process of conversion from ammonia to nitrate is sometimes found as a tertiary treatment in sewage works to enable the nitrate consent to be reached. The process typically occurs in trickling bed filters which have, over time, become populated with a *Nitrosomas* and *Nitrobacter* along with the usual flora and fauna which balance this ecosystem. Denitrification may then occur to release atmospheric nitrogen or the nitrate ion, released by *Nitrobacter*, may be taken up by plants or some species of anaerobic bacteria where it is reduced to ammonium ion and incorporated into amino acids and other nitrogen–carbon containing compounds. To complete the cycle, atmospheric nitrogen is then fixed by nitrifying bacteria, either free living in the soil or in close harmony with plants as described earlier in this chapter.

SECTION II

Environmental Biotechnology in Waste-water Treatment

Chapter 6

Biological Treatment Fundamentals

INTRODUCTION

Biological degradation of waste is a natural process that has occurred since the beginning of time. Controlled and uncontrolled biological systems are the major systems used to treat organic wastes. An understanding of the factors affecting the biological processes occurring in these systems is essential to the design and operation of treatment facilities for agricultural wastes. The systems may treat liquid or solid wastes, may be aerobic, anaerobic, or facultative, and may be within controlled structures or unconfined on the land. Examples of biological treatment processes include oxidation ponds, aerated lagoons, oxidation ditches, anaerobic lagoons, anaerobic digesters, composting, and land disposal.

Because the processes are biological, an understanding of the processes must be based upon the fundamentals of microbiology and on the transformations in biological waste treatment units. If this understanding can be achieved, rational predictions of performance become possible and the capabilities of a process can be better utilised. Without an understanding of the fundamentals, the processes can be treated only as 'black boxes' in which the performance is subject to parameters seemingly beyond our control. Lack of proper understanding means that successful design and operation of biological processes must be based only on prior performance which may be difficult to translate to different wastes and environmental conditions.

BIOCHEMICAL REACTIONS

In the biological systems, micro-organisms utilise the wastes to synthesise new cellular material and to furnish energy for synthesis. The organisms also can use previously accumulated internal or endogenous food supplies for their respiration and do so especially in the absence of external or exogenous food sources. Synthesis and endogenous respiration occur simultaneously in biological systems with synthesis predominating when there is an excess of exogenous food and endogenous respiration dominating when the exogenous food supply is small or nonexistent.

Regardless of the biological system utilised, the principles of energy, synthesis, and endogenous cellular respiration are basic. The rates at which these reactions occur are a function of the environmental conditions imposed by and/or on a given biological treatment process.

The general reactions that occur can be illustrated in Eq. 6.1.

Energy containing metabolisable wastes + micro-organisms $\longrightarrow$

$$\text{end products} + \text{more micro-organisms} \qquad \ldots (6.1)$$

Equation 6.1 represents energy-synthesis reactions in which the wastes are metabolised for energy and for the synthesis of new cells. The energy utilised in Eq. 6.1 is obtained during the metabolism of the wastes. Synthesis or growth is affected by the ability of the micro-organisms to metabolise and assimilate the food, the presence of toxic materials, the temperature and pH of the system, and the presence of adequate accessory nutrients and trace elements.

The wastes must contain sufficient carbon, nitrogen, phosphorus, and trace minerals to satisfy nutritional requirements. In a biological system, the indispensable nutrient that is present in the smallest quantity needed for microbial growth will become the limiting factor. With most organic wastes, adequate nutrients are available and the biological reactions proceed at a rate constrained only by environmental factors such as temperature, pH, and inhibitory compounds.

When growth becomes limited, the micro-organisms die and lyse releasing the nutrients of their protoplasm for utilisation by still living cells in an autoxidative or endogenous cellular respiration process:

$$\text{Micro-organisms} \longrightarrow \text{end products} + \text{fewer micro-organisms} \qquad \ldots (6.2)$$

Endogenous respiration proceeds in the presence as well as in the absence of an external food source. The rate of cellular oxidation and endogenous respiration is related to the mean time the cells have undergone treatment, i.e. solids retention time. In the presence of waste material (food), microbial metabolism will occur to produce new cells and energy and the microbial solids will increase. In the absence of food, endogenous respiration will predominate and a reduction of the net microbial solids will occur. The microbial mass will not be reduced to zero even with a long endogenous respiration period, however. A residue of about 20 to 25 per cent of synthesised microbial mass will remain. Even in a long term biological treatment system there will be a minimum rate of solids accumulation. Any inert solids in the raw waste will increase the rate of solids build-up in the unit. Eventually these solids must be removed from the units. When the organic matter is metabolised and converted into microbial cells, the waste is only partially stabilised. As indicated in Eq. 6.2, the microbial cells are capable of further degradation. Only when the microbial cells are oxidised or removed does a stabilised effluent result. It is possible to design and operate a biological treatment unit to function in any portion of a synthesis-endogenous respiration relationship. The specific design will depend on the characteristics of the desired effluent. If the treated wastes are to be discharged to surface waters, a high quality effluent will be required. This can be attained by operating well into the endogenous region and removing residual solids from the effluent before it is discharged. If the land is the ultimate disposal point, a high quality effluent may not be necessary. In this case the treatment unit can be operated without separation of the solids since further degradation will take place on the soil.

Basic Biological Processes

Biological processes can be defined by the presence or absence of dissolved oxygen, i.e. aerobic or anaerobic, by their photosynthetic ability; or by the mobility of the organisms, i.e. suspended or adherent growth. Common examples of processes that are utilised for waste treatment are shown in Table 6.1. Since the terms are not mutually exclusive, some processes can be defined in more than one manner.

Table 6.1. Common biological treatment processes.

Aerobic	Anaerobic
Activated sludge units	Anaerobic lagoons
Trickling filters	Digesters

(Contd ...)

Oxidation ponds	Anaerobic filters
Aerated lagoons	
Oxidation ditch	Photosynthetic
	Oxidation ponds
Suspended growth	
Activated sludge	Adherent growth
Aerated lagoons	Trickling filters
Mixed digesters	Rotating biological contractors
Oxidation ditch	Anaerobic filters
	Denitrification columns

Aerobic

As used with biological waste treatment processes, the term refers to processes in which dissolved oxygen is present. The oxidation of organic matter using molecular oxygen as the ultimate electron acceptor is the primary process yielding useful chemical energy to micro-organisms in these processes. Microbes that use oxygen as the ultimate electron acceptor are aerobic micro-organisms.

Anaerobic

Some micro-organisms are able to function without dissolved oxygen in the system. Such micro-organisms can be called anaerobic organisms or anaerobes. Certain anaerobes cannot exist in the presence of dissolved oxygen and are obligate anaerobes. Examples of these are the methane bacteria commonly found in anaerobic digesters, anaerobic lagoons, and swamps. Anaerobes obtain their energy from the oxidation of complex organic matter but utilise compounds other than dissolved oxygen as oxidising agents. Oxidising agents are defined broadly as electron acceptors.

Oxygen is not necessary to have an oxidation reaction. Oxidising agents other than oxygen that can be used by micro-organisms include carbon dioxide, partially oxidised organic compounds, sulphate, and nitrate. The process by which organic matter is degraded in the absence of oxygen frequently is called fermentation.

Facultative

Only a few species of organisms are obligate anaerobes or aerobes. A large number of organisms can live either in the absence or presence of oxygen. Organisms that function under either anaerobic or aerobic conditions are facultative organisms. When oxygen is absent from their environment, they are able to obtain energy from degradation of organic matter by nonaerobic mechanisms but, if dissolved oxygen is present, they metabolise the organic matter more completely. Organisms can obtain more energy by aerobic oxidation than by anaerobic oxidation.

Biological waste treatment units may be designed to be either aerobic or anaerobic. There are occasions when anaerobic conditions occur in units that are designed to be aerobic. Examples of these conditions are organic matter that has settled to the bottom of oxidation ponds and streams, i.e. benthic deposits, when aerobic systems are overloaded because of an increase in the strength of the raw waste, and in the interior of activated sludge floc particles and trickling filter growths. The majority of the organisms in biological waste treatment processes are facultative organisms.

Photosynthetic

Photosynthesis is the utilisation of solar energy by the chlorophyll of green plants for the incorporation of carbon dioxide and other inorganic constituents in the production of cellular material. In this process molecular oxygen is formed. The photosynthetic organisms of interest in biological treatment systems are algae and rooted or floating plants. Examples of such biological treatment systems include oxidation ponds, streams, reservoirs, lakes, and high rate algal production systems to recover the nutrients in wastes.

Suspended growth

This term refers to mixtures of micro-organisms and the organic wastes. The micro-organisms are able to aggregate into flocculant masses and are able to move with the liquid flow. Agitation of the liquid keeps microbial solids in suspension. Suspended growth processes may be either aerobic or anaerobic. Anaerobic suspended growth units can be agitated by mechanical mixing and gas diffusion. Activated sludge units, aerated lagoons, oxidation ditches, and well-mixed anaerobic digesters are suspended growth processes.

Adherent growth

Microbial growth is adherent when the micro-organisms grow on a solid support medium and the wastes flow over or come in contact with the organisms. The support media can be large stones, rocks, slag, corrugated plastic sheets, or rotating disks. Commonly the organic wastes flow over or through the openings of the supporting media. Although the vast majority of adherent growth systems currently used for waste treatment are aerobic, a few are anaerobic. Examples of adherent growth units are trickling filters, rotating biological disks, and anaerobic filters.

ENERGY RELATIONSHIPS

Knowledge of the energy relationships of microbial cells permits an understanding of energy available for synthesis and respiration, of production of microbial cells in biological waste treatment units, and of the nature of the expected end products under certain conditions. All cells, whether animal, plant, or microbial, use similar fundamental mechanisms for their energy transforming activities. These activities involve transferring chemical energy from food to the processes which utilise energy for the functions and survival of living cells. In both aerobic and anaerobic cells, the energy of the food material is conserved chemically in the compound adenosine triphosphate (ATP). ATP is the carrier of chemical energy from the oxidation of foods, either aerobic or anaerobic, to those processes of the cells which do not occur spontaneously and can proceed only if chemical energy is supplied. These processes are involved in the performance of osmotic, mechanical, or chemical work. The food for the cells would be organic wastes of agriculture.

During the oxidation in the cells, ATP is formed from adenosine diphosphate (ADP). ATP is the high energy form of the energy transporting system and ADP is the lower energy form. A portion of the energy of the oxidation thus is conserved as the energy of the ATP. This process operates in a continuous dynamic cycle, receiving energy during the oxidation of foods and releasing energy during the performance of cellular work. A molecule of inorganic phosphate (P_i) is released when ADP is formed and incorporated in ATP when the ATP is formed. The principle of the cellular energy cycle is shown in Fig. 6.1. Although ATP is not the only energy carrying compound in every cellular reaction, it is the common intermediate in the energy transformation in the cells.

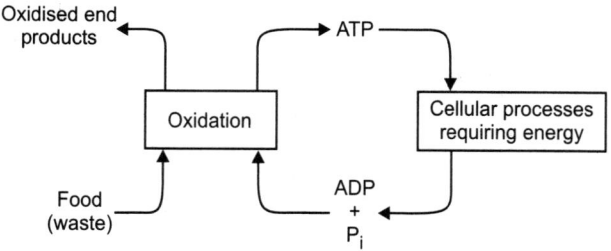

Fig. 6.1. Schematic pattern of energy transfer in the ATP-ADP system.

The purpose of biological waste treatment is to stabilise or oxidise the organic wastes of man, industry, and agriculture. Oxidation is the process in which a molecule or compound loses electrons. Reduction is the process in which a molecule or compound gains electrons. Examples of these processes are noted below. In the first case ferrous iron is oxidised to ferric iron with the release of an electron. In the second case carbon dioxide is reduced to methane. The carbon gains electrons and is reduced.

$$Fe^{2+} \xrightarrow{\text{Oxidation}} Fe^{3+} + e^-$$
$$\text{(Ferrous)} \qquad\qquad \text{(Ferric)}$$

$$CO_2 \xrightarrow{\text{Reduction}} CH_4$$
$$(C^{4+}) \qquad\qquad (C^{4-})$$

The general oxidation-reduction relationship can be indicated by:

$$AH + B \longrightarrow A + BH \qquad\qquad\qquad ... (6.3)$$

where, B is the electron (hydrogen) acceptor and is being reduced and A is the compound being oxidised. Although all the reactions involve oxidation, they sometimes are referred to in terms of the type of hydrogen acceptor. Transformations in which oxygen is the hydrogen acceptor are called oxidation; when nitrate is the hydrogen acceptor, denitrification; when sulphate is the hydrogen acceptor, sulphate reduction; and with carbon dioxide as the hydrogen acceptor, the transformation is methane fermentation. Oxidation and reduction reactions do not occur independently but as coupled reactions. When a compound is oxidised, another compound must be reduced.

The reducing agent is an electron donor and an oxidising agent is an electron acceptor. Each electron donor has a characteristic electron pressure and each electron acceptor has a characteristic electron affinity. Electron donors may be arranged in a series of decreasing electron pressures. The tendency will be for electrons to flow from compounds having the highest electron pressure to compounds lower in the series. A schematic diagram of the electron flow in the aerobic oxidation of an organic compound illustrates the oxidation-reduction sequence (Fig. 6.2). In each step, two electrons are passed along. The electrons flow from compounds having the highest electron pressure with the oxidised forms of the electron carriers serving as electron acceptors. The electron carriers noted in Fig. 6.3 are NAD, nicotinamide adenine dinucleotide; FAD, flavin adenine dinucleotide; CYT b, c, a, cytochromes; CYT a_3, cytochrome oxidase. The cytochromes are iron-containing enzymes. The iron is reduced and oxidised as the oxidation-reduction reactions occur. The respiratory sequence involving the cytochromes is the final common metabolic pathway by which all electrons derived from the oxidation of different organics flow to oxygen, the final oxidant, or acceptor of electrons in aerobic cells.

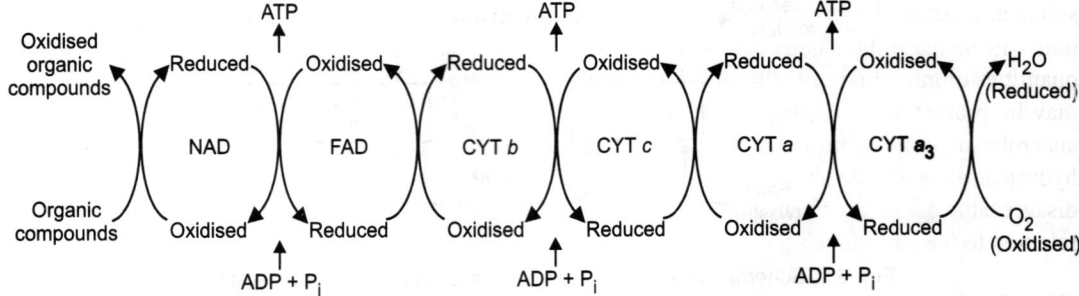

Fig. 6.2. Schematic diagram of the oxidation of organic compounds.

In anaerobic cells, the cytochrome pathway does not exist. The energy conserving steps of the cytochrome system are not available to organisms that do not use oxygen as the terminal electron or hydrogen acceptor. An example of the difference in relative energy conversions by aerobic and by anaerobic cells can be illustrated by the metabolism of glucose (Fig. 6.3). Anaerobic cells obtain energy from the conversion of glucose to lactate which then leaves the cell as a metabolic waste. The energy available to anaerobic cells from this conversion is only about 7 per cent of the amount that would be available if glucose were oxidised aerobically. Aerobic organisms can conserve for themselves a greater portion of the available energy from the metabolism of organic matter than can anaerobic organisms. Thus, anaerobic organisms must process a greater quantity of food to obtain the same amount of energy.

This information is useful in predicting the products and the efficiency of aerobic and anaerobic biological treatment processes. The synthesis of organisms per molecule of ATP should be the same for most bacteria since once the substrate energy is converted to ATP or biological energy, the growth of organisms follows generally similar biochemical pathways. Both aerobic and anaerobic bacteria have essentially the same composition and both contain ATP. The concept of ATP as an energy resource permits the formulation of a general relationship between substrate and growth. Because the energy recovery per unit of food is so small for anaerobic organisms, it follows that the amount of microbial cells synthesised per unit of food metabolised will be significantly less than for aerobic organisms.

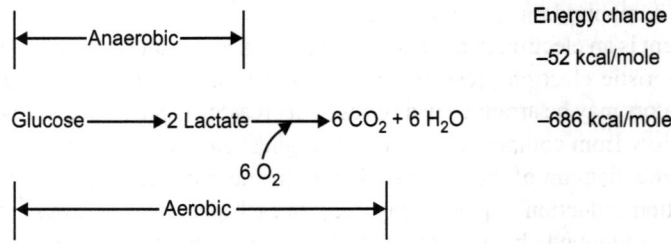

Fig. 6.3. Aerobic and anaerobic metabolism of glucose.

Figure 6.3 shows the end products of aerobic metabolism in the most oxidised state, carbon dioxide and water. The end products of anaerobic metabolism are in a partially oxidised state and, if oxygen were available, would have an oxygen demand.

For a given organic loading, aerobic conditions will produce a more oxidised end product or effluent than will anaerobic conditions and will permit synthesis of a greater quantity of microbial cells. These additional cells are an asset because it is, thus, possible to have a larger amount of active microbial solids to increase the removal of organic wastes. The greater synthesised microbial cells in an aerobic unit will increase the sludge disposal problem, however. Anaerobic conditions will produce smaller quantities of microbial cells for ultimate disposal but because of the decreased rates of synthesis, there may be problems in maintaining adequate microbial solids in anaerobic units. The end products of anaerobic units are in the partially oxidised state. Some of the end products, i.e. methane, carbon dioxide, hydrogen, and nitrogen gases, can be exhausted to the atmosphere without problems. Others can produce disagreeable odours, i.e. mercaptans, amines, or volatile acids, and will exert an oxygen demand when released to the environment.

MICRO-ORGANISMS

Biological waste treatment processes contain a mixture of micro-organisms capable of metabolising organic wastes. Within limits, they can adjust to varying organic loads and environmental influences, such as temperature and pH, that may be imposed. Extreme temperature, high concentrations of metal ions, or toxic chemicals can decrease or eliminate the activity of the micro-organisms. The micro-organisms in various biological treatment systems include bacteria, fungi, algae, protozoa, rotifers, crustacea, bacteriophage, worms, and insect larvae depending upon environmental conditions.

Bacteria

Bacteria are the most important group of micro-organisms in waste treatment systems. The diverse biochemical activities of bacteria, as a group, enable them to metabolise most organic compounds found in municipal, industrial, or agricultural wastes. Aerobes and facultative bacteria are active in all aerobic treatment units. Facultative and obligate anaerobic bacteria are active in anaerobic treatment units. Bacteria are single cell micro-organisms that metabolise soluble food. Insoluble foods are converted into soluble food by microbial enzymes. The bacteria exist in a variety of forms, usually some modification of a cylinder or ovoid, with dimensions on the order of a few micrometers. They exist in waste treatment processes in agglomerations of varying arrangements and species.

A microbe is a complex organised system. A representative formula for bacterial cells is $C_5H_7O_2N$ or $C_{75}H_{105}O_{30}N_{15}P$. The composition of bacteria is not constant and varies according to the stage of growth and the particular substrate utilised. Storage of reserve materials can occur during the growth phase and will alter the representative composition of bacterial protoplasm. This empirical formula expresses only the average proportions of the principal constituents in a bacterial cell. The cell contains many other elements in small amounts.

Bacteria can be divided into groups depending upon their source of carbon used for synthesis of protoplasm. Organisms that use organic carbon as their carbon source are heterotrophic organisms while organisms that utilise carbon dioxide for cellular carbon are autotrophic organisms. Heterotrophs are the most numerous and important group of organisms in the common biological waste treatment processes.

The microbial species having the fastest growth rate and the ability to utilise most of the available organic matter will be the predominant species. Shifts in microbial predominance occur in waste treatment systems as environmental conditions such as temperature, pH, available dissolved oxygen, ultimate hydrogen acceptor, or available food vary in the system.

A useful characteristic of some bacteria is their ability to flocculate. Such flocculation permits the removal of microbial solids in a subsequent solids separation unit and assists in the production of a good quality effluent.

Fungi

Fungi are non-photosynthetic, multicellular, aerobic, branching, filamentous micro-organisms that metabolise soluble food. Both bacteria and fungi can metabolise the same kinds of organic material. The environmental conditions will determine which group of organisms will predominate. Fungi will predominate at low pH levels, low moisture content, in low nitrogen wastes, and when certain nutrients are missing. The composition of fungal cells can be represented empirically by $C_{10}H_{17}O_6N$.

Fungi are not active in anaerobic systems. Since fungal cells contain less nitrogen than bacterial cells, fungi may compete more favourably in wastes having a lower nitrogen content than required for bacterial synthesis. Many fungi grow well at pH levels of 4 to 5, levels at which it is difficult for bacteria to compete.

The filamentous nature of the fungi make them less desirable in biological waste treatment units because they do not settle well.

Under the normal environmental conditions that exist in most waste treatment processes, the fungi will not predominate. Fungi will be of secondary importance in common, properly operating aerobic biological treatment units.

Algae

Algae are photosynthetic autotrophs. The composition of algal cells can be represented by $C_{106}H_{180}O_{45}N_{16}P$. Since the nutritive requirements of algal species are different, this formula is an empirical average. Algae obtain their energy from sunlight and utilise inorganic materials such as carbon dioxide, ammonia or nitrate, and phosphate in the synthesis of additional cells. In photosynthesis molecular oxygen is formed. It is released to the environment and utilised by bacteria as the bacteria metabolise available organic matter. The design and management of oxidation ponds attempts to balance and exploit both groups of organisms.

Algae obtain carbon dioxide from the following sources in water or waste-water: (i) absorption from the atmosphere, (ii) respiration of aerobic and anaerobic heterotrophic organisms, and (iii) bicarbonate alkalinity. As the carbon dioxide is removed from a waste-water by growing algae, the pH will increase. pH values as high as 10 are not uncommon in active algal systems such as oxidation ponds and similar units. Although algal growth can be controlled by carbon limitation, carbon from alkalinity and bacterial carbon dioxide production provides an ample amount of carbon for algal growth. Carbon in natural systems rarely limits algal growth.

Algae are of consequence only where sufficient sunlight can penetrate the liquid. Algae will not predominate where there is high turbidity as in activated sludge units and aerated lagoons, where sunlight is excluded, or where the liquid is dark in colour.

In the absence of sunlight, photosynthesis ceases and the endogenous respiration of the algae continues in the same manner as it does with bacteria. The algae, thus, present an additional oxygen demand on the unit in which they exist.

After 0.5–1 year of aerobic decomposition, an average of 50 per cent of the initial nitrogen and phosphorus remained in the undecomposed algal fraction while the other 50 per cent was regenerated. Under anaerobic conditions 40 per cent of the nitrogen and 60 per cent of the phosphorus were regenerated. Nutrients from dead algal cells are released to surface waters for a long period of time. To accomplish a high degree of organic carbon, nitrogen, and phosphate removal in biological treatment units utilising algae, the algal cells must be removed from the unit effluent before discharge.

Protozoa

Protozoa are single-celled organisms that can metabolise both soluble and insoluble foods. The protozoa found in aerobic treatment systems include flagellates, free-swimming ciliates, and stalked ciliates which are attached to solid particles by stems. Protozoa reduce the concentration of bacteria and non-metabolised particulate organic matter in a treatment system and assist in producing a higher quality and clearer effluent. Activated sludge units free of protozoa produced effluents of high turbidity. The turbidity was caused by the presence of large numbers of dispersed bacteria. As a result, effluent BOD and nonsettleable solids were high. The addition of ciliated protozoa to these units increased effluent quality and decreased bacterial numbers. The succession of protozoa types in aerobic systems can be related to the degree of treatment in the system.

Protozoa generally have more complex nutritional requirements than do bacteria or fungi. Because of their utilisation of particulate organic matter and their need for dissolved oxygen, protozoa will exist in well-stabilised systems in which the soluble food has been converted to microbial cells and in which the oxygen supply exceeds the oxygen demand. Since they are sensitive to dissolved oxygen changes, they can serve as indicators of the status of aerobic biological waste treatment.

Protozoa have been observed in anaerobic treatment of sewage solids and in systems treating animal wastes, especially ruminant wastes. The role of protozoa in these systems is unknown, but it is postulated as the same as in aerobic systems, i.e. metabolism of particulate material and bacteria, and clarification of the resultant effluent.

Rotifers

Multicellular organisms that can metabolise solid food, such as rotifers, are found in highly stabilised systems having dissolved oxygen at all times. Rotifers metabolise solid particles some of which the protozoa cannot use and also assist in producing a nonturbid effluent.

Crustacea

Crustacea are multicellular organisms with hard shells. They grow in well-stabilised systems using smaller organisms as their major source of food. In doing so, they assist in producing a clarified effluent and are indicative of a high quality effluent from aerobic treatment systems.

Thus, the predominance of the various forms of micro-organisms in biological systems may at times be indicative of the performance and environmental conditions in the systems. Microscopic examination of the biological system can be utilised as a tentative guide to the quality of the effluent, the degree of treatment that has been accomplished, and changes occurring in the systems. Knowledge of the environmental factors affecting the typical micro-organisms can be useful in understanding and operating biological waste treatment units. Many biological treatment units will have their individual peculiarities and with experience the observer can learn to relate the microscopic pattern in a unit with trends in effluent quality and process performance.

BIOCHEMICAL TRANSFORMATIONS

A number of changes take place in biological units. Some of the transformations affect the constituents of the wastes undergoing treatment, thus, affecting the quality of the unit effluent. Others affect the properties and the quantity of microbial solids. Many of the important transformations in biological waste treatment systems are discussed in this chapter. These are by no means the only ones but they are fundamental transformations in a variety of treatment systems.

Carbon

The oxidation of organic carbon-containing compounds represents the mechanism by which heterotrophic organisms obtain the energy for synthesis. The process is called respiration. The general relationships were noted in Eq. 6.1. In aerobic treatment systems organic carbon is transformed, via many steps, to synthesised microbial protoplasm, $C_5H_7O_2N$, and carbon dioxide.

$$\text{Organic carbon} + O_2 \longrightarrow C_5H_7O_2N + CO_2 \qquad \qquad ... (6.4)$$

The uptake of oxygen and formation of carbon dioxide represent the effects of respiration.

In anaerobic systems, molecular oxygen cannot be the terminal electron acceptor and all of the respired carbon will not be transformed to carbon dioxide. Under anaerobic conditions, organic carbon is converted to microbial solids, carbon dioxide, methane, and other reduced compounds. Anaerobic metabolism leading to the formation of methane occurs in a series of steps. For simplicity these can be summarised as the conversion of complex organics to simpler compounds:

$$\text{Organic carbon} \longrightarrow \text{microbial cells} + \text{organic acids, aldehydes, alcohols, etc.} \qquad ... (6.5)$$

and the conversion of the simpler compounds to gaseous end products:

$$\text{Organic acids} + \text{oxidised organic carbon} \longrightarrow$$
$$\text{microbial cells} + \text{methane} + \text{carbon dioxide} \qquad ... (6.6)$$

Little stabilisation of organic matter occurs in the first step (Eq. 6.5). Stabilisation of the organic matter occurs in the second step (Eq. 6.6) in which the carbon compounds, carbon dioxide (CO_2) and methane (CH_4), are released to the atmosphere and removed from the substrate. The oxygen demand of the waste is, thus, reduced. At standard conditions, the production of 5.6 ft^3 of methane results in the stabilisation of 1 lb of ultimate oxygen demand.

Nitrogen

Nitrogen is an important nutrient in biological systems. Nitrogen is about 12 per cent of bacterial protoplasm and 5 to 6 per cent of fungal protoplasm. In waste matter, nitrogen will be present as organic and ammonia nitrogen, the proportion of each depending upon the degradation of organic matter that has occurred. In biological systems, organic nitrogen compounds can be transformed to ammonium nitrogen and oxidised to nitrite and nitrate nitrogen.

$$\text{Organic N} \longrightarrow \text{ammonium N} \longrightarrow \text{nitrite N} \longrightarrow \text{nitrate N} \qquad ... (6.7)$$

The oxidation of ammonia to nitrite and nitrate is termed nitrification and occurs under aerobic conditions. A more basic definition of nitrification is the biological conversion of inorganic or organic nitrogen compounds from reduced to a more oxidised state. In waste treatment the term usually is used to refer to the oxidation of ammonia. A residual dissolved oxygen concentration of about 2 mg/litre has been found necessary to have optimum nitrification. Autotrophic bacteria, such as *Nitrosomonas* which obtain energy from the oxidation of ammonia to nitrite and *Nitrobacter*, which obtain energy from the oxidation of nitrite to nitrate, are organisms that in combination can accomplish the complete oxidation of nitrogen.

Ammonia nitrogen is the main soluble nitrogen end product in anaerobic units. The release of ammonia nitrogen to aerobic treatment units or to receiving streams creates an added oxygen demand to these systems. The oxidation of 1 lb of ammonia nitrogen to nitrate nitrogen will require 4.57 lb oxygen. The oxygen demand of ammonia is significant and requires consideration when evaluating the effect of discharging wastes to the environment and when evaluating the design of adequate biological treatment processes. Denitrification is the process by which nitrate and nitrite nitrogen are reduced to nitrogen gas and gaseous nitrogen oxides under anoxic conditions. This process requires the availability of electron donors (reducing agents). The necessary donors can be organic material, such as methanol, addition of untreated wastes, unmetabolised organic matter, or the endogenous respiration of microbial cells.

Denitrification offers the opportunity to reduce the nitrogen content of waste effluents by having a fraction of the nitrogen exhausted to the atmosphere as an inert gas. Because of the role nitrogen plays in the eutrophication and oxygen demand of surface waters, control of nitrogen by denitrification in biological waste treatment systems will play a larger role in the future.

Phosphorus

The sources of phosphorus in waste-waters include organic matter, phosphates originating in cleaning compounds used for process clean-up, and the urine of man and animals. The organic phosphorus is transformed to inorganic phosphorus during biological treatment.

Condensed phosphates constitute a substantial portion of the phosphorus in municipal sewage. The form of phosphates in waste-waters is of interest since phosphate removal techniques generally are evaluated on their ability to remove orthophosphates. The hydrolysis of condensed phosphates to orthophosphate (Eq. 6.8) is affected by environmental conditions such as temperature and microbial concentration.

$$\text{Tripolyphosphate } (P_2O_{10}^{5-}) + H_2O \longrightarrow \text{orthophosphate } (PO_4^{3-}) + H^+ \qquad \text{... (6.8)}$$

The rate of hydrolysis of condensed phosphates in the following systems decreases in the order given: activated sludge, untreated waste-water, algal cultures, and natural waters.

Aerobic biological treatment will convert condensed phosphates to orthophosphates. Anaerobic treatment will result in other changes. A primary step in anaerobic treatment is the liquefaction of organic matter and inorganic phosphorus compounds will be released from organic compounds. The effluent from an anaerobic unit can contain a greater concentration of soluble phosphorus compounds than the influent.

The release of such effluents to other parts of a waste treatment facility or to the environment can complicate and/or negate phosphorus removal processes at the facility.

Sulphur

Microbial transformations of sulphur are similar to those of nitrogen. Both sulphide and ammonia are decomposition products of organic compounds. Both are oxidised by autotrophic bacteria, as are other incompletely oxidised inorganic sulphur and nitrogen compounds. Sulphate and nitrate are reduced by micro-organisms under anaerobic conditions.

Inorganic unoxidised sulphur compounds and elemental sulphur are oxidised by photosynthetic and chemosynthetic bacteria as well as by certain heterotrophic micro-organisms. Under anaerobic conditions, sulphide is the reduced end product and under aerobic conditions, sulphate is the oxidised end product.

All organisms contain sulphur and are involved in the transformations of sulphur to some degree. The assimilation of sulphur into cellular protoplasm is the primary reaction of heterotrophic organisms. With other organisms, sulphur transformations can provide the energy for metabolism and sulphur compounds can be hydrogen donors or acceptors. Because of these reactions, certain bacteria are designated as sulphur bacteria. These bacteria are autotrophic, can utilise sulphur or incompletely oxidised inorganic sulphur compounds as reducing agents, i.e. direct or indirect hydrogen donors, and can assimilate carbon dioxide as their sole source of carbon.

Food and Mass

The primary purpose of biological waste treatment is to oxidise the organic content of the waste, i.e. the food for the micro-organisms. The waste concentration decreases as the microbial mass increases. In aerobic systems, approximately 0.7 lb of cell mass is synthesised for every 1.0 lb of food, as BOD, that is oxidised. Following extensive endogenous respiration, or aerobic digestion of the cells, the 0.7 lb of cells will be reduced to about 0.17 lb of residual cellular material that remains for ultimate disposal. The actual residual cellular solids in a system will be somewhere between the latter two values depending upon how the aerobic system is operated, i.e. the degree of endogenous respiration that takes place. Changes similar to these also occur in anaerobic systems.

Engineers generally use the volatile suspended solids concentration of a biological treatment unit as an estimate of the concentration of active micro-organisms in the unit. While this parameter is an imperfect measure of the active mass, it has been a useful design and management parameter. Other parameters have been explored as better measures of both biomass and bioactivity in treatment units. These include dehydrogenase enzyme activity to measure overall rates of cellular oxidation reactions, specific enzymes involved in intermediary metabolism, and DNA concentration. ATP is a specific measure of microbial activity and can be used to estimate viable micro-organism concentrations in a biological treatment unit.

Oxygen

Oxygen plays a critical role in biological systems since when it serves as an ultimate hydrogen acceptor, the maximum energy is conserved for the micro-organisms. Minimum dissolved oxygen concentrations of from 0.2 to 0.6 mg/litre are necessary to maintain aerobic systems. The dissolved oxygen concentrations in aerobic treatment units should be kept above about 1.0 mg/litre if oxygen limitations are to be avoided.

pH

Biological activity can alter the pH of a treatment unit. Photosynthesis, denitrification, organic nitrogen breakdown, and sulphate reduction are examples of biological reactions that can cause an increase in pH. Sulphate oxidation, nitrification, and organic carbon oxidation are examples of biological reactions that can cause a decrease in pH. The relative changes in pH will be affected by the buffer capacity of the liquid and amount of substrate utilised by the micro-organisms.

NUTRIENT NEEDS

To achieve satisfactory biological treatment of wastes, the wastes must contain sufficient carbon, nitrogen, phosphorus, and trace minerals to sustain optimum rates of microbial synthesis. In most wastes, nutritional balance is not a problem since there usually is more than enough nitrogen, phosphorus, and trace minerals with respect to the carbon used in cell synthesis. These excess nutrients can be a cause of eutrophication in surface waters when the treated effluent is discharged. Methods to control or manage these excess nutrients are becoming required before discharge of the treated effluents.

Certain wastes, such as some food processing wastes, may have a deficiency of specific nutrients which need to be added in proper amounts to accomplish satisfactory biological waste treatment. Knowledge is required of the amount of nutrients that are needed both to assure that adequate nutrients are available and to avoid excess nutrients in the resultant effluent. Besides being uneconomical, added nutrients appearing in the effluent have the potential of causing environmental quality problems. Inadequate quantities of nutrients, such as nitrogen and phosphorus, tend to decrease the rate of microbial growth, decrease the rate of BOD removal, and impair the settling characteristics of the sludge.

The common approach of avoiding nitrogen or phosphorus limitations is to add nutrients to obtain a BOD:N:P ratio of 100:5:1. This ratio is satisfactory if one wishes to assure no nutrient deficiency but is of little use if the purpose is to have the nitrogen and phosphorus levels be low in the effluent. The above ratio was designed to assure adequate nutrients in high rate biological treatment. Studies with nutrient deficient wastes established that 3–4 lb N/100 lb BOD_5 removed and 0.5–0.7 lb P/100 lb BOD removed would avoid nutrient deficient conditions. This results in a BOD:N:P ratio of 100:3:0.6. Other studies with food processing wastes have noted that a BOD to nitrogen ratio of 100:2 or 100:1.5 was satisfactory in treating cannery wastes without a decrease in process efficiency.

The actual nutritional needs will be related to the manner in which the biological treatment process is operated. A high rate process will have a high rate of microbial synthesis and a higher nutrient requirement. However, for a stationary or declining growth biological treatment system, such as most treatment systems, a lower rate of microbial synthesis and nutrient requirement will prevail. With the long solids retention time, a matter of days in the common treatment systems, endogenous respiration of the microbial cells will release nutrients to the system. These nutrients will be used in the synthesis of new microbial cells. Approximately 0.11 lb of nitrogen will be released from the oxidation of 1 lb microbial cells. The required nutrients should be added in relation to the rate of cell synthesis. Practically, when wastes are nutrient deficient, the nutrients should be added to the system in proportion to the nutrients in the microbial solids that are lost in the effluent and/or wasted from the system.

Nutrients will not need to be added to animal wastes or meat and poultry processing wastes since nutrients are in excess of the amounts required for synthesis. Wastes having excess nutrients such as domestic sewage or animal processing wastes can be combined with nutritionally deficient carbonaceous wastes for mutual benefit.

OXYGEN DEMAND MEASUREMENTS

Biochemical Oxygen Demand

The BOD test is one of the most widely applied analytical methods in waste treatment and water pollution control. The test attempts to determine the pollutional strength of a waste in terms of microbial oxygen demand and is an indirect measure of the organic matter in the waste. It evolved as an estimate of the oxygen demand that a treated or untreated waste will have on the oxygen resources of a stream. The acceptable BOD test is described in Standard methods.

Experience with a number of organic wastes have indicated that the change in the oxygen demand of a waste (BOD) can be characterised by a first-order equation:

$$\frac{dC}{dt} = -kC \qquad \qquad ... (6.9)$$

where C is the waste concentration and k is a proportionality constant referred to as the BOD rate constant. Expressing the waste concentration in terms of the amount of oxygen required to biologically oxidise the waste, Eq. 6.9 can be written as:

$$Y = L\,(1 - e^{-kt}) \qquad \qquad ... (6.10)$$

in which, Y is the oxygen or BOD exerted in time t and L is the ultimate amount of oxygen to biologically oxidise the carbonaceous waste or the ultimate first-stage BOD (Fig. 6.4a). The BOD test is conducted as a batch aerobic experiment in BOD bottles. Other oxygen demand determinations can be conducted in manometric respirometers and similar large containers.

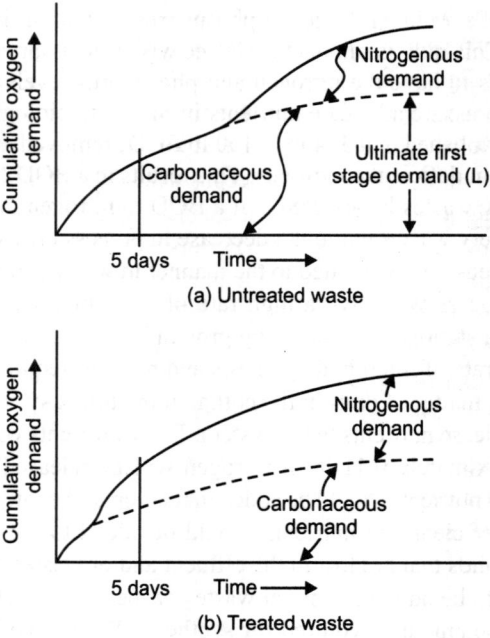

Fig. 6.4. Generalised oxygen demand patterns for heterogenous untreated and treated wastes.

Micro-organisms can oxidise both carbon-containing compounds (carbonaceous demand) and nitrogen compounds (nitrogenous demand). The nitrogen-oxidising bacteria are autotrophs, normally not in large concentrations in untreated waste-waters. These organisms can be present in well-oxidised waste-waters such as aerobically treated waste-water effluents from activated sludge and trickling filter plants, and in streams. If a low concentration of nitrifying organisms is present in a BOD bottle, a lag period can exist before the nitrifiers are present in large enough numbers to exhibit a noticeable nitrogenous demand. In waste-waters containing a number of organic compounds, such as agricultural waste-waters, a two-stage oxygen demand frequently can be observed if the oxygen demand is measured over a long enough period.

The BOD test is standardised at a 5-day period at 20°C using prescribed quality dilution water to permit comparison of results. The test does not provide an absolute measure of the oxygen-consuming organic matter in the waste. Unless otherwise noted, results reported as BOD indicate that the test has been conducted under standard conditions.

BOD values are affected by time and temperature of incubation, presence of adequate numbers of micro-organisms capable of metabolising the waste, and toxic compounds. In practice a constant temperature of 20°C does not occur and water is not in a state of rest for five days in the dark. The bacteria used In the test are the real link with practice.

The k value in Eqs 6.9 and 6.10 changes with temperature, increasing with increasing temperatures. Relationships are available to determine k at temperatures other than 20°C:

$$k_T = (k_{20}) \, \theta^{(T-20)} \qquad \qquad ... (6.11)$$

Experiments have shown that θ can vary from 1.016 to 1.077. Theta (θ) is commonly used as 1.047. The maximum or total oxygen demand is not affected by temperature since it is a function only of the quantity of organic matter available.

With heterogenous wastes, the five-day period frequently occurs before the beginning of significant nitrification. With adequately treated wastes, the carbonaceous demand is caused primarily by microbial cells and is low. In addition, a significant population of nitrifiers could be present. Under these conditions, the nitrogenous demand can occur early and before the five-day test period (Fig. 6.4b). Because of these conditions, a treated waste-water may exhibit both a carbonaceous and nitrogenous demand while an untreated waste-water may exhibit only a carbonaceous demand. When this occurs, evaluation of the BOD removal at a waste-water treatment facility will be in error since the oxygen demand of the influent and effluent samples does not measure the same materials.

The maximum oxygen demand (OD_m) will occur if all of the unoxidised organic and inorganic matter is oxidised completely. In most biological treatment units, this means that the organic carbon in a waste is oxidised to carbon dioxide and all of the organic and ammonia nitrogen is oxidised to nitrate. Mathematically, this can be expressed as:

$$OD_m = 2.67\ C + 4.57\ N \qquad \ldots (6.12)$$

where, C is the organic carbon concentration and N is the sum of the organic and ammonia nitrogen expressed as nitrogen. In practice not all of the organic carbon in a waste may be oxidised, not all of the organic nitrogen in the waste may be converted to ammonia, not all of the ammonia may be oxidised, and a portion of the synthesised microbial cells will not be completely oxidised. Thus, Eq. 6.12 will not determine the actual oxygen demand of a waste in a treatment system or a stream. It can, however, be used to estimate the maximum oxygen demand that could occur. The BOD rate constant, k, is a function of the oxidisability of the waste material. Wastes having a high soluble organic content, such as milk wastes, will exhibit a higher k than a waste having a high particulate organic content, such as a cellulosic waste.

Micro-organisms must first solubilise particulate organic material before it can be metabolised while they can metabolise soluble wastes more rapidly. The first-order equations expressed in Eqs. 6.9 and 6.10 represent a best estimate of the rate of oxygen demand and have been the subject of considerable discussion over the years. Because of the heterogeneous nature of most waste mixtures, the different waste constituents can have varying reaction rates. For a specific waste, the oxygen demand may be better described by a second-order equation or a composite exponential equation. Heavy reliance should not be placed on the monomolecular or first-order oxygen demand relationship since it is only an estimate of the complex reactions that are taking place in the biological reactor and frequently reflects only the carbonaceous demand. A nitrogenous demand and in some wastes an initial chemical oxygen demand also can occur. The small quantity of oxygen present in the BOD test bottle, 2–3 mg, means that high strength wastes, such as many food processing waste-waters and animal wastes, must be diluted prior to analysing the waste. Prior to BOD analysis, animal wastes may require dilutions of 1:100 to 1:000 or more. The difficulty of diluting wastes that are neither physically nor chemically uniform decreases the precision of the standard BOD test which is estimated to have a precision of ±20 per cent.

In spite of the problems associated with the BOD test, it remains an important analytical tool in water pollution control work since it is one of the few analyses that attempts to measure the effect of a waste under conditions approximating natural stream conditions.

Chemical Oxygen Demand

The lengthy analytical time of the BOD test as well as a desire to find a more precise measure of the oxygen demand of a waste led to the development of the COD test. The COD, chemical oxygen demand, test is a wet chemical combustion of the organic matter in a sample. An acid solution of potassium dichromate is used to oxidise the organic matter at high temperatures. Various COD procedures, having reaction times of from 5 minutes to 2 hours, can be used.

The use of two catalysts, silver sulphate and mercuric sulphate, are necessary to overcome a chloride interference and to assure oxidation of hard to oxidise organic compounds, respectively. Animal wastes and certain food processing wastes such as those from sauerkraut, pickle, and olive processing can contain high chloride concentrations and will require the use of the mercuric sulphate in COD analyses or a chloride correction factor. Compounds such as benzene and ammonia are not measured by the test. The COD procedure does not oxidise ammonia although it does oxidise nitrite.

BOD and COD analyses of a waste will result in different values because the two tests measure different material. COD values are always larger than BOD values. The differences between the values are due to many factors such as chemicals resistant to biochemical oxidation but not to chemical oxidation, such as lignin; chemicals that can be chemically oxidised and are susceptible to biochemical oxidation but not in the 5-day period of the BOD test such as cellulose, long chain fats, or microbial cells; and the presence of toxic material in a waste which will interfere with a BOD test but not with a COD test.

In spite of the inability of the COD method to measure the biological oxidisability of a waste, the COD method has value in practice. For a specific waste and at a specific waste treatment facility, it is possible to obtain reasonable correlation between COD and BOD values. The method is rapid, more precise (± 8 per cent), and in most circumstances provides useable estimates of the total oxygen demand of a waste.

Changes in both the BOD and COD values of a waste will occur during treatment. The biologically oxidisable material will decrease during treatment while the nonbiological but chemically oxidisable material will not. The nonbiologically oxidisable material will exist in the untreated wastes and will increase because of the residual cell mass resulting from endogenous respiration. The COD/BOD ratio will increase as the biologically oxidisable material becomes stabilised.

The COD/BOD ratio can be used to estimate the relative degradability or oxidisability of a waste. A low COD/BOD ratio would indicate a small nonbiodegradable fraction. A waste with a high COD/BOD ratio such as animal wastes have a large nonbiodegradable fraction that will remain for ultimate disposal after treatment. Wastes that have been treated, such as waste activated sludge or waste mixed liquor from oxidation ditches, have a high COD/BOD ratio indicating that most of the organic matter has been metabolised and that further treatment might not be economically rewarding.

As with BOD rates, COD data must be used with caution and judgment. Both can be used, separately and together, to estimate the oxidisability of a waste and its effect on a stream.

Total Organic Carbon

Total organic carbon (TOC) is measured by the catalytic conversion of organic carbon in a waste-water to carbon dioxide. No organic chemicals have been found that will resist the oxidation performed by the equipment now in use. The time of analysis is short, from 5–10 minutes, permitting a rapid estimate of the organic carbon content of waste-waters.

The relationship of TOC values of wastes and effluents to pollution control results requires further understanding. A TOC value does not indicate the rate at which the carbon compounds degrade. Compounds analysed in the TOC test, such as cellulose, degrade only slowly in a natural environment. Values of TOC will change as wastes are treated by various methods.

BOD and COD utilise an oxygen approach. TOC utilises a carbon approach. There is no fundamental correlation of TOC to either BOD or COD. However, where wastes are relatively uniform, there will be a fairly constant correlation between TOC and BOD or COD. Once such a correlation is established, TOC can be used for routine process monitoring.

Total Oxygen Demand

The total oxygen demand (TOD) of a substance is defined as the amount of oxygen required for the combustion of impurities in an aqueous sample at a high temperature (900°C) using a platinum catalyst. The oxygen demand of carbon, hydrogen, nitrogen, and sulphur in a waste-water sample is measured by this method. The interpretation of TOD values to treatment plant efficiency or to stream quality requires further investigation but generally can be related to BOD and COD values. A portion of both TOC and TOD values will represent nonbiodegradable matter. TOD and TOC methods are rapid and can be incorporated in waste-water and treatment plant control systems.

TEMPERATURE

General

Temperature is an important factor affecting waste treatment since it influences the physical properties of the liquid under treatment, the rates of the biological and chemical treatment processes, and the waste assimilation capacity of land or water. Most investigations have concluded that, within specific temperature ranges, an equation of the form:

$$k = ae^{bT} \qquad \qquad \dots (6.13)$$

can be used to express the relationship of a reaction rate k and temperature $T(°C)$. The values of a and b are a function of the specific process and reaction. Reaction rates or coefficients are determined or known at a specific temperature and can be estimated at other temperatures by:

$$k_{T_2} = k_{T_1} e^{c(T_2 - T_1)} = k_{T_2} \theta^{(T_2 - T_1)} \qquad \qquad \dots (6.14)$$

where, T_1 is the temperature at which the reaction rate or coefficient is known (k_{T_1}) and T_2 is the temperature at which the rate or coefficient is desired.

Equation 6.14 is only an approximation since the temperature variation is theoretically exponential in nature. However, over a limited range, the above relationship can be utilised for practical purposes. The temperature effect is the alteration of the rates of specific enzyme activity. In general, only the overall effect of temperature is of engineering and design interest and Eq. 6.14 has proven adequate to describe the temperature effects on biological systems. The value of θ will be different for different treatment systems and different physical, chemical, and biological conditions. Table 6.2 summarises values of θ for a number of biological processes.

For simplicity, it is assumed that θ is not a function of temperature. The error introduced in assuming θ to be independent of temperature is in the range of 10–15 per cent which may be acceptable in most engineering work. Where more precise results are necessary, specific studies may be necessary.

Because temperature has an effect on many fundamental factors, i.e. viscosity, density, surface tension, gas solubility, diffusion, and enzyme activity, it is illogical to assume that θ should be constant over the entire temperature range affecting a treatment process. A number of investigations have demonstrated the interrelationship of θ with temperature. An example is shown in Fig. 6.5.

Table 6.2. Temperature coefficients (θ) for biological waste treatment processes.

Treatment	Temperature coefficients	
	Range	Average
Activated sludge	1.0–1.04	1.03
Aerated lagoon	1.085–1.1	–
Anaerobic lagoon	1.08–1.09	1.085
Trickling filter	1.035–1.08	–
Aerated lagoon	–	1.035
Aerated lagoon	–	1.05

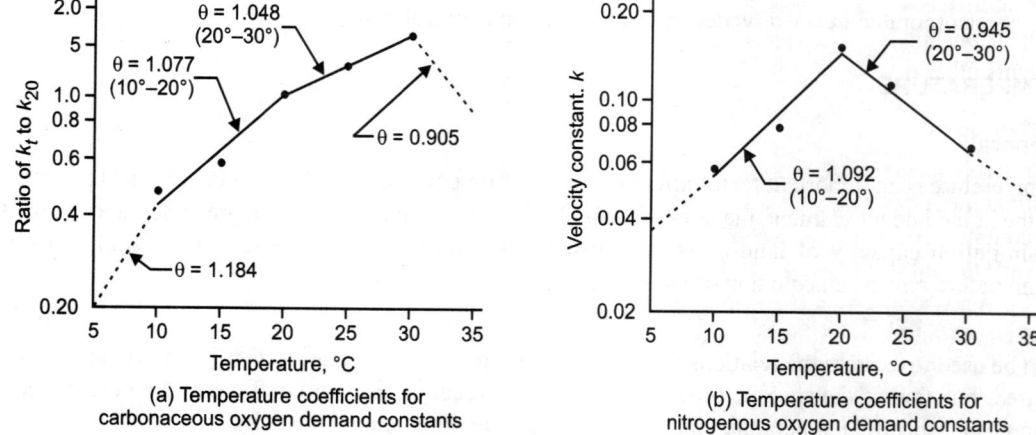

(a) Temperature coefficients for carbonaceous oxygen demand constants

(b) Temperature coefficients for nitrogenous oxygen demand constants

Fig. 6.5. Variation of carbonaceous and nitrogenous temperature coefficients with temperature.

After the optimum temperatures range for the specific micro-organisms, the reaction rate decreases and θ becomes negative.

If θ = 1.072, a reaction rate is doubled for an increase in temperature of 10°C. This value, 1.072, is in the same range of the coefficients for many processes and reactions and has led to the common phrase that, in general, biological reaction rates are doubled for each 10°C rise in temperature. This estimation generally is useful for only a given temperature range, around 20°C. Its use is less applicable at extreme temperature conditions.

In a biological treatment system, the reduction of the temperature of the biological unit by 10°C will require about double the active organisms in the unit to achieve equivalent process efficiencies. This can be accomplished by increasing the mixed liquor suspended solids (MLSS) concentration in the unit. Such an increase in MLSS may affect the viscosity of the liquid in certain cases and may reduce the solids settling rate. Although temperature variations of 10°C rarely occur abruptly, an uncovered unit can experience considerable temperature differences between winter and summer. Systems with solids recycle permit the operator to compensate for lower temperatures with increased microbial solids in the system. Systems without solids recycle do not have this flexibility. A knowledge of the effect of temperature on a biological system permits better design and operation of the system.

PROCESS EQUATIONS

General

The proper utilisation of biological treatment processes depends upon an understanding of the kinetics of the processes and the effects of environmental factors on the kinetics. If organic matter, i.e. waste is added at a constant rate to a continuous flow biological treatment unit, the unit eventually will reach equilibrium conditions. Until equilibrium conditions occur, the micro-organisms will respond to the waste addition and synthesise new organisms until the microbial mass is in equilibrium with the available food supply, i.e. waste. At equilibrium, the net microbial concentration is related to the available substrate and to the decay rate, or endogenous respiration of the organisms. At equilibrium the unit is a food-limited unit.

In this explanation, the substrate, i.e. the carbonaceous material, BOD, or COD is assumed to be the limiting material. The same relationship would be observed for cases where some other nutrient, i.e. nitrogen, phosphorus, or a trace metal, would limit the maximum reaction rates. For agricultural wastes, nutrients other than carbon rarely are the limiting nutrient.

Continuous Growth

The microbial cell concentration is a function of the substrate in the system. With a given and constant substrate input and a desired substrate effluent or removal efficiency, a continuous, nonrecycle process will contain a specific quantity of microbial cells. For this system the only factor that a design engineer can vary to produce different removal efficiencies and effluent quality is the hydraulic retention time (HRT). When a removal efficiency or an effluent substrate concentration is specified, there is only one set of conditions that will meet the specified removal efficiency.

The basic relationship for predicting microbial growth in a continuous flow system is:

Net microbial growth per unit time =
(waste utilised per unit time) × (microbial cell yield coefficient)
− (organism decay coefficient) × (microbial mass in the system)   ... (6.15)

The net microbial growth produced per unit time can be designated as dX/dT and the waste utilised per unit time as dS/dt. Equation 6.15 can be expressed as:

$$\frac{dX}{dt} = Y\frac{dS}{dt} - K_D X$$ ... (6.16)

where, Y is the microbial cell yield coefficient, K_D is the organism decay coefficient, and X is the microbial mass in the system. Equation 6.16 can be rearranged to yield:

$$\frac{1}{SRT} = YU - K_D$$ ... (6.17)

where, SRT equals $X/(dX/dt)$ and U equals $(dS/dt)/X$.

These parameters, SRT and U, and Eq. 6.17 are key factors in the understanding, design, and operation of biological treatment systems. The solids retention time (SRT) is sometimes referred to as MCRT (mean cell residence time) or θ_c by various authors. SRT is the time that the microbial mass is retained in the biological system. U is the rate that the wastes are removed from the system per unit of microbial mass. It usually is referred to as the food to micro-organism ratio or F:M.

As noted (Eq. 6.17), the microbial growth in a biological system is related to both SRT and *U*. However, these parameters are interrelated and if one is controlled, the other will reach an equilibrium level and also be controlled. While both parameters can be used for process control, process control using SRT is an easier approach.

Fundamentally, SRT is:

$$\text{SRT} = \frac{\text{Weight of micro-organisms in the system}}{\text{Weight of micro-organisms leaving the system/time}} \qquad \ldots (6.18)$$

and is the time that the micro-organisms are retained in the system to stabilise the wastes. As SRT increases, removals of unstabilised wastes in the system such as volatile solids, COD and organic nitrogen will increase (Fig. 6.6). The level of unstabilised wastes in a biological treatment system can be controlled by regulating SRT.

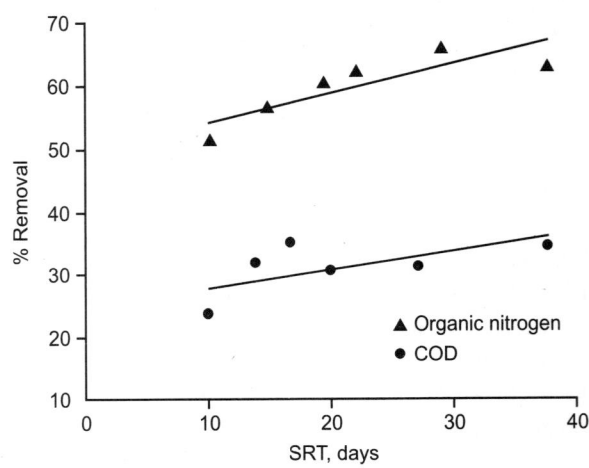

Fig. 6.6. COD and organic nitrogen removal in an oxidation ditch stabilising poultry manure as related to SRT.

Fundamentally, SRT should be determined using the quantity of active micro-organisms in the system. However, measuring the active microbial mass in biological treatment systems is difficult. Fortunately, other parameters can be used to determine the SRT of a system.

Assuming that complete mixing results in a uniform distribution of the active micro-organisms and other solids in a biological treatment system, SRT can be determined by using the quantity of other forms of solids in the system, i.e. volatile suspended solids, total suspended solids, or total solids. In practice, the SRT of the system can be determined by:

$$\text{SRT} = \frac{\text{Weight of solids in the system}}{\text{Weight of solids leaving the system/time}} \qquad \ldots (6.19)$$

The solids in the system are those in the aeration unit and those in any secondary solids separation unit used to clarify the mixed liquor from the aeration basin.

The actual SRT of a biological treatment system must be greater than the minimum time it takes for the micro-organisms to reproduce in the system. If this does not occur, the micro-organisms will be removed from the system at a faster rate than they can multiply and failure of the system will result. The critical SRT or cell washout time can be written as:

$$\frac{1}{SRT_c} = YU_{max} - K_D \qquad \qquad \dots (6.20)$$

U_{max} is the maximum substrate (waste) removal rate per unit of micro-organisms. SRT_c is the minimum microbial residence time at which a stable microbial cell population can be maintained. Because the yield coefficient, Y, is smaller for anaerobic metabolism than for aerobic metabolism, the value of SRT_c for anaerobic processes is larger than for aerobic processes.

The concept of a minimum SRT is important in all biological waste treatment systems, especially in anaerobic treatment systems. In aerobic treatment systems, the energy relationships are such that micro-organisms can reproduce rapidly, a matter of hours or less, depending upon the specific system and its management. It is extremely rare to note an aerobic treatment system that failed because its SRT was less than the minimum time necessary for microbial reproduction.

In anaerobic systems, the micro-organisms reproduce less rapidly and a longer minimum SRT is required to accommodate the slower net growth rate. An example of the relationship between the SRT and the efficiency of substrate removal is shown in Fig. 6.7. Values for these parameters that have been obtained for agricultural and other waste treatment systems are presented in Tables 6.3 and 6.4.

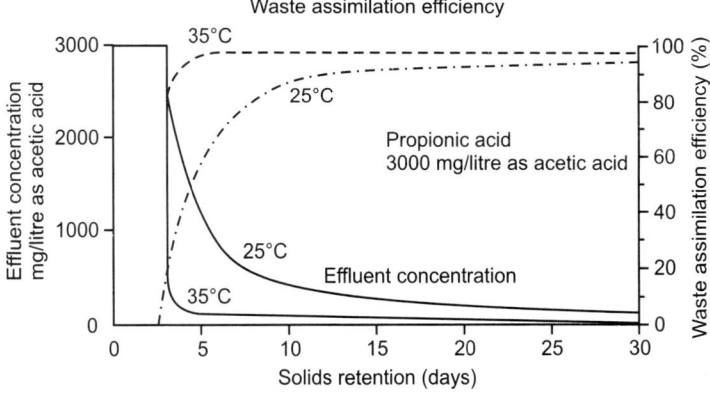

Fig. 6.7. Process efficiency as related to SRT in an anaerobic treatment unit.

Table 6.3. Ranges of kinetic coefficients for aerobic and anaerobic treatment processes.

Coefficient	Units	Treatment	
		Aerobic	Anaerobic
Y	lb volatile suspended solids/lb BOD_{ult}	0.3–0.4	0.03–0.15
K_D	day^{-1}	0.02–0.06	0.01–0.04
U	lb/BOD/day/lb volatile suspended solids	4–24	4–20
SRT_c	days	0.1–0.3	2–6

Many biological treatment systems used with agricultural wastes can be considered as completely mixed, no recycle biological treatment systems (Fig. 6.8). Examples of such systems include aerated lagoons, oxidation ditches, and mixed anaerobic digestion units. A characteristic of these systems is that no solids are recycled back to the biological units to increase the microbial solids concentration. The microbial solids concentration in these units is directly related to the concentration of waste (food) in the unit.

Table 6.4. Types of waste.

Waste
Packinghouse waste
Synthetic milk waste
Synthetic carbohydrate and protein wastes
Ammonia oxidation
Nitrite oxidation
Pear processing
Peach processing
Apple processing
Potato processing
Field extended aeration system
Municipal waste-water

In such systems, the hydraulic retention time (HRT) is equal to the SRT because the systems are considered completely mixed and because the liquids and solids stay in the system the same length of time. HRT is the theoretical time that a volume of liquid remains in the system:

$$\text{HRT} = \frac{\text{Volume of system}}{\text{Volume of liquid leaving the system/time}} = \frac{V}{Q} \qquad \qquad ...(6.21)$$

The degree of stabilisation can be regulated by controlling either the SRT or HRT of such a system. A substrate balance for a nonrecycle system (Fig. 6.8) will yield:

$$S_o - S_i = X_1 U(\text{HRT}) \qquad \qquad ...(6.22)$$

Therefore, for a specific influent waste concentration, the amount of substrate removed and stabilisation efficiency is a function of the liquid detention time, the microbial cells in the system, and the substrate removal rate per micro-organism.

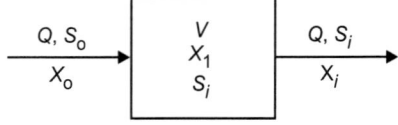

Q = Flow
S = Substrate (waste) concentration
X = Microbial concentration
V = Reactor volume

Fig. 6.8. Completely mixed, no recycle biological treatment system.

The waste removal rate, U, is a system loading rate and has been used as a design loading rate, i.e. quantity of substrate added per unit of micro-organisms per unit time. Such rates are generally in terms of pounds of BOD or COD/day/pound of mixed liquor suspended solids.

A mass balance for the nonrecycle system will yield Eq. (6.17) assuming that the microbial mass entering the system, X_0, is small compared to the microbial mass, X_1, in the system. For simplicity, the term YU can be replaced by μ, the microbial growth rate. The term $\mu - K_D$ is the net growth rate of the microbial solids in the system which is important since it estimates the accumulation of microbial solids that ultimately must be removed from the system. Equation 6.17 also verifies an earlier statement that synthesis and respiration occur simultaneously in biological systems with synthesis predominating when food is in excess ($\mu > K_D$) and respiration predominating when food, or essential nutrient, is limited, ($K_D > \mu$).

The net microbial solids production is inversely related to SRT:

$$\frac{dx}{dt} = \frac{X}{\text{SRT}} \qquad \text{... (6.23)}$$

Thus, a biological unit with a long SRT will have less net microbial solids for wasting than will a unit with a shorter SRT. The amount of microbial solids to be wasted can be varied by controlling the SRT of the unit. A long SRT biological unit is less effective in removing inorganic nutrients because net microbial solids production and incorporation of the nutrients into microbial cells is less. Biological systems with high microbial solids production, i.e. high rate synthesis systems, should be utilised where high rates of inorganic nutrient removal by micro-organisms are desired.

The total quantity of solids that will accumulate or require removal will include the excess microbial solids and the relatively stable organic and inorganic solids contained in the untreated waste and which are not altered in the treatment process. The total quantity of excess solids can be estimated by:

$$\frac{dX_s}{dt} = \frac{dX}{dt} + \frac{dX_i}{dt} \qquad \text{... (6.24)}$$

where, dX_s/dt represents the rate of total sludge solids produced, dX/dt represents the rate of net microbial solids produced, and dX_i/dt represents the rate of stable inorganic and organic solids accumulation.

The value for dX_i/dt varies with the type of waste. Agricultural wastes can have values of dX_i/dt ranging from close to zero for wastes such as milk processing wastes to large values with wastes having large quantities of nonbiodegradable material such as cattle wastes.

The rate at which solids will accumulate in a biological treatment system is dependent upon the waste loading rate, the rate at which solids are lost from the system, the rate at which inert solids enter the system, the rate at which volatile waste solids and microbial solids are oxidised in the system, and the rate at which the waste is being converted into microbial cells.

In aerobic systems, the above equations can be used to estimate the oxygen requirements. The quantity of oxygen required will be a summation of that required for substrate removal (synthesis) and that required for respiration. For a process such as in Fig. 6.8,

$$V\frac{dO}{dt} = aQ(S_o - S_i) + bK_D X_1 V \qquad \text{... (6.25)}$$

where, dO/dt is in terms of mg/litre time, a is a constant used to convert substrate units to oxygen units utilised in synthesis (units of oxygen/unit of BOD or COD), and b is a constant, used to convert cell mass units to oxygen units (unit of oxygen/unit of cell mass). Cell mass generally is expressed as volatile suspended solids although this parameter is an inadequate measure of the active micro-organisms. The rate of oxygen utilisation is:

$$\frac{dO}{dt} = \frac{(S_o - S_i)a}{\text{HRT}} + bK_D X_1 \qquad \text{... (6.26)}$$

The oxygen requirement varies directly with the substrate to be removed and inversely with the hydraulic residence time of the system. The longer the detention time of the biological system, the lower the rate of oxygen demand in the system and the greater the total oxygen utilisation. The constants *a* and *b* and Eq. 6.26 normally do not include the oxygen required for nitrification. The oxygen requirement for nitrification is a function of the amount of ammonia that is nitrified and the equations can be modified by including the following term:

$$\frac{4.5 \cdot \Delta NH_3}{HRT}$$ ... (6.27)

where, ΔNH_3 is the ammonia oxidised in the unit during aerobic treatment.

Solids Recycle

For a given substrate removal rate, a larger quantity of waste can be treated if the mass of organisms in the system is greater. Systems with solids recycle (Fig. 6.9) can increase the concentration of active organisms in a biological unit and can provide engineers and operators with additional alternatives to obtain satisfactory performance and to decrease the size of the biological unit.

The solids separator, generally a sedimentation unit, plays an important role in such systems since the quantity of recycled solids and the effluent quality depends on the efficiency of the solids separator. The microbial solids must be separated easily otherwise the system will approximate a system without recycle (Fig. 6.8), the advantages of recycle will be lost, and the system may not produce an effluent of the desired quality.

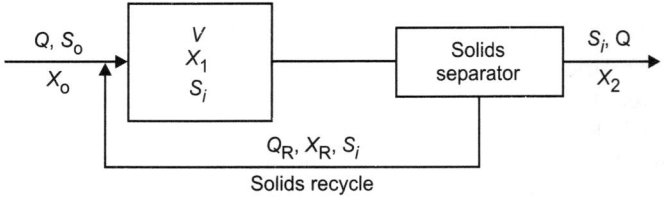

Q = Flow
S = Substrate (waste) concentration
X = Microbial concentration
V = Reactor volume

Fig. 6.9. Completely mixed biological treatment system with recycle.

A substrate, microbial mass, and oxygen requirement balance can be made for the recycle system in the same manner as was done for the nonrecycle system. A microbial mass balance on the entire system operating at equilibrium and assuming the influent solids concentration to be negligible illustrates that:

$$\mu - K_D = \frac{QX_2}{VX_1} = \frac{1}{(HRT)(r)} = \frac{1}{SRT}$$ ... (6.28)

where, *r* is the mixed liquor to effluent cell ratio, X_1/X_2 and is numerically greater than 1.0. The relationship between the cell mass in the system, X_1, and the substrate removed, $S_o - S_i$, for the system in Fig. 6.10 can be expressed by substituting (HRT)(*r*) for SRT to yield:

$$X_1 = \frac{Yr(S_o - S_i)}{1 + K_D(SRT)}$$ ... (6.29)

which indicates that the microbial mass in the system will be a function of both the substrate removal and the cell ratio. The microbial mass in a biological system with recycle is greater than one without recycle all other factors being equal. The effluent substrate concentration can be expressed as

$$S_i = S_o = \left(\frac{X_1[1 + K_D(\text{SRT})]}{Yr} \right) \qquad \ldots (6.30)$$

The oxygen requirements for a system with recycle also can be described by Eq. 6.31 which results from combining several previous equations:

$$\frac{dO}{dt} = (S_o = S_i) \left(\frac{a}{\text{HRT}} + \frac{bK_Dr}{U(\text{SRT})} \right) \qquad \ldots (6.31)$$

For a biological system with recycle, the oxygen requirement is related to both HRT and SRT. The oxygen requirement for substrate removal for synthesis is a function of hydraulic residence time while the oxygen requirement for respiration is related to the microbial cell residence time.

The HRT of a system with recycle would be less than one without recycle to achieve a specific substrate removal efficiency. When design values are used in these equations, the oxygen demand rate for a system with recycle will be greater, because of a shorter HRT and a larger quantity of microbial solids in the system, than for a system without recycle used to treat the same wastes.

As indicated by Eq. 6.28, the SRT of the system is a function of both the HRT and the mixed liquor to effluent cell ratio of the system. This permits the system to have a long SRT to obtain a high treatment efficiency, low S_i with a short HRT, and a smaller size biological unit. Solids recycle also offers the opportunity to maintain a SRT greater than the minimum required for cell growth with an HRT which could be less than the minimum SRT.

A system with cell recycle offers greater flexibility for design and operation than a system without recycle. When a treatment process is subject to variable waste loads, the microbial solids in the biological unit can be varied by changing the recycle ratio to adjust to the waste loads and produce a consistent effluent. This requires a qualified operator, a consideration when deciding to use a system with or without recycle.

A system without recycle will require a longer HRT and a larger biological unit than will a system with recycle to obtain the same quality of waste effluent. A large biological unit can dampen the surges caused by variable waste load and may provide adequate time for the microbial solids to adjust to an increased waste concentration in the unit. For many agricultural wastes, the decision to use a system with or without solids recycle will hinge on the availability of an operator to manage a system with recycle. Because many facilities producing agricultural wastes are located where land costs are not excessive, treatment systems without recycle, such as oxidation ponds, aerated lagoons, and oxidation ditches are common.

Application to Agricultural Wastes

While fundamental to all biological systems, the mathematical relationships and equations noted above rarely have been applied to systems treating agricultural wastes. The use of these relationships offers an opportunity to those who wish to develop better biological processes for agricultural wastes and to better understand the processes currently handling these wastes. Because agricultural wastes are organic wastes, some type of biological treatment will be utilised prior to ultimate disposal on the land or to surface waters. The current biological treatment processes for agricultural wastes rest almost entirely on uncoordinated empirical approaches that offer little hope of success when utilised with wastes and under conditions different from those where success has been obtained.

The design engineer can utilise the mathematical relationships to obtain satisfactory performance. The actual design of a waste treatment facility will include an estimation of possible overloads to the system, temperature effects, operator ability and interest, differences in waste characteristics, and allowance for incalculable risks.

Some of the specific differences that are involved with agricultural wastes include the solids concentration in the raw waste, long detention time, nonhomogeneity in the biological system, and the oxygen requirements. With municipal wastes and certain industrial wastes, the quantity of solids in the untreated waste is small compared to the quantity of solids in the treatment system. Such an assumption cannot be made for agricultural wastes, especially food processing and animal wastes. These wastes contain a high concentration of solids which must be considered in all mass balance and mathematical relationships. These wastes frequently have a large nonbiodegradable fraction which will not be removed in a biological treatment unit and will remain for ultimate disposal. In most of the previous mathematical relationships, the effect of an influent non-biodegradable fraction was not considered. The total solids for disposal will include the net increase in microbial solids and the non-biodegradable solids.

Because of the high concentration of BOD in agricultural wastes, long detention times are necessary to produce an effluent suitable for discharge to surface waters. Where discharge on land is used, long detention times in storage units prior to disposal are common. Detention times can range from days with dilute waste where discharge to surface water is contemplated to weeks and months where storage and land disposal is practiced. The long detention times will have an obvious effect on the quantity of active organisms in the system. The active mass will be a minor fraction of the suspended solids in the biological unit. The long detention times permit accommodation of decreased reaction rates caused by lower temperatures or by microbial inhibition caused by materials in the wastes.

One of the basic assumptions made in developing the basic equations was that the biological treatment process was completely mixed. This is not always the case with processes treating agricultural wastes. The solids content and particle size of some of the wastes preclude complete mixing and solids sedimentation and accumulation in the quiescent areas of the biological unit can occur. In evaluating the performance of biological units treating agricultural wastes, this possibility should be closely checked.

The oxygen requirements are based upon maintaining an excess of dissolved oxygen, generally at least 1–2 mg/litre. When lesser amounts of dissolved oxygen exist in the system, the system is oxygen limited and the microbial reaction rates and treatment efficiency decrease. In long detention time units having a residual dissolved oxygen content, a population of nitrifying organisms can be established and an oxygen demand caused by nitrification can result.

For most agricultural wastes, especially those disposed of on the land, a residual dissolved oxygen concentration is not required. The minimum input oxygen requirement would be to avoid the odours that are produced under highly reduced conditions.

The mathematical relationships described in this chapter assume that the rate at which organic matter is utilised by micro-organisms is a function of a limiting nutrient. In most waste treatment systems the organic waste itself is the limiting nutrient, i.e. substrate-limited. With certain food processing wastes, inorganic nutrients such as nitrogen and phosphorus can be limiting and may have to be added to achieve optimum rates of treatment and desired treatment efficiency.

Chapter 7

Biological Treatment of Waste-water

INTRODUCTION

The function of biological treatment processes is to remove organic matter and at times ammonia from waste-water through the metabolic means of oxidation and cell synthesis. Although several physical and chemical approaches have been proposed as substitutes, biological treatment remains the only proven means of economically abating the oxygen depletion caused by the discharge of waste-water contaminated with low concentrations of a mixture of biodegradable organic compounds.

If this organic matter were to reach the receiving body of water, bacteria would oxidise it and thereby reduce the oxygen resources upon which aquatic life is dependent. Biological treatment processes are basically an accelerated form of these natural water purification mechanisms. Organics causing problems in addition to oxygen depletion also are economically removed, e.g. materials toxic to fish and odourous in water supplies. The fit of biological processes into overall waste-water treatment sequences is shown in Fig. 7.1.

ENVIRONMENTAL REQUIREMENTS

In order that the bacteria and higher microbial forms in the biological treatment unit may stabilise the waste organics at a suitably high rate, key environmental conditions must be maintained at near optimum levels.

The conditions which are basic to all aerobic treatment processes include:
1. Oxygen availability.
2. pH near neutral.
3. Available nitrogen and phosphorus.
4. Absence of toxic materials.
5. Adequate mixing.

Since anaerobic processes utilise materials other than molecular oxygen as acceptors for the hydrogen atoms removed from the organics during oxidation, oxygen availability can be omitted from the above list for these processes.

Most industrial biological treatment processes are aerobic, however, since aerobic processes can stabilise organics faster at lower temperatures and have less potential for odour problems. Some of the pollutants that make pretreatment necessary before the wastes can be handled in the biological unit are listed in Table 7.1.

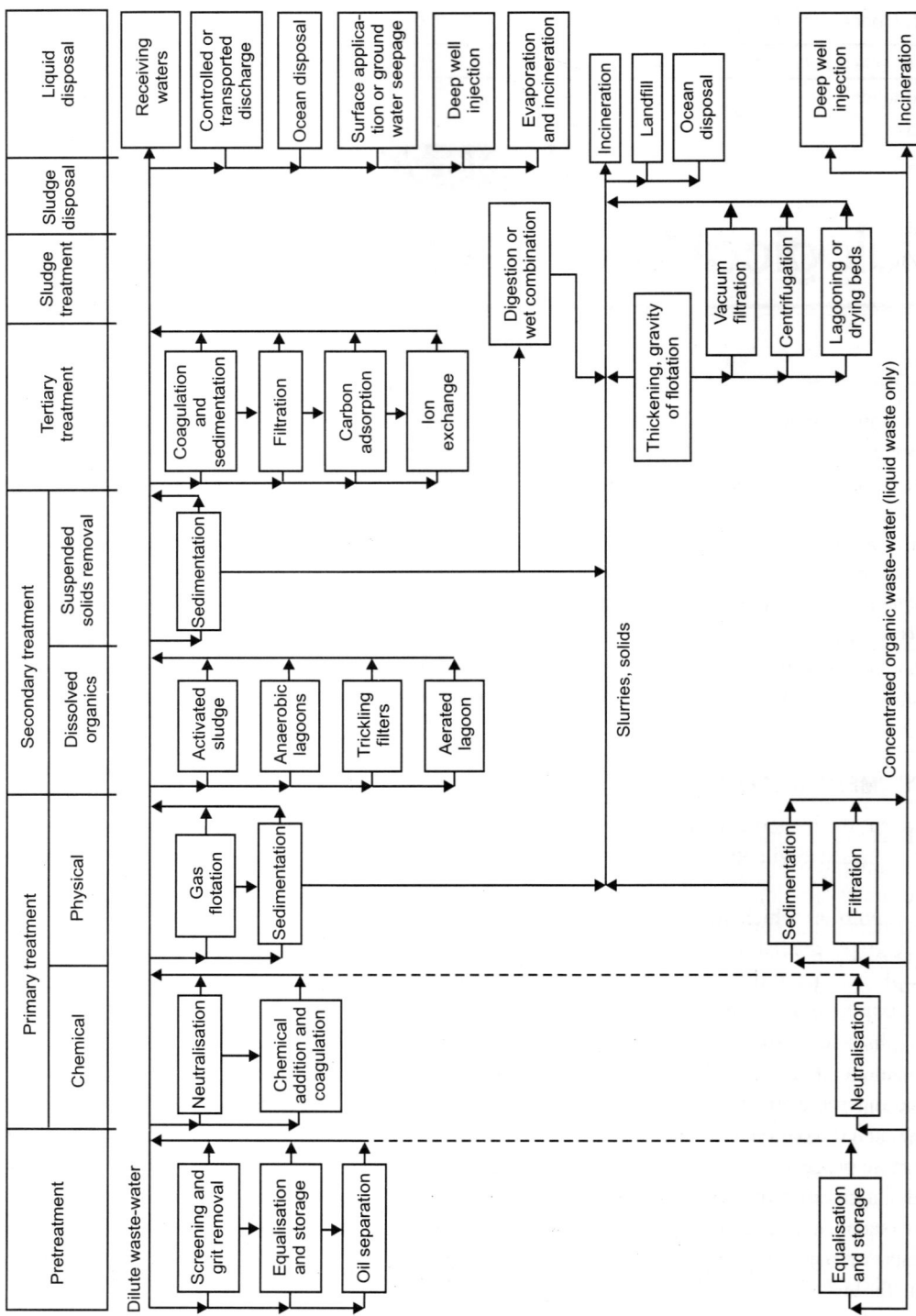

Fig. 7.1. Fit of biological treatment into overall waste-water treatment sequences.

Table 7.1. Concentration of pollutants that make prebiological or primary treatment desirable.

Pollutant or system condition	Limiting concentration	Kind of treatment
Suspended solids	>50–125 mg/l	Sedimentation, flotation, lagooning
Oil or grease	>35–50 mg/l	Skimming tank or separator
Toxic ions		Precipitation or ion exchange
Pb	≤0.1 mg/l	–
Cu + Ni + CN	≤1 mg/l	–
Cr^{+6} + Zn	≤3 mg/l	–
Cr^{+3}	≤10 mg/l	–
pH	6–9	Neutralisation
Alkalinity	0.5 lb alkalinity as $CaCO_3$/lb BOD removed	Neutralisation for excessive alkalinity
Acidity	Free mineral acidity	Neutralisation
Organic-load variation	>2:1–4:1[a]	Equalisation
Sulphides	>100 mg/l	Precipitation or stripping with recovery
Phenols	>70–300 mg/l[b]	Extraction, adsorption, internal dilution
Ammonia	>1.6 g/l	Dilution, ion exchange, pH adjustment and stripping
Dissolved salts	>10–16 g/l	Dilution, ion exchange
Temperature	13°–38°C in reactor	Cooling, steam addition

[a] Higher level if constituents remain in same ratio.
[b] Up to at least 1500 mg/l if bacterial acclimation is maintained.

In addition to the basic environmental factors, biological processes are specifically designed to operate efficiently by proper manipulation of these rate-controlling variables:

1. Micro-organism concentration.
2. Bacterial acclimation or adaptation.
3. Temperature level.
4. Contact duration and mode.
5. Organic feed concentration.

The rate at which organic matter is stabilised, and to some degree the extent of degradation, is dependent upon the concentration of active bacteria in the system. Unless the organic matter is of natural origin, waste stabilisation often is delayed until the bacteria in the system have been allowed either to develop adaptive enzyme systems or to undergo shifts in species mix in order to oxidise the organic material at a high rate. The oxidation rate increases with increasing temperature until a maximum level is attained either based on metabolic or solids-retention considerations; the optimum temperature varies for each type of system. The minimum allowable contact time is dictated by the rate of conversion of the organic matter to carbon dioxide, water, new cells, and stored or adsorbed products. The conversion obtained in a given time also is dependent upon whether the system is completely mixed or has reactors in series (staged). The maximum time is governed by the extent to which the stored organics and synthesised cells are allowed to be oxidised in turn, since excess oxidation can cause problems in retention of viable cells. The organic feed concentration governs the rate at which food can be supplied to the biological system while still maintaining the minimum desirable contact with the bacteria; it also affects the equilibrium level achievable. The function of the various types of biological units is to utilise these rate-controlling factors to the best advantage. These qualitative statements will be expressed as mathematical relationships in subsequent sections to aid in their being understood and used.

MICROBIAL METABOLISM AND BIODEGRADABILITY

Familiarity with a few selected terms and concepts regarding microbial life should allow the engineer or chemist to realise better the full potential of biological systems for treating industrial waste-waters.

Protista

The microbial life of interest in treatment systems belongs to the Protista Kingdom; the members of which, as opposed to plants and animals, do not have similar cells arranged in a tissue structure. Among the Protista, the classes of micro-organisms described in Table 7.2 are of most importance.

Table 7.2. Characteristics of microbial classes important in waste treatment systems.

1. Bacteria
   Unicellular
   Prokaryotic (no distinct nucleus)
   Absorb soluble nutrients
   Primarily binary-fission reproduction
   Cylindrical, spherical, or helical
   0.5 to 3.0 μm (cylinders or rods)
2. Fungi (true fungi or moulds)
   Multicellular
   Generally reproduce by spore formation
   Nonphotosynthetic
   Low nitrogen requirement
   Survive at low pH
   Most are strict aerobes
   Heterotrophic (organic carbon source)
3. Algae
   Photosynthetic
   Unicellular or multicellular
   Autotrophic (inorganic carbon source)
   Types:
      Green algae (*Chlorella*)–chloroplasts, eukaryotic (nuclear membrane)
      Motile green (*Eugelena*)-flagellated
      Yellow green or golden brown-diatoms
      Blue green unicellular, dispersed chlorophyll, prokaryotic
4. Protozoa
   Unicellular
   Eucaryotic
   Majority aerobic

(Contd ...)

Types in treatment systems:

Amoebae-pseudopods for movement and particulate food engulfment

Flagellates-phytoflaggelates (chloroplasts) and zooflagelates (absorb food)

Ciliates–cilia for motion and capturing solid food, free-swimming (e.g. *Paramecium*), and stalked (e.g. *Vorticella*)

Tentacles-capture other protozoa and draw out protoplasm

5. Rotifers

Multicellular

Aerobic

Heterotrophic

Two sets of rotating cilia for mobility and capturing food

6. Other

Yeasts

Unicellular

Eukaryotic

Reproduce by budding

Viruses

Obligate parasites, i.e. redirect invaded cells to produce viral cells

Bacteria are the primary organisms which serve to stabilise organic and certain inorganic constituents in waste-waters. The structural components of a hypothetical bacterial cell are shown in Fig. 7.2. The functions of each component also are indicated. The wide range of chemical transformations capable of being conducted at a fast rate by these organisms will be discussed in later sections.

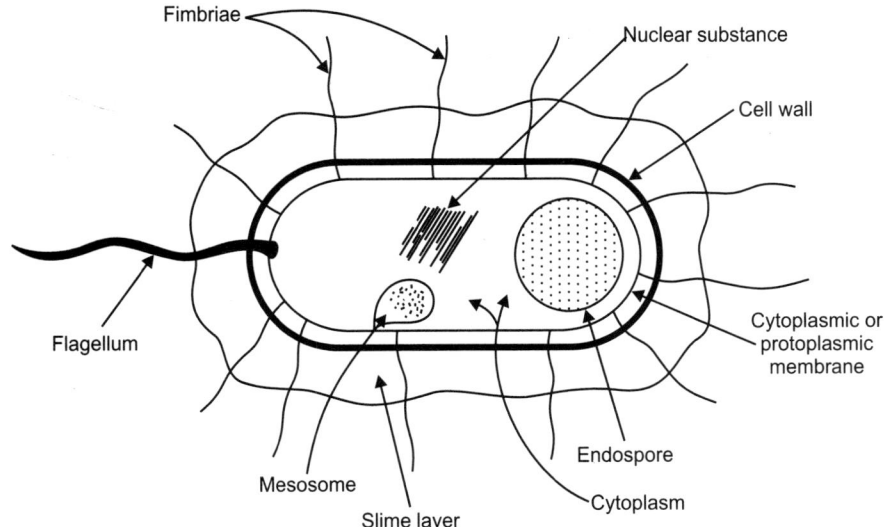

Fig. 7.2. Hypothetical bacterial cell.

Fungi occur in liquid waste treatment systems, usually when nitrogen is deficient or the pH is low. Except when they are needed to degrade certain large molecules, fungi are undesirable as they cause problems during separation of the biomass from the effluent liquor. Fungi are important in composting.

Algae are important in lagoon-type waste treatment systems where they photosynthetically convert carbon dioxide and water to oxygen and cellular material. Their growth often is stimulated in receiving waters rich in nitrogen and phosphorus.

Protozoa and rotifers play an important role in biological waste treatment systems by feeding on bacteria. A clearer effluent is produced, and additional organic material is converted to carbon dioxide and water. The maturity or state of the system can be determined by the rotifers and types of protozoa present; as the system reaches a higher degree of conversion, growth of the protozoan classes and rotifers progresses as follows:

Sarcodina (amoebae).
Phytoflagellates.
Zooflagellates.
Free-swimming ciliates.
Suctoria (tentacled).
Stalked ciliates.
Rotifers.

1. Cell wall: 10–40 per cent of cell weight, provides rigidity to protect against osmotic pressure changes.
2. Cytoplasm: Colloidal suspension of proteins, lipids, carbohydrates; granular in appearance; contains ribonucleoprotein structures (ribosomes) which are the site of protein synthesis. Inclusions found in various bacteria under various conditions include glycogen, lipid, and volutin granules, and sulphur droplets.
   (a) Glycogen granule: Polysaccharide granules formed from excess organic matter if the medium is N deficient.
   (b) Lipid granule: Natural fats or poly-β-hydroxybutyric acid (an ester polymer formed from excess organic material if N is deficient in the medium).
   (c) Volutin granule: Polyphosphate accumulation, also termed metachromatic granule, often due to nutrient deficiency impeding nucleic acid synthesis.
   (d) Sulphur globule: Associated with sulphur as an end product.
3. Cytoplasmic or protoplasmic membrane: A semipermeable lipoprotein complex which controls material passage in and out of the cell by passive (equilibrium) and active transport.
4. Endospore: Some bacteria have the ability to transpose into small spheres which are highly resistant to environmental factors such as heat, etc. and can germinate to vegetative cells.
5. Fimbriae (Pili): Employed by the bacterium for attachment; implicated in conjugation, DNA (deoxyribonucleic acid) transfer.
6. Flagellum: Responsible for motility, visible with special stain. Flagella may be disposed in a polar or peritrichous (many all around) fashion, and are macromolecular protein structures appearing as rope-like spirals.
7. Mesosomes: Involved in cross-wall formation during cell division.
8. Nuclear substance (chromatinic area): Not enclosed by nuclear membrane; contains the genetic information of the cell and is composed of a circular, double helical strand of DNA.
9. Slime layer: Generally polysaccharide, called a capsule if of a regular thickness and too viscous to diffuse away. Microscopic examination of the system under low power magnification is an effective tool to visualise the succession of these forms during treatment.

Growth

In order for the bacteria and other Protista to accomplish the desired stabilisation (energy-reduction) reactions at optimum rates, proper growth conditions need to be maintained. These conditions are summarised in Table 7.3.

Table 7.3. Factors influencing bacterial growth

Nutritional requirements

    Energy source

        Oxidise chemical compounds (chemotrophs)

            Organics-organotrophic (heterotrophs)

            Inorganics-lithotrophic (autotrophs)

        Employ radiant energy (phototrophs)

            Bacterial photosynthesis–sulphur bacteria

    Carbon source (~50 per cent of cell on dry weight basis)

        Organics (saphrophytic heterotrophs)

        Carbon dioxide as sole source (autotrophs)—usually oxidise reduced, S, N, Fe forms

    Nitrogen source (~12 per cent of dry cells)

        Inorganic-N suitable for algae, most bacteria

    Phosphorus and sulphur (2.6 and 0.7 per cent)

        Phosphorus—usually supplied as PO_4

        Sulphur—some bacteria require inorganic, some organic, some elemental

    Trace metals

$$\underbrace{Na, K, Ca, Mg, Fe, Mn, Zn, Cu, Co}_{2.5\%}$$

    Vitamins and vitamin-like compounds

        Some bacteria can manufacture all; others need one or more in the growth media

    Water–nutrients must be in solution

    Hydrogen acceptor (oxidant)

        Respiration

            Molecular oxygen

            Nitrate, nitrite, sulphate ions—in the absence of oxygen

            Carbon dioxide

        Fermentation

            Oxidised organics

Physical conditions

    Temperature

	Range (°C)	Best (°C)
Psychrophiles	7–35	20–30
Mesophiles	25–40	30
Thermophiles	25–75	40–60

(Contd ...)

Growth rate: generally doubles per 10°C rise (up to denaturing temperature)

Gaseous requirements

Aerobic—grows in presence of free oxygen

Anaerobic—grows in absence of free oxygen

Facultatively anaerobic—grows in either case

Microaerophilic–obligate aerobes which grow best under low partial pressures of oxygen

pH

6.5–7.5 optimum for most (6–8 at outside)

5–9 minimum to maximum for growth-most systems

Light (phototrophs)

Salt (obligate halophiles)

Oxidation-reduction potential (ORP) influences anaerobic reactions

Lack of toxicants

Organic (concentration, ratio to enzyme level, and organism acclimation state influence degree of toxicity)

Heavy metals

High cation, ammonia, and sulphide levels

The time interval required for the bacterial cell to divide is termed the generation time; it ranges from 10 to 60 minutes for some heterotrophs, about 20 hours for one nitrite oxidiser, and 3 days for some methanogenic bacteria. As the cells divide, the population doubles (1,2,4,8,16, etc.) until nutrients become limiting or end-product inhibition occurs. A typical growth progression for a batch-fed system starting with a low level of seed micro-organisms is shown in Fig. 7.3. In a steady-state treatment system, an overall growth state in the declining growth phase is desirable. In actuality, various species are likely in different growth states due to the inherent variability of the system.

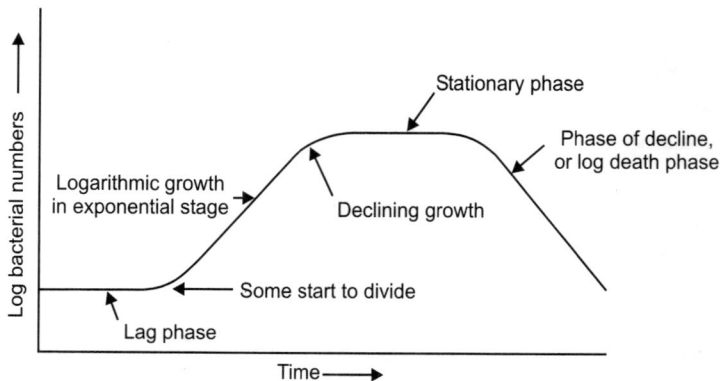

Lag phase—enzyme development (catalysts), new protoplasm (elongation), adjustment to physical factors.

Log growth—divide at rate according to generation time, excess food: stored, adsorbed, soluble.

Declining growth—food supply becoming limited.

Stationary—nutrients limiting, toxicants produced, division balanced with death, endogenous growth (utilises stored and lysed nutrients).

Log death—lack of nutrients, end products toxic rapid die-off, auto oxidation.

Fig. 7.3. Typical bacterial growth curve.

The complex chemical transformations resulting in the growth of micro-organisms can occur at ambient temperatures and pressure levels due to the catalytic action of enzymes produced by the micro-organisms. A given species will have a set of enzymes always available to conduct both energy-yielding (catabolic) reactions and cell-synthesis (anabolic) reactions, while others are produced only upon the external stimulation of a new substrate. The former enzymes are termed constitutive and the latter adaptive. The transfer of energy released in the catabolic reactions to the energy-consuming anabolic reactions is accomplished through the linkage of the adenosine-triphosphate/adenosine disphosphate (ATP/ADP) couple (Fig. 7.4).

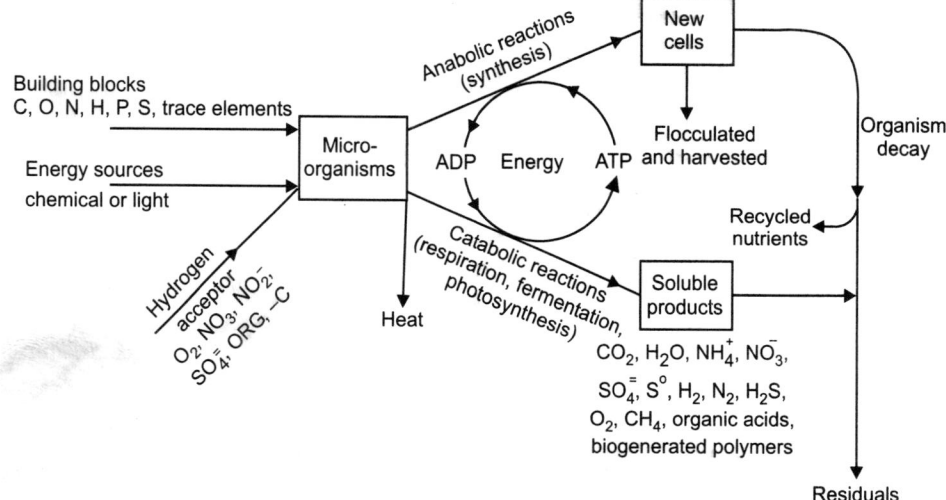

Fig. 7.4. Biological transformations.

Hydrolysis of large molecules to facilitate transport across the cellular membrane is accomplished by extracellular enzymes; while intracellular enzymes are responsible for oxidative and synthesis reactions. The transformation of an organic molecule to carbon dioxide, water, and cellular constituents involves a sequence or chain of single steps of the removal or addition of atoms or electrons. Each step is catalysed by an enzyme and has its own rate of reaction. One of the steps becomes rate limiting. The enzymes have three components:

1. Apoenzyme: High molecular weight organic compound, a protein, determines where reaction occurs on substrate molecule.
2. Coenzyme: Smaller organic molecule, determines what reaction occurs, not always required.
3. Metal activator: Helps to line up enzyme and substrate, not always required.

Familiarisation of engineers and chemists with these concepts and terms should aid in a deeper understanding of the biosystem involved.

Energy Metabolism

The basic features of bacterial metabolism are summarised in Fig. 7.4. The inputs are the cellular building blocks, chemical or light energy, and a final acceptor of the hydrogen atoms or electrons. The catabolic reactions yield the energy used for synthesis, as well as the indicated soluble products. Typical reactions are listed in Table 7.4. The reactions shown for organic matter oxidation are of an overall nature. The actual process involves transforming the waste constituent into a form which upon entering the terminal respiratory cycle (tricarboxylic acid or TCA cycle) yields carbon dioxide, water, cellular building blocks, and energy.

Table 7.4. Typical biological treatment reactions.

Anaerobic nonphotosynthetic reactions (molecular oxygen absent)

Nitrate reduction (denitrification)

$$5CH_3COOH + 8NO_3^- \rightarrow 10CO_2 + 4N_2 + 6H_2O + 8OH^-$$

$$5S + 6NO_3^- + 2H_2O \rightarrow 5SO_4^= + 3N_2 + 4H^+$$

Sulphate reduction

$$2CH_3CHOHCOOH + SO_4^= \rightarrow 2CH_3COOH + H_2S + 2OH^-$$

$$4H_2 + SO_4^= \rightarrow 2H_2O + H_2S + 2OH^-$$

Organic carbon reduction (fermentation)

$$CH_3COOH \rightarrow CH_4 + CO_2$$

$$4CH_3OH \rightarrow 3CH_4 + CO_2 + 2H_2O$$

$$C_6H_{12}O_6 \xrightarrow{\text{bacteria}} 3CH_3COOH$$

$$C_6H_{12}O_6 \xrightarrow{\text{yeast}} 2CH_3CH_2OH + 2CO_2$$

Carbon dioxide reduction

$$2CH_3CH_2OH + CO_2 \rightarrow 2CH_3COOH + CH_4$$

$$4H_2 + CO_2 \rightarrow CH_4 + 2H_2O$$

$$4H_2 + 2CO_2 \rightarrow CH_3COOH + 2H_2O$$

Aerobic nonphotosynthetic bacterial reactions

Oxygen limited systems

$$CH_3CH_2OH + O_2 \rightarrow CH_3COOH + H_2O$$

$$2CH_3CHO + O_2 \rightarrow 2CH_3COOH$$

$$2CH_3CHOHCH_3 + O_2 \rightarrow 2CH_3COCH_3 + 2H_2O$$

Complete oxidation

$$CH_3COOH + 2O_2 \rightarrow 2CO_2 + 2H_2O$$

$$2H_2 + O_2 \rightarrow 2H_2O$$

$$CH_4 + 2O_2 \rightarrow CO_2 + 2H_2O$$

Nitrification

$$2NH_3 + 3O_2 \rightarrow 2NO_2^- + 2H^+ + 2H_2O$$

$$2NO_2^- + O_2 \rightarrow 2NO_3^-$$

Sulphur oxidation

$$2H_2S + O_2 \rightarrow 2S + 2H_2O$$

$$2S + 2H_2O + 3O_2 \rightarrow 2SO_4^= + 4H^+$$

$$S_2O_3^= + H_2O + 2O_2 \rightarrow 2SO_4^= + 2H^+$$

Nitrogen fixation

$$N_2 \rightarrow \text{Nitrogenous organics}$$

Photosynthetic reactions

$$CO_2 + 2H_2S \xrightarrow{\text{light}} (CH_2O) + H_2O + 2S$$

$$3CO_2 + 2S + 5H_2O \xrightarrow{\text{light}} 3(CH_2O) + 4H^+ + 2SO_4^=$$

$$CO_2 + 2H_2O \xrightarrow{\text{light, algae}} (CH_2O) + H_2O + O_2$$

(Contd ...)

$$9CH_3COOH \xrightarrow{\text{light}} 2CO_2 + 4(C_4H_6O_2) + 6H_2O$$

$$CO_2 + 2H_2 \xrightarrow{\text{light}} (CH_2O) + H_2O$$

$$2CH_3COOH + H_2 \xrightarrow{\text{light}} (C_4H_6O_2) + 2H_2O$$

Conversion of organic waste constituents to simple acids, mainly acetic, generally is needed as a first step to enter the TCA cycle. The preliminary reactions for a range of organic classes are shown in Fig. 7.5. Familiarity with these steps should allow judgments to be made concerning the amenability to biodegradation of some of the waste constituents encountered.

1. Carbohydrates
    (a) Hydrolyse to at least disaccharide stage before transfer through cell wall.
        Starch (alpha linkage) to glucose
        Cellulose (beta linkage) anaerobically to glucose
        Hemicellulose to glucose and xylose (pentose)
        Sucrose to glucose and fructose
        Lactose to glucose and galactose
        Maltose to glucose
    (b) Convert to pyruvic acid

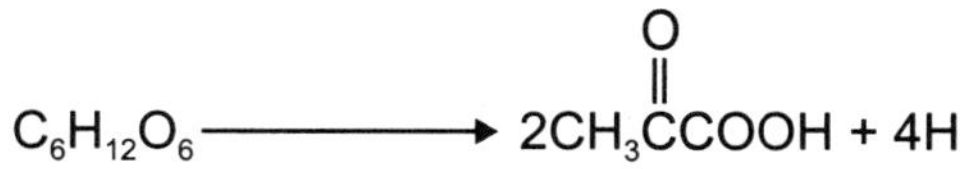

$$C_6H_{12}O_6 \longrightarrow 2CH_3\overset{\displaystyle O}{\overset{\|}{C}}COOH + 4H$$

(c) Convert to CO_2, H_2O, organic acids, ethanol

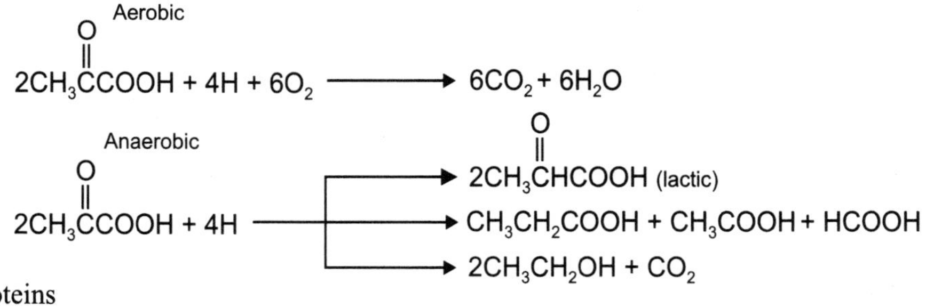

Aerobic

$$2CH_3\overset{\displaystyle O}{\overset{\|}{C}}COOH + 4H + 6O_2 \longrightarrow 6CO_2 + 6H_2O$$

Anaerobic

$$2CH_3\overset{\displaystyle O}{\overset{\|}{C}}COOH + 4H \longrightarrow \begin{cases} 2CH_3\overset{\displaystyle O}{\overset{\|}{C}}HCOOH \text{ (lactic)} \\ CH_3CH_2COOH + CH_3COOH + HCOOH \\ 2CH_3CH_2OH + CO_2 \end{cases}$$

2. Proteins
    (a) Hydrolysis

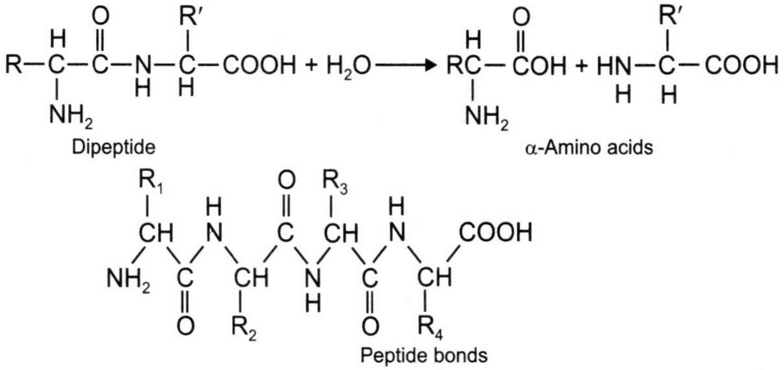

Dipeptide → α-Amino acids

Peptide bonds

Fig. 7.5. Preliminary biochemical reactions *(Contd ...)*.

(b) Deamination

Aerobic

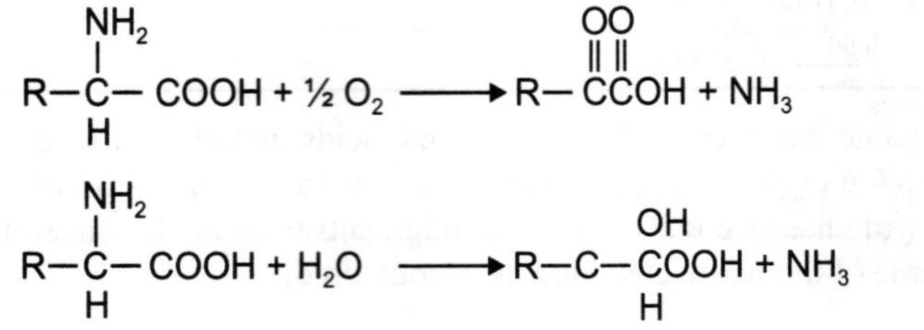

$$R-\underset{\underset{H}{|}}{\overset{\overset{NH_2}{|}}{C}}-COOH + \tfrac{1}{2}O_2 \longrightarrow R-\overset{\overset{OO}{||\ ||}}{CC}OH + NH_3$$

$$R-\underset{\underset{H}{|}}{\overset{\overset{NH_2}{|}}{C}}-COOH + H_2O \longrightarrow R-\underset{\underset{H}{|}}{\overset{\overset{OH}{|}}{C}}-COOH + NH_3$$

Anaerobic

$$R-\underset{\underset{H}{|}}{\overset{\overset{NH_2}{|}}{C}}-COOH + H_2 \longrightarrow R-CH_2-COOH + NH_3$$

$$R'-CH_2-\underset{\underset{H}{|}}{\overset{\overset{NH_2}{|}}{C}}-COOH \longrightarrow R'-\overset{\overset{H}{|}}{C}=\overset{\overset{H}{|}}{C}-COOH + NH_3$$

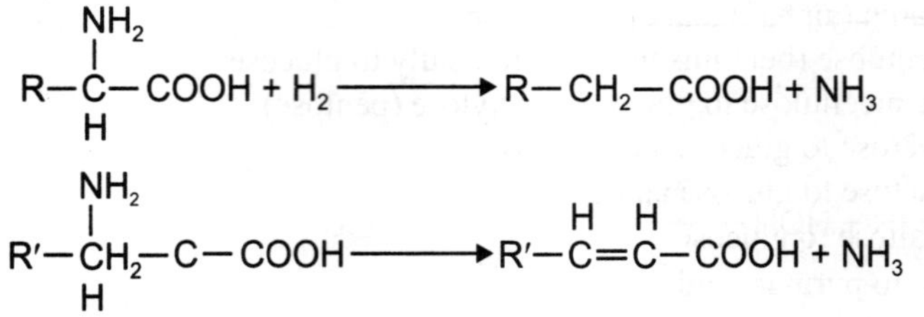

3. Fats and oils

Hydrolysis

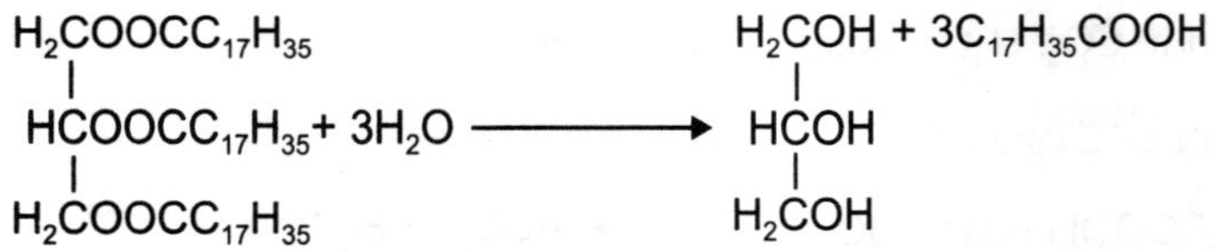

$$\begin{matrix} H_2COOCC_{17}H_{35} \\ | \\ HCOOCC_{17}H_{35} + 3H_2O \\ | \\ H_2COOCC_{17}H_{35} \end{matrix} \longrightarrow \begin{matrix} H_2COH + 3C_{17}H_{35}COOH \\ | \\ HCOH \\ | \\ H_2COH \end{matrix}$$

Stearin   Glycerol   Stearic acid

4. Acids (β oxidation with coenzyme A)

Aerobic

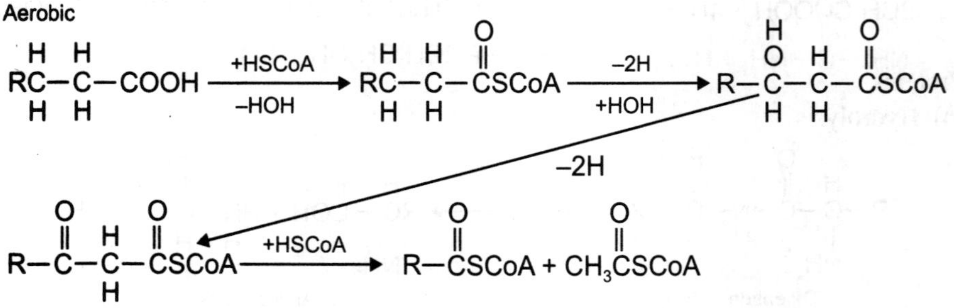

$$RC\underset{\underset{H}{|}}{\overset{\overset{H}{|}}{}}-\underset{\underset{H}{|}}{\overset{\overset{H}{|}}{C}}-COOH \xrightarrow[-HOH]{+HSCoA} RC\underset{\underset{H}{|}}{\overset{\overset{H}{|}}{}}-\underset{\underset{H}{|}}{\overset{\overset{H}{|}}{C}}-\overset{\overset{O}{||}}{C}SCoA \xrightarrow[+HOH]{-2H} R-\underset{\underset{H}{|}}{\overset{\overset{H}{|}}{C}}-\underset{\underset{H}{|}}{\overset{\overset{OH}{|}}{C}}-\overset{\overset{O}{||}}{C}SCoA$$

$$R-\overset{\overset{O}{||}}{C}-\underset{\underset{H}{|}}{\overset{\overset{H}{|}}{C}}-\overset{\overset{O}{||}}{C}SCoA \xrightarrow{+HSCoA} R-\overset{\overset{O}{||}}{C}SCoA + CH_3\overset{\overset{O}{||}}{C}SCoA$$

(−2H arrow)

$$4H + O_2 \longrightarrow 2H_2O$$

$$CH_3COSCoA + 2O_2 \longrightarrow 2CO_2 + 2H_2O \text{ (via TCA cycle)}$$

Anaerobic

$$CH_3COOH + 8/5NO_3^- \longrightarrow 8/5HCO_3^- + 4/5N_2 + 2/5CO_2 + 6/5H_2O$$

$$CH_3COOH + SO_4^= \longrightarrow 2CO_2 + 2H_2O + S^=$$

Fig. 7.5. Preliminary biochemical reactions *(Contd ...).*

$$CH_3COOH \longrightarrow CO_2 + CH_3$$

Also, $4H + 1/2CO_2 \longrightarrow 1/2CH_4 + H_2O$

5. Other aliphatics

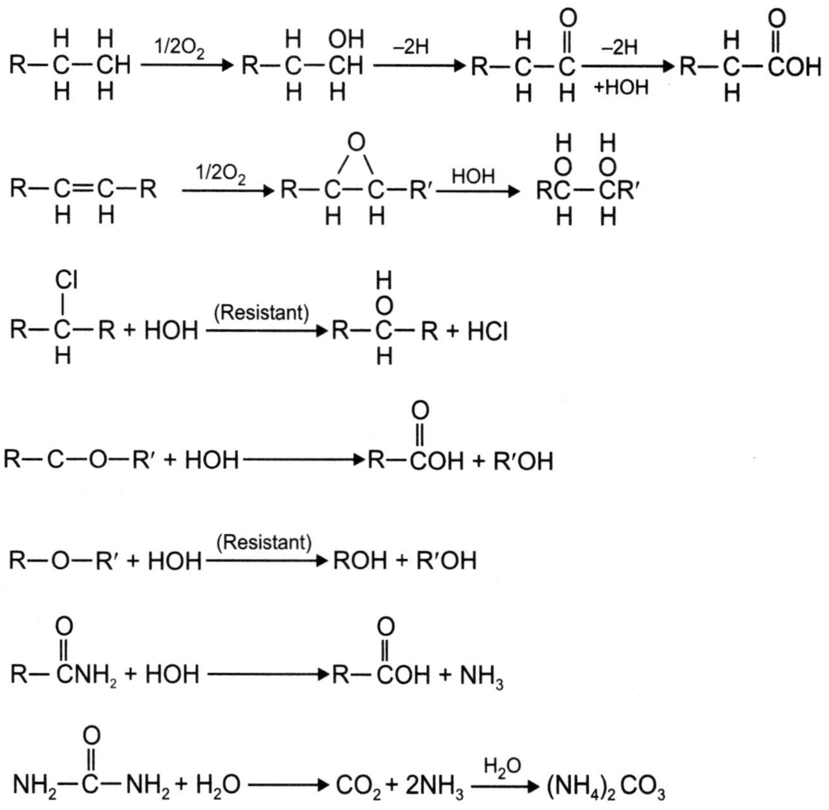

$$R-\underset{\underset{H}{|}}{\overset{\overset{H}{|}}{C}}-\underset{\underset{H}{|}}{\overset{\overset{H}{|}}{CH}} \xrightarrow{1/2O_2} R-\underset{\underset{H}{|}}{\overset{\overset{H}{|}}{C}}-\underset{\underset{H}{|}}{\overset{\overset{OH}{|}}{CH}} \xrightarrow{-2H} R-\underset{\underset{H}{|}}{\overset{\overset{H}{|}}{C}}-\overset{\overset{O}{\|}}{C}\overset{}{\underset{H}{|}} \xrightarrow[+HOH]{-2H} R-\underset{\underset{H}{|}}{\overset{\overset{H}{|}}{C}}-\overset{\overset{O}{\|}}{C}OH$$

$$R-\underset{\underset{H}{|}}{\overset{}{C}}=\underset{\underset{H}{|}}{\overset{}{C}}-R \xrightarrow{1/2O_2} R-\overset{\overset{O}{\triangle}}{C}-C-R' \xrightarrow{HOH} RC-CR'$$

$$R-\underset{\underset{H}{|}}{\overset{\overset{Cl}{|}}{C}}-R + HOH \xrightarrow{\text{(Resistant)}} R-\underset{\underset{H}{|}}{\overset{\overset{H}{O}}{C}}-R + HCl$$

$$R-C-O-R' + HOH \longrightarrow R-\overset{\overset{O}{\|}}{C}OH + R'OH$$

$$R-O-R' + HOH \xrightarrow{\text{(Resistant)}} ROH + R'OH$$

$$R-\overset{\overset{O}{\|}}{C}NH_2 + HOH \longrightarrow R-\overset{\overset{O}{\|}}{C}OH + NH_3$$

$$NH_2-\overset{\overset{O}{\|}}{C}-NH_2 + H_2O \longrightarrow CO_2 + 2NH_3 \xrightarrow{H_2O} (NH_4)_2CO_3$$

6. Aromatics

Phenol $\xrightarrow{1/2O_2}$ Catechol $\xrightarrow{O_2}$ Cis, cis-muconic acid $\xrightarrow{+HOH}$ β-keto adipic acid

$$CH_3COOH + \underset{CH_2-COOH}{\overset{CH_2-COOH}{|}} \longleftarrow \text{β-keto adipic acid}$$

Acetic acid   Succinic acid

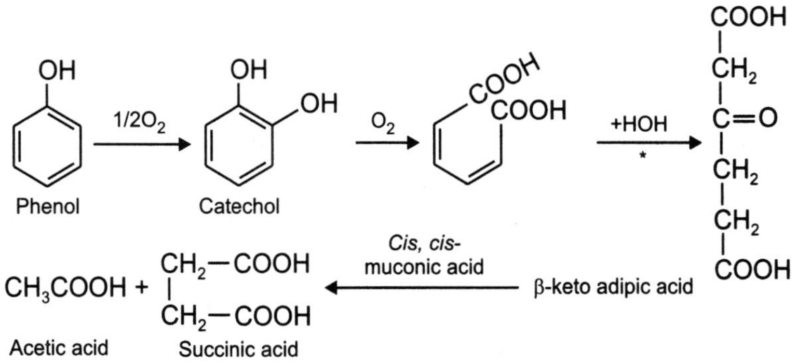

*Via (+)—muconolactone and β-keto adipic enol lactone

Fig. 7.5. Preliminary biochemical reactions.

Biodegradability

The resistance of certain organic materials to rapid degradation in a given situation can be related to several mechanisms:

Nonexistence of an active organism or enzyme

Violation of comparative biochemical sequences

Violation of enzyme specificity

Lack of sufficient energy or carbon for growth

Lack of an essential nutrient

Exceeding microbial tolerance to environmental factors

Toxicity of substrate or products of its metabolism

Inhibition or inactivation of an extracellular enzyme

Failure of a chemical to penetrate a cell

Concentration of substrate in aqueous solution being too low

Lack of induction of a requisite enzyme

Need for extracellular enzymes from different organisms

Inaccessibility of a substrate to a micro-organism

Complexing of a substrate with a polyaromatic or with other resistant organic compounds

Inaccessibility of the site on substrate to be acted on enzymatically

Consideration of these factors can lead to improvements ranging from slight modifications in problem molecules for increased biodegradability to the addition of a trace nutrient required by specific bacterial species. While only a few naturally occurring chemicals are resistant to rapid biodegradation, e.g. polyaromatics such as lignin, problems are encountered in degrading many synthetic organic chemicals. Foremost examples of resistant synthetic materials are certain compounds within the classes of chlorinated hydrocarbon pesticides, polychlorinated biphenyls, synthetic polymers, and surfactants. Other compounds which need special consideration when planning treatment approaches are listed in Table 7.5.

Table 7.5. Example organic compounds potentially resistant to rapid degradation.

Acetylethanolamine	2,2-Dimethyl-1, 3-propanediol
Acetyl morpholine	2,2-Dimethylsuccinic acid
Aminobenzenesulphonic acids	Dinitrobenzenes
tert-Amyl alcohol	Dioxane
Anthraquinone sulphonic acid	bis-2-Ethoxy ethyl ether
tert-Butanol	Ethylenediamine tetraacetic acid
Chloroanilines	Methoxyanilines
Chloronitrobenzenes	Morpholine
Chlorophenols, meta-substituted	Nitroanilines
Diaminobenzenes	Nitroanisoles
2,6-Dibromohexanoic acid	Nitrobenzenesulphonic acids
Dichloroacetic acid	Nitrotoluenes
2,3-Dichloropropionic acid	Pentaerythritol
Diethylaniline	tert-Pentanol
Diethylene glycol	Phenoxyalkyl carboxylic acids,
Diethyl ether	α-substituted

(Contd ...)

3,3-Diethylglutaric acid	2-Phenylbutyric acid
3,3-Dimethyl-1-butanol	Poly(ethylene glycol)400
2,2-Dimethylglutaric acid	Tetraethylene glycol
1,1-Dimethylhexanol	Toluene sulphonic acid
Dimethylmalonic acid	Triethanolamine
2,2-Dimethyloctanoic acid	Triethylene glycol
1,1-Dimethyl-1-pentanol	Trimethylacetic acid
2,2-Dimethyl-1-pentanol	

Note: Omitted from list are certain members of the chlorinated-hydrocarbon pesticide, polychlorinated-biphenyl, synthetic-polymer, and surfactant classes.

Many techniques available for the experimental determination of biodegradability have been described by Waggy, Price, Conway, and others. Test methods include:

1. Biochemical oxygen demand (BOD) by dilution bottle method.
2. Oxygen uptake by respirometry or oxygen electrode.
3. Die-away under river water conditions.
4. Shake culture tests.
5. Techniques simulating biological treatment systems.
6. Tests in soil environment.
7. Techniques for photochemical and chemical alteration.

Results from BOD tests on a range of synthetic organic chemicals are presented in Table 7.6.

Table 7.6. BOD determinations on typical synthetic organic chemicals.

Product tested	Water solubility, g/100 ml of solution	Theoretical oxygen demand, mg/mg	Measured COD mg/mg	Biooxidation, per cent							
				Nonacclimated				Acclimated			
				Days				Days			
				5	10	15	20	5	10	15	20
Acetic acid (neutralised)	C	1.07	1.09	76	82	85	96	–	–	–	–
Acetone	C	2.20	2.00	56	76	83	84	–	–	–	–
Benzene	0.17	3.10	1.40	24	27	24	29	58	67	76	80
n-Butanol	7.7	2.59	2.45	68	87	92	92	–	–	–	
n-Butyl acetate	0.68	2.20	2.32	58	68	70	83	–	–	–	–
Cumene	0.05*	3.50	1.13	40	62	63	70	–	–	–	–
Di-decylphthalate	0.2	2.69	2.50	1	1	1	0	7	10	3	7
Diethanolamine	95	1.52	1.47	17	72	81	88	–	–	–	–
Diethylene glycol	C	1.50	1.49	5	8	13	30	43	55	61	67
Diethylene glycol monoenthyl ether	C	1.90	1.74	17	71	75	87	–	–	–	–
Diethylenetriamine	C	1.55	1.57	4	4	4	0	23	46	51	70
Di-2-ehtyl-hexyl phthalate	0.2	2.58	2.74	0	0	–	0	13	0	6	23
Diisobutyl ketone	0.05	2.93	2.88	4	39	57	88	–	–	–	–

(Contd ...)

Product tested	Water solubility, g/100 ml of solution	Theoretical oxygen demand, mg/mg	Measured COD mg/mg	Biooxidation, per cent							
				Nonacclimated Days				Acclimated Days			
				5	10	15	20	5	10	15	20
Epoxidised soyabean oil	0.03*	–	2.24	1	1	0	0	4	–	13	24
Ethanol	C	2.10	1.99	74	74	95	84	–	–	–	–
Ethyl acetate	8.5	1.82	1.69	62	62	69	69	–	–	–	–
Ethyl acrylate	2	1.92	1.71	28	32	32	35	66	74	76	79
Ethylenediamine	C	1.33	1.30	24	44	55	47	36	45	56	70
Ethylene dichloride	0.81	0.97	0.025	0	18	–	–	–	–	–	–
Ehtylene glycol	C	1.30	1.29	34	86	92	100	–	–	–	–
Ethylene glycol monobutyl ether	C	2.30	2.25	26	74	82	88	–	–	–	–
Ethylene glycol monoethyl ether acetate	23	1.81	1.76	36	79	82	80	–	–	–	–
Ethylene glycol monoethyl ether	C	1.80	1.98	36	88	92	100	–	–	–	–
Ethylene glycol monomethyl ether	C	1.68	1.64	30	62	74	88	–	–	–	–
Ethyl hexanol	0.07	2.95	2.79	26	75	78	86	–	–	–	–
Ethyl hexyl acrylate	<0.01	2.60	2.48	0	24	29	30	9	15	23	40
Ethoxy triglycol	C	1.89	1.78	8	47	63	71	–	–	–	–
Formic acid (neutralised)	C	0.40	0.36	48	45	60	60	45	41	34	53
Hexylene glycol	C	2.30	2.11	2	29	47	48	55	85	88	90
Isobutanol	8.5	2.59	2.39	64	73	76	72	46	71	75	81
Isobutyl acetate	0.63	2.20	1.43	60	74	79	81	–	–	–	–
Isodecanol (mixed isomers)	0.04*	3.03	2.87	24	44	42	39	14	26	45	32
Isophorone	1.2	2.78	2.64	0	13	47	42	–	–	–	–
Isopropanol	C	2.40	2.30	28	77	80	78	–	–	–	–
Isopropyl acetate	2.9	2.04	1.67	61	72	74	76	47	53	54	62
Linear alkyl benzene	0.04*	3.18	2.31	–	–	–	–	16	5	5	11
Methanol	C	1.50	1.50	76	88	91	95	–	–	–	–
Methyl amyl acetate	0.13	2.44	2.36	20	87	62	69	–	–	–	–
Methyl amyl alcohol	0.62*	2.82	2.64	50	72	90	94	–	–	–	–
Methyl ethyl ketone	26.8	2.44	2.23	76	82	84	89	–	–	–	–
Methyl isobutyl ketone	1.9	2.70	2.40	56	66	69	69	–	–	–	–
Octyl epoxytallate	0.06*	–	2.25	–	–	–	–	1	1	3	6
Phenol	8.4	2.40	2.30	90	89	87	96	–	–	–	–
Primary amyl acetate	0.2	2.33	2.22	64	76	67	72	–	–	–	–
n-Propanol	C	2.40	2.18	64	76	81	75	–	–	–	–
n-Propyl acetate	1.03*	2.04	2.04	62	80	75	72	–	–	–	–

(Contd ...)

Product tested	Water solubility, g/100 ml of solution	Theoretical oxygen demand, mg/mg	Measured COD mg/mg	Biooxidation, per cent							
				Nonacclimated				Acclimated			
				Days				Days			
				5	10	15	20	5	10	15	20
Propylene glycol	C	1.68	1.63	62	68	75	79	–	–	–	–
Styrene	0.03	3.07	2.88	65	65	78	87	–	–	–	–
Tetrahydronaphthalene	0.035*	3.15	2.50	–	–	–	–	–	–	–	–
Tetraethylene glycol	C	1.65	1.64	4	10	15	22	9	58	71	88
Toluene	0.08*	3.13	1.40	53	62	70	80	73	74	80	86
Triethanolamine	C	1.61	1.52	8	9	45	66	–	–	–	–
Triethylene glycol	C	1.60	1.60	4	10	17	24	32	64	77	80
Vinyl acetate	2	1.67	1.39	34	34	31	32	62	70	66	72

* Solubility measured at 25°C in synthetic seawater. Other values are for distilled water. C = completely miscible. BOD tests run in standard dilution water not seawater.

Biological treatment processes are categorised according to the growth-phase of the bacteria, the method of contacting the organic food with the bacteria, and the presence or absence of molecular oxygen. The common types of systems are:

1. Activated sludge.
2. Aerated stabilisation.
3. Fixed film systems.
4. Anaerobic systems.
5. Stabilisation ponds.

The basic features of each system, along with experimental design approaches and process equipment descriptions will be covered in the remainder of this chapter.

ACTIVATED SLUDGE REACTION SYSTEMS

Flow Schemes and Reaction Kinetics

The activated-sludge process can stabilise soluble organic material to a low level in a short period because a high concentration of flocculant biological solids is maintained in the aerated or oxygenated tank in which the waste and bacteria are contacted. This concentration is maintained by routing the mixed liquor flowing from the aeration tank through a secondary clarifier, and recycling most of the settled solids back to the aeration tank. This concept is illustrated in Fig. 7.6 for three basic types of systems: staged or plug, completely mixed, and contact-stabilisation. The staged or plug-flow system has inherent kinetic advantages when the reaction rate is dependent upon the residual organic concentration; however, the effect of transient loads at the influent end of the basin may be more pronounced. The completely mixed system operates under more steady reactor conditions, but a lower driving force for the reactions is present. In a contact-stabilisation system the waste is contacted with the bacteria for only a brief period before flowing to the settling tank. The return biological solids are aerated for a relatively long period to allow oxidation of the adsorbed and stored organic matter to occur prior to re-entry of the cells into the contact chamber.

Evaluation of the activated sludge system for a particular application can be achieved best by first representing the system as a mathematical model, and then determining the necessary coefficients by running laboratory or pilot reactors at various loading rates while measuring organic reduction, biomass production, oxygen utilisation, and biomass settleability. Results from these determinations need to be tempered by practical engineering judgements before their application. All notations and symbols used are compliled in Appendix 7.1.

The rate of the biological reactions governs the selection of the key design parameters of the biological system, i.e. the detention time and the biomass concentration, or more basically, as will be discussed later, the cell residence time and food to micro-organism ratio. In order for the micro-organisms to grow and metabolise the waste constituents, they obviously must be left in the system long enough to reproduce. The kinetics of biological growth have been studied in great depth and many models are available. Only the key elements of two approaches are summarised herein without extensive derivation.

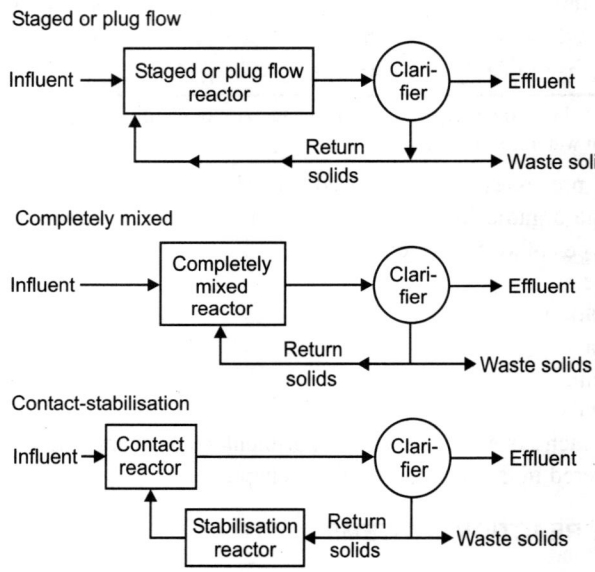

Fig. 7.6. Major activated sludge process variations.

The effluent quality in terms of soluble BOD from a completely mixed activated sludge system may be predicted under many conditions by using the relationship of liquid detention time and concentration of biological solids as developed by Adams.

$$\frac{S_e}{S_o} = \frac{1}{1 + KX_v t} \qquad \qquad ...\,(7.1)$$

where,

S_e = effluent dissolved BOD, mg/l

S_o = influent dissolved BOD, mg/l

K = reaction rate coefficient (independent of S_o in this model, l/mg-hr)

X_v = mixed liquor volatile suspended solids (MLVSS), mg/l

t = average liquid retention time, hr

While the relationship deals with the usually more important soluble BOD, organics in the form of large suspended solids in the waste-water are enmeshed in the floc; also, colloidal organics are flocculated and adsorbed. Their subsequent dissolution and assimilation needs to be considered in these models when concentrations are significant relative to soluble constituents. Also, refinements can be made to the above and subsequent relationships by expressing the MLVSS level as active biomass when the nonviable fraction is high due to contained nonliving volatile matter. Another limitation is that it applies best when treating to relatively low effluent levels. The relationship is Eq. 7.1 assumes an approximate first-order reaction rate. When considering the total amount of soluble substrate remaining at any time, however, the actual kinetic relationship is likely the simulation of multiple zero order reactions down to low substrate levels. This is not true when sequential reactions occur.

Although the Eckenfelder 'first-order' model has considerable utility, the trend seems to be toward modelling biological growth kinetics (growth and substrate removal) by procedures developed by Monod, based on the Michaelis-Menten hypothesis for rates of enzyme-catalysed reactions. Monod kinetics were related to waste treatment processes by Lawrence and McCarty and later a multiprocess biological treatment model was published by Christenson and McCarty. Their contribution was to incorporate removal and growth kinetics into a single approach. The Monod equations can be written as:

$$\mu = \frac{dX_a}{dt} \cdot \frac{1}{X_a} \qquad \qquad ...(7.2)$$

where,

μ = specific (per unit mass) growth rate in the system, hr^{-1} ... mg growth/mg biomass-hr
X_a = active biomass concentration usually approximated by MLVSS, mg/l
t = time, hr

also,

$$\mu = \mu_{max} \left(\frac{S}{K_s + S} \right) \qquad \qquad ...(7.3)$$

where,

μ_{max} = maximum specific growth rate under defined conditions or rate that a plot of μ vs S asymptotically reaches (see Fig. 7.7), hr^{-1}. Note that specific growth rate is directly proportional to specific rate of substrate utilisation.

S = substrate concentration in the reactor, mg/l.

K_s = half velocity constant or substrate concentration resulting in $\mu = 0.5\ \mu_{max}$ (see Fig. 7.7), mg/l.

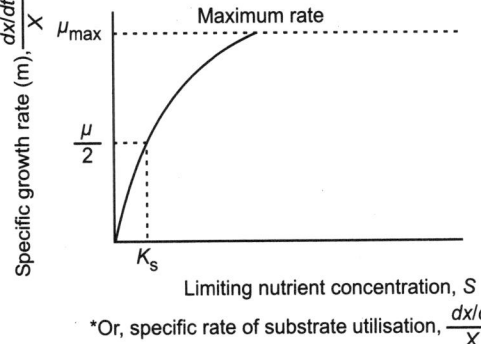

Fig. 7.7. Monod kinetic relationships.

If one assumes that cell yield can be defined as mass of cells produced per unit mass of substrate consumed, then the rate of substrate metabolism can be related to the specific growth rate via the constant of proportionality, Y:

$$Y = \frac{dX}{dS} \qquad \text{... (7.4)}$$

where,

Y = maximum cell yield coefficient, g bacteria synthesised/g BOD_L consumed.

therefore,

$$\frac{dS}{dt} = -\frac{\mu_{max} X_a}{Y}\left(\frac{S}{K_s + S}\right) \qquad \text{... (7.5)}$$

Division of μ_{max} by Y changes the expression to contain a substrate removal rate constant.

$$\frac{dS}{dt} = \frac{K'' X_a S}{K_s + S} \qquad \text{... (7.6)}$$

The net growth of active organisms is related to the rate of substrate utilisation:

$$\frac{dX_a}{dt} = Y\frac{dS}{dt} - bX_a \qquad \text{... (7.7)}$$

where, b is the cell auto-oxidation rate coefficient, day^{-1}. Equations 7.6 and 7.7 and a mass balance for a complete mixed reactor can be used to yield the expression:

$$\frac{1}{\theta_c} = \frac{YK''S}{K_s + S} - b \qquad \text{... (7.8)}$$

as

$$\mu = \frac{1}{\theta_c} \qquad \text{... (7.9)}$$

where,

θ_c = solids or cell retention time, days

Solving for S, which is the same as S_e for a completely mixed reactor, in Eq. 7.8, yields:

$$S = \frac{K_s(1 + b\theta_c)}{\theta_c(YK'' - b) - 1} \qquad \text{... (7.10)}$$

BOD levels preferably are expressed as those after long-term incubation. Monod relationships also can be used to predict sludge yield and oxygen requirements.

In cases where $K_s \gg S$, i.e. low levels of substrate in a reactor (same as effluent in completely mixed system), Eq. 7.6 becomes first order with respect to substrate level, i.e.

$$\frac{dS}{dt} = -kX_a S \qquad \text{... (7.11)}$$

Integration yields the first order relationship for a continuously fed, complete mixed system.

$$\frac{S_e}{S_o} = \frac{1}{1 + KX_a t} \qquad \text{... (7.12)}$$

which is identical to Eq. 7.1. In cases where $S >> K_s$, Eq. 7.6 becomes zero order:

$$\frac{dS}{dt} = -kX_a \qquad \qquad \text{... (7.13)}$$

or

$$\frac{S_0 - S_e}{X_a t} = k_{max} \qquad \qquad \text{... (7.14)}$$

as shown in Fig. 7.7, which means that substrate removal proceeds at a constant, linear rate. In cases where S_e is neither very high nor about an order of magnitude smaller than K_s (i.e. the central curved portion of Fig. 7.7) other techniques need to be used. This can be the case when feed BOD levels are high and/or removal efficiencies are low; a typical value of K_s for a mixed waste is 200 mg/l. Equation 7.10 covers the whole range of S levels in a continuous manner.

The application of these relationships along with calculative means of reactor design, solids production, and oxygen requirements have been published by Christenson and McCarty. Reaction kinetics for a plug flow system are included. A simplified mathematical model of the complete mix activated sludge system has been developed by McKinney. Field data have verified its applicability to design and operational evaluation.

Temperature Effects

The removal rates for BOD assume an adequacy of other nutrients, such as nitrogen and phosphorus, and optimum levels of pH, oxygen, and mixing. The reaction rate constant is temperature dependent according to:

$$K_2 = K_1 \theta_t (T_2 - T_1) \qquad \qquad \text{... (7.15)}$$

where,

K_2 = organic removal rate coefficient at T_2, day^{-1}
K_1 = organic removal rate coefficient at T_1, day^{-1}
θ_t = temperature coefficient
T_2, T_1 = temperature, °C

The value for θ_t typically ranges from 1.03 to 1.15. This coefficient appears to increase with increasing waste strength and with the content of synthetic organic compounds that are more difficult to degrade. At a high S_0 of 4500 mg/l with a synthetic organic chemical waste, a θ_t of 1.25 was measured. Experimental determination is made by operating parallel systems at ambient and cold-weather conditions, and inserting the rate coefficients obtained into Eq. 7.15. At high θ_t values and low temperatures, the effects on effluent quality are drastic. The temperature of an open reactor using surface-entrainment aerators can be predicted based on flow rate, influent waste-water temperature, ambient air temperature, and installed horsepower. With closed systems, such as those using pure oxygen, heat losses are less.

Temperature level has effects other than upon reaction rates. Protozoan and rotifier populations are less above a temperature of about 36°C and usually are very low above 40°C. Decreased water viscosity tends to enhance flocculation and settling at a higher temperature. However, at about 35°C deflocculation can start to occur. At temperatures below about 18°C effluent solids level often increases. Some evidence suggests that less sludge is produced at higher temperatures as the rates of the oxidation reactions increase more than that of the synthesis reactions. Values for K_s generally increase with decreasing temperature, unlike rate constants.

Feed Concentration Effects

The substrate removal rate also can be affected by the initial strength of the waste-water according to the Grau model as extended by Adams, Eckenfelder, and Hovious. For a completely mixed reactor the relationship is:

$$\frac{S_o(S_o - S_e)}{X_v t} = K'S_e$$

.. (7.16)

where,

K' = reaction rate coefficient dependent on S_o for completely mixed system, l/mg-hr.

while for batch or plug-flow systems, the relationship is:

$$\frac{S_e}{S_o} = e^{-kX_v t / S_o}$$

... (7.17)

where,

k = batch-fed reaction coefficient

These models, which are new and require additional evaluation, imply that as the concentration of organics remaining in the reactor decreases, the rate of removal also decreases since the organics remaining are progressively becoming more difficult to remove. The completely mixed model holds particularly when the influent level is varying with step increases in incoming strength.

In cases where either COD or TOC is used in the model and nonbiodegradable organics are present, Eq. 7.16 can be modified:

$$\frac{(S_o - Z)(S_o - S_e)}{X_v t} = K'(S_e - Z)$$

... (7.18)

where,

Z = concentration of nondegradable organics in mg/l

This relationship would apply where data are taken in terms of COD or TOC and the effect of influent concentration needs to be considered.

Reaction Rate Determination

The value of K is determined by operating reactors at different loading levels (varying feed concentration, mixed liquor suspended solids, and retention time as appropriate) and measuring the achieved effluent level. Equation 7.1 is rearranged:

$$\frac{S_o - S_e}{X_v t} = K(S_e)$$

... (7.19)

A plot on the ordinate (Y axis) and abscissa (X axis) respectively of $S_o - S_e/X_v t$ vs. S_e with slope = K (S_o independent) yields the desired rate coefficient. Some typical values are listed in Table 7.7. An example at the top end of the typical range cited is a high strength waste of 4000 mg BOD/l, containing mostly volatile acids in which K was measured to be about 10×10^{-4} l/mg hr; however, a value of 2.5×10^{-4} l/mg-hr does seem typical for many chemical wastes. Likewise, after rearrangement of Eq. 7.16 and appropriate plotting $S_o(S_o - S_e)/X_v t$ vs. S_e with slope = K' (S_o dependent) yields the rate coefficient when it is dependent on influent concentration.

A unique rate constant does not exist for a particular waste. In reality, rate constants vary considerably from day to day, primarily due to the feed variability. The extent of feed variability is indicated by the scatter in the above plots; a range encompassing a desired degree of confidence can be used. This is an alternative means of arriving at the variability portion of the approach.

Table 7.7. Typical coefficients and constants for activated sludge treatment of wastes from the chemical industry using the Eckenfelder model.

Systems	Range of values of one standard deviation	Average value
K, l/mg-hr	0.00012–0.00076	0.00024
a	0.31–0.72	0.52
a'	0.31–0.76	0.53
b, day^{-1}	0.02–0.18	0.07
b', day^{-1}	0.10–0.24	0.17
F:M, lb. BOD/ (lb. MLVSS) (day)	0.4–0.8	0.5

Similar calculative means are available using Monod kinetics in cases where first-order reaction rates do not apply.

System Limitations

One further point concerning the application of kinetic data needs to be kept in mind. In addition to materials which are nondegradable in a structural sense, the concept of a 'residual BOD' level should be considered. Biological systems treating relatively high strength waste-waters generally do not decrease the BOD to the low levels predictable from the kinetic models. This can be attributed to several factors, all of which are related to the fact that the sample collected under conditions in the biological treatment system reactor is tested in a BOD dilution bottle under simulated stream conditions:

1. Equilibrium established with the high level of reactor solids is shifted under the low level of seed in the BOD bottle.
2. Reseeding in the BOD bottle allows a culture to develop specific to the residual structures present.
3. Essential micronutrients (for specific species) depleted in the reactor are replenished in the BOD bottle.
4. Surface adsorption in the BOD bottle increases the effectiveness of the conversions.
5. Dilution of inhibitory end products allows reinitiation or acceleration of the reactions.
6. Growth of nitrifiers and higher microbial forms would be enhanced due to the dilution of inhibitory constituents.
7. Degradation of the residual materials requires the longer incubation periods afforded in the BOD test.

For these reasons, as well as the relationships developed by Grau, the models should not be extrapolated to achieve very low levels of BOD starting at a high strength, especially with synthetic organic waste-waters. Even with low strength industrial wastes, the lowest achievable levels seem to be about 10 to 15 mg/l. Some long-term effluent values measured under warm-temperature conditions for reasonably designed treatment systems at three petrochemical plants are plotted in Fig. 7.8. Data are also plotted for a single laboratory study of municipal wastes which had been concentrated by vacuum distillation. Practical achievable BOD removal efficiency in a single step system is on the order of 90 to 95 per cent.

The effect of feed variability on achievable effluent quality also needs to be emphasised. The data in Table 7.8 show that not only is the average effluent level increased by a factor of 8, but the range of effluent quality is increased by a factor of 15 under highly variable conditions.

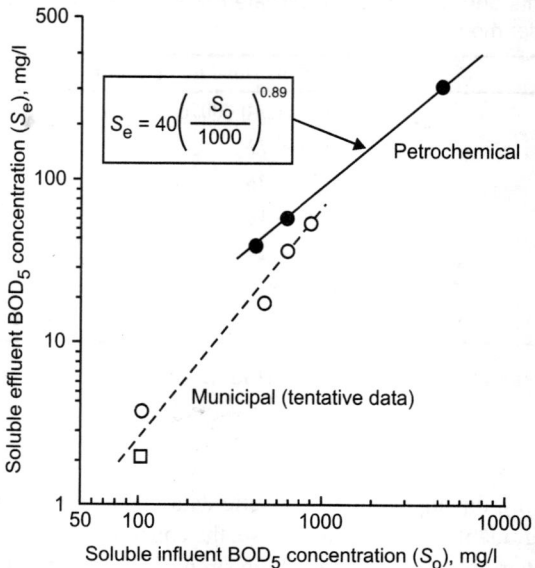

$$S_e = 40 \left(\frac{S_o}{1000} \right)^{0.89}$$

Fig. 7.8. Soluble effluent BOD values for biological treatment systems as a function of influent BOD.

Table 7.8. Summarised data from laboratory study of feed variability effects.

	Constant feed[b]	*Highly variable feed[b]*
Influent BOD, mg/l[a]		
Average	1400	1400
Standard deviation	120	850
Effluent BOD, mg/l		
Average	22	180
Standard deviation	16	240
BOD removal (average), per cent	98	87
Variability reduction, per cent of initial standard deviation on absolute basis	87	72

[a] All BOD data are on a soluble basis. Results shown are the average from duplicated reactors. Average F/M and MLVSS concentration were 0.72 d^{-1} and 2200 mg/l, respectively.

[b] Constant feed consisted of a mixture of 14 1-hour composite samples of petrochemical waste-water collected at random over a 3-day period. The units receiving this feed were subject only to a small degree of quantitative variability. Variable feed units were fed the hourly composite samples individually on a 12-hour cycle, i.e. the feed was changed between composites once every 12-hour. The variable-feed units, therefore, were subjected to a high degree of quantitative and qualitative variability, although on the average they received the same feed as the constant-feed units.

Biomass Production

The production of biomass is the net effect of growth due to substrate conversion and cellular autooxidation:

$$\Delta X_{vt} = aS_{rt} - bf_bX_{vt} \qquad \qquad \text{... (7.20)}$$

where,

ΔX_{vt} = change in MLVSS, lb/day (kg/day)

a = fraction of substrate removed converted to cells

S_{rt} = substrate removed in terms of BOD_5, lb/day (kg/day)

b = cell autooxidation rate coefficient, day^{-1}

X_{vt} = total weight of volatile suspended solids in aeration tank, lb (kg)

f_b = fraction of generated biomass that is degradable, decreases with sludge age, experimentally determinable or computable by:

$$f_b = \frac{aS_{rt} + bX_{vt}\sqrt{(aS_{rt} + bX_{vt})^2 - (4bX_{vt})(0.77\,aS_{rt})}}{2\,bX_{vt}} \qquad \qquad \text{... (7.21)}$$

The accumulation of solids, both organic and inorganic, from non-biological sources also needs to be considered when calculating excess solids which require disposal. Wood pulping fines and calcium carbonate are examples of materials accumulating in biological flocs.

$$\Delta X_t = rX_{ot} + \frac{\Delta X_v}{f_v} - X_{et} \qquad \qquad \text{... (7.22)}$$

where,

ΔX_t = total excess sludge, lb/day (kg/day)

X_{ot} = total influent suspended solids, lb/day (kg/day)

r = nondegradable fraction of influent suspended solids

f_v = ratio of MLVSS/MLSS

X_{et} = total effluent suspended solids, lb/day

A common value for f_v is 0.8.

When running the experimental units to determine substrate removal efficiency, biosolids production also is measured by a daily solids balance. Equation 7.20 is rearranged:

$$\frac{\Delta X_{vt}}{f_bX_{vt}} = a\left(\frac{S_{rt}}{f_bX_{vt}}\right) - b \qquad \qquad \text{... (7.23)}$$

Plot on the Y and X axes, respectively:

$$\frac{\Delta X_{vt}}{f_bX_{vt}} \text{ vs. } \frac{S_{rt}}{f_bX_{vt}}$$

$$\frac{\text{lb VSS produced}}{\text{lb biodegradable VSS-day}} \text{ vs. } \frac{\text{lb organics removed}}{\text{lb biodegradable VSS-day}}$$

Slope = a; Y intercept = $-b$.

The fraction of biodegradable solids can be determined by aerating without feeding a sample of mixed liquor and plotting the solids concentration versus time. Extrapolation of the plot will approach the nondegradable level. Published correlations indicate fractions about 0.74 at F/M of 0.8 day^{-1}, 0.36 at F/M of 0.4 day^{-1}, and 0.31 at F/M of 0.1 day^{-1}.

Typical values for other coefficients in the model are presented in Table 7.7; values for use when Monod relationships are used also are available.

Factors which influence cell yield have been reviewed by Ramanathan and Gaudy. Random variations in predominant species in the treatment system had the major effect. Various species have different partitioning of the synthesis and respiration pathways. Although the free energy of a given substrate can be used to predict available energy for synthesis, this concept was over-shadowed by species variations.

Oxygen Requirements

Requirements for oxygen to be supplied through aeration or pure oxygenation may be predicted from the additive effects of substrate removal and biomass autooxidation.

$$O_t = a'S_{rt} + b'f_b X_{vt} \qquad \qquad ... (7.24)$$

where,

O_t = total oxygen required, lb./day (kg/day)

a' = oxygen utilisation coefficient for substrate conversion, lb O_2 required/lb BOD_5 removed (kg/kg)

b' = oxygen utilisation rate for endogenous respiration, lb O_2/day-lb MLVSS (kg/day-kg)

When a chemical oxygen demand, such as for sulphite oxidation, must be supplied, that requirement needs to be added. Likewise, when the system converts ammonia to nitrate (nitrification), a requirement of up to 4.6 lb O_2/lb NH_3 oxidised is added. Nitrification requires long mean cell residence times for the slowly growing responsible species. The sensitivity of nitrifiers to pH, temperature, and chemical inhibitors reduces nitrification processes to a negligible rate in many industrial wastes.

Oxygen utilisation is followed in experimental units by measuring oxygen uptake rate under a range of conditions. Rearrangement of Eq. 7.24 yields:

$$\frac{O_t}{f_b X_{vt}} = a'\frac{S_{rt}}{f_b X_{vt}} - b' \qquad \qquad ... (7.25)$$

Plot on the Y and X axes, respectively:

$$\frac{O_t}{f_b X_{vt}} \text{ vs. } \frac{S_{rt}}{f_b X_{vt}}$$

$$\frac{\text{lb } O_2 \text{ required}}{\text{lb biodegradable VSS-day}} \text{ vs. } \frac{\text{lb organics removed}}{\text{lb biodegradable VSS-day}}$$

Slope = a'; Y intercept = $-b'$.

The sum of the biomass produced and oxygen utilised should be checked, on an oxygen equivalent basis, versus substrate removed according to the relationship:

$$O_t = (y)(S_{rt}) - 1.42 (X_{wt} + X_{et}) \qquad \qquad ... (7.26)$$

where,

y = lb BOD_L/lb BOD_5

BOD_L = BOD measurable through long-term incubation (or removable COD)

X_{wt} = total biological solids wasted, lb/day

X_{et} = total effluent biological solids, lb/day

1.42 is lb O_2 required to oxidise 1 lb of biomass of formulation $C_5H_7O_2N$

Loading Factor

One important parameter affecting design and operation is the food-to-micro-organism ratio:

$$F/M = \frac{S_a}{(X_{vt})} \qquad \qquad \dots (7.27)$$

where,

F/M = food-to-micro-organism ratio, day^{-1}

S_a = substrate (BOD$_5$) applied, lb/day (kg/day)

X_{vt} = average MLVSS in aeration tank, lb (kg)

The previously cited relationships infer that as F/M increases, the extent of soluble BOD removal decreases, the oxygen requirement decreases, and the biomass production increases for a given amount of waste treated.

An additional important effect of the F/M ratio is on the settleability of the biomass. Optimum settleability usually is achieved between values of about 0.1 to 0.8/day; presumably because at lower levels the polymeric materials enhancing cell flocculation are excessively degraded and at higher levels polymer production decreases due to high growth rates. Filamentous growths also are stimulated at high loadings.

When the experimental units are run to determine substrate reduction, oxygen requirements, and solids production, effluent solids levels should be measured and plotted versus F/M to indicate the levels achievable. Results from larger pilot units can be used with more confidence. Suspended solids levels in both the effluent from the test unit and the supernatant from settling tests of the mixed liquor in a slowly stirred graduated cylinder (simulates idealised settler) should be measured. Determinations of soluble and total BOD levels are made on effluent or supernatant samples collected at various loadings. A plot of mg BOD/mg VSS versus F/M is useful in calculating total effluent BOD levels when soluble effluent BOD and effluent suspended solids levels are known. A value of 0.3 mg BOD$_5$/mg VSS is common.

The initial settling velocity in the graduated cylinder test also should be plotted versus F/M to indicate the rates achievable. Sludge thickening rates may need to be noted for use in clarifier design by one method, as discussed in a later section. Levels of MLVSS usually are maintained between 1500 and 8000 mg/l, depending on an optimised balance between clarifier and reactor costs as well as upon operating and performance considerations.

Cell Residence Time or Sludge Age

Many kinetic models are expressed in terms of mean cell residence time (θ_c); this can be related to F/M by:

$$1/\theta_c = (a)(F/M) - b \qquad \qquad \dots (7.28)$$

Mean cell residence time is calculatable by this equation:

$$\theta_c = \frac{X_{at}}{X_{wt} + X_{et}} \qquad \qquad \dots (7.29)$$

where,

X_{at} = average weight of biological solids maintained in reactor, lb

X_{wt} = weight of biological solids wasted, lb/day

X_{et} = weight of biological solids in the effluent, lb/day

or, by this relationship,

$$\theta_c = \frac{X_{vt}}{\Delta X_{vt}} \qquad \qquad \dots (7.30)$$

The mean cell residence time or sludge age is a basic control parameter as it can be related to micro-organism generation time. When transformations involving slowly growing micro-organisms are involved (e.g. those involved in nitrogen oxidation and certain polymeric degradations) longer cell residence times must be provided. As with F/M, the settleability of the biological solids can be related to θ_c for various types of waste-waters (Table 7.9). Incidentally, adverse effects of high salt levels on settleability can overshadow θ_c effects.

Table 7.9. Example of sludge settling properties for various modifications of the activated sludge process with a synthetic, degradable feed.

Modification	Solids retention time (θ_c), days	Sludge settling properties
High rate (rapid assimilation)	0.25–2	Predominantly dispersed growth; practically no zone settling; SVI > 250
Conventional activated sludge	2–6	Well-formed floc; zone settling velocity between 2 and 6 ft. hr^{-1} ; SVI ranges from 580 (at 2 days) to 125 (at 6 days)
Extended aeration	6–30	Pinpoint floc; deflocculated particles; zone settling velocity averages 15 ft. hr^{-1}; SVI about 100

Nutrient Requirements

In order to support cell synthesis, nitrogen and phosphorus must be added if deficient in the waste stream. These are usually added at a level in proportion to the BOD removed.

$$\text{Nitrogen required in lb/day} = \frac{S_{rt}}{20} \qquad \qquad \dots (7.31)$$

$$\text{Phosphorus required in lb/day} = \frac{S_{rt}}{100} \qquad \qquad \dots (7.32)$$

Nitrogen usually is added as ammonia, and phosphorus as phosphoric acid. Organic sources in the wastes, such as degradable amines, need to be considered when calculating addition requirements.

Instead of using the average ratios given above, the consideration that while new cells average 12.4 per cent nitrogen and 2.6 per cent phosphorus, these levels will decrease after endogenous oxidation to 7.0 per cent and 1.0 per cent, can be taken into account.

$$\text{lb N/day} = \frac{0.124\,f\Delta X_{vt}}{0.77} + 0.07\frac{(0.77-f)\Delta X_{vt}}{0.77} \qquad \qquad \dots (7.33)$$

$$\text{lb P/day} = \frac{0.026\,f\Delta X_{vt}}{0.77} + 0.01\frac{(0.77-f)\Delta X_{vt}}{0.77} \qquad \qquad \dots (7.34)$$

In addition to nitrogen and phosphorus, the adequacy of other elements, such as iron, sulphur, magnesium, and manganese, needs to be established, especially for waste-water coming from a single manufacturing operation where contamination by a range of materials is less likely to have occurred. Trace, but not toxic, copper and zinc levels also should be checked. Sodium, potassium, calcium, and chloride are required in substantial quantities, but usually are present. Certain protists, especially higher forms, require boron, molybdenum, vanadium, cobalt, iodine, and/or selenium. Nutrient deficiencies affect not only substrate conversion but also biomass settleability. Proper floc formation seems to be hampered; and excessive filamentous organisms, which have a lesser nutrient requirement, can develop.

AERATION/MIXING

When air is used, the oxygen requirement (O_t) for activated sludge systems, calculated using Eq. 7.24, is supplied by one of several means:
1. Surface-entrainment aerators.
2. Diffused aeration.
3. Sparged turbine aeration.
4. Venturi (jet) aeration.
5. Static-mixer aeration.
6. Brush aerators.

The system selected also needs to provide adequate macro-turbulence to keep the biological floc in suspension and micro-turbulence to enhance substrate bacterial contact.

Transfer Efficiency

The oxygen transfer efficiency of the device can be specified as:

$$N_a = N_s \frac{\beta C_{sw} - C_L}{C_s} \alpha \theta_o{}^{T_w - 20} \qquad \ldots (7.35)$$

where,

N_a = O_2 transfer efficiency at application conditions in the field, lb. O_2/hp-hr (kg/joule $\times$ 5.92×10^6)

N_s = oxygen transfer efficiency under standard conditions (tap water at zero dissolved oxygen, 20°C, and 760 mm Hg), lb/hp-hr (kg/joule $\times 5.92 \times 10^6$)

β = ratio of dissolved oxygen level at saturation in reactor liquor to that in pure tap water

C_{sw} = dissolved oxygen saturation level calculated for reactor liquor at design pressure and liquor temperature, mg/l

C_L = design operating dissolved oxygen concentration, mg/l

C_s = dissolved-oxygen saturation concentration at standard conditions, mg/l

α = ratio of $K_L a$ of reactor liquor to that of pure water

$K_L a$ = overall oxygen transfer coefficient, mg O_2/mg O_2 deficit-hr

θ_c = temperature adjustment coefficient for oxygen transfer

T_w = design reactor temperature, °C

The standard transfer efficiencies usually are determined for the various types and sizes of aerators by the equipment manufacturers through reoxygenation rate tests either in large test tanks or in field installations as described by Conway and Kumke and by Nogaj.

The β factor is determined by aerating a sample of filtered mixed liquor (or effluent from a completely mixed reactor) and dividing the equilibrium level by that obtained with tap water at the same pressure and temperature. Salt content depresses the saturation level (0.1 mg/l by each 100 mg/l of chloride ion at 15°C) as do other materials. Typical values for β are 0.90 to 0.98. For surface-entrainment aeration, C_{sw} is obtained by multiplying the saturation value at the design temperature by $p/760$, where p is the design atmospheric pressure in mm mercury (kN/cm^2 $\times$ 7.50). Usually, C_L is selected at 2 mg/l for well-mixed, air-based systems. And, C_s equals 9.2 mg/l at the surface at 20°C. In the case of submerged aerators, the effect of increased pressure creates an average C_{sw} according to:

$$C_{sw} = C_{sa}\left(\frac{P_b}{29.4} + \frac{O_v}{42}\right) \qquad \text{... (7.36)}$$

where,

C_{sa} = oxygen saturation at one atmosphere pressure, mg/l

p_b = absolute pressure at depth of air release, psia (kN/m^2 × 0.145 or kgf/cm^2 × 14.2)

O_v = volume concentration of oxygen in gas leaving the test unit, per cent

An assumed value for O_v can be used for initial calculations; the correctness of C_s will be evident from the straightness of the plot of log oxygen-saturation deficit versus time.

The α factor usually is determined by following the reoxygenation rate in a test vessel aerated under conditions simulating those expected in the field, i.e. similar mechanism of transfer in terms of physical appearance of contact interface and similar mixing-power levels (same $K_L a$). Typical values for α are 0.70 to 0.90. The slope of a plot of $C_s - C_t$ on a log scale versus time in hours, on an arithmetic scale is $K_L a$:

$$K_L a = \frac{2.3 \log_{10}\left(\dfrac{C_s - C_{t_1}}{C_s - C_{t_2}}\right)}{t_2 - t_1} \qquad \text{... (7.37)}$$

where,

C_t = dissolved oxygen concentration at times t_1 and t_2, mg/l

which was derived from the first order relationship:

$$\frac{dD_o}{dt} = -K_3 D_o \qquad \text{... (7.38)}$$

where,

D = dissolved-oxygen deficit

K_3 = proportionality constant

This relationship is used in determining performance of aeration equipment.

$$N_a = \frac{(K_L a)(D)(W)}{P} \qquad \text{... (7.39)}$$

where,

W = weight of aerated water, millions of pounds (kg × 2.21 × 10^6)

P = power, horsepower (kW × 1.34)

The power needs to be specified either as line horsepower to the aeration device or input (brake) horsepower to the rotor after motor and gear efficiencies are considered. In the case of compressed air, motor, gear, and fan, efficiencies are involved. Due to the effects on diffusivity and viscosity, the oxygen transfer coefficient is influenced by temperature; a value for θ_o of 1.024 is typical. The value for θ_o can range from about 1.01 to 1.04 depending upon the type of system.

An in-depth coverage of all aspects of oxygen transfer testing is found in a report by Boyle and Brenner on a 1978 ASCE-EPA workshop toward an oxygen transfer standard.

Power and Mixing

The total horsepower required is calculated by:

$$hp = \frac{O_t}{(N_a)(24 \text{ hr/day})} \qquad \qquad ...(7.40)$$

This value needs to be checked for adequacy of mixing; at least 0.1 hp/1000 gallons (0.02 kW/m^3) is required. Surface aerator size selection and placement are critical as interactions occur which adversely affect mixing (Fig. 7.9), as described by Price, Conway, and Cheely. A rather strict limitation on minimum spacing exists for a given combination of aerator type, horsepower, and basin depth to avoid adverse interactions as regards both oxygen transfer and biosolids suspension. For one type of 1000 hp (75 kW) stationary aerator, an aerator spacing of 70 ft (21 metres) provided adequate mixing to a depth of 15 ft (4.6 metres); at closer spacing, the level of oxygen transfer and macromixing would be reduced. A horizontal velocity of 0.4 to 0.5 ft/sec (0.12 to 0.15 m/sec) measured under viscosity conditions in a functioning biological system is a reasonable minimum value for allowing up to a biosolids level of about 5000 mg/l to be maintained in suspension. Deep tanks require bottom mixers or draft tubes on the aerators.

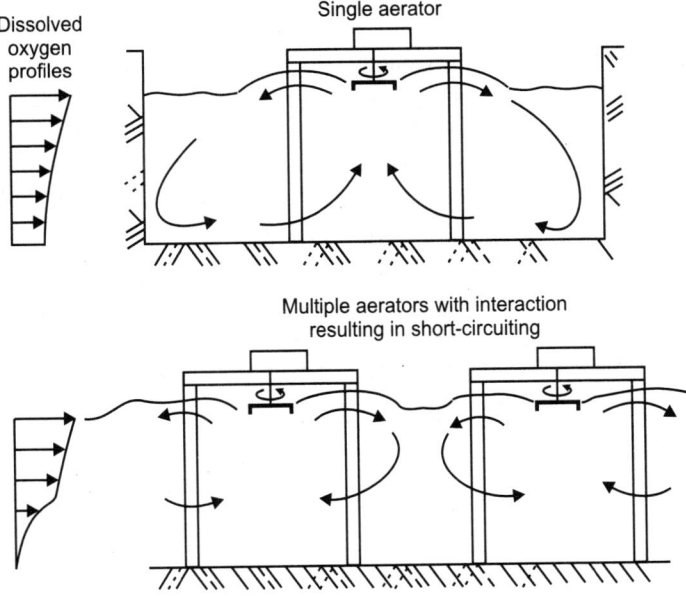

Fig. 7.9. Conceptual representation of aerator mixing patterns.

Aeration Equipment

The basic types of surface-mechanical aerators which have been developed include:
1. Submerged propeller driving water upwards against a diffuser cone at the top of the unit.
2. Impeller rotating at the surface of the water.
3. Combination of a surface impeller with a submerged impeller on the same shaft.
4. Spiral-vaned rotating cone with a draft tube or scooped impeller.
5. Downward-pumping impeller in a draft tube with radial inlet troughs at the surface.

6. Plate-type surface aerators with horizontally vaned impellers.
7. Combination aerators employing surface or subsurface impellers, or both, with the addition of compressed air.
8. Submerged, sparged turbine for satisfying high oxygen demand rates.
9. Paddle wheel, brush, or disks on a horizontal axis revolving with partial submergence.

Diffused aeration equipment utilising compressed air includes:

1. Porous ceramic plates or tubes.
2. Ceramic tubes with integral cast-iron caps and orifices.
3. Plastic-cord-wrapped metal cores with integral end-caps and orifices.
4. Flexible plastic cloth on a metal frame with integral end-cap and orifice.
5. Porous plastic media with a plastic pan holder.
6. Perforated, weighted hosing for lagoon installation.
7. Stainless steel or plastic nozzles with check valves.
8. Tubular grid located 1.5 to 3 ft (0.5 to 0.9 m) below the surface.
9. Shear type nozzle with control orifice.
10. Adjustable nozzle with 4 to 12 openings.
11. Bronze, aluminium-magnesium, or plastic multiple orifice.
12. Metal valve with a moving plastic ball.

The jet aeration system consists of a submersible pump for circulating the mixed liquor, air compressors, and a cluster of air-liquid jets operating on a Venturi principle. In the static mixer system air is conveyed in a tubing arrangement to the base of a vertical mixing element.

In the case of surface aerators an evaluation of two additional options needs to be made: Floating versus fixed installation and direct drive versus gear reduced. Factors to be considered include the trade off between the decreased capital costs of floating and/or direct-drive units and the considerations of oxygen transfer capacity, mixing capabilities, maintenance costs, and available space. Typical oxygen transfer efficiencies in terms of power requirements are presented in Table 7.10.

Table 7.10. Aerator oxygen transfer properties.

	Typical standard transfer capacity (N_S) with air, lb O_2/hp-hr
Surface aerators	
Low speed	
<<30 hp rating	5.0
>30 hp rating	3.5
Floating, high-speed	
< 30 hp rating	3.0–3.5
>30 hp rating	2.5–3.0
Diffused aeration	
Porous diffusers	3.7[a]
Nonporous diffusers	1.2[b]
Sparged turbine	2.0–3.0

[a] At 12 per cent oxygen transfer efficiency.

[b] At 4 per cent oxygen transfer efficiency.

The surface aerators and diffusers with air are capable of satisfying demands of up to about 100 to 140 mg O_2/l-hr due to limitations on minimum aerator spacing and depth. Sparged turbines can supply at least 250 mg O_2/l-hr. In diffused air systems the efficiency of oxygen transfer is reduced by two major components of the system: (i) air compression is an inefficient process, and (ii) horsepower loss due to head loss in the piping system cannot be used in the aeration process. In addition, many diffusers require filtered air to reduce problems of internal clogging. External or surface clogging is also a problem when using many types of diffusers, and periodic removal for cleaning is considered normal maintenance.

CLARIFICATION/THICKENING

Thickener Analysis

In order for the activated sludge system to function, the desired biological transformations must take place in the reactor. Equally important is that the produced biomass be separated from the mixed liquor in the following clarifier, be thickened, and then be either returned to the reactor or wasted. An analysis of the thickening performance of final settling tanks has been performed by Dick and Young. Activated sludge settling rate data except at very low solids levels were found to fit the relationship:

$$v_i = a_s C_i^{-n} \qquad \qquad ...(7.41)$$

where,

v_i = settling velocity of sludge, ft/hr (m/hr × 3.28)
C_i = suspended solids concentration, mg/mg (mg/l × 10^{-6})
a_s, n = constants depending on sludge properties; values in the order of $a_s = 4 \times 10^{-5}$, $n = 2.23$ are typical

Taking the natural logarithum of both sides:

$$\ln v_i = -n \ln C_i + \ln a_s \qquad \qquad ...(7.42)$$

Plot on the Y and X axes, respectively (Fig. 7.10).

$$\ln v_i \text{ vs. } \ln C_i$$

$$\text{Slope} = -n = -\frac{\ln(v_1/v_2)}{\ln(C_1/C_2)}$$

theoretical intercept (a_s) is calculated from v_1/C_1^n.

where,

v_1 = velocity at any concentration C_1 as related by the straight line
v_2 = velocity at any concentration C_2 as related by the straight line

The settling properties of activated sludge at various initial concentrations are determined by observing the subsidence of the liquid-solids interface in transparent columns, as a function of time. Sludge samples for the lower concentrations are obtained by diluting mixed liquor with clarifier effluent. Intermediate concentrations are obtained by blending varying fractions of mixed liquor and clarifier underflow. The highest concentrations are obtained directly from the clarifier underflow. All tests used for developing a given plot of v_1 versus C_1 should be made on the same day.

Either a 2-litre graduated cylinder or larger settling column, such as a 6-inch diameter plexiglass column with 9-ft sludge depth, may be used. Either should be equipped with slow speed stirring devices to minimise the artificial conditions encountered in laboratory settling tests. In the larger column, solids should be redistributed after the column is full by plunging the stirring device up and down.

The interrelationship between these process parameters and settler performance, as derived from flux analysis, assuming negligible loss in the effluent is:

$$X_r = k_s / [(R/Q)(OR)]^{1/n} \qquad \ldots (7.43)$$

$$k_s = \frac{n}{n-1} [180(n-1)a_s]^{1/n} \times 10^6 \qquad \ldots (7.44)$$

where,

k_s = constant dependent upon a_s and n

X_r = recycle sludge solids concentration, mg/l

R/Q = recycle flow fraction

OR = overflow rate or flow volume/clarifier area, gal./sq ft-day (m³/m² day × 24.5)

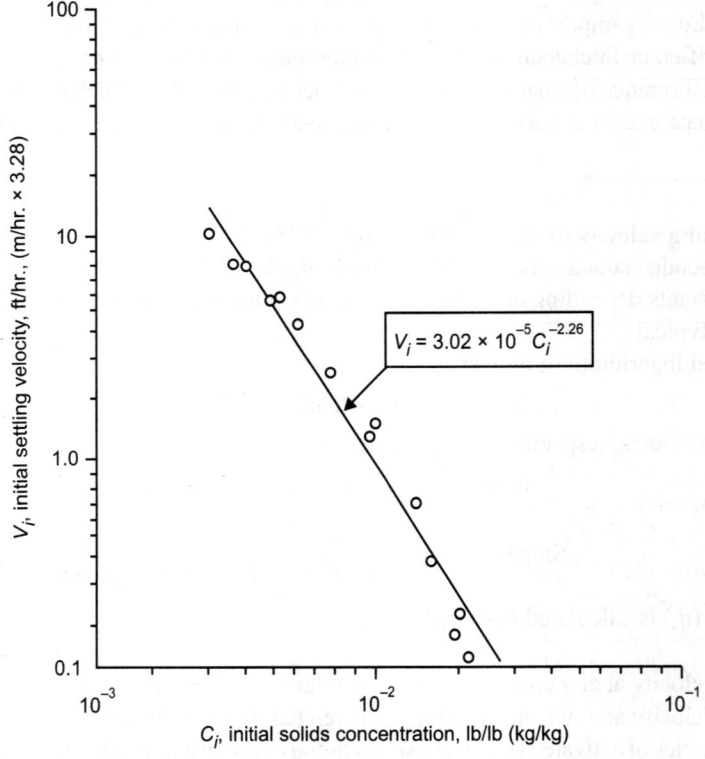

Fig. 7.10. Typical correlation of biological solids settling data.

For existing plants, where the overflow rate is known, the predicted level of return sludge concentration can be calculated for various recycle ratios. For planned installations, an optimum balance between recycle solids (affects reactor size) and overflow rate (controls-clarifier size) can be established, and the required recycle fraction calculated.

Appropriate scale-up factors can be applied, depending either on the variability expected as defined by Nyer and Hovious or on the factor of safety desired.

The observation that larger-scale performance at times exceeds predictions from cylinder tests also needs to be considered. An alternative approach for separately relating initial settling rates and thickening rates to clarifier sizing has been described by Adams and Eckenfelder. Either the clarification or thickening function can control clarifier sizing.

The reactor solids can be calculated directly from X_r and R/Q, ignoring solids entering the basin with the influent flow and solids synthesised in the basin:

$$MLSS = \left(\frac{R/Q}{1 + R/Q} \right) X_r \qquad \qquad ... (7.45)$$

This demonstrates the dependence of MLSS on settling tank underflow concentration, an obvious factor often overlooked due to over attention to reactor design. On the other hand, the dependence of clarifier design on reactor loading conditions is illustrated in Table 7.9. Some typical hydraulic design levels for secondary clarifiers are presented in Table 7.11. A common underflow solids level for air activated sludge is 0.7 to 1 per cent.

Table 7.11. Typical design parameters for secondary clarifiers.

Type of treatment	Overflow rate (OR), (gallon/sq. ft-day)	
	Average	*Peak*
Settling following activated sludge (excluding extended aeration)	400–800	1000–1200
Settling following extended aeration	200–400	800
Settling following trickling filtration	400–600	1000–1200
Conversion: m^3/m^2-day $\times$ 24.5 = gallon/ft^2-day		

Settling Problems

The models for clarifier design are aimed at removing and thickening the bulk of the biological solids for recycle and wasting. The phenomena of colloidal growth, pinpoint floc, rising sludge, and bulking sludge also need to be considered. Colloidal biomass can be attributed to high salt levels, shock loadings, lack of protozoa and rotifers, and too high a loading rate. Pinpoint, or nonsettling floc, usually is due to too high or too low a loading rate or sludge age (Table 7.9). Less frequent causes of nonsettling floc include adsorbed oils and other immiscible liquids, floc breakup due to high shear rate in the reactor, and flotation due to adsorption of gas bubbles in the reactor. Rising of once-settled sludge usually is due to the biological reduction of nitrate ions (denitrification) to nitrogen gas, which buoys up the sludge; faster sludge removal from the clarifier is indicated. Bulking sludge or poorly settling and compacting sludge, is attributable to either filamentous organisms or bound water which swells the floc and reduces its density.

The control of filamentous organisms involves many interrelated factors. Influent waste-water characteristics, such as fluctuating strength, low pH, extreme temperatures, high carbohydrate level, high sulphide levels, and low nitrogen or phosphorus levels can contribute. Operating parameters such as oxygenation level, solids retention time in the clarifier, and high organic loading or low cell residence time also can be involved.

The best means to handle this problem is to detect it early and search out the cause before the ratio of filamentous organisms to floc-forming organisms in the biomass becomes large. However, treatment with chlorine or hydrogen peroxide to kill the filamentous organisms is effective at times; addition of inert materials also can help.

Clarification Equipment

Secondary clarifiers can either be circular or rectangular, although the former seem to have wider application. Sludge take-off is either by the suction type or the plow type, as with primary clarifiers. The suction type reportedly can remove the sludge in a denser and more oxidised condition. Weir placement and loading is critical to prevent upwelling. Scum collection is desirable.

OXYGENATED ACTIVATED SLUDGE AND OTHER MODIFICATIONS

Direct Oxygenation

Activated sludge treatment can use direct oxygenation in contrast to air oxygenation by means of the Unox system (Union Carbide Corp.) and other proprietary processes. The Unox system reduces area requirements for treatment of municipal and industrial wastes through a high-rate, high-solids approach in a staged, covered reactor (Figs 7.11, 7.12). Either surface aerators or sparged turbines can be used. Design of the Unox system is keyed to maintaining a higher biomass concentration in the reactor, and at times loading the system at a higher rate. Most air-operated plants use $F:M$ loading ratios of 0.3 to 0.5 day^{-1}, while operations where oxygen is not limiting can use ratios up to 0.5 to 0.8 day^{-1} as in the Unox system, perhaps because a larger fraction of the volatile solids are aerobically active. BOD removals range generally over 87 to 97 per cent. Mixed-liquor direct-oxygenation levels vary over 4 to 8 mg/l, as compared to 1 to 2 mg/l (at best) for conventional air systems.

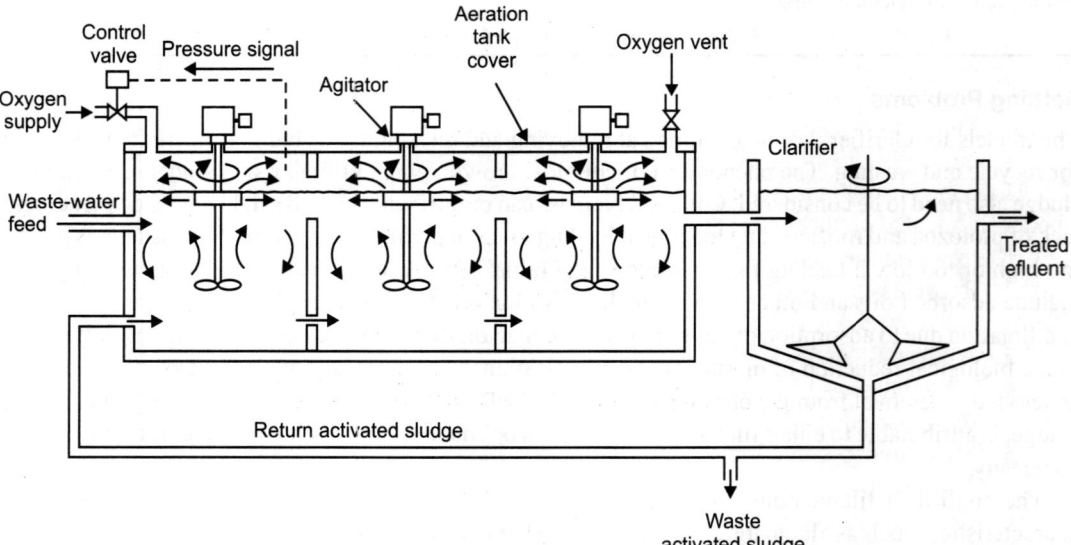

Fig. 7.11. Three-stage Unox pure oxygenation system.

The mixed liquor suspended-solids (MLSS) concentrations for the Unox system range from 4500 to 8000 mg/l, compared to 1500 to 4000 mg/ litre common for air systems. Recycle-sludge ratios (R:Q) are typically 0.2 to 0.5 for the Unox system, compared to 0.3 to 1.0 for air systems. Sludge production per pound of BOD removed ranges from 0.4 to 0.55 for direct oxygenation, compared to 0.5 to 0.75 for air systems.

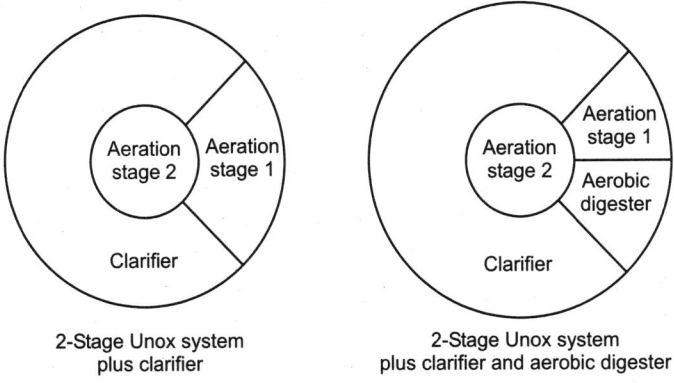

2-Stage Unox system
plus clarifier

2-Stage Unox system
plus clarifier and aerobic digester

Fig. 7.12. Unox two-stage modular system with integral clarifier.

The basic features of the Unox pure-oxygen system rest in these considerations:

1. The high dissolved oxygen levels that can be practicably achieved can satisfy the high oxygen demand rates by large bacterial flocs without imposing mass-transfer limitations.
2. The concurrent staging of both gas and liquid allows high efficiency of oxygen utilisation and has kinetic advantages with noninhibitory substrates when reactions are first order.
3. The covered system prevents discharge of problem vapours and aerosols; odour control on the low volume of effluent gas is possible.
4. The compact biomass that often develops results in a higher MLSS level upon recycle.
5. A statistically significant lesser level of net biosolids generation exists, which is believed to be due to increased endogenous respiration.
6. More oxygen can be supplied per unit reactor volume at reasonable shear levels due to the higher differential between saturation level and operating level of dissolved oxygen.

These factors of higher biochemical oxidation rates per unit aerated volume, low gas feed rate, and better flocculated biomass have many ramifications:

1. Lowered aeration-basin volume; less space needed.
2. Recycle capacity can be lower, and wasted solids can be of lower volume and easier to thicken and dewater.
3. A covered, compact system has aesthetic (and perhaps health) advantages in congested locations.
4. Less sludge is wasted when net synthesis is less, which saves on disposal costs but increases oxygen needs.
5. More compressible biomass tends to lower clarifier area, but higher recycle solids tends to increase it.
6. If short cell-residence times are used, the development of micro-organisms having relatively long generation times could be hampered, especially if environmental conditions such as pH and temperature were suboptimal.
7. For some types of inhibition (i.e. dependent on concentration only and not on ratio of inhibitor to enzyme level), low volume and staging can enhance susceptibility to shock loading. However, maintenance of dissolved-oxygen 'buffer' level in all parts of the aeration tank can lessen the variability of effluent quality as adverse effects of shock loadings, nutrient shortages, pH variations, and temperature changes, are heightened at marginal DO levels.

8. Power requirements, including air separation and oxygen transfer, are at least competitive and many times are lower.
9. Oxygen supply can be tailored to demand by a simple pressure control.
10. Higher carbon dioxide content in the gas phase can internally neutralise alkaline wastes, but otherwise can result in a pH less than neutral.
11. Heat loss is less, which is advantageous at least in cold weather.
12. Monitors are needed to detect any flammability hazards and to initiate air purging of the gas space; however, problems are normally precluded by pre-treatments for immiscible liquid removal and by the elimination of ignition sources.

As with other alternatives, an evaluation of all cost-performance factors is needed for system selection and design. Considerable pilot plant and plant-scale data in a range of applications are available for such an evaluation. Other pure-oxygen-based systems more recently have been commercialised. These include the Oases system (air products), Marox diffuser units (FMC Corp.), and the forced-free fall oxygen system (Airco).

The Oases system is a gas-tight closed reactor that provides positive vent control. The Marox system involves fine-bubble diffusion in deep tanks, usually with active fluid flow against the diffuser or with rotation of the diffuser. The underlying principle is to achieve high utilisation of oxygen in a single pass of the process gas through the mixed liquor in an uncovered unit; produced carbon dioxide is stripped out. In the forced free fall oxygen (F^3O) system, oxygen is mixed in a turbulent waste-water fall zone inside a reinforced concrete module. The mixed liquor is forced down a duct by an impeller, flows up an annular space and over a weir, from which it falls into the oxygen chamber. The modules may be installed in open tanks. Several oxygen supply options are available: liquid oxygen transport, pipe line transport from a central air separation plant, on-site cryogenic processing plant, or on-site generation by a pressure-swing-absorption process using molecular sieves which preferably absorb nitrogen. The choice depends on the oxygen usage rate and facility location.

Other Process Modifications

The activated sludge process is most versatile. Discussed in prior sections have been the concepts or operating modes of:

1. Completely mixed reaction systems.
2. Staged or plug-flow reaction systems.
3. Contact stabilisation.
4. Extended aeration.
5. Pure oxygen systems.

Many other modifications have been developed:

1. Addition of powdered activated carbon to reactor primarily for the purpose of increasing removal of bioresistent materials (e.g. Pact process, Du Pont company).
2. Phosphorus removal process involving inducement of high uptakes and subsequent anaerobic stripping of phosphorus from the recycle sludge (Phostrip process, Union Carbide Corp.).
3. Nitrification in a second step system with separate clarifier and sludge recycle.
4. Denitrification in a third step using methanol as a carbon source.
5. Two step system for carbonaceous BOD removal (e.g. Zurn Attisholz process).
6. Oxidation ditch in which the liquor is forced around an oval path using an axially mounted cage rotor.

7. Deep-shaft concept in which introduced air reaches a high pressure during its flow down the shaft (ICI).
8. Integral aerator-clarifier in package units.

AERATED STABILISATION

Aerated stabilisation is accomplished using a dispersed-growth system without biological-solids recycle. This process sometimes is termed 'aerated lagooning' since the simplest prototype consists of one or more aerators installed in a large pond with the accomplishment of only partial mixing. However, full advantage of this approach can be realised by installing sufficient aeration capacity to keep the system completely mixed, and to satisfy the oxygen requirements of the system. Some typical operating data from a facility which treated a waste flow of 3700 gal./min. (230 litres/sec) of fairly concentrated waste-water (2100 mg BOD/l) are presented in Table 7.12. Due to the already dispersed nature of the culture, the aerated-stabilisation approach does not require as close control over variations in temperature, pH, and organic loading as does the activated sludge process. A disadvantage of the aerated-stabilisation process is a practical limitation in maximum BOD removal of about 75 per cent, primarily due to the dispersed bacteria in the effluent and inhibition of the biological reactions at cold temperatures.

Table 7.12. Aerated stabilisation of a synthetic organic chemical waste.

	Summer	Winter
Temperature, °C	35	15
Dissolved oxygen, mg/l	Nil	2.0
Power, bhp/1000 gallon^a	0.077	0.062
Detention time, days	2.9	2.3
BOD removal, %	54	48
COD removal, %	41	39

^{a} hp/1000 gallon × 0.197 = kW/m^3.
bhp is brake horsepower (power input to motor).

Aerated Stabilisation Applications

Due to the limitations of this type system and the increasing strictness of effluent quality standards, the main applications for aerated stabilisation are:
1. Pretreatment of waste-water prior to another biological system to gain the overall removal efficiency possible with systems in series.
2. Pretreatment prior to another biological system to level out fluctuating loads and/or reduce problem constituents.
3. Pretreatment to achieve levels permitting discharge into municipal facilities.
4. Interim treatment until upgrading becomes necessary to meet anticipated future standards.
5. Treatment of dilute wastes or activated-sludge effluents where suitable final effluent quality can be achieved directly or through a subsequent unaerated stabilisation pond.

Process stability and relatively low cost make this process attractive, despite its efficiency limitations.

System Design

One model for the aerated-stabilisation process is similar to the relationship developed for the completely mixed activated-sludge process, as derived from a simulated first-order reaction, except that the level of biomass maintained is not considered:

$$\frac{S_e}{S_o} = \frac{1}{1 + K_a t_d} \qquad \qquad ... (7.46)$$

where,

S_e = effluent soluble BOD, mg/l
S_o = influent soluble BOD, mg/l
K_a = reaction rate constant, day^{-1}
t_d = liquid retention time, days

A typical range of K_a at 20°C, according to Eckenfelder and Ford, is 0.5 to 1.0; although values of up to 1.8 have been experienced with high strength chemical wastes. The lowest level of BOD concentration that this process can reach is subject to the same limitations as discussed for the activated-sludge process, i.e. the conditions in the treatment system are such that the reactions slow as low BOD levels are reached, even though this near-equilibrium level is reflected as degradable organics when measured under more favourable conditions in the BOD test procedure. The reaction rate constant is adjusted to the temperature levels expected in the system under winter and summer conditions using Eq. 7.15. A typical θ_t value is 1.04; however, measurement of θ_t for the particular waste being treated is desirable. Relationships for predicting basin temperature levels have been developed. Basins in series have the advantage of maintaining a higher temperature in the initial basin. Reaction rates may be of zero order (constant), i.e. independent of reactor substrate level, with wastes of high initial concentration. An alternative kinetic model has been developed using Monod kinetics; Eq. 7.10 applies for the calculation of the effluent substrate level. In addition to soluble organic removal, the level of biosolids in the basin is important as it also appears in the effluent. These can be predicted using:

$$X_v = X_{ov} + aS_r - bX_v t_d \qquad \qquad ... (7.47)$$

where,

X_v = volatile suspended solids (VSS) in reactor and effluent, mg/l
X_{ov} = influent degradable VSS, mg/l
a = fraction of S_r converted to cells
S_r = BOD removed ($S_o - S_e$), mg/l
b = cell autooxidation rate, day^{-1}
t_a = liquid retention time, day

Upon rearrangement,

$$X_v = \frac{X_{ov} + aS_r}{1 + bt} \qquad \qquad ... (7.48)$$

Application of Eqs 7.46 to 7.48, including typical values for coefficients and experimental means to determine constants, is discussed in the section covering the activated sludge process. Monod-based expressions for biosolids level and oxygen requirements also are available.

Another alternative means of modelling the basin logically takes into account the level of biological solids, although it is in one sense an artifact of the system and cannot be controlled. Adams and Eckenfelder show that:

$$\frac{S_o}{S_e} = \frac{1}{1 + K_{ax} X_v t_d} \qquad \qquad ... (7.49)$$

After rearrangement and combination with Eq. 7.47 (assuming X_{ov} is nil), the following relationship for S_e is achieved.

$$S_e = \frac{1}{aK_{ax}t_d} + \frac{b}{aK_{ax}} \qquad \qquad \dots (7.50)$$

The slope of a plot of S_e (Y axis) versus $1/t_d$ (X axis) is $1/aK_{ax}$, and the Y intercept is b/aK_{ax}. Substitution of values for a and b yields K_{ax}. Some indications are that K values derived from activated sludge results can be used in this relationship, after converting from hr^{-1} to day^{-1}.

In cases in which the power used for aeration is insufficient to keep the solids in suspension throughout the whole basin, solublisation of BOD from the deposited solids through anaerobic decomposition can be significant, especially in the summer when the contribution can reach 20 to 40 per cent of that calculated from Eq. 7.46. Any feedback also needs to be considered when calculating oxygen requirements. A minimum value of 0.01 hp/1000 gallon (0.002 kW/m^3) typically is used when evaluating adequacy of mixing, although the level required is dependent upon the solids level and liquid properties. Procedures for calculating oxygen requirements are discussed already; aeration equipment alternatives and capacity determinations are outlined already.

Nutrient requirements are as discussed already in this chapter. The basic consideration is that cells are 12.6 per cent nitrogen and 2.6 per cent phosphorous and that the net increase in cell weight needs to be provided with the proper nutrient quantities.

In cases in which the effluent from the aerated-stabilisation process needs to be settled before being discharged, either a partially mixed second basin in series with a completely mixed first basin or a large quiescent settling basin can be used. In the latter case the development of algae and odours from the stored sludge can be minimised by maintaining liquid retention times from 1 to 2 days.

FIXED FILM SYSTEMS

Applications

While the activated-sludge and aerated-stabilisation systems involve biomass suspended in an aerated or oxygenated reactor, fixed growth systems employ biomass attached to surfaces which are contacted with the waste-water. The main attractions of this type system are:
1. Process stability not closely tied to settleability of the biomass; able to pass shock loads.
2. Relatively simple operation.
3. Relatively low power requirements.

The disadvantages include:
1. Lower practically achievable efficiency than activated sludge.
2. Performance markedly decreased in cold weather (covering lessens this problem).
3. Scale-up using available evaluation and design procedures is less rational.
4. Potential for nuisance conditions odours, insects.
5. Relatively high capital costs and large space requirements.

These considerations result in many of the applications for fixed film systems being either to pretreat waste-water before a final biological treatment step or to handle low-volume wastestreams.

Trickling Filters

The trickling filtration process utilises biological growth on a contact medium over which the waste-water flows. Sufficient void space in the 'filter' is provided to maintain aerobic conditions. The micro-organisms are cultivated usually either in a packed bed of crushed stone or on a system of vertical plastic sheeting. Other packings are available, such as flexirings. The waste is fed at such a hydraulic rate that a portion of the attached growth is continuously sloughed from the filter. A clarifier is provided after the filter; and a portion of the supernatant can be recycled for additional treatment, to maintain adequate hydraulic loading, and to equalise the constituents in the influent stream. Figure 7.13 depicts the mass transfer operations involved. Nitrification can be achieved at low loadings.

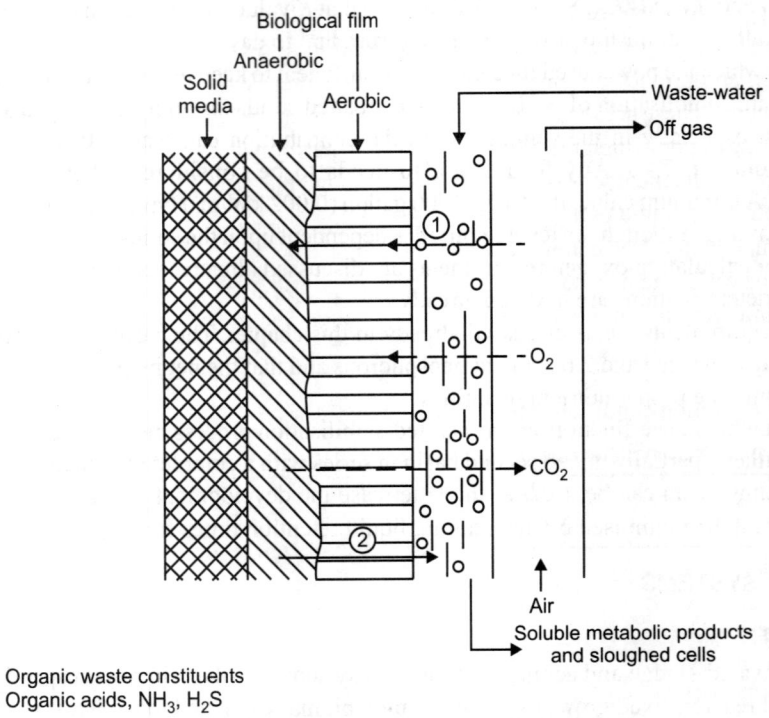

1 Organic waste constituents
2 Organic acids, NH_3, H_2S

Fig. 7.13. Trickling filter mass transfer operations.

Filter construction

Trickling filter construction is quite diverse. Design details are governed by available land area, volume and strength of the wastestream, extreme temperatures, and local construction costs. Periodic dosage of the influent flow over the filter surface without flooding the system, which would prevent oxygenation of the film, usually is accomplished by using commercially available rotating distribution arms. The arms consist of tapered pipes connected to a rotating stilling well. Orifice holes are drilled along the arm's length, and deflector plates are attached to the arm below each orifice. As an alternative special nozzles are available which fasten directly to the arm, thus eliminating the orifices and deflection plates. The reaction of the escaping waste-water causes the arm to rotate. Fixed nozzle flow distribution is sometimes used to supply waste to rectangular or irregular filters. The nozzles are connected by piping to a dosing siphon which periodically discharges the waste to the filter. Waste may also be supplied to the nozzles directly by the use of pumps. Stone ranging from 2 to 4 inches (5 to 10 cm) in diameter installed in beds from 6 to 8 ft (1.8 to 2.4 metres) deep commonly is used as a filter packing, although other coarse materials such as slag or coal can be employed in addition to the plastic sheeting alternatives.

Filters up to 30 to 40 ft (9 to 12 metres) in height have been constructed by using commercially available synthetic media. In general, synthetic filter media consist of flat or corrugated sheets of rigid material assembled in self-supporting modules having the appearance of a honeycomb; void space is about 94 per cent, as compared to about 45 per cent for stone filters. Contact between the biomass and waste-water is maximised, and space is provided for unimpeded ventilation and liquid flow. Specific surface areas of synthetic media range from 20 to 35 ft²/ft³(66 to 115 m²/m³), while rock packing ranges from 10 to 25 ft²/ft³ (33 to 82 m²/m³).

The floor of a filter needs to be designed to support the filter media, drain the treated waste-water from the filter, and provide air circulation through the filter. Vitrified clay filter block is available for floor construction. These are rectangular in cross-section and hollow in the centre. The upper face of the block, the surface upon which the filter media rest, is perforated. Waste-water and air flow in opposite directions through the tile; the waste-water passes through the perforations and is directed by the hollow blocks to centralised liquid collection galleries.

Where temperatures drop below freezing for prolonged periods of time, filters are sometimes covered. Feeds also can be preheated. Filters have been constructed using forced or induced fans for air circulation, although natural ventilation induced by density differences usually is sufficient.

Filter design

Some typical operating conditions are shown in Table 7.13.

Table 7.13. Typical trickling filter operating conditions.

	Nominal filter rate		
	Low	*High*	*Super*
Hydraulic loading			
gal./ft²-day	25–100	200–1000	1400–8500
Organic loading			
lb BOD/1000 ft³-day	5–25	25–300	130–1500
BOD removal efficiency, %			
Single-stage	60–70	40–50	50
Two-stage	90+	85	–
Conversion: gal./ft²-day × 0.0408 = m³/m²-day			
lb/1000 ft³-day × 6.0 = g/m³-day			

Several models for trickling filters have been developed; one described by Thackston and Eckenfelder that seems to apply best to industrial wastes is:

$$\frac{S_e}{S_a} = e^{-K_f(D_f / Q_h^m)} \qquad \qquad ... (7.51)$$

where,

S_e = effluent BOD concentration, mg/l

S_a = BOD concentration applied to the filter, mg/l

e = constant (2.72)

K_f = product of the reaction rate constant (gal./ft²-min) and the specific surface area (ft²/ft³) of the packing; reportedly 0.09 is typical, min⁻¹

D_f = media depth, ft (m × 3.28)

Q_h = hydraulic loading (including recycle), gpm/ft² (m³/m²-min × 24.5)

m = constant (reportedly 0.5 is common, can range from 0.4 for some random packings to 1.0 for some vertical sheets)

This equation is similar to that developed for a batch or plug-flow activated sludge system:

$$\frac{S_e}{S_o} = e^{-kX_v t} \qquad \qquad ...(7.52)$$

The retention time is proportional to the ratio of the depth to the hydraulic loading, and the biomass level is proportional to the specific surface of the filter medium.

Calculation of S_a is by mass balance.

$$S_a = \frac{S_o + (R/Q)S_e}{1 + R/Q} \qquad \qquad ...(7.53)$$

where R/Q = recycle ratio, recycle flow/influent flow

The variables may be evaluated by collection of pilot-scale performance data at several surface loading rates and media depths. Data are reduced by plotting ln ($100\ S_e/S_o$) versus D at various hydraulic loadings; the slope is K/Q_h^m. The slope of a ln-ln plot of KQ_h^m versus Q_h is b. Then the slope of a plot of ln (S_e/S_o) versus D/Q_h^m (m is known) is K; K is adjusted for expected temperatures using Eq. 7.15. A typical θ_t value is 1.035. By multiplying by the ratio of the specific surface areas, K can also be adjusted to similar packings. Perhaps the broader utility of these equations is for the estimation of allowable surface loadings with and without recirculation in order to achieve desired efficiencies at a given temperature. In this case, a reasonable value of the coefficients is assumed.

Oxygen transfer capabilities limit the waste concentration that can be applied to the filter without recirculation; 500 mg BOD/l is a limiting guide for readily degradable wastes.

Rotating Biological Contactors and other Modifications

As opposed to passing the waste-water over a fixed medium, a newer development is a rotating biological contactor. The biological growth is developed on a set of partially submerged, rotating disks. During rotation, the growth is alternately exposed to the waste-water and to air to provide a means of both contacting the growth with the organic impurities and aerating the culture. Rotational speed is adjusted according to waste strength. Successive units can be used to upgrade efficiencies. Shearing forces cause excess biomass to slough into the mixed liquor, which is kept mixed by the disks. Treated wastes flow to a clarifier, where the solids are separated for ultimate disposal without recycle.

Low power requirements are a particularly cited advantage from among the list of considerations previously presented for fixed-film systems. Housing can be provided for protection from inclement weather. In addition to the rotating disks (e.g. bio-surf process), another approach is to use a rotating cage-like drum (biodrum) filled with hollow plastic balls.

Another development, termed activated bio-filter process, is a two-stage system employing both fixed film and activated sludge. The fixed film unit consists of stacked racks made of wooden laths attached to supporting rails. The laths and rails are sized to permit free transfer to liquid and air in all directions. The incoming waste-water flows to the fixed film reactor along with recycled biological solids from a final clarifier. A portion of the effluent from the fixed-film reactor is recycled and a portion flows to an aeration tank and then to the final clarifier.

ANAEROBIC SYSTEMS

Anaerobic Treatment Basics

Although the stepwise chemical reactions for the metabolism of organic chemicals by anaerobic and aerobic bacteria are complicated, more simple, overall equations familiar to chemists and engineers may be written that describe the initial reactants and the final products (Table 7.4). The anaerobic reactions, known as fermentation and anaerobic respiration, occur in closed reactors or in the bottom of open lagoons, and typically involve the reduction of sulphates, nitrates, and organic molecules. Biological cycles of interest in anaerobic systems are shown in Fig. 7.14.

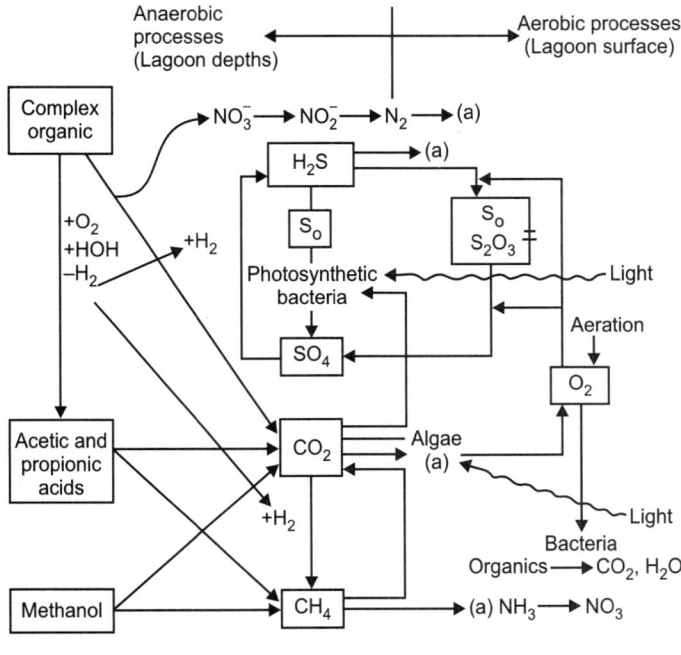

(a) Possible gaseous emission to atmosphere

Fig. 7.14. Anaerobic reactions coupled with cycles at aerobic surfaces.

Several important economic and technical advantages inherent in the anaerobic treatment process along with potential problem areas are as follows:

Advantages

1. No aeration equipment is required for organic reduction. Associated capital, power, and maintenance costs are avoided. System loading is not limited by oxygen transfer.
2. Cellular material is produced in lower quantity and more stable form. Savings in nutrients and in flocculants, equipment, and labour costs for dewatering and final disposal can be realised.
3. Some problem organic chemicals difficult to degrade aerobically will degrade anaerobically. The oxygen in sulphate (and nitrate) ions can be utilised for organic oxidation. Methane in off-gas potentially can be utilised.

Potential problems

1. High temperatures are needed for maximum rates.
2. High biomass concentration is required for reasonable rates at short retention times.
3. Generation time for methane bacteria is long (2 to 11 days at 37°C), thereby requiring long solids retention and acclimation times.
4. Methane bacteria are very sensitive to shock loads, toxic materials, and environmental conditions.
5. Effluents low in BOD (<50 mg/l) with good aesthetic properties are difficult to produce.
6. Odour emission potential is high.

In some instances, significant savings can result if the anaerobic and aerobic processes are joined to utilise the best features of both to compensate for some of the problems of each. This could involve utilising a roughing anaerobic treatment followed by an aerobic treatment step for polishing of the waste-water.

Toxicity

As shown in Fig. 7.14, for most substrates the anaerobic process proceeds in two steps, i.e. conversion of the organic material to volatile organic acids by one set of bacteria, and then conversion of the acids to methane and carbon dioxide by the methanogenic bacteria. The methane bacteria are sensitive to high levels of alkali and alkaline earth cations (1000 to 10,000 mg/l), ammonia (1500 to 3000 mg/l), sulphide ion (100 to 200 mg/l), ionised heavy metals, dissociated volatile acids (~2000 mg/l), and various synthetic organic chemicals. Toxic effects can be lessened through acclimation in the case of organics and sulphides, through addition of antagonistic ions in the case of cation toxicity, through pH adjustment in the case of ammonia, and through precipitation of heavy metals by controlled sulphide generation. Using a Warburg respirometric procedure, Hovious, Waggy, and Conway identified the following organic materials (and concentrations which produced a 50 per cent decrease in the activity of an unacclimated biomass) as inhibitory: acrolein (20 to 50 mg/l), formaldehyde (50 to 100 mg/l), 2-ethyl-1-hexanol (500 to 1000 mg/l), methyl isobutyl ketone (100 to 300 mg/l), diethylamine (300 to 1000 mg/l), acrylonitrile (100 mg/l), 2-methyl-5-ethylpyridine (100 mg/l), ethylene dichloride (150 to 500 mg/l), ethyl acrylate (300 to 600 mg/l), and phenol (300 to 1000 mg/l). A typical test run is shown in Fig. 7.15. Inhibitory effects were more severe at high volatile acid concentrations.

Acclimated cultures were developed in mixed digesters for crotonaldehyde, phenol, and to some degree for ethyl acrylate. No acclimation was observed for sodium acrylate. Cultures acclimated to crotonaldehyde and ethyl acrylate were able to degrade the material, while phenol was not degraded with acclimation but was no longer inhibitory. Additional acclimation studies were made in continuously fed anaerobic filters. A filter was acclimated to a crotonaldehyde concentration of 600 mg/l as compared to the 50 to 100 mg/l level found inhibitory in Warburg studies. Treatment of formaldehyde, ethyl acrylate, phenol, and acrylonitrile indicated synergistic inhibitory effects. These mixed inhibitors were treated satisfactorily at low concentrations in two series anaerobic filters; however, increasing inhibitor concentrations resulted in failure of both filters. The amenability of organic materials to treatment in anaerobic systems is highly dependent upon the nature of the system to be employed.

Anaerobic Reactors

The basic types of anaerobic systems used in treating industrial waste-water and residues are described in Table 7.14.

Table 7.14. Basic anaerobic systems.

System type	Submerged filter	Contact digester[a]	Open lagoon
Reactor	Packed column	Completely mixed vessel	Basin with considerable stratification
Flow pattern	Plug flow	Backmixed	Some wind and wave mixing, thermal turnovers
Biosolids level	High biomass through attached growths	High biomass through settling and return	Low suspended solids, bottom sludge layer
Metabolic pathways	Fermentation and anaerobic respiration	Fermentation and anaerobic respiration	Fermentation, anaerobic respiration, sulphur oxidation, photosynthesis, some aerobic respiration
Retention times	1 to 3 days	1 to 10 days	10 to 100 days
Gas collection	Normally collected	Collected	Gas is released, although a plastic covering with peripheral collection tiles is possible
Temperature control	Not normally practiced	Usually practiced	Unfeasible

[a]As opposed to a standard digester, which is only partially mixed and has biomass return only if two digesters are operated as stages with the second unmixed.

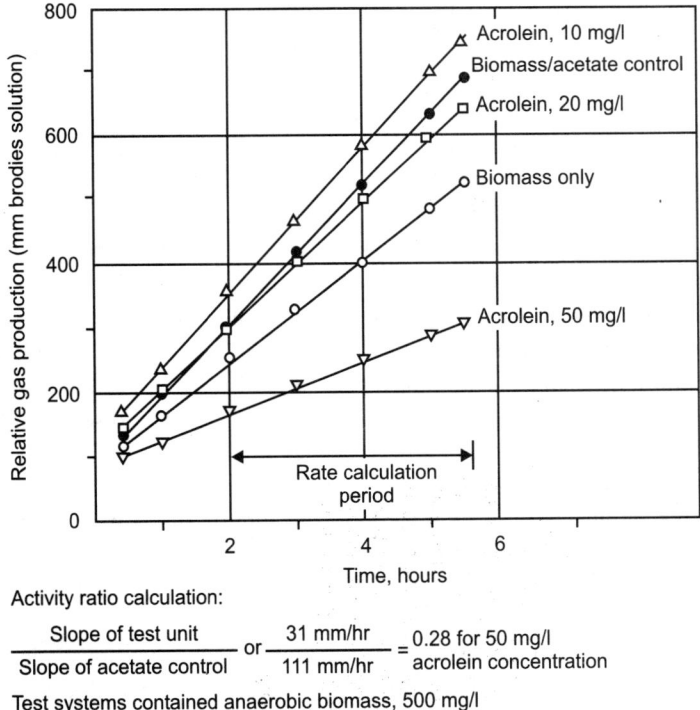

Activity ratio calculation:

$$\frac{\text{Slope of test unit}}{\text{Slope of acetate control}} \quad \text{or} \quad \frac{31\ \text{mm/hr}}{111\ \text{mm/hr}} = \frac{0.28\ \text{for 50 mg/l}}{\text{acrolein concentration}}$$

Test systems contained anaerobic biomass, 500 mg/l
Acetic acid, buffer–nutrient water, and acrolein

Fig. 7.15. Typical Warburg respirometer data measuring methanogenesis in anaerobic systems.

Contact reactor

The contact reactor employs solids separation and recycle to increase the organism concentration and the biomass retention time within the digestion system. The increased solids retention time (θ_c) compensates for the long generation time of the methanogenic bacteria. Solids separation usually is accomplished by gravity settling, but if carried out in open clarifiers it would have the problem of attached gas bubbles associated with the decreased partial pressures; this may be alleviated by a vacuum degassing step. The digester gas also may be used in flotation separation of solids. Other means which can be used to increase organism separation efficiency are addition of flocculants or weighting agents.

Filter

Anaerobic filters utilise both the tendency of methane bacteria to grow on surfaces and the filtering capacity of a flooded, packed bed to overcome the long generation time of the methanogenic culture. The low solids production of the anaerobic system slows filter clogging if a low solids feed is used. High recycle is the key to stable operation in a system.

Lagoon

Anaerobic lagoons operate at low suspended micro-organism concentrations and, therefore, require a relatively long retention time for adequate reduction of waste constituents. The retention time required in a system is primarily a function of temperature and the amenability of the waste material to transformation by the various types of organisms involved. The key pathways are illustrated in Fig. 7.14.

The anaerobic lagoon has the potential to utilise additional organic removal pathways not found in the other anaerobic processes. For example, an uncovered lagoon which is not excessively loaded will develop an algal culture, which may result in a shallow aerobic surface layer. This aerobic layer can account for a significant aerobic oxidation of wastes.

Another process which may function in a lagoon is re-oxidation of reduced sulphur forms. In the conventional digester, sulphates are reduced by *Desulphovibrio* to sulphides with a conversion of complex substrates to volatile acids. If the sulphides remain in the system, no net reduction in COD accompanies this reaction. In an enclosed type of anaerobic system, the sulphides may be lost in part as hydrogen sulphide in the produced gas or may be precipitated with heavy metals. In the anaerobic lagoon, any sulphides lost in the produced gas usually constitute an air pollution problem. Fortunately, additional biological processes may exist in a lagoon to oxidise the produced sulphide. The anaerobic, photosynthetic sulphur bacteria, *Chlorobacteriaceae* and *Thiorhodaceae*, utilise light as an energy source to oxidise sulphides. Aerobic bacteria such as *Beggiatoa* and *Thiobacillus*, which oxidise sulphides, can live in the upper layers of the lagoon. Direct oxidation of sulphides by molecular oxygen in the aerobic upper lagoon layers is also a possibility.

Experimental work on anaerobic lagoons is most meaningful when performed with actual plant waste-water, outdoors under the full spectrum of expected operating conditions and removal processes. Besides organic removal efficiency, the key aspects needing evaluation are inhibition of methanogenesis and emission of sulphide and other odours.

Anaerobic digesters can be designed in a manner analogous to that previously described for aerobic systems. In an approach described by Eckenfelder and Ford, experimental systems are operated at various retention times and data are taken regarding biomass levels and organic matter (COD) reduction. Graphical reduction of the data using Eq. 7.19 is used to determine the reaction rate constant and the nondegradable fraction. Other design constants are defined using relationships of specific removal versus retention time and methane production versus COD removal. Alternative procedures have been described by Christenson and McCarty using Monod-type kinetics. Constants for synthesis and other relationships (Eq. 7.20) have been developed for various substrates by Speece, Lawrence, and McCarty.

A design procedure which takes into account feed organic concentration, hydraulic loading, and temperature has been developed by Hovious, Conway, and Ganze for anaerobic lagoon pretreatment of petrochemical wastes relatively low in sulphates. Also for lagoons a relationship similar to that in Eq. 7.46 can be used with a reaction rate constant of 0.030 to 0.055.

STABILISATION PONDS

Pond Applications

Stabilisation ponds rely upon surface reaeration and algal photosynthesis for the oxygen used in the biological processes. However, most industrial waste ponds are anaerobic in their lower levels and aerobic near the surfaces. In this type pond, termed facultative, methane formation in the lower levels also is a means for organic removal, as can be sulphate reduction. Depths range from 3 to 8 ft (0.9 to 2.4 metres); however, 4 to 6 ft (1.2 to 1.8 metres) is more common. Often in series operations of ponds, the first one will be virtually all anaerobic, the next facultative, and the last aerobic. The allowable loadings for facultative ponds range from 15 to 80 lb BOD/acre-day (170 to 900 kg/hectare-day).

The factors that affect the capacity of the pond, as described by Gloyna and Hermann, include: air and waste temperature, wind velocity, orientation of pond with respect to prevailing winds, rainfall, horizontal and vertical movement of the water in the pond, infiltration, evaporation, seepage, depth of the pond, length of daylight, hours of overcast and sunshine, sulphate level, and types of predominating micro-organisms. Pond systems are sometimes designed to provide for recirculation to increase treatment efficiencies. Stabilisation ponds have primary application in situations when adequate land area is available at reasonable cost and the waste discharge is relatively small. The potential reactions involved are depicted in Fig. 7.14; design is set to allow the aerobic reactions to predominate to a considerable depth.

The conditions which favour the use of stabilisation ponds are:

1. Low land costs.
2. Low flow rate to be treated.
3. Turbid effluent allowable.
4. Warm climate.
5. Low latitude and minimum cloud cover (for light).
6. Steady winds (for reaeration).
7. Need for impoundment or equalisation.
8. Low sulphate level in waste.
9. Low percolation rate.
10. High power costs.
11. Minimum operating capabilities

Often lagoons are used in series with other systems to provide polishing treatment for further removal of soluble organics, nutrients, or suspended solids; however, either algal growth needs to be controlled or a final solids-removal step provided to meet effluent quality standards. In reality, however, the effect of a small amount of algal discharge can be beneficial to fish life in the receiving water.

Design of Ponds

Design of ponds often is based on allowable surface loading of BOD, based on experience with similar waste-waters and climatic conditions. An alternative approach is to apply the first-order kinetic relationships previously described for anaerobic lagoon systems to stabilisation ponds using procedures described by Eckenfelder and Ford. For single ponds the relationship is:

$$\frac{S_e}{S_o} = \frac{1}{1 + K_p t_d} \qquad \ldots (7.54)$$

where, K_p = the rate constant coefficient for ponds, day^{-1}, which for multiple ponds is:

$$\frac{S_e}{S_o} = \frac{1}{(1 + K_p t_{d1})(1 + K_p t_{d2})(1 + K_p t_{d3})} \qquad \ldots (7.55)$$

where, t_d = hydraulic retention time in days for Ponds 1, 2, and 3. Design data can be collected in large field pilot units, or with some risk, in laboratory units equipped with suitable baffling, lighting, and simulated wind action. Data reduction proceeds as described for the other biological systems.

Adjustment of the reaction rate coefficient needs to be made for temperature effects using Eq. 7.15 with a constant (θ_t) of 1.06 to 1.09; 1.085 is typical. The design approach needs to consider the depth of light penetration, as this affects photosynthesis. Higher loadings create turbid conditions, which limit the depth of aerobic operation. Many pond operations in the southwestern United States are based on a design loading of 50 to 60 lb. BOD$_5$/acre-day (560 to 670 kg/ha-day), while in northern areas of the USA loadings down to 10–15 lb. BOD$_5$/acre-day (110–170 kg/ha-day) have been used. Rubber, plastic, or asphaltic liners are available to prevent seepage; the use of soil sealants is an alternative approach. Various aeration devices have been developed especially for usage in this type of lightly loaded biological system.

Pond Upgrading

Due either to increased loads or to more strict effluent quality standards, upgrading of stabilisation ponds frequently needs to be considered. The general problems are excessive algae, offensive odours, and seasonal variations. Alternatives which should be considered would be to:

1. Deepen ponds (or final portion of pond system) to increase detention time, and more importantly, to allow sedimentation of algae; wind scour is lessened.
2. Pretreat wastes by aerated stabilisation or other means to decrease loading.
3. Add another pond in series; utilise interpond and/or intrapond recirculation.
4. Consider multiple-entry and multiple-exit approaches for fuller utilisation of volume.
5. Install mechanical or compressed-air aeration.
6. Remove algae by staged: (i) chemical coagulation, flocculation, and gravity sedimentation, followed by, and (ii) multimedia, rapid-sand filtration (pressure operation).
7. Remove algae by staged: (i) coagulation and dissolved-air flotation, followed by and (ii) polishing multimedia filtration.
8. Remove algae by a dike-type, submerged-rock filter.
9. Remove algae by intermittent, slow sand filters (Fig. 7.16).
10. Use effluent for spray irrigation.
11. Use microstrainers.
12. Use parallel ponds, make into one and discharge from another which is quiescent. Benemann terms this the pond-isolation process.

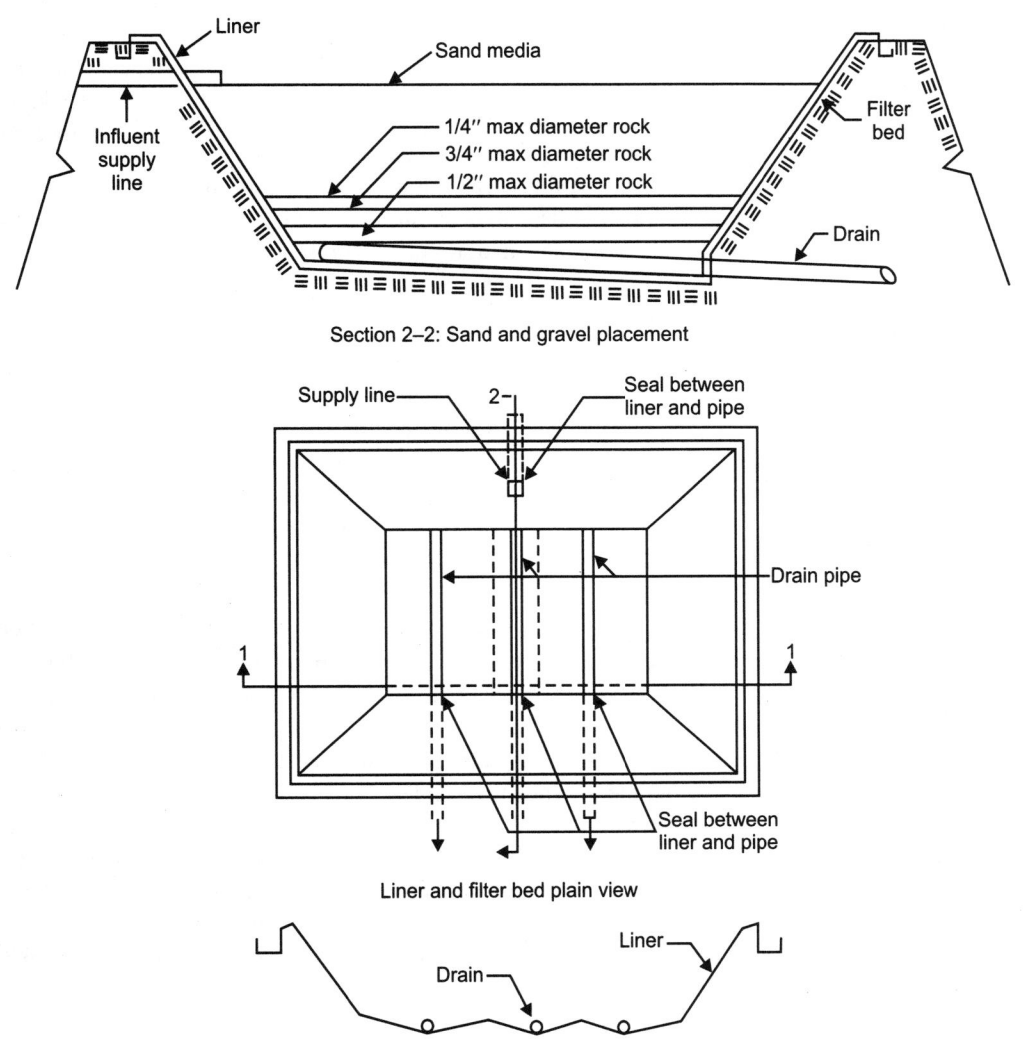

Fig. 7.16. Intermittent sand filter for upgrading stabilisation ponds.

In the intermittent sand-filtration approach, filters operated by Middlebrooks at 6,00,000 gallons/acre-day (5600 m³/ha-day) reduced the effluent suspended solids from an average of 26 mg/l (10 to 70 mg/l) to less than 7 mg/l during a 26-day run before plugging required them to be cleaned; some nitrification and BOD reduction also occurred.

Natural Systems

Passing waste through a balanced ecosystem, which includes plants and higher animal forms, has been indicated to be an effective, low-cost treatment technique. Reeds and bullrushes (or bacteria acting in symbiosis with them), as well as Daphnia, shellfish, and brine shrimp in conjunction with algae are involved in various types of these natural systems.

BIOLOGICAL EXPERIMENTAL TECHNIQUES

General Approach

Experimental programmes to develop design data for biological treatment processes must be developed individually according to waste-water characteristics, feasible treatment processes, and effluent-quality requirements. Typical approaches are presented in this section; references to comprehensive coverages of the details of experimentation and process-design theory are provided. Considerable information as to collection of process feasibility and design information has been presented along with the discussions of the individual treatment processes in prior sections.

Basic factors in the design of an activated sludge system, as an illustration, are shown below:

Independent variables	*Dependent variables*
Hydraulic detention time	Organic removal efficiency
F/M ratio or θ_c	Oxygen uptake rate
Biological solids concentration	Solids synthesis rate
Temperature level	Sludge settling rate
pH level	Oxygen transfer characteristics
Oxygen residual	Foaming and other nuisances
Nutrient supplementation	

The complexity of the experimental work can be minimised by holding several independent variables at near steady state during the initial test period, e.g. temperature at about 16° or 35°C depending upon predicted extreme conditions, pH at 6 to 8, oxygen residual at 0.5 to 2 mg/l or 5 to 8 mg/l depending on whether air or oxygen is to be used, and the ratio of available nitrogen and phosphorus to BOD removed at 1:20 and 1:100, respectively. The system then is operated at two or three detention times and biological-solids concentrations while measuring the dependent variables.

The mathematical relationships previously cited are used to relate organic removal efficiency to detention time and biomass concentration through development of a reaction rate constant. Oxygen utilisation and solids synthesis rates are similarly determined from the experimental data. The influence of loading factor (F/M ratio) or cell retention time (θ_c) on these rates and upon effluent suspended solids levels and biomass settling rates is measured. Oxygen transfer characteristics, excessive foaming, stripping of volatiles, and other factors of concern are examined.

Equipment

Laboratory studies of activated sludge processes are conducted with either semi-continuous (batch) feed or continuous feed. Batch-fed systems are somewhat easier to operate, provide clearer mass balances, and generate meaningful feasibility data. Their use for design purposes is possible only if shock feeding of waste does not inhibit the system. The laboratory units shown in Fig. 7.17 can be used in screening the responses of completely mixed systems to various loading and environmental stresses. For more refined studies, external clarification and pumped sludge return are desirable. Frequently fabrication of a small pilot unit, such as that shown in Fig. 7.18, is warranted. Operation of units with on-line feed experiencing any variability of the waste-water under study is most desirable toward achieving meaningful results, as demonstrated by Conway, Hovious, and Macauley.

Detailed procedures for the design and operation of laboratory and pilot units have been published along with techniques for developing design criteria from the experimental data. These references contain apparatus and procedural descriptions for evaluating fixed-film systems, aerated stabilisation, and anaerobic systems, as well as many ways of evaluating the activated sludge approach. Techniques for evaluating auxiliary physical-chemical systems are also presented. Relative data on fixed film processes can be achieved using a rotating tube biological filter (Fig. 7.19); design studies need to be made in fairly large systems simulating the actual configurations being considered.

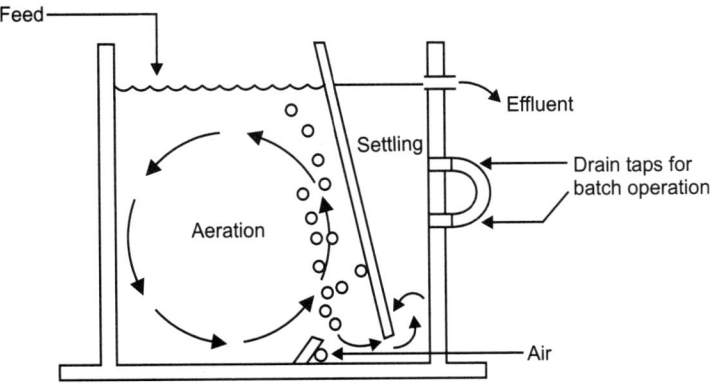

Fig. 7.17. Laboratory activated sludge unit.

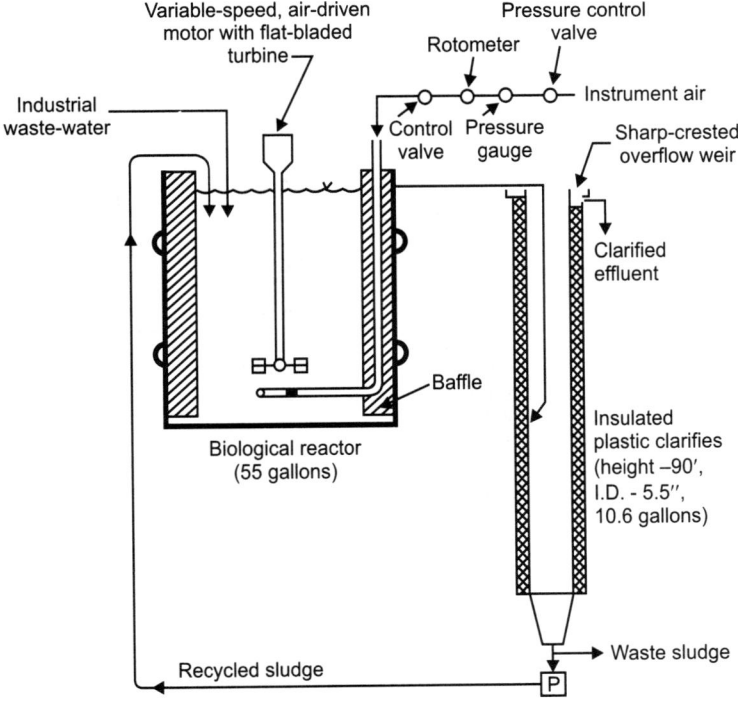

Fig. 7.18. Pilot activated sludge system.

An apparatus of general utility in evaluating metabolic rates of micro-organisms under a range of feed and environmental conditions is the Warburg respirometer. Figure 7.20 depicts this investigative tool as used for aerobic standards; anaerobic systems can also be followed by gas evolution. Microbiological response to a range of conditions can be examined in a single test as the Warburg apparatus accommodates 18 to 20 respirometers. A simplified means of using sealed serum bottles to follow anaerobic degradation (and inhibition) has been described by McCarty.

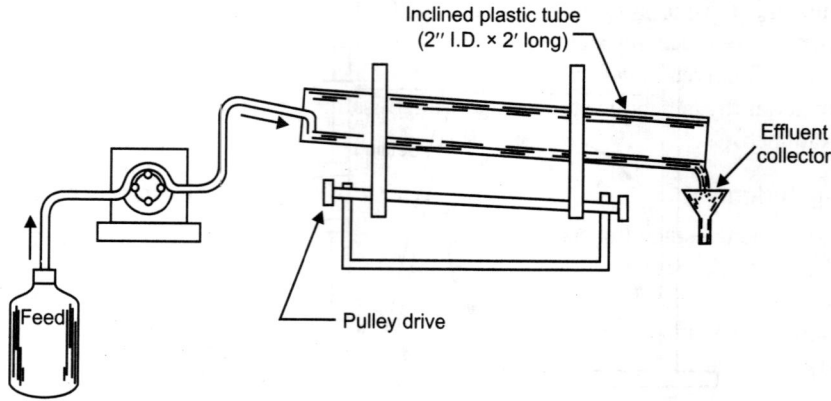

Fig. 7.19. Rotary-tube trickling filter.

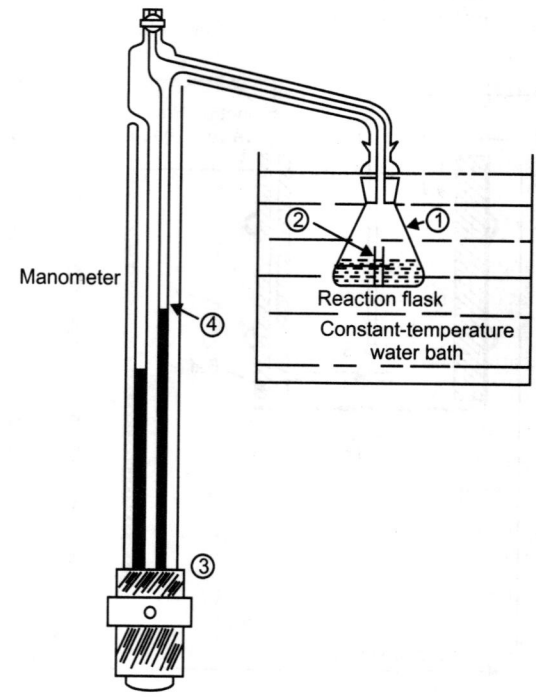

Fig. 7.20. Warburg constant-volume respirometer. (1) Main compartment containing waste-water and micro-organisms. (2) Centrewell containing KOH to absorb evolved CO_2. (3) Fluid reservoir with screw clamp for volume adjustment as O_2 is used by micro-organisms. (4) Reference level of closed leg of manometer.

Analysis

Thorough analysis of the performance of the biological system is essential. A first step usually is to measure the BOD_5 removal across the system. Since this measurement reflects only a portion of the biodegradable material, longer term incubations in analysing the BOD level in feed and effluent samples shed more insight into the system, as do tests of COD and TOC removal efficiency. Frequently, measurement of the removal of specific organic compounds or classes of compounds also is essential in understanding the involved transformations. The fate of heavy metals should be checked. The modes of removal of materials by metabolic processes, by volatilisation, or by incorporation in the waste biomass should be examined.

Engineering Judgment

Results of experimental studies should be applied to design using considerable engineering judgment. With virtual certainty, the assumption can be made that the volume and composition of the industrial waste-water studied in laboratory or in field pilot units is going to change, even before start-up of the treatment facility, as manufacturing plant operations are modified. Effluent goals also will change according to societal needs. Consequently, the experimental information should be viewed as a guide in making decisions, not as the dictator of the decision. A considerable effort should be spent on conceptual engineering work before proceeding to the process and detailed design phases. Process design work should include a least-cost analysis; one such means was described by Middleton and Lawrence.

APPENDIX 7.1

Biological Terms and Notation

a	:	Fraction of S_r converted to cells.
a'	:	Oxygen utilisation coefficient for substrate conversion, lb O_2 required/lb BOD_5 removed (kg/kg).
α(alpha)	:	Ratio of $K_L a$ of reactor liquor to that of tap water.
a_s	:	Biological solids settling rate constant.
B	:	Conversion factor, mg BOD_5/mg effluent suspended solids.
b	:	Cell autooxidation rate coefficient, day^{-1}.
b'	:	Oxygen utilisation rate for endogenous metabolism, lb O_2/day-lb. MLVSS (kg/day-kg).
β(beta)	:	Ratio of dissolved oxygen level at saturation in reactor liquor to that in pure tap water.
BOD_L	:	Long-term biochemical oxygen demand (~20-day incubation period), mg/l.
BOD_5	:	5-day biochemical oxygen demand (5-day incubation period), mg/l.
c	:	Exponent for feed concentration effect.
C_i	:	Supended solids concentration to be clarified, mg/l.
C_L	:	Design DO level, mg/l.
COD	:	Chemical oxygen demand, mg/l.
C_s	:	DO saturation at standard conditions, mg/l.
C_{sa}	:	DO saturation at one atmosphere pressure, mg/l.
C_{sw}	:	DO saturation level calculated for reactor liquor at design pressure and liquor temperature, mg/l.
C_t	:	DO at times t_1, t_2, etc. mg/l.
C_1	:	Suspended solids concentration at settling velocity v_1, lb./lb. or mg/mg or mg/l $\times 10^{-6}$.

C_2	:	Suspended solids concentration at settling velocity v_2, lb/lb or mg/mg or mg/l $\times$ 10^{-6}.
D_f	:	Biological filter depth, ft (m $\times$ 3.28).
DO	:	Dissolved oxygen concentration, mg/l.
D_o	:	DO deficit, mg/l.
f_b	:	Fraction of generated biomass that is degradable.
F/M	:	Food-to-micro-organism ratio, lb BOD_5/lb MLVSS-day.
f_v	:	Ratio of MLVSS/MLSS.
K	:	Reaction rate coefficient independent of S_o, l/mg-hr.
K'	:	Reaction rate coefficient dependent on S_o for complete mixed system, l/mg-hr.
K''	:	Maximum rate of substrate utilisation per unit weight of micro-organisms, g BOD_L/day-g bacteria
k	:	Batch-fed reaction rate coefficient, l/mg-hr.
K_a	:	Reaction rate constant for aerated stabilisation basins when level of biosolids is not considered, day^{-1}.
K_{ax}	:	Reaction rate constant for aerated stabilisation basins when level of biosolids is considered, l/mg-day
K_f	:	Overall reaction rate constant for a biological filter taking into account actual reaction rate constant (gal./ft^2 -min) and specific surface area (ft^2/ft^3), min^{-1}.
K_La	:	Overall oxygen transfer coefficient, mg/l O_2 per mg/l DO deficit-hr (or hr^{-1}).
K_p	:	Reaction rate coefficient for unaerated stabilisation ponds, day^{-1}.
K_s	:	Half velocity constant or substrate level resulting in $\mu = 0.5$ μ_{max}, mg/l.
K_1	:	Reaction rate coefficient at T_1, l/mg-hr.
K_2	:	Reaction rate coefficient at T_2, l/mg-hr.
K_3	:	Oxygen transfer proportionality constant.
k_1	:	Thickening constant dependent on a_s and n.
m	:	Packing constant for biofilter.
MLSS	:	Mixed liquor suspended solids in aeration tank, mg/l.
MLVSS	:	Mixed liquor volatile suspended solids, mg/l.
μ(mu)	:	Specific growth rate, mg growth/mg biomass-hr (or hr^{-1}).
μ_{max}	:	Maximum specific growth rate attainable with a given type substrate, hr^{-1}.
n	:	Biological solids settling rate exponent.
N_a	:	O_2 transfer efficiency at field conditions, lb./hp-hr (kg/joule $\times$ 5.92 $\times$ 10^6).
N_s	:	O_2 transfer efficiency at standard conditions (20°C, 760 mm, pure tap water, nil DO), lb/hp-hr (kg/joule $\times$ 5.92 $\times$ 10^6).
OR	:	Overflow rate (flow volume/clarifier area), gal./sq ft-day ($\times$ 24.5 = m^3/m^2-day).
O_t	:	Total oxygen required, lb./day (kg/day).
O_v	:	Volume concentration of oxygen in gas leaving the test unit, %.
P	:	Power hp (KW $\times$ 1.34).
p	:	Design atmospheric pressure mm Hg (atm $\times$ 760, psia $\times$ 51.7, kN/cm^2 $\times$ 7.50, Kgf/cm^2 $\times$ 735).
p_b	:	Absolute pressure at depth of air release, psia (kN/m^2 $\times$ 0.145).
Q	:	Influent flow rate not including recycle, gal./day (or litres/day).
Q_h	:	Hydraulic loading to biofilter, gpm/ft^2 (m^3/m^2-min $\times$ 4.5).
R	:	Recycle flow rate, gal./day (or litres/day)

r	:	Nondegradable fraction of influent suspended solids.
R/Q	:	Recycle flow fraction.
S	:	Substrate level, mg/l.
S_a	:	BOD concentration applied to the biosystem (after dilution by recycle), mg/l.
S_{at}	:	Total substrate applied, lb. BOD_5/day (kg/day).
S_e	:	Effluent soluble BOD_5, mg/l.
S_{ea}	:	Long-term average soluble BOD_5 achievable with a single biological system in the field for a typical petrochemical S_o of 1000 mg/l, mg/l.
S_{em}	:	Predicted effluent BOD level for high month, mg/l.
S_o	:	Influent soluble BOD_5, mg/l.
S_r	:	BOD concentration reduction, mg/l.
S_{rt}	:	Total BOD_5 removed, lb./day (kg/day).
SVI	:	Sludge volume index, ml/gm.
T	:	Temperature, °C.
t	:	Average liquid retention time, hr.
θ_a(theta)	:	Temperature coefficient for long-term effluent quality adjustment.
θ_c	:	Mean cell residence time, days.
θ_t	:	Coefficient for temperature adjustment of reaction rate for BOD removal.
TOC	:	Total organic carbon, mg/l.
t_d	:	Retention time, days.
T_w	:	Design reactor temperature, °C.
t_1, t_2	:	Time, hr.
V	:	Adjustment factor for effluent variability to convert long-term average S_{ea} to maximum month S_{em}.
v_i	:	Initial biosolids settling rate at c_i, ft/hr (m/hr × 3.28).
v_1	:	Settling velocity at concentration c_1, ft/hr (m/hr × 3.28).
v_2	:	Settling velocity at concentration c_2, ft/hr (m/hr × 3.28).
W	:	Weight of aerated water, millions of pounds (kg × 2.21 × 10^6).
X_a	:	Active biological solids concentration in the reactor, mg/l.
X_{at}	:	Active biological solids weight in the reactor, lb. (kg × 2.21).
X_{eh}	:	Effluent suspended solids in high month, mg/l.
X_{et}	:	Total effluent biological solids, lb./day (kg/day).
X_{ot}	:	Total influent suspended solids, lb./day (kg/day).
X_{ov}	:	Influent degradable VSS, mg/l.
X_r	:	Recycled sludge solids concentration, mg/l.
ΔX_t	:	Total excess sludge, lb./day (kg/day).
X_v	:	MLVSS, mg/l.
X_{vt}	:	Total weight of VSS in aeration tank, lb. (kg).
ΔX_{vt}	:	Change in MLVSS, lb/day (kg/day).
X_{wt}	:	Total biological solids wasted, lb./day (kg/day).
Y	:	Maximum cell yield coefficient, g bacteria synthesised/g BOD_L consumed.
y	:	Conversion coefficient for BOD_5 to BOD_L, lb. BOD_5/lb BOD_L (kg/kg).
Z	:	Concentration of nonbiodegradable organics, mg/l.

Chapter 8

Biological Treatment of Solid Wastes

INTRODUCTION

Biological treatment involves using naturally occurring micro-organisms to decompose the biodegradable components of waste. If left to go to completion, this process will result in the production of gases (mainly carbon dioxide, methane and water vapour) plus a mineralised residue. Normally the process is interrupted when the residue still contains organic material, although in a more stable form, comprising a compost-like material.

The garden compost heap is the simplest form of biological treatment. With some care and regular turning, this can transform vegetable scraps and garden refuse into a rich and useful garden compost. Garden compost heaps are a valuable method for valorising part of the household waste at source, but are limited to more rural and sub-urban areas where space and gardens are plentiful. The alternative method to treat organic waste not composted at source (in particular from urban areas), involves centralised biological treatment plants.

Almost any organic material can be treated by this method. It is particularly suitable for many industrial wastes from such sources as breweries, fruit and vegetable producers and processors, slaughter-houses and meat processors, dairy producers and processors, paper mills, sugar mills, and leather, wool and textile producers. At the local community level, it is widely used to treat sewage sludges and organic wastes from parks and gardens.

Household waste is also rich in organic material, consisting of kitchen and garden waste. According to geography, this accounts for between 25 per cent and 60 per cent of municipal solid waste by weight, with levels of organics particularly high. If one adds to this the paper fraction, which is also of organic origin and suitable for biological treatment, some 50–85 per cent of the municiple solid waste (MSW) can be treated by such methods. The suitability of biological treatment for wet organic material contrasts markedly with other treatment methods, such as incineration and landfilling, where the high water content and putrescible nature can be a source of major problems, by reducing overall calorific value and increasing the production of leachate and landfill gas. This potential of biological treatment is being exploited in some countries, but almost ignored in others.

Numerous variants of biological treatment exist, differing according to the feedstock used (Table 8.1) and the process employed. Feedstocks range from highly mixed wastes, e.g. MSW, which require extensive treatment to remove the non-organic fractions prior to, or occasionally after, biological processing, to the separately collected and more narrowly defined biowaste, VFG (vegetable, fruit and garden) and green wastes. Although there are many different types of plant available, there are two basic process types, aerobic and anaerobic. In aerobic treatment, usually known as composting, organic material decomposes in the presence of oxygen to produce mainly carbon dioxide, water and compost. Considerable energy is released in the process, which is generally lost to the surroundings. Anaerobic processes are variously described as anaerobic fermentation, anaerobic digestion or biogasification. Throughout this chapter, the term biogasification will be used. As the name implies this produces biogas, a useful product consisting mainly of methane and carbon dioxide, plus an organic residue which can be stabilised to produce compost, but differs somewhat from aerobically produced composts.

Table 8.1. The range of possible inputs to biological treatment plants.

Category	Description
Mixed wastes	
MSW	Municipal solid waste, commingled solid waste collected from households, commerce and institutions
HW	Household waste, commingled waste collected from households only
Centrally sorted waste	
RDF sort fines	Putrescible material sorted mechanically from mixed waste during the production of refuse derived fuel (RDF)
Separately collected waste	
Wet waste	Household waste from which dry recyclables have been removed
Biowaste	This term is widely misused, ranging in meaning from garden waste only, to VFG material or to VFG plus paper; here it refers to separately collected organic and non-recyclable paper waste only
VFG	Separately collected vegetable, fruit and garden waste only
Greenwaste (GW)	Separately collected garden waste only

BIOLOGICAL TREATMENT OBJECTIVES

Both composting and biogasification can fulfil several functions, and it is necessary to identify the key objective(s) required of the process. They can either be considered as pre-treatments for ultimate disposal of a stabilised material (normally in a landfill) or as a valorisation method.

Pretreatment for Disposal

Volume reduction

Breakdown into methane and/or carbon dioxide and water results in the decomposition of up to 75 per cent of the organic material on a dry weight basis. From wet biowaste to normal compost the weight loss is generally around 50 per cent. As organics and paper represent the two largest fractions of the household waste stream this is a significant reduction. Additionally there is considerable loss of water, either by evaporation (in composting) or by pressing of the residue (biogasification). The moisture content of the organic fraction of household waste is around 65 per cent, whilst for compost made from biowaste, it is around 30–40 per cent and for material from biogasification 25–45 per cent.

The breakdown and moisture loss together result in a marked volume reduction in material for further treatment and disposal. Removal of water will also reduce the formation of leachate if the residues are subsequently landfilled.

Stabilisation

As much of the decomposition has occurred during biological treatment, the resulting materials are more stable than the original organic inputs, and thus more suitable for final disposal in a landfill. The cumulative oxygen demand of the organic material, a measure of biological activity and thus inversely related to stability, can decrease by a factor of six during biological treatment (Table 8.2). Similarly, the carbon/nitrogen (C/N) ratio, which gives a measure of the maturity of a compost (high C/N ratio indicates fresh organic material, low C/N ratio indicates mature, stable material), falls markedly during biological treatment processes.

Table 8.2. Compost quality.

Description	Fresh organic fraction	Windrow composting (after 6 weeks)	Biogasification (after 6 weeks)
C/N ratio	30	15	12
Cumulative oxygen demand (mg O_2/g organic matter over 10 days)	250–300	150–160	50–60
Pathogen destruction (colonies/g dry wt.)			
Faecal coliforms	3×10^3	2×10^2	0
Faecal streptococci	2×10^5	4×10^4	0

Sanitisation

Both composting and biogasification are effective in destroying the majority of pathogens present in the feedstock. Aerobic composting is a strongly exothermic process, and temperatures of 60°–65°C are built up and maintained in composting piles or vessels over an extended period of time, sufficient to ensure the destruction of most pathogens and seeds (Table 8.2). Biogasification processes are only mildly exothermic, but may be run at temperatures of 55°C (thermophilic process) by the addition of heat. The combination of this temperature and anaerobic conditions is sufficient to destroy most pathogens (Table 8.2), though if lower process temperatures are used (mesophilic process), further heat treatment during the final aerobic stabilisation stage may be required to produce sanitary residues.

Valorisation

In contrast to the above, the main objective of most biological treatment is to produce useful products (biogas/energy, compost) from organic waste, i.e. to valorise part of the waste stream.

Biogas production

Biogasification produces a flammable gas with a calorific value of around 6–8 kWh (21.6–28.8 MJ) per m³, which can be sold as gas, or burned on-site in gas engine generators to produce electricity. Some of the biogas will be burned to provide process heating on site, and some electricity will be consumed, but there can be a net export of either gas or electrical power from the plant. There will normally be a market for this product, at least for the electricity.

As the gas can be stored between production and use for power generation, electricity export into the national grid can be timed to coincide with peak consumption times, and thus highest energy prices. This economic advantage is increased further where additional premium prices are paid for electricity generated from non-fossil fuel sources.

Compost production

Both composting and biogasification produce a partly stabilised organic material that may be used as a compost, soil-improver, fertiliser, filler, filter material or for decontaminating polluted soils. Alternatively, the material can be considered as a residue and landfilled. The only point that determines whether the material is a useful product, and hence of value, or a residue to be disposed of at a cost, is the presence of a market.

Markets for compost will differ widely across Europe. In southern Europe, the lack of organic matter in the soil creates a large need for additional organic material. There is, therefore, a strong market for compost made from any feedstock, provided that the compost is safe for use, even though the level of contamination may be high. The same compost, if produced in Holland or Germany, however, would be considered only for landfill cover material or as a residue for disposal. As it would not meet the relevant quality guidelines, there would be no market for such a product, although markets do exist for higher quality composts. Since the main determinants of compost quality are the composition of the feedstock and the process used, production of compost for sale in such countries may require the use of restricted feedstocks involving separate collection (biowaste, either with or without paper; VFG; green waste), or the use of more sophisticated processing techniques. There is a grey area, however, around the distinction between product and residue, as in many cases, waste-derived compost is freely distributed.

The need to define the objective of any biological treatment process bears repeating. If the aim is to produce a quality compost for sale, then a restricted input (e.g. VFG, or biowaste) is preferable, and the necessary source separated collection schemes must be put in place. If, however, the objective is to maximise diversion from landfill, while still producing a quality compost, the biowaste definition can be widened to include paper as well as organic materials so long as there is a market for the resulting compost. If the objective is to pre-treat waste prior to final disposal, then treating a mixed waste stream will be effective.

In biogasification, where there are two possible products, biogas and compost, it is also necessary to decide which should be optimised. The digested residue produced in Germany cannot be marketed as compost, as the quality is too low due to the presence of hazardous materials. In contrast, a biogas plant in Belgium, using a different process, produces a humus-like product for which there is a viable market.

BIOLOGICAL TREATMENT PROCESSES

A classification of the types of biological treatment processes is given in Fig. 8.1. Each consists of a pre-treatment stage followed by a biological decomposition process.

Pretreatment

Pretreatment has two basic functions, the separation of the organic material from other fractions in the feedstock, and the preparation of this organic material for the subsequent biological processing. Clearly, the amount of pre-treatment will depend on the nature of feedstock; the more narrowly defined the incoming material, the less separation will be required, although pre-treatment for size reduction, homogenisation and moisture control will still be needed.

Where the plant input is mixed waste, e.g. MSW, the non-organic material (plastic, glass, metal, etc.) needs to be removed at this stage (unless the overall objective is volume reduction alone). In some plants, part of this material can be recovered for use as secondary materials. In the Duisburg-Huckingen composting plant in Germany, for example, incoming mixed waste is passed under a magnet to remove ferrous metals, and then along conveyor belts where glass bottles, non-ferrous metals and plastic items are hand picked and recovered (Fig. 8.2).

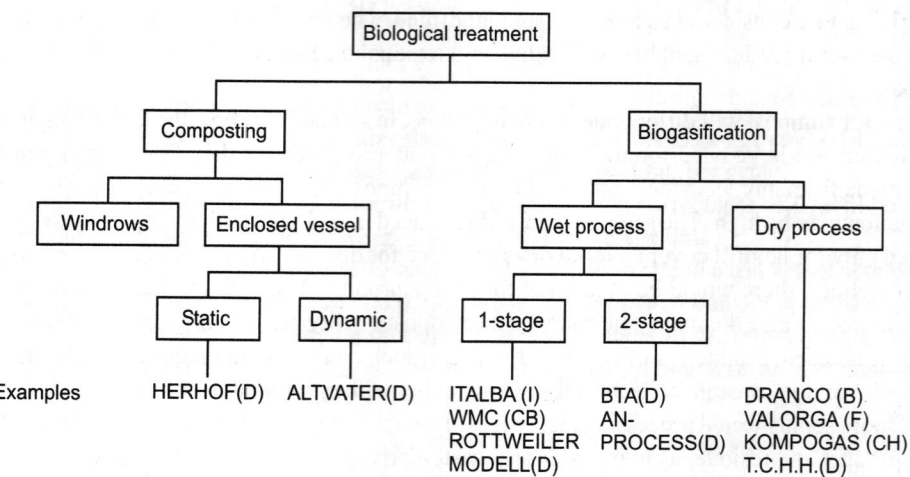

Fig. 8.1. Classification of biological treatment.

Preparation for the actual composting or biogasification usually involves some form of screening to remove oversize items, size reduction and homogenisation. For biogasification, it is necessary to produce a pumpable feedstock. Size reduction and mixing are achieved either by shredding the feedstock in a mill, or by the use of a large rotating drum.

Shredding the feedstock removes the need for a screening stage prior to processing, but means that nuisance materials are also shredded. This makes them much more difficult to separate from the compost in the later refining stage. A drum achieves some degree of size reduction and homogenisation as it rotates, but does not shred nuisance materials. These can then be removed intact by a screen (which can be incorporated into the rotating drum) prior to the biological process, so that the later refining stages can be simplified.

Nuisance materials can, therefore, be removed either before or after the biological treatment stage. There is an advantage in removing them as early as possible, since the longer they are in contact with the organic material, the greater the likelihood of cross-contamination.

Additionally, it reduces the amount of material entering the biological treatment process, by removing material that would not be degraded.

The amount of nuisance material removed in the pre-treatment stage depends on the waste used as feedstock. Even where the feedstock arises from source-separated collection of biowaste, separation of nuisance material during pre-treatment is advisable, especially if the feedstock comes from urban areas. A biogas plant in Brecht, Belgium, for example, using a feedstock of separately collected VFG plus paper (Table 8.1) discards up to 19 per cent of its input during the pre-treatment stage (Fig. 8.3).

Aerobic Processing: Composting

Biological treatment can be described as the biological decomposition of organic wastes under controlled conditions; for composting, these conditions need to be aerobic and elevated temperatures are achieved due to the exothermic processes catalysed by microbial enzymes. Three main groups of micro-organism are involved in the composting process: bacteria, actinomycetes and fungi. Initially bacteria and fungi predominate, and their activity causes the temperature to rise to around 70°C in the centre of a pile. At this temperature, only thermophilic (heat-tolerant) bacteria and actinomycetes are active. As the rate of decomposition and hence temperature subsequently falls, fungi and other heat-sensitive bacteria become active again. Temperature, therefore, is one of the key factors in composting plants that needs to be constantly monitored and controlled.

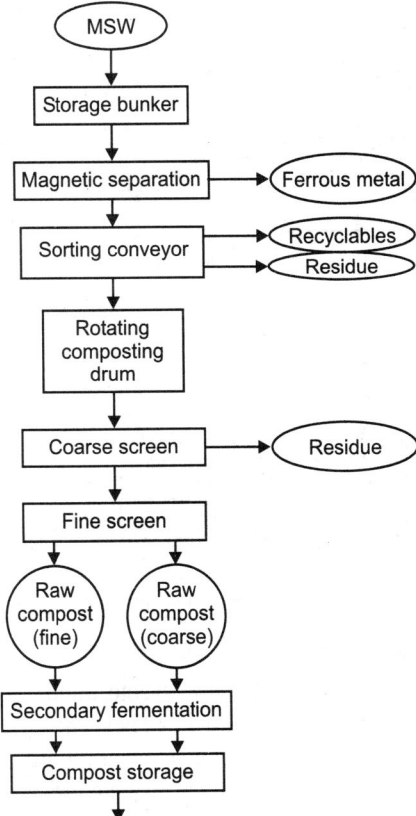

Fig. 8.2. Simplified flow chart for composting process for commingled municipal solid waste.

To maintain the high rate of decomposition, oxygen must be constantly available. In the simplest process type, as with a garden compost heap, this is achieved by regular turning of the composting material in long piles or windrows.

The alternative method is forced aeration, whereby air is forced through a static pile using small vents in the floor of the composting area. Air can either be forced out of the vents, or drawn down through the composting pile by applying a vacuum to the vents. The former method aids dispersion of the heat from the centre of the pile to the outside, making for a more uniform process. The latter helps in controlling odours as the air passing through the pile is effectively filtered to reduce many odours before release. Aeration also helps remove carbon dioxide and volatile organic compounds, such as fatty acids, and buffers the pH.

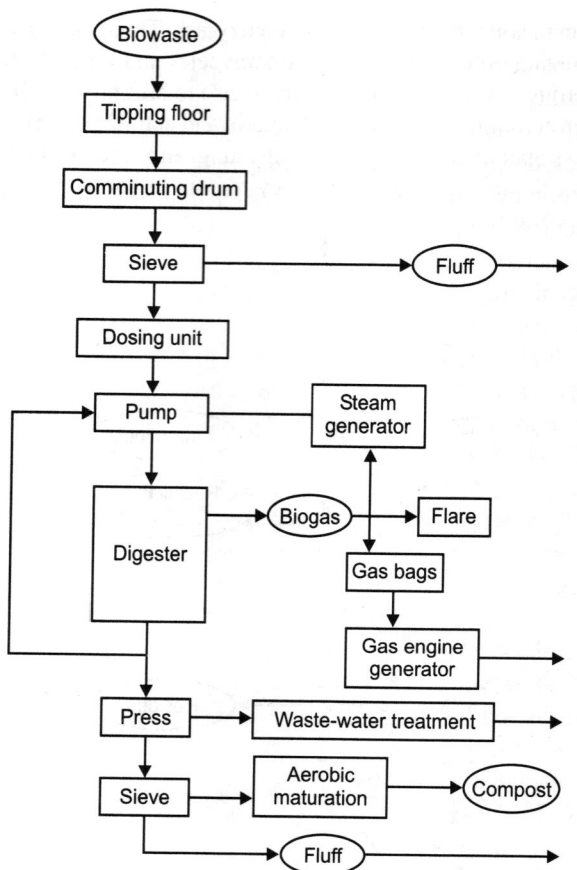

Fig. 8.3. Flow chart for dry biogasification process.

Percolation of composting piles by air depends on the structure and water content of the input material. The water content for aerobic composting needs to be over 40 per cent, otherwise the rate of decomposition will start to fall, but if it is too high the material will become waterlogged and limit air movement. If the input material is too wet, water-absorbing and bulking agents such as woody garden waste, wood chips, straw or sawdust can be added to improve the structure, and increase the air circulation.

Windrow composting is the most common technology used, being least capital intensive. However, when it is open to the elements, control over moisture content, temperature and odour emissions is limited. One way round this is to have the entire area enclosed, and the exhaust air filtered. In the Netherlands, open air composting is generally not allowed for plants with a capacity exceeding 2000 tonnes/year, but due to the expense, Fricke and Vogtmann recommend this only for plants in excess of 12,000 tonnes/year. Further control over both composting conditions and emissions are possible in more advanced technologies, using a variety of enclosed vessels (boxes and drums) for totally enclosed processing. Open or semi-enclosed windrows are often still used in these systems, for the maturation stage.

The duration of the composting process varies with the technology employed, and the maturity of the compost required. Compost maturity can be assessed by the carbon/nitrogen (C/N) ratio of the material, which falls from around 20 in raw organic waste to around 12 in a mature compost after some

12–14 weeks. Application to soils of immature composts with high residual microbial activity and high C/N ratios can result in uptake of the nitrogen from the soil by the compost, which will reduce, rather than enhance the soil fertility.

Before marketing of the compost, further maturation and refining are needed. Additional maturation may be necessary to break down complex organic materials toxic to some plants, which may still be present in the compost. Refining involves size classification of the compost particles and the removal of nuisance materials by sieving, ballistic separation or air classification, ready for the chosen end use. Nuisance materials may include oversized material, stones, metal fragments, glass, plastic film and hard plastic. Oversize organic fragments can be recycled into the composting process, but the rest of the residue will need to be incinerated or landfilled.

An alternative way to both mature and refine compost has been developed using earthworms. The beneficial effects of earthworms in garden compost heaps has long been recognised, but recent research in France has developed 'lumbricomposting' or 'vermicomposting' into an industrial process to deal with household waste. The plant takes in mixed waste and the pre-treatment stage involves removal of glass, plastic and metal for materials recovery. The remaining waste is graded, but not shredded, and then composted aerobically to start off the decomposition process and kill off pathogens. At this stage, the immature compost material is added to vertical cages known as 'lumbricators' containing cultures of earthworms. Various species have been tested for their suitability, but due to its prolific reproduction. *Eisenia andre* (Bouche) is the species usually cultured. The earthworms eat and partially digest the organic material, leaving any contaminants intact as residue. Part of the eaten organic material is metabolised by the worms and converted into worm biomass, the rest is eliminated as worm faeces, which are collected at the base of the lumbricators. The worms are particularly efficient at eating all of the biodegradable material, but will not ingest any of the inert and contaminating material. The resulting compost has a very fine and consistent particle size, and so can be separated from the residual inert material with relative ease, using a 5 mm sieve. This is facilitated by the fact that the feedstock is not shredded in the pre-treatment stage.

Anaerobic Processing: Biogasification

Conditions for biogasification need to be anaerobic, so a totally enclosed process vessel is required. Although this necessitates a higher level of technology than some forms of composting, containment allows greater control over the process itself and also of emissions such as noxious odours. Greater process control, especially of temperature, allows a reduction in treatment time when compared to composting. Since a biogas plant is usually vertical, it requires less land area than a composting plant.

Biogasification is particularly suitable for wet substrates, such as sludges or food wastes, which present difficulties in composting as their lack of structural material will restrict air circulation. The anaerobic process has been used for some time to digest sewage sludges and organic industrial wastes, and this has been extended more recently to fractions of household solid waste.

The various biogasification processes can be classified according to the solids content of the material digested, and the temperature at which the process operates. Dry anaerobic digestion may be defined as taking place at a total solids concentration of over 25 per cent; below this level of solids, the process is described as wet digestion. With regard to temperature, processes are either described as mesophilic (operating between 30° and 40°C) or thermophilic (operating between 50° and 65°C). It has been well established that different anaerobic micro-organisms have optimum growth rates within these temperature ranges. In contrast to aerobic processing (composting), the biogasification process is only mildly exothermic. Thus, heat needs to be supplied to maintain the process temperature, especially for thermophilic processes. The advantage of the higher temperature, on the other hand, is that the reactions will occur at a faster rate, so shorter residence times are needed in the reactor vessel.

Wet anaerobic digestion

In its simplest form, this process consists of a single stage in a completely mixed mesophilic digester, operating at a total solids content of around 3–8 per cent. To produce this level of dilution, considerable water has to be added (and heated), and then removed after the digestion process. This method is routinely used to digest sewage sludge and animal wastes, but has also been used to treat household waste in Italy and Germany. During a retention time of 12–30 days, the organic materials are broken down in a series of steps that first hydrolyse them into more soluble material, then break these down into short chained organic acids before converting them to methane and carbon dioxide (Fig. 8.4).

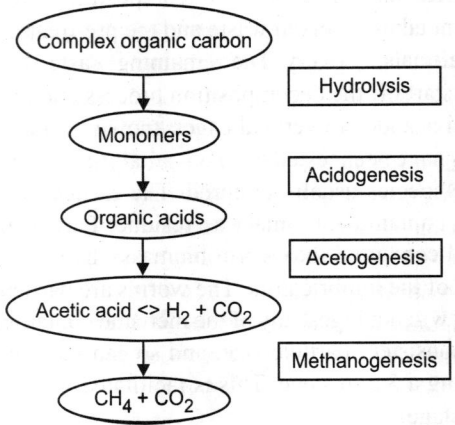

Fig. 8.4. Metabolic stages in the biogasification of organic wastes.

The single stage wet process can suffer from several practical problems, however, such as the formation of a hard scum layer in the digester, and difficulty in keeping the contents completely mixed. A basic deficiency is that the different reactions in the process cannot be separately optimised. The acidogenic micro-organisms will act to lower the pH of the reaction mixture, whereas the methanogens, which reproduce more slowly, have a pH optimum around 7.0.

This problem has been solved by the development of the two-stage process. Hydrolysis and acidification are stimulated in the first reactor vessel, kept at a pH of around 6.0. Methanogenesis occurs in the second separate vessel, operated at a pH of 7.5–8.2. Variations of the two-stage wet (mesophilic) digestion process have been developed and implemented in Germany. The whole process can be run with a retention time of 5–8 days.

Dry anaerobic digestion

Several processes have been developed that digest semi-solid organic wastes (over 25 per cent total solids) to produce biogas in a single stage. The processes can be either mesophilic, or thermophilic, and can use organic material from mixed wastes such as MSW, or separated biowaste. The dry fermentation process means that little process water has to be added (or heated). No mixing equipment is necessary and crust formation is not possible due to the relatively solid nature of the digester contents. This anaerobic process usually takes from 12–18 days, followed by several days in the post-digestion stage for residue stabilisation and maturation.

Maturation and refining

The residues of both wet and dry biogasification processes require further treatment before they can be used as compost. They contain high levels of water; even the dry process residue contains around 65 per cent water, compared to German maximum recommended water levels for compost of 35 per cent and 45 per cent for bagged and loose compost respectively organic reclamation and composting association (ORCA). Excess water can be removed by filtering or pressing, to produce a cake-like residue; further drying can be achieved using waste beat from the gas engines if the biogas is burnt on site to produce electricity. Some of the waste-water can be re-circulated and used to adjust the water content of the digester input, the rest represents an aqueous effluent requiring treatment prior to discharge.

The digested residue, initially anaerobic, will also still contain many volatile organic acids and reduced organic material. This needs to be matured aerobically to oxidise and stabilise these compounds, in a process similar to the maturation of aerobic composts, prior to sale as compost, or disposal as a residue.

COMPOST MARKETS

It is the presence or absence of a viable market that determines whether the composted output from biological treatment represents a valued product or a residue for disposal. Consequently much effort has been put into the definition and development of markets for waste-derived composts both in Europe and the United States by organisations such as the organic reclamation and composting Association (ORCA) and the solid waste composting council (SWCC), respectively.

Compost can fulfil one or more of four basic functions:

1. Soil conditioner or improver: By adding organic matter to the soil, compost will improve the structure of the soil and replace the organic material lost during sustained intensive cultivation.
2. Soil fertiliser: The actual value of compost as a fertiliser will depend on its content of nutrients in general and of nitrate and phosphate in particular. This is normally much lower than for inorganic fertilisers, and because these nutrients are bound to the organic matter, their release is slow and sustained. This is an advantage that is becoming increasingly important in countries such as Denmark, Belgium, the Netherlands and Germany where strict limitations on nitrate application are being implemented to reduce ammonia emissions and possible groundwater contamination.
3. Mulch: Compost can be applied to the soil surface to reduce evaporation losses and weed growth.
4. Peat replacement: Use of peat is facing growing public opposition, being seen as the exploitation of an irreplaceable natural biotope. In both the UK and Germany, some sectors of the trade have specified that no peat be used in products for home gardening. Whilst the use of waste-derived composts instead of peat may be limited in the potted plant industry due to very strict phytosanitary regulations in Europe, to control the spread of plant diseases, there appears to be a market as a peat replacement in the home gardening and landscaping sectors.

As well as fulfilling different functions, composts from biological treatments come in different forms. Many processes produce more than one grade of compost (e.g. coarse and fine) at the final refining stage.

The essential marketing step is to match up these products to the market requirements. In some cases, new markets may need to be developed; for example, where composting plants produce a novel product, such as the very fine textured and uniformly graded compost produced by the lumbri-composting process. The market potential can be assessed by considering both current and potential future usage of composts.

Surveys of current compost consumption show that, in Switzerland, 46 per cent compost is used in agriculture and vineyards, 30 per cent in horticulture and tree nurseries, 13 per cent in hobby gardening and 11 per cent in recultivation. A more detailed analysis of German usage is given in Table 8.3. Several assessments undertaken of market potential suggest that there is considerable potential for increasing this level of usage. Penetration of these new market areas will depend on effective marketing of waste-derived compost as a quality product, i.e. that it is safe and fit for use, and gives clear benefits compared to competing products at an affordable cost. Whilst these are general pre-conditions, there are additional specific compost quality requirements that will vary between different compost uses (Table 8.4).

Table 8.3. Utilisation of compost in Germany.

	Compost from biowaste (%)	Compost from green waste (%)
Hobby gardening	30	25
Commercial horticulture	10	13
Departments of parks and cementeries	12	29
Roads departments	1	7
Landscape gardening	29	13
Viniculture	1	1
Agriculture	10	8
Technical use	2	–
Landfill cover	5	4
Total	100	100

Table 8.4. Market requirements for compost quality in France[a].

Market outlet	Impurities (glass, plastic)	Maturity	Organic material	Particle size	Salinity	Humidity
Agriculture	1	3	2	4	6	5
	xxx		xxx			
Market gardening	1	1	3	5	3	6
	xxxx	xxxx	xxx		xxx	
Produce farming	1	2	3	5	4	6
	xxxx	xxxx	xxx		xxx	
Viniculture	1	2	2	4	6	5
	xxx					
Arboriculture	1	2	2	4	6	5
	xxx		xxx			
Mushroom farms	2	1	4	5	6	2
	xxx	xxxx				xxx

[a] Numbers 1–6 give quality criteria in descending order of importance; xxx/xxxx, customers sensitive/very sensitive to this criterion.

The failure to obtain widespread acceptance of waste-derived composts, especially in the agricultural sector has most likely been due to concerns over its safety and quality. Failure of many early plants to completely separate visual contaminants (e.g. plastic film) from the final compost reinforced the idea of waste-based composts as inferior products. The connotation of waste also raises concerns over safety, in particular the possible presence of pathogens, although these should be effectively destroyed in the biological treatment process. More recently, the level of heavy metals in waste-derived composts has become a concern. The high levels of some heavy metals in some fractions of household waste can result in contamination of the final compost, if biological treatment of mixed wastes is used. What are needed, if waste-derived composts are to become fully accepted and used more extensively, are: (i) widely accepted quality standards that can reassure potential users that the compost is both safe and fit for use, especially with repeated applications, and (ii) plant growth studies demonstrating a commercial benefit from the application of compost or compost-based products.

COMPOST STANDARDS

Compost market development would be facilitated by the application of consistent quality standards across Europe, but present standards vary widely between countries both in approach and detail. Of these, 9 countries (Austria, Belgium, Denmark, France, Germany, Greece, Italy, the Netherlands and Switzerland) have implemented or proposed standards, Sweden and the UK are in the process of drafting standards while Spain uses standards relating to fertilisers. In countries such as Germany, these criteria take the form of marketing standards, whereas in other countries they actually comprise a legally defined standard.

The objective of the standards is to protect land from contamination and to ensure that the composts marketed are fit for use. Since there are many uses for compost, however, different compost quality criteria need to be applied for each separate application. Several countries, such as the Netherlands and Austria, define several different grades of compost with different maximum levels of contaminants for each (Table 8.5). Belgium also specifies which grades can be used for different applications such as growing food or fodder crops.

Most standards relate to the physical and chemical properties of the compost, although there is normally more emphasis on what should not be in the compost (i.e. contaminants) rather than what should be in the compost (e.g. nutrients). Heavy metal levels come in for close scrutiny, but as Table 8.5 demonstrates, limit levels vary widely between countries. To a large extent, this reflects differences in the interpretation of the available scientific data on the heavy metal levels that constitute a significant health or environmental risk. Another cause for variability, however, is the use to which the compost may be put. Many of the most restricted heavy metal limits refer to composts that can be freely applied; some of the more relaxed standards are supplemented by restrictions on their level or time of use, frequency of application, application during wet weather, soil type or proximity of water supply plants. Measured levels for contaminants such as heavy metals will also depend on the analytical methods used. Whilst most national standards include details of the analytical methods required, some, such as Switzerland, do not. Clearly this lack of uniformity can only hinder the development of free markets for compost across Europe.

Not all standards systems even take the same basic approach. Since the quality of a compost is largely determined by the feedstock used and the processing method, some standards set criteria for these rather than the quality of the resulting compost itself. Criteria for some of the high quality composts specify that unsegregated household waste cannot be used as a feedstock. Criteria for compost processing methods are commonly used to determine microbiological safety. Several standards include both the temperature that must be achieved and its duration for destruction of pathogens during aerobic composting.

Table 8.5. Limit values for elements in compost, in current standards (mg/kg dry matter).

Country	A	A Class 1	A Class 2	B Agricultural land	B Parkland	DK	F NF Urbain	D RAL	I	NL Compost	NL Clean compost	E	CH
Arsenic	–	–	–	–	–	–[a]	–	–	10	25	15	–	–
Boron	100	–	–	–	–	–	–	–	–	–	–	–	–
Cadmium	4	0.7	1	5	5	1.2	8	2	10	2	1	40	3
Chromium	150	70	70	150	200	–	–	100	–[c]	200	70	750	150
Cobalt	–	–	–	10	20	–	–	–	–	–	–	–	25
Copper	400	70	100	100	500	–	–	100	600	300	90	1750	150
Lead	500	70	150	600	1000	120[b]	800	150	500	200	120	1200	150
Mercury	4	0.7	1	5	5	1.2	8	1.5	10	2	0.7	25	3
Molybdenum	–	–	–	–	–	–	–	–	–	5	–	–	–
Nickel	100	42	60	50	100	45	200	50	200	50	20	400	50
Selenium	–	–	–	–	–	–	–	–	–	–	–	–	–
Zinc	1000	210	400	1000	1500	–	–	400	2500	900	280	4000	500

[a] 25 for private gardens.
[b] 80 for private gardens.
[c] 500 for chromium(III) and 100 for chromium(VI).

The French compost standard takes yet another approach. Rather than set criteria in terms of compost/ composting conditions considered safe and fit for use, the criteria reflect the engineering capabilities of existing plants. In this case, some plants should be capable of meeting the requirements, but elsewhere the problem of compost not meeting quality criteria seems widespread. Taking a sample of 27 biowaste composting plants in Germany, for example, Smith calculated that the output of 25 per cent of them would not meet the German Bundesgütesgemeinschaft quality limits, and almost 70 per cent would not meet the stricter proposed Dutch limits.

In the United States, the Environmental protection agency (EPA) has taken yet a different approach, based on a risk assessment of soil to which compost has been added. This approach is related to the US (and UK) approach towards application of sewage sludge to fields, and does have a certain scientific logic.

In conclusion, criteria are needed to provide reassurance that marketed composts are fit and safe for use, but such criteria should be set uniformly across Europe on the basis of good scientific data, considering all aspects of compost usage. Such standards should define the quality and quantity of compost that can be used for different applications ranging from horticulture and agriculture to the reclamation of derelict land and erosion control.

ENVIRONMENTAL IMPACTS: INPUT-OUTPUT ANALYSIS

Defining the System Boundaries

The system boundaries for biological treatment are defined here as the physical boundaries of the plant. Thus, both the pre-sorting treatment and the biological process are included. Materials enter the system as waste inputs and leave as compost, recovered secondary materials, residues (from sorting and composting), or as air or water emissions (Figs 8.5 and 8.6). Energy enters the system as either electrical energy from the national grid, or as fuels (e.g. diesel). In the case of biogasification, some of the energy recovered in the biogas is consumed on site for process heating, and it is assumed that the rest of the biogas is burned on site in a gas engine-powered generator to produce electricity. Again some of this is used on site, but the rest is exported from the site as electrical energy.

Inputs

Waste input

The feedstock for biological treatment can arise from at least three different sources: separately collected organic/paper material, mechanically separated putrescibles from an RDF process or mixed and unsorted MSW.

The current trend in Europe is towards a separated collection of organic material from households. The exact composition of this feedstock will vary according to the definition of 'green waste' or 'biowaste' used by the collection scheme, but will generally consist of kitchen and garden waste, plus in many cases non-recyclable soiled paper and paper products. Even in narrowly defined feedstocks there will always be a level of nuisance materials, requiring a pre-sorting stage. Such nuisance materials arise from the inclusion of: (i) bags (often plastic) used to contain organic material, (ii) other materials which form a small part of otherwise organic materials, and (iii) materials included in the biowaste by mistake. There will also be some organic material not suitable for biological treatment, e.g. woody garden waste. Mixed waste inputs, such as MSW will need extensive pre-sorting to remove all of the non-organic material, which is not suitable for biological treatment. In contrast, finely sorted putrescible feedstock from an RDF type process will have already undergone a sorting stage, so will not require another pre-sort prior to the biological treatment process.

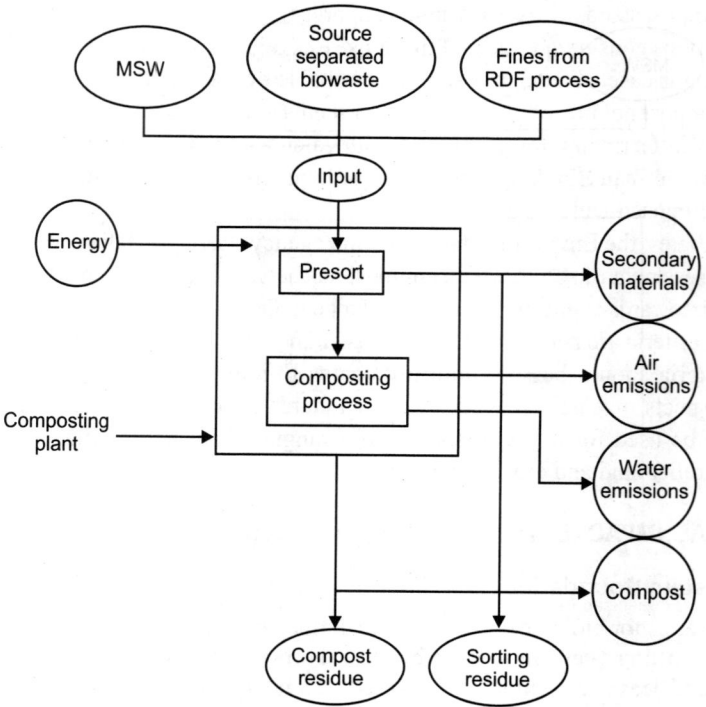

Fig. 8.5. Flow diagram for typical composting plant.

Energy consumption

The energy consumption of the pre-treatment process will depend on the feedstock used. Mixed feedstocks, such as MSW will need more extensive sorting per tonne of input, with associated energy requirements, than more narrowly defined feedstocks or those that have already been mechanically sorted as part of an RDF process, irrespective of the subsequent method of treatment. The energy consumption of the biological treatment process itself will depend on the technology employed.

Composting

Composting involves a net consumption of energy, consuming process energy and not producing any energy in a usable form. The German Government report a typical energy consumption of from 20 to 50 kWh (electrical energy) per input tonne for plants capable of processing 10,000 tonnes of biowaste per year, and suggest a range from 18 to 50 kWh (electrical) per tonne of input. This variability will reflect both the different feedstocks used, the different sizes of the composting plants, and also the maturity of the compost produced.

Kern looked at several different composting methods and calculated an average energy consumption of 21 kWh/tonne input; for plants producing less mature compost (rotte grades I–II) the average consumption was 18.3 kWh/tonne, whilst for plants producing mature compost (rotte grades III–IV) the average was 30.7 kWh/tonne.

For the purposes of the LCI model, an energy consumption of 30 kWh of electrical energy per tonne of input to the composting plant is assumed.

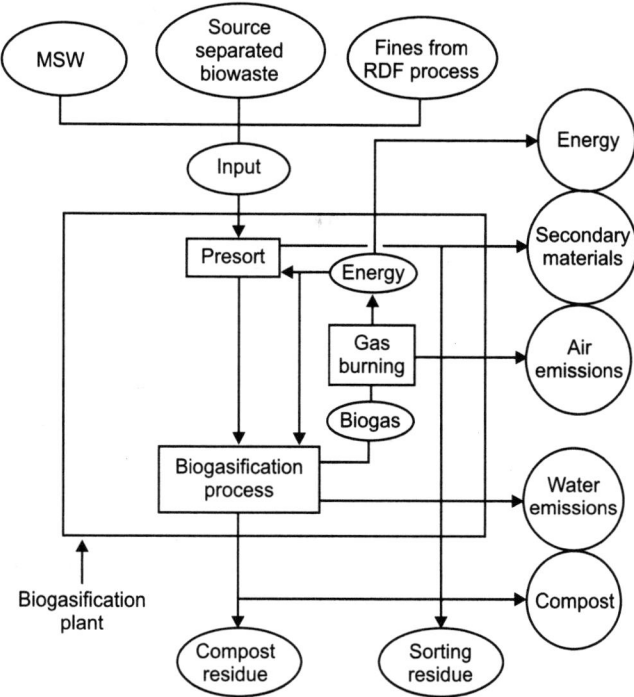

Fig. 8.6. Flow diagram for typical biogasification plant.

Biogasification

Biogasification involves both consumption of energy during processing, and the production of useful energy as biogas. Since some of the biogas can be burned to produce steam to heat the digester, and more can be burned in a gas engine to produce electricity, the energy requirement for the process can be met from within the biogas produced. The remaining biogas can either be exported as biogas (i.e. as fuel) or burned on-site to provide heat or to generate electricity (both for export). For the purposes of the present study, it is assumed that the biogas is burned on-site for power generation, and that surplus energy is exported as electrical energy.

The electrical energy requirement for biogasification has been reported as 50 kWh and 54 kWh per input tonne for two different processes. This represents around 32–35 per cent of the gross electricity produced by the plant. In another example, a biogas plant operating using the dry process consumes from 30 to 50 per cent of the electricity produced.

Thermal energy is also required for the process, but this can be obtained by using waste heat left after electricity generation, or by burning some of the biogas. Therefore, no additional energy needs to be imported into the site for this.

In the LCI spreadsheet, biogasification is assumed to consume 50 kWh of the generated electricity, for every input tonne (including nuisance materials and recoverable materials).

Outputs

Mass balances for both aerobic and anaerobic processing plants are given in Figs 8.7–8.9.

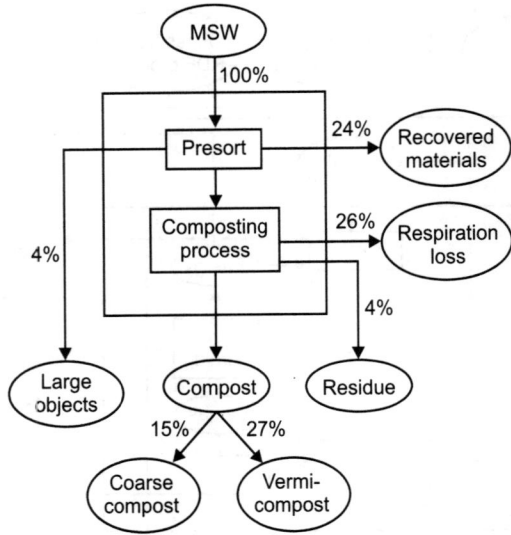

Fig. 8.7. Typical mass balance (on the basis of dry weight) for a lumbricomposting plant.

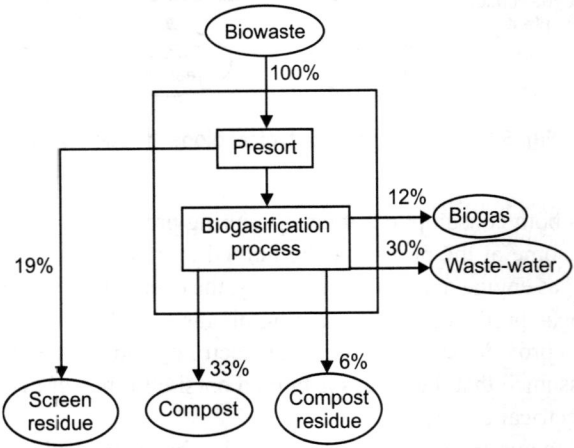

Fig. 8.8. Mass balance (on the basis of wet weight) for a dry process biogasification plant.

Secondary materials from pre-sorting

The amount of secondary materials that will be produced by a composting plant depends on the composition of the input stream, and on the pre-sorting equipment installed. A narrowly defined input, such as biowaste or VFG will contain a certain level of contamination, but this material would not be suitable for recovery. A mixed waste stream input (MSW or household waste) will contain considerable amounts of glass, plastic and metal that could be recovered for use as secondary materials, but levels of contamination are likely to be high, and the quality of the material recovered is likely to be lower than that from source-separated collection of recyclables. Recovery of recyclables from the input requires suitable sorting equipment or manual sorting; in most cases this is limited to magnetic separation, which can remove up to 90 per cent of incoming ferrous material.

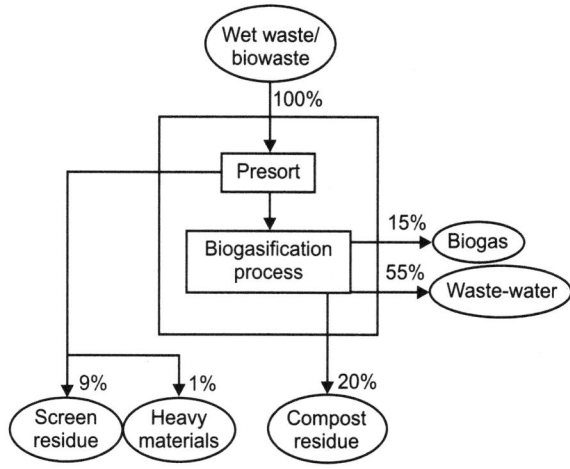

Fig. 8.9. Mass balance (on the basis of wet weight) for a two-stage wet biogasification plant.

Biogas/energy

The amount of biogas produced during anaerobic digestion will depend on the nature of the organic material used as feedstock, as well as the process used. Biogasification of a range of industrial organic wastes from vegetables to dairy and brewing wastes in Switzerland produce from 200 to 600 Nm^3 per tonne of input (dry weight).

Biogas from household wastes is normally expressed per tonne as received (i.e. wet weight); grass clippings, for example, may be expected to produce 100 Nm^3 per input tonne. Putrescible material mechanically sorted has been shown to produce 130–160 m^3 of biogas per tonne.

Production figures for the different processes reflect the amount of organic decomposition that is achieved. The more complex two-stage process converts more organic material to biogas (around 65–70 per cent by dry weight) than single stage processes (around 45 per cent by dry weight), giving typical production rates of 115 and 75 m^3 per tonne of biowaste, respectively. Biogas composition, especially methane content, also varies with process type, again being generally higher in the two-stage process. The methane content generally varies from 50 to 75 per cent, the rest of the biogas comprising carbon dioxide and some trace components (Table 8.6).

If it is assumed that 100 Nm^3 of biogas are produced per tonne of input to the digestor (i.e. after nuisance materials have been removed in the pre-treatment stage), with a methane content of 55 per cent (methane has a calorific value of 37.75 MJ/Nm^3, this will give a gross energy potential of 2076 MJ thermal energy per tonne digested.

If this is burned in a gas engine to produce electricity with an efficiency of around 30 per cent, this will give a gross electricity production of 173 kWh per tonne digested.

Compost

The quantity and quality of the compost produced by biological treatment are clearly not independent. The more the product is refined to improve the quality, the less the final quantity (and hence the greater the residue). In many cases, different grades of compost will be produced, the important factor being the existence of a market for the material. Put simply, if there is no market for the compost, regardless of its quality, it will be a residue rather than a valuable product.

Table 8.6. Biogas composition.

Source	Biogas	Biogas	Biogas after combustion
	Lentz	BTA	IFEU
% Volume			
CO_2	26.8%	45%	
CH_4	71.4%	54%	
N_2	1.4%		
O_2	0.3%		
mg/m^3			
NO_x			100
SO_x			25
Sum chlorine	0.6	0.9	11
Sum fluorine	0.1		0.021
HCl			
HF			
H_2S	700	420	0.33
Total HC		<1.5	0.023
Chlorinated HC		<1.5	7.3 E – 3
Dioxins/furans (TEQ)			1.0 E – 7
Ammonia			
Arsenic			
Cadmium			9.4 E– 6
Chromium			1.1 E–6
Copper			
Lead			8.5 E–6
Mercury			6.9 E–8
Nickel			
Zinc			1.3 E–4

Compost quantity

For composting, the final amount of compost produced (wet weight) is in the region of 50 per cent of the input of organic material (organics plus paper). The other 50 per cent is lost due to evaporation and respiration. Where further refining of the compost occurs, the amount of compost actually marketed may be considerably less than this. For biogasification, the amount of final compost-like material will depend on the extent to which the organic material is broken down into biogas. Production can account for 33 per cent by weight of a plant's input (equivalent to 41 per cent of the input to the digester after the pre-sort). By contrast, the two-stage wet process produces more biogas with a higher methane content than the dry process, leaving around 20 per cent of the plant input (22 per cent of the digester input) as composted residue (Fig. 8.9).

For the purposes of the LCI spreadsheet, it is assumed that in composting, the final compost accounts for 50 per cent of the input to the composting process (i.e. after any pre-sorting); for biogasification, an average figure of 30 per cent is used.

Compost quality

Compost quality is the key factor that determines whether the output from biological treatment processes is a valuable product or a residue. A valuable material is one that has a market, hence the need to develop markets for different grades of compost. Producers will then either be able to produce large amounts of lower grade composts, or smaller amounts of higher grade material.

Compost quality is determined by the feedstock type, technology used and level of process control. The physical characteristics, plant nutrient and heavy metal contents of a range of composts derived from different feedstocks are given in Tables 8.7 and 8.8. These can be compared with the standards discussed above. It can be seen that the major variability occurs in the heavy metal content. Not surprisingly, the more mixed the feedstock, the higher the heavy metal content of the compost. So, while it is possible to make compost from mixed waste streams, the high level of contamination may mean that no market for this material can be found. It is accepted in Germany, for example, that the composted residue from biogasification is not marketable as compost and that it needs to be disposed of.

Table 8.7. Physical characteristics and plant nutrient contents of different types of compost produced by aerobic process.

	Biowaste compost	Biowaste with paper compost	Green waste compost	Wet waste compost[a]	Total waste compost
H$_2$O% wet wt.	37.7	45.0	34.8	44.2	35.6
pH value	7.6	7.5	7.6	7.5	7.3
Salt (g/l wet wt.)	3.9	3.6	2.3	5.8	7.3
OS (% dry wt.)	33.3	42.0	32.5	55.4	39.7
C/N ratio	17.0	21.8	20.0	18.8	17.8
N total (% dry wt.)	1.2	1.1	0.8	1.7	1.1
P$_2$O$_5$ (% dry wt.)	0.6	0.6	0.4	0.9	0.9
K$_2$O (% dry wt.)	1.0	0.9	0.8	1.2	0.6
MgO (% dry wt.)	0.8	0.8	0.6	2.0	0.7
CaO (% dry wt.)	4.0	4.1	3.0	10.0	4.9

[a]Fraction remaining after separate collection of dry waste (e.g. recyclables like glass, paper, metal, wood, etc.).

Table 8.8. Heavy metal content of different composts produced by aerobic process (mg/kg dry wt.).

Element	Biowaste compost	Biowaste with paper compost	Green waste compost	Wet waste compost	Total waste compost	BGGK limits[a]
Based on material as produced						
Pb	77.6	78.6	60.8	449	513	
Cd	0.8	0.7	0.7	2.6	5.5	
Cr	33.7	31.7	27.0	72	71.4	
Cu	43.2	58.2	32.7	228	274	
Ni	19.1	16.1	17.5	30	44.9	
Zn	232.8	273.8	167.8	850	1.570	
Hg	0.3	0.4	0.3	1.0	2.4	

(Contd ...)

Element	Biowaste compost	Biowaste with paper compost	Green waste compost	Wet waste compost	Total waste compost	BGGK limits[a]
Based on standardised organic matter content of 30% (dry wt)						
Pb	83.1	116.2	63.1	705	596	150
Cd	0.8	1.0	0.7	4.1	6.4	1.5
Cr	35.8	39.8	28.4	113.0	82.9	100
Cu	46.8	76.2	34.5	357.8	318	100
Ni	20.5	21.4	18.6	47.1	52.1	50
Zn	249.1	350.3	176.9	1334	1823	400
Hg	0.4	0.5	0.3	1.6	2.8	1.0

[a] BGGK, Bundesgütesgemeinschaft Kompost.

Residues

Sorting residue

This will consist of two types of materials: (i) non-biodegradable materials arriving as nuisance materials in biowaste, or materials in mixed waste that have not been recovered as secondary materials, and (ii) degradable material (organic or paper) that is either unsuitable for biological processing (e.g. too large) or is removed adhered to nuisance materials. There is little data available that distinguish between these types, however. Where the feedstock is source-separated biowaste, a nuisance level of around 50 per cent is typical. Where the feedstock is mixed waste such as MSW then the level of sorting residue is likely to be much higher, although where recovery of other materials occurs (Fig. 8.7) residue rates as low as 5 per cent may be found.

In the LCI spreadsheet, it is assumed that all of the categories other than paper and organics are removed as residue during the pre-sort. In addition, 5 per cent of the organic and paper fractions are added to the residue to account for material that is not readily biodegradable, or that adheres to the nuisance materials as they are removed.

Compost residue

This represents the composted/digested output that is not marketed. The amount will range from zero, if a use can be found for all of the compost, to 100 per cent of the output if no market can be found.

Air emissions

The major air emission by volume from biological processing will be carbon dioxide, which is a contributor to the greenhouse effect. In aerobic processing, the organic material is broken down directly to carbon dioxide and water. In anaerobic processing, biogas containing methane and carbon dioxide is produced, of which the methane also forms carbon dioxide when burned. The amount of emissions per tonne of process input will depend on the moisture content of the incoming material. In the following calculations, an average moisture content of 50 per cent is assumed. The actual level will depend on the ratio of paper to wet organic material present, but Smith suggest that 50 per cent is the optimum moisture content level for composting feedstocks.

For composting, the dry weight loss during composting is around 40 per cent, giving a dry weight loss of 200 kg per wet input tonne. Assuming that most of the organic material decomposed is cellulose, with a carbon content of 44 per cent (from formula), composting will evolve approximately 323 kg of CO_2 (164 Nm^3) per tonne of wet organic feedstock.

For biogasification, the dry weight loss varies with process type, and reports vary from 45 per cent to 70 per cent. Assuming a mid-range dry weight loss of 55 per cent, means that 275 kg of organic matter are converted into gas. If all this was converted to carbon dioxide the total emitted would be 444 kg (226 Nm^3) per tonne of digester input. Given the composition of biogas in Table 8.6, combustion will convert the methane to carbon dioxide and water in the reaction

$$CH_4 + 2O_2 \rightarrow CO_2 + 2H_2O$$

Complete combustion of the biogas will, therefore, produce 0.982 Nm^3 of CO_2 per Nm^3 of biogas burned, equivalent to 1.93 kg of CO_2. Given a production of around 100 Nm^3 of biogas per tonne of organic material feedstock, this produces a CO_2 emission of 193 kg per input tonne, considerably less than that predicted from the dry weight loss during the process.

This discrepancy probably reflects some process losses, and more importantly, the aerobic maturation stage that follows the anaerobic stage. During this stage, the material needs to be aerated and heats up, demonstrating considerable aerobic microbial activity, during which further carbon dioxide is likely to be released.

For the purposes of the LCI spreadsheet, overall carbon dioxide emissions are assumed to be 320 kg and 440 kg per tonne of wet organic material, for composting and biogasification, respectively.

No reliable data were found on other air emissions from composting processes, although the odour problems that can occur around compost plants demonstrate that other air emissions do occur. Air emissions resulting from the combustion of biogas are given in Table 8.6.

Water emissions

The aqueous effluents reported for biological treatment vary widely in both amounts and composition, depending on both the process used and the feedstock. In composting, considerable evaporation will take place during the process. Any run-off collected is often sprayed back onto the composting material to maintain sufficiently high moisture contents. If waste paper is included in the feedstock, this will absorb much of the water, and so little or no leachate is actually produced.

In biogasification, water is produced when the digested material is pressed or filtered. Large amounts will be produced, especially in the wet (low solids) process type. Some of this water will be recirculated to adjust the water content of the incoming feedstock, the rest needs to be treated prior to discharge. Typical amounts and compositions of the leachates produced by both composting and biogasification are given in Table 8.9.

Other Considerations

Land usage

Table 8.10 compares the land usage of composting and biogas processing. Whilst there is likely to be an effect of plant capacity on land usage (larger plants will have proportionately less free space at any time than smaller plants), it can be seen that generally composting is a more space intensive process than biogasification.

This is because biogas plants are built vertically, whilst composting plants are built horizontally. Also, in composting, a greater percentage of the input is produced as compost, which requires maturing, and so occupies space for some time.

Table 8.9. Water emissions from biological treatment processes.

Process	Composting					Biogasification			
	Worm composting	Box composting	Drum composting	Tunnel reactor	Dry 1-stage	Dry 1-stage	Dry 1-stage	Wet 2-stage	
Amount (litres/tonne)	0	300	–	–	290	490	540	500	
Composition (mg/l)									
BOD₅	–	270–485	50–600	3300–7050	<65	–	740	60	
COD	–	458–808	150–7000	6200–15100	<250	–	1400	200	
NH₄	–	48–117	–	–	<100	–	250	100	
N total	–	0–1	6–36	0–3	<100	–	6	–	
pH	–	7.9	7.1–7.8	7.1–8.1	–	–	8.0	–	

Table 8.10. Space requirements for biological treatment plants.

	Composting			Biogasification					
	Windrow	*Drum*	*Tunnel reactor*	*Dry 1-stage*	*Dry 1-stage*	*Wet 2-stage*	*Dry 1-stage*	*Wet 2-stage*	*Dry 1-stage*
Space m²/t capacity	1.45	0.6	0.5	0.12	0.4	0.32	0.23	0.57	0.14

ECONOMIC COSTS

Data on the economic costs of biological treatment are not always reported on a consistent basis, so comparisons are difficult to make. In many cases, biological treatment is considered as a final disposal option, and consequently costs given are as an all-inclusive 'gate fee' or 'tip fee'. This cost will include allowance for any revenues collected from the sale of recovered materials, compost, and energy from biogas utilisation, and include disposal costs for any residues requiring incineration or landfilling. The problem with this level of accounting is that the cost of biological treatment will vary with the market prices of energy, compost and recovered materials and the cost of landfill. Alternatively, cost data for biological treatment can refer to the biological processing itself. This is more useful when modelling the economics of the overall waste management system, since it is independent of the cost of other parts of the system, but this type of data is not widely available.

These costs and revenues are inserted by user to calculate the overall cost of biological treatment. Note the revenue from sale of biogas/electricity is only applied to the surplus of biogas, after the amount used to run the process has been subtracted.

Chapter 9

Biomethanation Systems for Energy Recovery from Urban and Industrial Waste-water

INTRODUCTION

The selection of an appropriate bioreactor configuration is a critical factor determining the successful implementation and sustained operation of a total biomethanation system.

Several bioreactor designs and configurations have been utilised in the implementation of biogas systems operating in the country. Engineering know-how for the full-scale plant design has been acquired through technical collaborations with leading international organisations.

Engineering companies, consultants, institutional experts and R & D personnel together can offer total expertise necessary for turnkey execution of biomethanation projects.

Conventional anaerobic digestion process has been successfully developed for the generation of biogas from municipal sewage sludge with several plants operating worldwide. A heterogeneous consortium of anaerobic bacteria feed on the organic fraction of sewage sludge forming biogas and the solid residue is utilised as a low-grade fertiliser. In India, sewage sludge digestion units are in operation in the municipal corporations of Mumbai, Delhi and in some industrial townships.

Anaerobic processes have been increasingly adapted in full-scale installations for the treatment of several process waste-waters. Proprietary anaerobic bioreactors have been developed for the recovery of biogas from process waste-waters generated by distillery, paper, dairy, pharmaceuticals (fermentation), leather, poultry, yeast, starch, rayon, rubber, abattoir, food processing, dairy farm, etc. besides domestic sewage. The opportunities for energy recovery as biogas by anaerobic treatment and the tangible savings through fuel and power requirements have been largely responsible for the successful implementation of biomethanation plants during the nineties in India. Biomethanation systems represent the most mature and proven processes that convert waste-to-energy efficiently achieving the following goals:

1. Pollution prevention/reduction.
2. Reduction of uncontrolled methane emissions and odour.
3. Recovery of bio-energy potential as biogas.
4. Production of stabilised residue for use as low-grade fertiliser.

PRINCIPLES OF BIOMETHANATION

The anaerobic microbial conversion of organic substrates to methane is a complex biogenic process involving a number of microbial populations, linked by their individual substrate and product specificities. The overall conversion process may be described as involving both direct and indirect symbiotic associations between different groups of micro-organisms as given in Table 9.1. The methanogenic bacteria are crucial for the anaerobic stabilisation of a variety of substrates, since they constitute the final step leading to the generation of biogas. The conversion possibilities shown in Fig. 9.1 serve as a convenient basis for emphasising some important biochemical and environmental requirements of anaerobic microbial treatment of municipal, agricultural and industrial wastes substrates and for directing the development or selection of substrate-linked process configurations.

Table 9.1. Core biochemical steps in anaerobic digestion.

Step	Core reactions	Process	Type of bacteria
1	Hydrolysis	Fermentation of complex organics to soluble organics	Fermentative
2	Acidogenesis	Soluble organics converted to volatile fatty acids (VFAs) and alcohols	Acidogenic
3	Acetogenesis	VFAs and alcohols converted to acetic acid (i.e. ethanoic acid), carbon dioxide and hydrogen	Acetogenic
4	Methanogenesis	Acetic acid converted to methane and carbon dioxide	Methanogenic
		Carbon dioxide and hydrogen converted to methane and water	

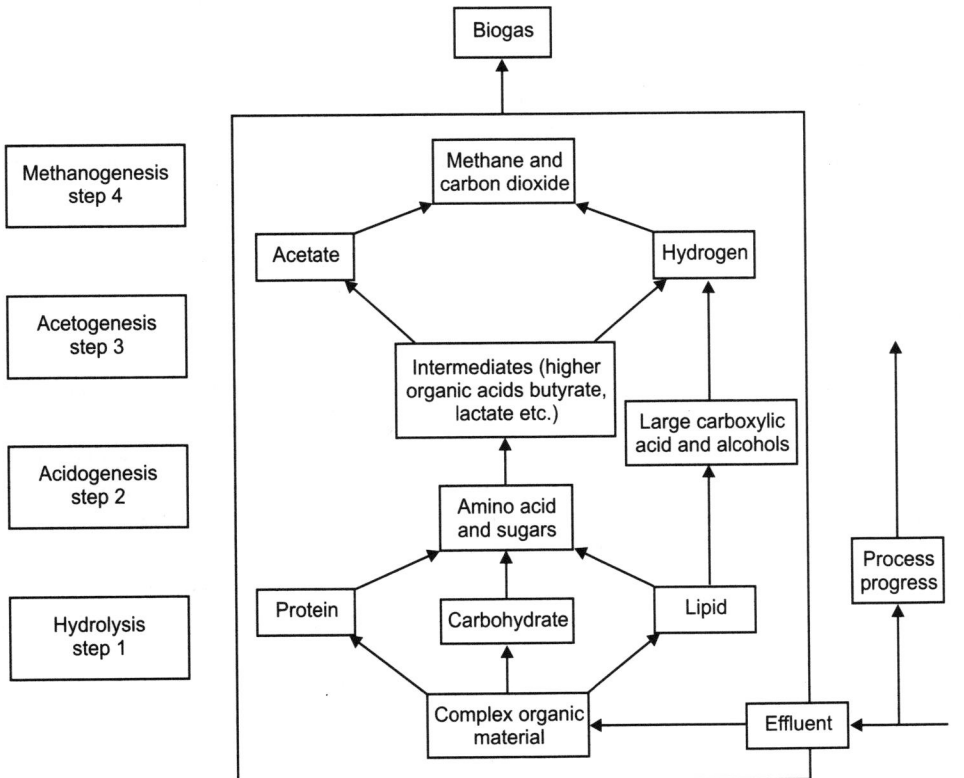

Fig. 9.1. Biochemical reaction steps in anaerobic digestion system.

The solubilisation of particulate material is relatively slow and accomplished by providing long contact time between the substrate and an anaerobic microbial consortium. Thus, for waste-waters containing particulate organic material, hydrolysis becomes the rate-limiting step. Solids retention time (SRT) of four to ten days may be required at mesophilic temperatures to prevent the washout of bacterial biomass. Factors to be considered for screening the anaerobic treatment systems include: source and nature of waste-water, flow rate, concentration of organic pollutants (BOD, COD) and suspended solids, temperature, toxicants and biogas and sludge generation potentials. Wastes containing mainly soluble organics require short anaerobic reactor retention times for good treatment efficiency since the kinetic rates of the acidogenic and methanogenic bacteria are relatively rapid. The growth rate of acetotrophic methanogenic bacteria is the rate-limiting step for anaerobic fermentation of soluble waste-waters containing acetate as the primary organic contaminant.

Process Parameters

The rates of methanogenesis in anaerobic microbial conversion processes depend primarily upon substrate availability and viable microbial population, besides environmental factors like pH, temperature, ionic strength or salinity, nutrients, and toxic or inhibitory substances.

pH

Most anaerobic processes operate best at neutral pH. Deviations from this optimum, if not introduced with the influent substrate, usually results in excess production and accumulation of acidic or basic conversion products such as organic fatty acids or ammonia, respectively. pH also affects the solubility and reaction behaviour of other potentially influencing substances, including both organic and inorganic species. pH should range between 6.6 to 7.6 and sufficient alkalinity should be present to ensure that pH does not drop below 6.2. When the reaction is progressing well, the alkalinity normally ranges between 1000 to 5000 mg/l, and the volatile fatty acid concentration is less than 250 mg/l. Gas production and pH levels are good indicators of the satisfactory performance of biomethanation processes and pH below 6 indicates digester upset. Low pH and excessive acid production and accumulation are considered inhibitory to methanogens than fermentative bacteria.

Temperature

Methanogenesis reactions are strongly temperature-dependent. Two optimal temperature ranges used are mesophilic (near 35°C) and thermophilic (55° to 60°C), with decreased rates between these optima, due to a lack of adaptation. With more complex microbial consortia, including sulphate and nitrate reducers, temperature influences may become more significant and will be advantageous to certain species and detrimental to others. Although methane-forming micro-organisms are active at temperatures as low as 8°C, most full-scale anaerobic treatment systems have been designed for operation at the optimal mesophilic temperatures range of 35°–40°C or 55°–60°C for thermophilic operation. Anaerobic systems at sub-optimal temperatures require longer start-up times. A drop in gas production indicates that the process is upset and one of the reasons for the upset could be too low a temperature.

Ionic strength and salinity

Sulphate ions exert a significant control on the viability of methanogenesis in the presence of certain substrates, primarily because of the competition between sulphate-reducing bacteria (SRB) and methanogens. The ionic strength of the medium also affects chemical activity and therefore, the possible effect of other chemical species in terms of inhibition. Salinity up to 0.2 M NaCl is reported to have minimal effects on mixed methano-genic populations, but higher salinity is inhibitory.

Nutrients

The organic constituents of the waste usually supply the macronutrients such as carbon and nitrogen. The inability of many anaerobes to synthesise some essential vitamins or amino acids often necessitates supplementation of the culture medium with specific nutrients like nitrogen and phosphorus for growth and metabolism. As a thumb-rule, the nutrient requirements are met by maintaining BOD:N:P ratio of 100:0.5:0.1. Other trace elements considered as necessary for various conditions of active methanogenesis include iron, nickel, magnesium, calcium, sodium, barium, tungstate, molybdate, selenium and cobalt. Many waste-waters from industrial processes do not represent a balanced nutrient status and the treatment of these wastes also poses many other process limitations such as nutrient deficiency, toxicity, and shock loading.

Toxicity

Toxicity or inhibition of methanogenic processes can be attributed to a variety of circumstances, including the generation of intermediary products such as volatile fatty acids, hydrogen sulphide and ammonia besides some heavy metals and cyanide present in process waste-waters. For instance, many industrial waste-waters contain excess sulphate that is toxic to the micro-organisms. The range of effluents and wastes that can be treated by anaerobic digestion has increased substantially over the last ten years due to greater understanding of microbiological processes, development of new methods of process control, better reactor designs and development of strategies to overcome problems caused by utrient imbalance and toxicity, such as nutrient dosing.

BOD (COD) concentration

Anaerobic treatment alone can give 80–90 per cent of BOD (biochemical oxygen demand) removal efficiency, leaving a relatively high residual of undergraded organics in treated effluents. With very dilute waste-waters, such as municipal sewage, this value may be closer to 50 per cent. Conversely, with very concentrated wastes, the total BOD removal efficiency achieved may be much higher, but the residual BOD concentration could still exceed several thousand mg/l. For an application requiring a high degree of BOD removal, waste-water concentration has a major impact on the energy recovery potential and the higher concentration levels would entail the recovery of a higher quantum of biogas necessary for power generation. Aerobic processes predominate for waste-waters with BOD or biodegradable COD below 2000 mg/l. Anaerobic process can be applied in either low or high rate forms between 1000 and 30,000 mg/l. For very concentrated wastes containing more than 30,000 mg COD/l, or for high concentrations of suspended solids, low-rate anaerobic digestion is more appropriate.

Suspended solids

Anaerobic digestion is well known as a treatment process for sewage sludges and manures that contain elevated levels of suspended solids. When the majority of the organic material is insoluble, lengthy digestion periods are required to allow for the relatively slow biological process of hydrolysis and solubilisation of the insoluble materials. Once solubilised, the dissolved organics can undergo further conversion to volatile organic acids and methane fairly rapidly. To permit anaerobic digestion of particulates, total digester retention times of at least 10–30 days are normal. In contrast, high-rate anaerobic treatment technologies are intended for waste-waters in which the organic pollutants are soluble. Since hydrolysis of organics is not required with soluble waste-waters, much faster conversion rates to methane can be obtained. This is one factor that has permitted the operation of high-rate anaerobic processes at retention times of less than eight hours for some applications.

Two rules of thumb are useful for establishing practical limits on suspended solids in the raw waste-water. The first one indicates that for high-rate UASB processes, the influent suspended solids should be less than 10 per cent of the waste-water total COD. Above this level, pretreatment may be required. It is reported that higher levels of suspended solids could be treated anaerobically, but only at reduced organic loading rates. The second rule of thumb hints that with low-strength wastes containing up to 50 per cent of the total COD in particulate form, it may be more economical to utilise anaerobic treatment at a loading of 1–4 kg COD/m³ d, than to construct a pre-treatment step.

Design of Biomethanation Reactors

There are basically three reactor configurations for biomethanation processes currently in use for full-scale applications for urban and industrial waste-waters.
1. Suspended growth reactors.
2. Fixed film reactors.
3. Hybrid reactors.

The suspended biomass growth processes are advantageous for the treatment of sludges or waste-waters containing high proportions of particulate biodegradable material. The fixed film processes on the other hand, are well suited to waste-waters that contain primarily soluble organic substrates. The hybrid processes falling in the middle, can be applied to waste-waters with intermediate levels of particulates, although performance is usually better with soluble waste-waters. A comparative analysis of the process design features of various bioreactor configurations is given in Table 9.2.

Suspended growth systems

Completely mixed anaerobic digester

The simplest form of suspended growth anaerobic digester is the completely mixed digester (Fig. 9.2), using either mechanical impeller-type or gas recirculation mixers. In a completely mixed digester, the concentration of suspended solids remaining in the effluent after treatment is a function of the influent composition and the degree of treatment provided. The effluent quality is reduced by the presence of biological suspended solids and non-biodegraded particulate material. Completely mixed digestors are particularly suitable for waste-waters containing high concentrations of particulates or extremely high concentrations of soluble biodegradable organic materials. The process is susceptible to toxics and shock loadings with relatively low biomass concentrations and short operating SRTs.

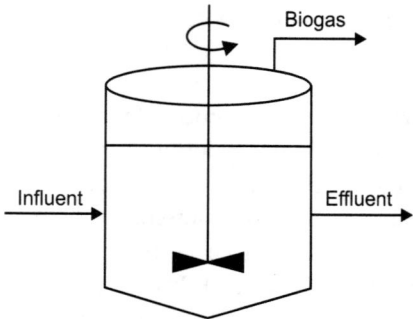

Fig. 9.2. Completely mixed suspended growth anaerobic digester.

Table 9.2. Comparative process design features of various bioreactor configurations.

Type of process	Advantages	Disadvantages	Loading^a	HRT(days)	SRT(days)	Suitable waste
Suspended growth systems						
Lagoon	Retain and decompose suspended solids over a period—months/years influent waste-water equalisation. Simple in operation and lower capital and operating costs	Large land area required. Periodic removal of settled sludge. No methane recovery	0.02–0.04^b	8–40		Low organic waste like sewage
Completely mixed digestion process	Long contact time. Degradation of suspended material	High space and energy requirement. Poor sedimentation of biomass. Washout of active bacterial biomass	1	20–30	20–40	Excess sludge from anaerobic plants
Anaerobic contact process (CSTR)	Smaller tank volume. High concentration of biomass. High retention of microbes	Poor biomass settlability. Need for vacuum degasification. Limited equalisation capacity	5	2–8	20–36	Effective on medium organic strength waste-water
UASB process	Higher loading capacity. High concentration of sludge. No clogging. Natural mixing. No mechanical mixing or support media is required	Require effective gas-liquid-solid separator (GLSS). Needs efficient feed distribution system at the bottom of the digester. Generally require effluent recycle for high strength waste-water	2–50	0.25–1	20–36	Effective on low to high organic strength waste-water
Fixed film systems						
Anaerobic filter	Operation simple. Suitable for waste-waters with low to high COD	Occurrence of scaling due to inorganic precipitation. Greater possibility for clogging of filter especially when waste-water has high suspended solids. Short	5–15	0.25–1	20–36	Effective on low to high organic wastes with low suspended solids concentration

(Contd ...)

Type of process	Advantages	Disadvantages	Loading[a]	HRT(days)	SRT(days)	Suitable waste
		circuiting/channeling and reduced contact between biomass and waste-water. Higher cost of packing material. Increased pressure drop during operation due to biomass accumulation				
Fluidised bed	Good contact between biomass and waste-water. High loading capacity and load variation can be absorbed	High capital and operating cost. Maintenance is more difficult. Support media may washout, damaging pumps and other equipment	2–50	0.25–1	20–36	Effective on high organic wastes with high SS[c] concentration
Hybrid systems UASB/AF	High loading capacity Have benefit of both fixed film and UASB High biomass concentration Problems related to media plugging and the associated hydraulic and mass transfer are low compared to AF	On long term, leading to clogging or even damaging of the filter part. Methanogenic activity is highest at the bottom part which generally lead to gas withdrawal problems through the filter	2–50	0.25–1	25–40	Effective on low to high organic strength waste-water
Anaerobic sequencing batch reactor (ASBR)	A single reactor for biological treatment and clarification. Low capital and operating costs. Less land required. Better resistance to sludge bulking	Poor sedimentation of biomass. Low loading capacity	1–6	0.25–2	25–40	Effective on low to medium organic strength waste-water
Anaerobic baffled reactor (ABR)	Long contact time Advantages when plug flow conditions accelerate the anaerobic conversion process	Low loading capacity. Little full scale experience	0.02–0.04	8–40	8–40	Low organic waste like sewage

[a] Achievable loading rates in kg COD/m³ day treating moderate strength waste-waters at removal efficiencies of more than 80 per cent.
[b] Sum of volume for anaerobic and facultative lagoons; in anaerobic lagoons only, more than 80 per cent treatment efficiency will not be achieved.
[c] SS, suspended solids.

The system offers several process advantages:

1. Process can provide uniform substrate, temperature, and pH.
2. Good mixing can minimise dead pockets and flow channeling.

The only disadvantage is the large reactor volumes required to provide necessary SRTs.

Anaerobic contact reactor

The anaerobic contact reactor configuration can overcome some of the disadvantages of the conventional digester by separating and recycling effluent suspended solids to the reactor (Fig. 9.3). The biomass separation system used in the anaerobic contact process retains both active micro-organisms and undigested influent suspended solids, thus promoting biodegradation of waste-water particulates. The anaerobic contact process retains most of the advantages of a conventional digester with the extra benefits of increased SRTs and smaller reactor volumes. Anaerobic contact systems that utilise gravity settling for anaerobic flocs usually entrain biogas. Solids settleability can often be problematic, and can be improved by gas stripping, vacuum degasification, inclined plate or lamella settlers and the addition of coagulants and flocculants to promote floc formation.

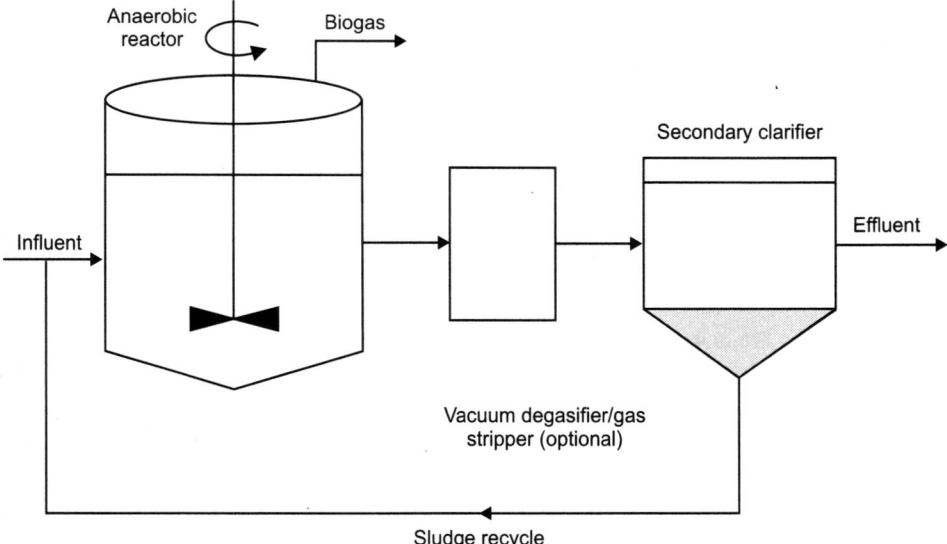

Fig. 9.3. Anaerobic contact reactor system.

The treatment efficiency of an anaerobic contact process is usually much greater than that of a completely mixed digester. Total COD reduction of 80–90 per cent is possible for highly biodegradable waste-waters with COD concentration 2000–10,000 mg/l.

Some of the major advantages of the contact system are:

1. Suitable for wastes with high concentration of soluble organics.
2. Uniform substrate concentration, temperature, and pH conditions.
3. Relatively high quality effluent.
4. Aerobic post-treatment sludge can be wasted to the anaerobic reactor for stabilisation.
5. Can handle waste with low to medium concentration of suspended solids.

Disadvantages are:
1. Poor biomass settling behaviour.
2. Vacuum degasification to promote settling.
3. Limited equalisation capacity for shock inputs.

Anaerobic lagoon (covered)

A low-rate anaerobic treatment process that has gained acceptance is an advanced version of anaerobic lagoon (Fig. 9. 4). The system can be constructed as a rectangular, excavated, and lined lagoon. Waste is introduced at one end of the reactor through a distribution system to maximise contact between the waste-water and a bed of anaerobic biosludge at the inlet zone of the tank.

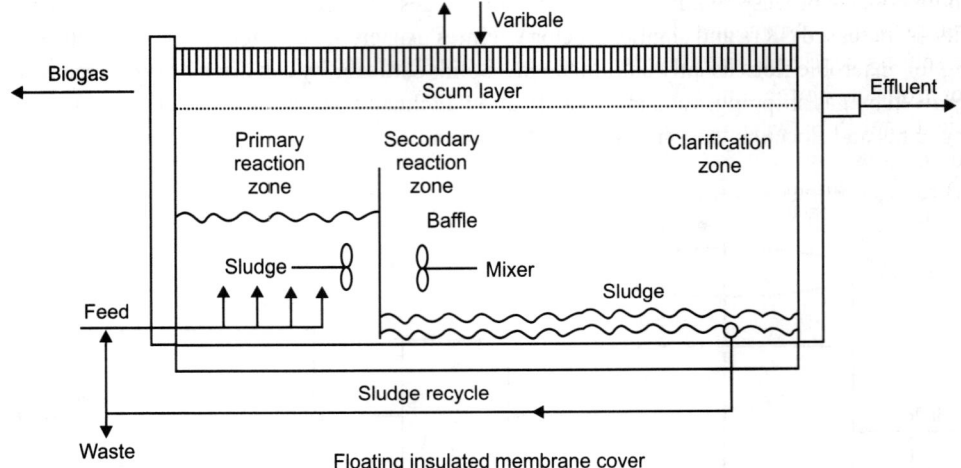

Fig. 9.4. Covered anaerobic lagoon (bulk volume fermenter).

The biogas evolved at the inlet zone contributes significantly for internal mixing, along the length of the tank. Near the outlet end of the lagoon, where biogas production is minimal, a relatively quiescent clarification zone is maintained to reduce the suspended solids content of the treated effluent. In the most modern systems of this type, internal mixers and sludge recycle are often used to improve contact between the waste-water and the anaerobic sludge. The entire reactor is covered with a floating insulated membrane that conserves process heat and permits the collection and utilisation of the evolved biogas.

Some of the advantages of the system include:
1. Simple and relatively economical construction.
2. Suitable for wastes with high concentrations of suspended solids and organics (BOD, COD).
3. Toxicants and shocks can be equalised in large reactor volume.
4. Significance of sludge settleability characteristics is reduced.
5. Relatively high quality effluent achievable.
6. Very long SRTs reduces waste sludge production.

The major disadvantages are:
1. Large tank volume may lead to inefficient internal mixing and waste-water flow distribution and large land area requirement.

Up-flow anaerobic sludge blanket (UASB reactor)

UASB reactor incorporates multiple functions of presedimentation, anaerobic treatment, final sedimentation and stabilisation in a single unit making it the most attractive high rate waste-water treatment option. It produces relatively high value by-products like treated waste-water for reuse, methane enriched biogas and mineralised excess sludge as manure for agricultural purpose.

The basic principle is to develop *in situ* flocculants or granular sludge in the reactor that would settle under gravity and get retained when applying moderate upward velocities in the reactor. Anaerobic bacteria are developed in the reactor and held in the sludge blanket zone for a sufficient time. Organic compounds present in the waste-water are absorbed or adsorbed on the sludge granules in the reaction zone during its passage through the sludge bed. Biogas can be used as an energy source and is collected separately.

An integral three phase gas-liquid-solids separator (GLSS) is provided to dislodge sludge particles from entrapped biogas bubbles. The sludge particles carried along with the waste-water flow are settled in the settling zone and slide down into the biological reaction zone. Waste-water enters the UASB reactor from the bottom and travels through the reactor in the upward direction. In order to ensure sufficient contact between the incoming waste-water and the anaerobic bacterial mass present in the reactor, the waste-water is fed uniformly all over the bottom of the reactor. A cross-sectional view of the UASB reactor system is given in Fig. 9.5.

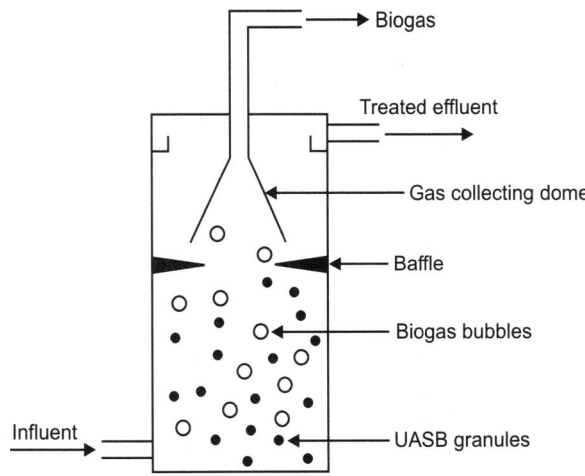

Fig. 9.5. Upflow anaerobic sludge blanket (UASB) reactor.

Some of the advantages of the UASB process are:

1. Low energy requirements.
2. Reduced excess stabilised sludge with good dewatering characteristics.
3. Low nutrient requirements.
4. Production of biogas containing methane.
5. High rate process with high volumetric loading.
6. NPK useful as fertilisers are conserved.
7. Anaerobic sludge can be preserved, unfed for many months without any serious quality deterioration and low land requirement.
8. Cost effective in removing bulk of the pollution.

Some of its limitations are:

1. Anaerobic bacteria particularly methane producing bacteria are very susceptible to inhibition by a large number of toxic compounds present in industrial waste-water and require feasibility studies for complex waste-waters;
2. Start-up of the process is relatively slow if seed sludge is not available.
3. Post-treatment is necessary to meet the final desired effluent standards.

Fixed film systems

Biofilm reactors utilise a fixed film for the development of high concentrations of required biomass for efficient anaerobic treatment. An inert medium is placed in the vessel and the process is operated to favour the growth of micro-organisms on the medium surface. The media is fully submerged and waste-water flow can be in upflow or downflow mode. As the waste-water passes through the media filled reactor, the attached anaerobic biomass converts both soluble and particulate organic matter in the waste-water to biogas. The most common anaerobic fixed film systems are anaerobic filter and fluidised bed reactors.

Anaerobic upflow/downflow filters

In an anaerobic upflow filter (Fig. 9.6), the waste stream is passed upward through a bed of medium. The growth of biofilm on the surface of the media contributes to the short hydraulic retention time and high organic loading rates.

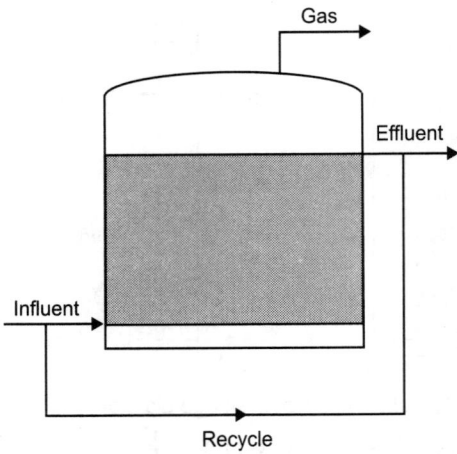

Fig. 9.6. Upflow anaerobic filter.

The early stone media designs of low voids have largely been replaced today by synthetic packing with open structures and high void volumes (95 per cent). The large voids maximise the available reaction volume and provide space for accumulation of nonattached biomass. Random loose-fill packings such as plastic rings and stacked modular media formed from plastic sheets have both been used in full-scale applications. The specific surface-to-volume ratios of these packings provide 100–150 m^2m^{-3} inter-facial area for biofilm development. The anaerobic filter has the ability to trap and hold settleable influent suspended solids and is suitable for the treatment of wastes with some biodegradable suspended material. However, a waste of this type increases the requirement of solids removal.

The downflow reactor (Fig. 9.7) utilises ordered modular packing which provides relatively straight vertical flow channels of approximately 40 mm in diameter. By operating the reactor in a downflow mode, influent suspended solids and sloughed biofilm solids are carried down with the liquid flow and out of the reactor. This may result in lower quality in some circumstances, particularly when the influent contains a large proportion of insoluble material.

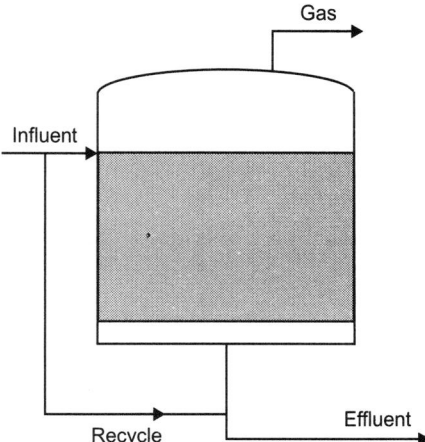

Fig. 9.7. Downflow anaerobic filter.

Fixed bed anaerobic treatment processes are applicable to waste-waters with COD upto 1,00,000 mg/l. For higher strength waste-waters, it has been recommended that effluent recycle be used to maintain the reactor inlet COD concentration between 8000 and 12,000 mg/l. In general, fixed bed processes provide a stable and easily operable form of anaerobic treatment technology.

The advantages are: .
1. High biomass concentrations and long SRT.
2. Smaller reactor volumes due to high organic loading rates.
3. Relatively stable operation under variable feed conditions or toxic shocks.
4. Suitable for wastes with low suspended solids concentrations.
5. No mechanical mixing required.
6. Biogas evolution and effluent recycle ensure relatively uniform temperature, pH and substrate concentrations in reactor.
7. Land area required is relatively small.

The disadvantages are:
1. Suspended solid accumulation may adversely affect reactor hydraulics and internal mass transfer characteristics.
2. Not suitable for high suspended solids waste-waters.
3. Relatively short anaerobic reactor HRT results in reduced equalisation capacity for shock inputs.
4. High costs of packing material and support.

Fluidised bed bioreactors

Attempts have been made to improve mass transfer characteristics in the anaerobic fluidised bed processes (Fig. 9. 8) by the utilisation of small media particles (like sand) with very high surface-to-volume ratio.

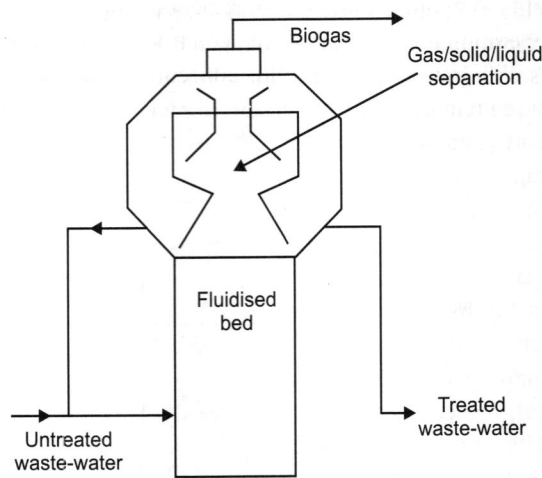

Fig. 9.8. Anaerobic fluidised bed reactor.

With such small diameter media, the interstitial void spaces in a settled bed would normally become plugged very rapidly. However, by applying high liquid upflow velocities, the media can be expanded to produce a substantial increase in bed voidage.

In expanded bed systems, sufficient flow is applied to increase the settled bed volume by 15 to 30 per cent and the individual particles are supported partly by the fluid flow and partly through contact with adjacent particles. The higher upflow velocities utilised in the fluidised bed produce 25 to 100 per cent bed expansion. In the fluidised state, the media particles are supported entirely by the flowing liquid and are therefore able to move freely in the bed. The energy required for effluent recycle for bed expansion or fluidisation is one of the most significant disadvantages of these systems.

In both processes, an anaerobic biofilm is developed on the surface of the media particles. The inert medium increases the average density of the biomass particle and prevents washout of the bed even under very high flow rate conditions. The large upflow velocity increases turbulence at the biofilm/liquid interface and promotes good mass transfer across the biofilm and exerts sufficient shear to prevent the development of thick biofilms on the media. The high upflow velocity in expanded and fluidised systems allows the reactors to be designed with relatively large height/diameter ratios and smaller land area requirements. In fluidised bed processes, the combination of thin biofilms and high turbulence prevents capture and retention of influent suspended solids within the reactor. Sloughed biofilm solids are also rapidly washed out of the reactor.

This makes the fluidised bed a classical fixed film process that is best suited to the treatment of waste-waters containing only soluble contaminants. Maximum dilution of waste-water is provided at the reactor inlet by very high effluent recirculation ratios required for media fluidisation. This enables the expanded and fluidised bed processes to accommodate a wide range of waste-water with COD concentration upto 1,00,000 mg/l. Organic loading rates of upto 21 kg COD/ m^3/d are typical of these systems.

Advantages are:
1. High biomass concentrations and long SRT.
2. Excellent mass transfer characteristics.
3. Compact reactor volumes due to high organic loading rates.

4. Better effluent quality than other anaerobic treatment options.
5. Relatively stable operation under variable feed conditions or toxic shocks.
6. Suitable for wastes with low suspended solids concentrations.
7. No mechanical mixing required.
8. Biogas evolution and extensive effluent recycle ensure relatively uniform temperature, pH, and substrate concentrations in reactor.
9. Small land area required.

Disadvantages are:

1. Lengthy start-up periods.
2. Power requirements for bed expansion or fluidisation are high.
3. Control of media and biomass inventories can be difficult.
4. Accidental washout of media can damage downstream components.
5. Not suitable for high suspended solid waste-waters.
6. Relatively short HRT results in reduced equalisation capacity for shock inputs.
7. Mechanical system design is relatively complex.
8. Cost of carrier medium is high.

Hybrid systems

The recent trend in design of anaerobic systems is towards the use of a 'hybrid' reactor. The removal of the lower 50–75 per cent of the media in anaerobic filters could produce a hybrid reactor configuration consisting of a lower sludge blanket zone and an anaerobic filter on the top. The resulting hybrid design has the potential of substantially reducing the media plugging and the associated hydraulic and mass transfer problems found in fixed bed reactors, while realising the advantages of both fixed film and upflow sludge blanket treatment besides a reduced volume of the costly filter medium. The packed zone at the top of the reactor also serves as a gas-liquid-solid separator that assists in the retention of biomass.

Detailed information relating to the biomethanation systems for handing distillery spentwash are given in Table 3 and Figs 9.9 and 9.10.

Table 9.3. Spentwash characteristics of batch and continuous fermentation processes.

Parameter (mg/l)	Batch process	Continuous process
Volume (l/l alcohol)	14–15	10–12
Colour	Dark brown	Dark brown
pH	3.7–4.5	4.0–4.3
COD	80000–1,00,000	1,10,000–1,30,000
BOD	45000–50000	55000–65000
Total solids	90000–1,00,000	1,30,000–1,60,000
Total volatile	60000–70000	60000–75000
Inorganic dissolved	30000–40000	35000–45000
Chlorides	5000–6000	6000–7500
Sulphates	4000–8,000	4500–8500
Total nitrogen	1000–1200	1000–1400
Potassium	8000–12000	10000–14000

(Contd ...)

Parameter (mg/l)	Batch process	Continuous process
Phosphorus	200–300	300–500
Sodium	400–600	1400–1500
Calcium	2000–3500	4500–6000

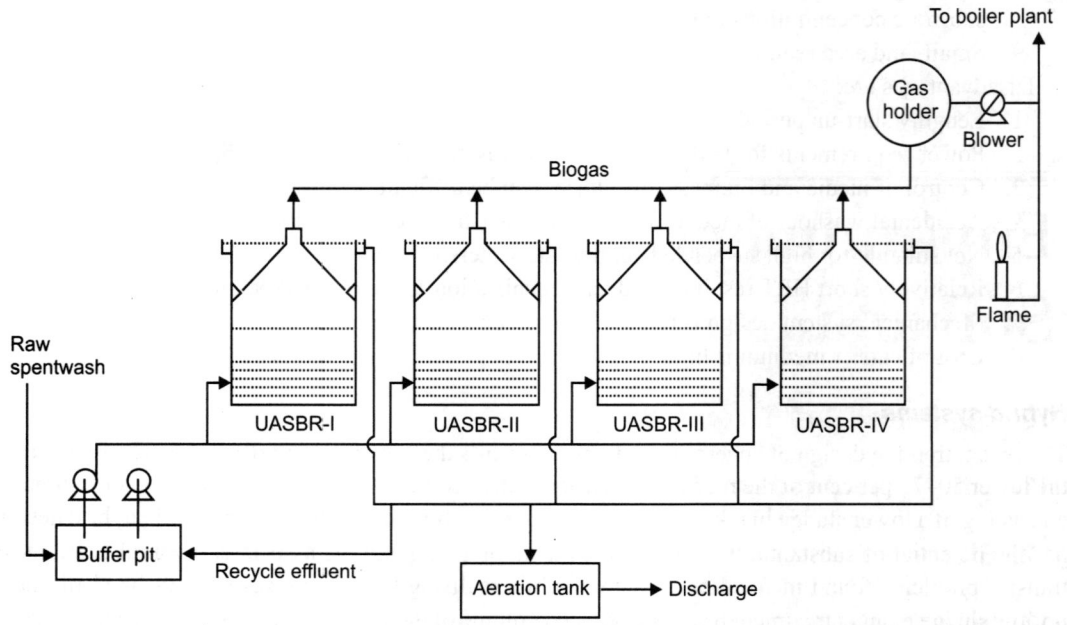

Fig. 9.9. Schematic of UASB system.

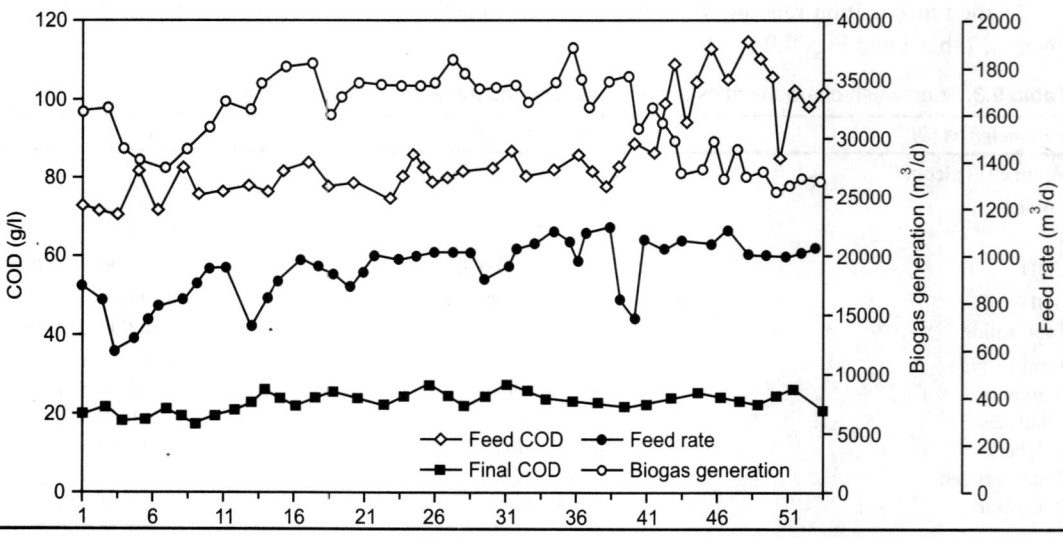

Fig. 9.10. Profiles of weekly average feed and final values, feed rate and biogas generation rates.

SECTION III

Environmental Biotechnology in Soil and Landfill

Chapter 10

Biological Soil Treatment

INTRODUCTION

Environmental protection over the past few decades has meant primarily the protection of air and water. Only with the increasing use of land in industrialised societies and the highlighting of possible hazards from contaminated soil did the public become aware of soil protection in the early 80s. This has also prompted industry to take up this market segment. Engineers and scientists have thus been spurred on to look for technically optimised, ecologically sound and economically appropriate solutions.

For more than a century natural biochemical processes (nature's self-cleaning forces) have been utilised to treat effluent, and reactors and plant systems had been adapted with increasing effect to cope with the difficult conditions.

FUNDAMENTALS

In biological processes, use is made of the capacity of micro-organisms to consume organic substances as a nutrient (substrate) and to convert them to harmless natural materials, such as CO_2, water and biomass. For degradation of noxious substances in contaminated soils, bacteria and fungi are of foremost importance,

The attack of organic substances in soils by micro-organisms results either in full degradation (mineralisation) or in a partial degradation process producing metabolites which may be used by other members of the biocenosis or which remain in the soil. Furthermore, the original substance and the metabolites can be cycled to the soil's carbon depot. This is called humification. The decisive point in that case is that the noxious matter or the resulting metabolite is incorporated into the soil matrix, which reduces sharply their availability for biochemical reactions. This phenomenon is used at present in comprehensive development work aimed at a conversion of the pollutants by microbiological attacks so they are converted to natural substances, such as humic compounds, which involve no further environmental risk. Detoxification can also be obtained by cometabolism using non-growth substances as co-substrate.

NECESSARY PRELIMINARY INVESTIGATIONS

The decision in favour of a biological decontamination process depends on the following pre-requisites:

1. Degradability of the contaminants.
2. Bioavailability of contaminants in the soil matrix.
3. Adjustability of the biological, physical and chemical conditions required for biological degradation in the soil.

Degradability of Contaminants

Laboratory methods for the evaluation of biological soil clean-up processes have been developed by a Smith, allowing finding out thoroughly about the microbial degradability of contaminants. However, it has to be considered that .the assessment of degradability of soil contaminants requires investigation on the original soil, either in suspension or by means of naturally moist samples.

Bioavailability

In many cases it is not the actual microbial degradability but physico-chemical parameters, such as adsorption/desorption, diffusion, and solution properties of the contaminants found in the soil, frequently in solid phase, which are decisive for degradation and the degradation rate. The availability of contaminants in the soil to the micro-organisms, the bioavailability, is decisively influenced by the configuration of the soil matrix, i.e. its material composition and particle size distribution, and also by the history of contamination. For these cases, suitable bioavailability assessment methods are on hand.

Figure 10.1 shows a sequence pattern for close-to-practice preliminary investigations. When following that scheme we arrive—with relatively low expenditure—first at the important decision whether biological decontamination is possible at all. If there is no bioavailability of contaminants in the soil, or if a contamination, which is toxic to micro-organisms, cannot be eliminated, this means that the soil concerned is out of question for a microbiological treatment.

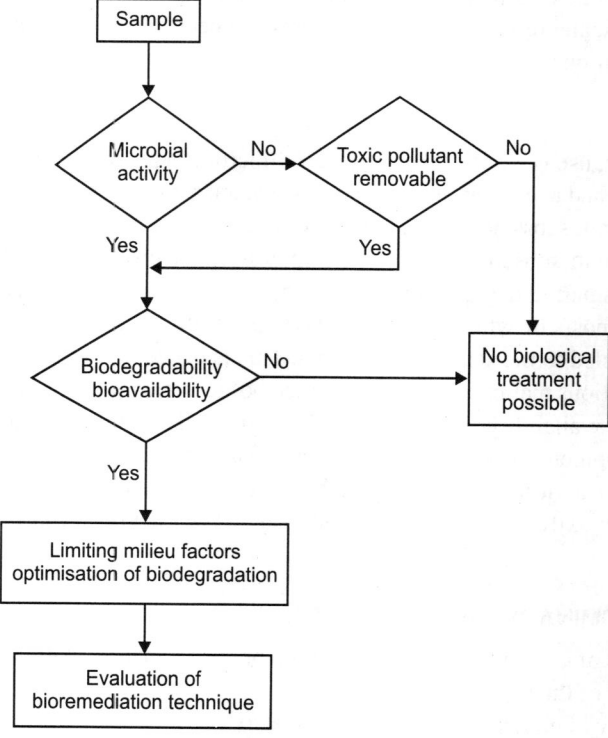

Fig. 10.1. Evaluation of the biodegradability of a pollutant.

Adjustability of the Biological and Physico-Chemical Conditions for Biological Degradation in the Soil

The physico-chemical and of course, also the geological properties of the soil are decisive for the choice of methods for bioremediation.

Figure 10.2 shows the sequence of investigations in view of the selection of methods. The decision in favour of an *in situ* or an *ex situ* method generally depends on the hydro-geological configuration of the soil, the permeability coefficient k_f, the soil's homogeneity, and its silt and fines content. The k_f value is regarded as orientation parameter. Experience has shown that with k_f values $< 10^{-5}$ m/s, *in situ* treatment is out of question. Only in relatively few cases, favourable conditions for a microbiological *in situ* decontamination prevail.

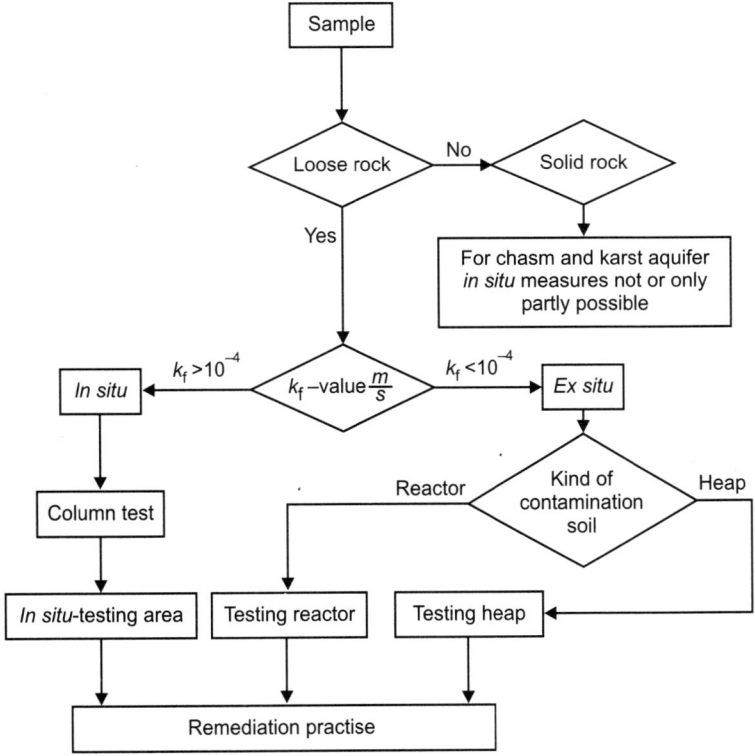

Fig. 10.2. Evaluation of bioremediation techniques.

Table 10.1 contains a list of the substance groups, which count as relevant in terms of contaminated sites, together with an assessment of their microbial degradability. It is not possible to define in general terms a concentration range within which microbial degradation is possible, but rather this differs according to the substance class. Similarly it is not possible to fix a generally applicable value for an achievable residual concentration, since this depends on the type and starting concentration of the pollutants and the adjustable ambient conditions.

To date the soils most frequently cleaned have been those contaminated with oil. The degradability of aliphatic hydrocarbons, such as petrol, diesel and other oil derivates, can be described as good.

Table 10.1. Biodegradability of soil contaminants.

Class of contaminants	Basically well degradable	Basically hard degradable
Aliphatic hydrocarbons (HC), petrol-HC and derivates	+	–
Monocyclic aromatic (e.g. BTEX) and heterocyclic (e.g. pyridin, chinolin) HC	+	–
Polycyclic aromatic HC (PAH)	+[a]	+[b]
Volatile halogenated, especially chlorinated hydrocarbons (VOCHs)	+	–
Alicyclic VOCH and derivatives (e.g. HCH)	+	
Polychlorinated biphenyls (PCBs)	–	+*
Polychlorinated dibenzodioxins and dibenzofurans (PCDDs resp. PCDFs)	–	+*
Pesticides and derivatives	–	+*
Heavy metals	Not degradable	

* Some low chlorinated congeners are principally degradable/dehalogenable, degradation of highly chlorinated congeners cannot be demonstrated at present: [a] up to 4-Ring-PAH; and [b] 5- and 6-Ring-PAH.

The persistence increases with the chain length and the degree of branching, and so for compounds with more than 25 carbon atoms the degradation rate slows down, if it does not come to a complete standstill. It is more difficult to clean soils from the coal by-product domain (gas works, coking plants), where the contamination is mainly in the form of BTEX aromatics (benzene, toluene, ethylbenzene, xylenes) and polycyclic aromatic hydrocarbons (PAHs).

Whereas 4-ring PAHs can now be described as being highly degradable, it is not always possible to degrade PAH with 5 and more aromatic rings. If degradation is encountered here, then this is due to co-metabolism, which means that the micro-organisms do not use these aromatics as the sole source of carbon and energy, but can only use them jointly in the presence of other hydrocarbons (co-substrates).

In many cases success is experienced with the biological treatment of soils contaminated by highly volatile halogenated hydrocarbons (VOCHs).

In contrast the degradation of polychlorinated biphenyls (PCBs) and polychlorinated dibenzodioxins and dibenzofurans (PCDDs/PCDFs) should be regarded in principle as very difficult. To date it has not been possible to provide a scientific verification of the complete dehalogenation of polychlorinated dioxins.

Heavy metals are in principle not degradable by microbial means. Under certain conditions they can be adsorbed on biomass by biosorption or taken up by plants from the soil.

BIOREMEDIATION TECHNIQUES

Figure 10.3 shows the generally practicable process options. After the required preliminary investigations and balancing of the microbial degradation processes to the greatest extent possible, a decision in favour of an *ex situ* or *in situ* method is made.

Ex Situ Processes

These processes require excavation of the contaminated soil masses and their treatment either in bio-heaps or in reactors, either on-site or off-site in a soil decontamination plant, which requires transport capacity.

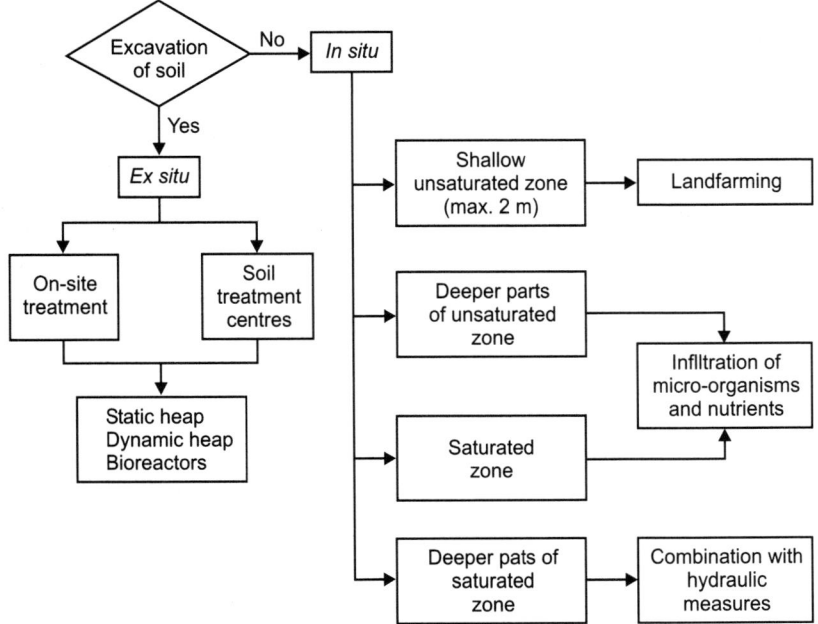

Fig. 10.3. Bioremediation techniques.

Bio-heap treatment

As to heap treatments, difference is made between static and dynamic ones. In static bio-heap methods, irrigation and aeration networks are installed for ensuring the necessary environment conditions.

In the case of dynamic heap methods the deposited soil masses are, in specified intervals, turned over, homogenised, and spread. During these turning-over cycles, further water and nutrients are added, if necessary.

Reactor processes

Reactor techniques are made use of for shortening the time for the treatment of soils with high fines portions and high rates of contamination as well as for better process control with respect to exhaust air and waste-water treatment. According to the water content of the soil, difference can be made between solid state and slurry state methods.

Solid-state processes

In solid-state processes, the soil is treated at a humidity rate corresponding approximately to 50 to 70 per cent of its maximum water capacity. The treatment is run in rotary reactors or in static reactors equipped with internal mixing systems. The principle of these methods is largely identical to the one of the dynamic heap processes. In both cases the biological degradation .of noxious substances contained in the soil is arrived at by agitation and aeration of the naturally moist soil. Also the treatment of soil/compost blends is to be categorised as solid-state process. These dry processes are advantageous in that the treated soil does not need to be dewatered.

A reactor, which is mainly used for mobile application allows the treatment of various amounts of soil by connecting together the appropriate number of container-like reactors to the necessary length respectively reactor volume (each reactor with a dimension of 5 × 1 metre). A horizontal driven mixing device realises a sufficient mixing and a homogeneous distribution of nutrients in the soil. The system is operated automatically controlled and allows either aerobic or anaerobic treatment as well as alternating combinations.

Slurry state processes

Extremely fine-grained or cohesive soils, or sludge, e.g. products from pre-treatment steps such as soil washing, cannot be purified by heap or solid-state reactor techniques. Accordingly, slurry state techniques are run for treatment of those soils. The soil portion per weight of slurries ranges between 30 and 50 per cent by weight. Processes run in impeller-type mixing vessels, airlift or fluidised-bed reactors, which provide sufficient and homogeneous nutrient and oxygen supply, are particularly suitable.

The key criteria for these processes read:
1. The particle sizes are less than 1000 μm.
2. All soil particles must be in full contact with the aqueous phase.
3. In particular for PAH, long residence times are to be catered for.
4. Due to the long residence times the energy requirement must be low and the solids portion of a reactor fill must be high.

Slurry-state bioreactor decontamination process

Technology of a series of tapered aerated slurry bioreactors is shown in Fig. 10.4.

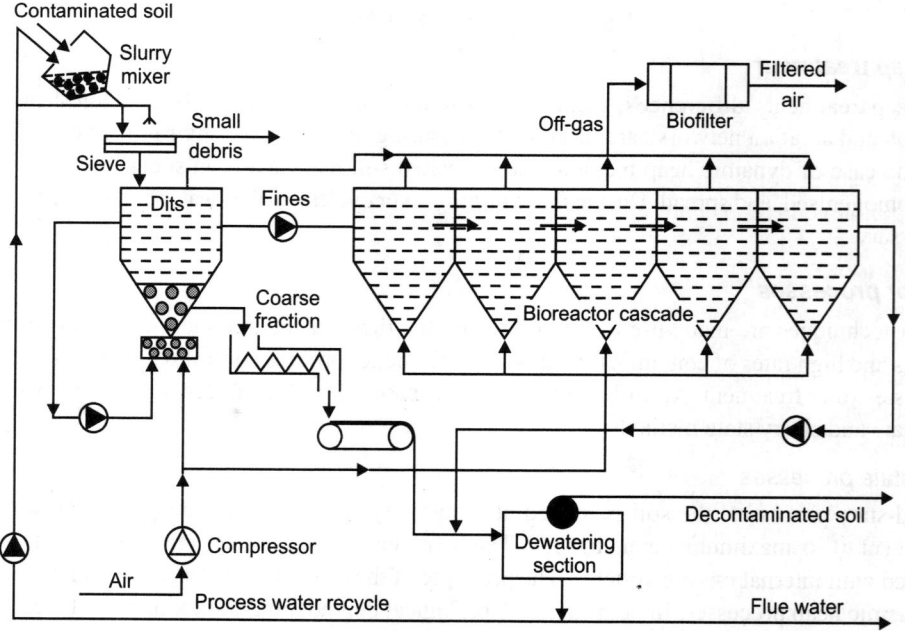

Fig. 10.4. Example for a slurry-slate bioreactor (SDP process).

The SDP-process consists of six steps:
1. Mixing of soil with water to produce the slurry.
2. Wet sieving of the slurry, the coarse fraction normally not contaminated is being separated.

3. Treatment in the dual injected turbulent separation (DITS) reactor, a combination of separation and decontamination. The coarse soil fraction can be separated, washed and removed to this first reactor. The fines are fed into the ISB-cascade.
4. Further treatment in the interconnected suspension bioreactor (ISB)cascade. Here the less available part of pollutants is degraded.
5. In the dewatering step the outgoing flow of treated soil are pressed to a filter cake or dewatered by other means.
6. Off-gas treatment by activated carbon filter or biofilter.

At the present time, a prototype plant with a reactor volume of 700 m³ to process 15,000 tonnes a year (8–10 days residence time) is in operation.

Another fluidised bed process has been developed by DMT. The fine-grained material is brought into suspension in a hydraulically run fluidised-bed reactor. Due to the necessary long residence times, e.g. for PAH degradation, the process is run batch wise. The larger cross-section in the reactor's top zone assures the sizing effect and a reduction of the solid's concentration in the slurry. Besides external aeration, also an internal aeration can be activated on option to cater for increased oxygen consumption. The inflow velocity relative to the reactor cross-section in the centre zone of the reactor is of roundabout 10^{-3} m/s. This allows .suspension of an approximately 4 to 8 metres high bed and a solids concentration of approximately 50 per cent by weight. These data also allow corresponding scaling up. A commercial plant with a reactor volume of 400 m³ is in operation in Sweden to clean PAH-contaminated soil.

The advantages of the application of bioreactors summarised below:
1. Decontamination takes place under well-controlled conditions easy to optimise.
2. Treatment of all kinds of soils even with high ratios of fines.
3. Treatment of soil contaminated with hazardous substances.
4. Aerobic and anaerobic as well as alternating aerobic/anaerobic treatment possible.
5. Increasing of bioavailability especially in slurry reactors.
6. Optimum emission control.

In Situ Methods

The decisive viewpoint for an *in situ* treatment is that no soil masses need to be removed and that the saturated or unsaturated zone of a contaminated site itself is used as integral reactor for the microbial degradation of contaminants. Figure 10.5 shows the typical features of an old pollution. The contaminants enter the soil and migrate downwards. The amount of contaminants remaining in the unsaturated zone is controlled by sorption and diffusion into the soil pores and retention by capillary forces. Generally the contaminants may form—when they reach the groundwater table—a separate phase on top of the groundwater so-called NAPLs (non-aqueous phase liquids) or at the basis of the aquifer groundwater zone) DNAPLs (dense non-aqueous phase liquids). Minor amounts of the contaminants are dissolved in the groundwater and are transported with the natural groundwater flow forming the contaminated plume. The spatial extent of the plume and the level of the contaminant concentrations depend on the age of the pollution, the sorption and transport characteristics as well on the efficiency of the natural degradation. Depending on the features of the contamination and of the site different technologies may be chosen. The technologies are subdivided into technologies for the treatment of the unsaturated and the saturated zone. A further subdivision comprises highly active technologies (bioventing, bioslurping, biosparging and hydraulic circuits) as well as active and passive technologies (funnel and gate, bioscreen and natural attenuation).

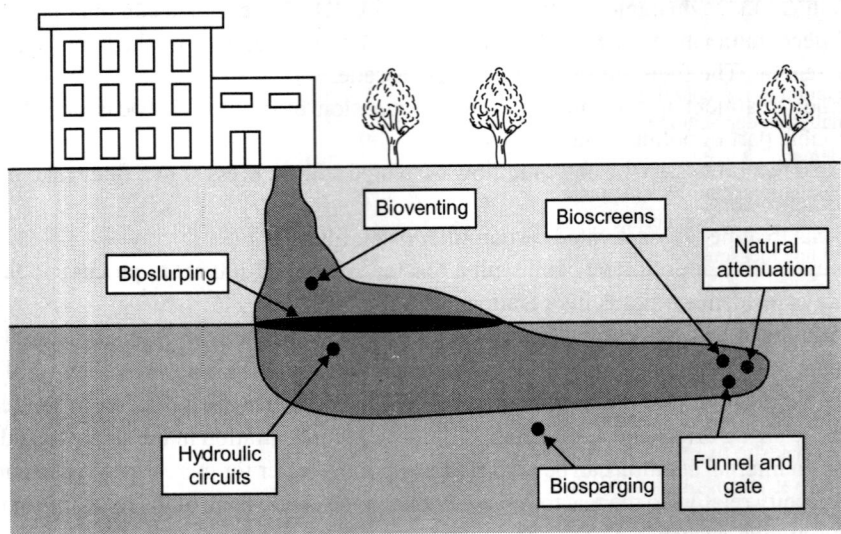

Fig. 10.5. Bioremediation alternatives.

For shallow unsaturated zones, land farming is possible, which allows addition of nutrients and the adjustment of the environment conditions. In deeper unsaturated zones and in parts of the saturated zones, infiltration of micro-organisms (bioaugmentation) and nutrients by a flushing circuit, sometimes combined with hydraulic measures is practised. The availability of molecular oxygen—dissolved in water and in this way cycled to the process—is decisive for rapid aerobic degradation. In such a process configuration, the addition of an oxygen carrier (such as hydrogen peroxide or industry grade oxygen) may be advantageous.

For decontamination under anoxic or anaerobic conditions (e.g. in the unsaturated zone) another electron acceptor (such as nitrate) is necessary to be used for the microbiological metabolism. The main features of biological soil remediation are summarised in Table 10.2.

Table 10.2. Comparison of *ex situ* and *in situ* bioremediation techniques.

Characteristics	Treatment	
	Ex situ	*In situ*
Removal of bioavailable contaminants by mineralisation to CO_2 and H_2O	+	+
Use of indigenous micro-organisms	+	+
Pre-investigations needed for evaluation of biodegradability and remediation techniques	+	+
Operation time depends on kind and concentration of contaminants	+	+
Prediction of remediation success is difficult		+
Treatment of large amounts of soil possible,		
If suitable areas are available	+	
If there are no remediation time limit,		+

(Contd ...)

Characteristics	Treatment	
	Ex situ	*In situ*
Flexible adaptation to site conditions e.g. remediation under buildings or on built-up areas		+
Low energy demand	+	+
Control of degradation conditions required during the total remediation period	+	+
Suitable for ad hoc measures, e.g. accidents		+

RE-USE OF THE SOIL

A major aspect of biological soil remediation is the re-use of the treated soil. Structural use includes, for example, backfilling noise baffle embankments, roadside fortification or ditches and landfill measures. The vegetation-related use ranges from roof greening and parks to agricultural use. The latter requires prior testing on large areas with grass as the test seed. Already a number of positive results have been obtained where it is possible to recultivate corn and potatoes after such a test.

BIOASSAYS FOR SOILS

A crucial factor for the re-use of soils is a toxicological/ecotoxicological assessment. For this purposes use is made of bioassays to measure the impact of contaminated or treated soils. Biological tests have proven especially beneficial if chemical or environmental samples of complex composition have to be tested with respect to their hazard potential. They integrate the effects of all acting substances, including those not considered or recorded in chemical analysis. A Dechema Working Group has reported the state-of-the-art of scientific development and experience and has recommended an assessment strategy which meets practical requirements such as:

1. Preliminary assessment of contaminated sites. Recognition of ecotoxicological effects, caused by contaminants, which might not have been detected by chemical analysis.
2. Ecotoxicological process control during biological soil clean up.
3. Evaluation of a possibly residual toxic/ecotoxic potential of treated soils before their further use.

PERSPECTIVES

The euphoria that has accompanied soil decontamination in the last few years has now given way to a realistic attitude of more appropriate proportions. The discussion on the equivalence of securing and decontamination techniques must not lead to a clean up on a low level, but rather to ecologically and economically appropriate solutions.

The original objective of multifunctional use through the restoration of a 'natural' soil is not feasible in most cases for technical and financial reasons. In view of this biological clean-up techniques still have to be improved and optimised in order to provide cost-effective, technically simple and near-natural processes.

Development Trends

Solutions attempted for *ex situ* processes, for example, are the combination of fixed-bed and liquid-phase bioreactors, which provide a great degree of flexibility in adapting the required ambient conditions to the relevant contaminant and also the special features of the soil matrix, or for *in situ* measures the dosing of tensides and heating of the soil by radio waves, for example, by which means it is possible to enhance the biological availability and hence the degree of degradation.

The treatment principle of humification is currently the subject of current attention in since with the clean-up of contaminated armaments sites, primarily the contaminant TNT. To eliminate TNT the only reasonable approach is cometabolic transformation with the subsequent binding of the products arising in the soil matrix. Both certain bacteria and fungi are capable of the cometabolic transformation of TNT to reduced metabolic products, such as aminonitrotoluenes. These are then partly degraded, mineralised or bound to the soil matrix in a process similar to natural humification. Both *ex situ* and *in situ* technologies are being studied. For example, anaerobic/aerobic combination processes (modified composting) are being tested as an *ex situ* technique. In the development of suitable *in situ* methods, an investigation is being conducted into whether an accumulation of TNT in the rhizosphere of plants and undergrowth can be economically exploited. This method, known as phytoremediation, is being researched mainly in the USA, Britain and Germany with a view to the further development of near natural, *in situ* clean-up processes for the accumulation of metals and organic compounds.

Successful research has also been conducted into the activation of natural biocenoses in the clean-up of sediments and acidic waters from uranium mining, as is demonstrated by the three-year-long operation of a pilot plant for heavy metal leaching. Since all biological clean-up processes are based on nature's own self-purification forces, they are the subjects of increasing attention and methods are being propagated under the names of 'intrinsic bioremediation' or 'natural attenuation'.

The USEPA policy directive defines monitored natural attenuation as 'the reliance of natural attenuation processes (within the context of a carefully controlled and monitored site clean-up approach) to achieve site-specific remediation objectives within a time frame that is reasonable compared to that offered by more active methods'.

In neither case are the terms used to mean that nothing is done and everything is left up to nature, which would not be acceptable anyway in the case of an actual hazard. Rather they involve more research work than is necessary for an engineering solution. The solution to the following questions is implied:

How can suitable micro-organisms most effectively be incorporated and distributed in the soil (bioaugmentation) and stimulated to optimum activity (biostimulation) and how must the groundwater be guided in order to render an *in situ* treatment possible and effective? With regard to the latter, in addition to the common techniques for groundwater treatment (pump and treat), techniques propagated in the USA under the names funnel and gate systems and reactive barriers are being tested increasingly. The most important restriction of such near-natural processes is the time span available to clean up the site.

FUTURE PERSPECTIVES

Suitable and sustainable solutions require a greater interdisciplinary approach, in other words the involvement of microbiologists, geneticists, chemists, hydrogeologists, soil scientists and process engineers.

A suitable and sustainable strategy for avoiding environmental contamination can also only be achieved by an interdisciplinary collaboration between all protagonists in research and industry. The wide ranging experience accumulated with respect to the contamination of soils and groundwater must be provided special impetus for testing the environmental impact of new chemical products before they are introduced, thus preventing subsequent contamination. A benign by design chemistry would therefore have to concentrate its research on identifying forms of bonding which facilitate the development of biodegradable and environmentally sound substances in the circulation of chemical products.

Chapter 11

Life Cycle Assessment in Soil Bioremediation Planning

INTRODUCTION

In several cases, life cycle assessment has been used as one supplementary tool in the planning of soil remediation. Three life cycle assessment based software tools for soil remediation planning are compared. One example of soil treatment in a bioreactor is investigated by using the software 'Umweltbilanzierung von Altlastensanierungsverfahren'.

The decision support tool 'risk reduction—environmental merit—costs' combines risk analysis, cost analysis with an approach, which is similar to life cycle assessment. The software 'Umweltbilanzierung von Altlastensanierungsverfahren' (environmental balancing of soil remediation measures) of the German state Baden-Württemberg compares the environmental burdens of the remediation with the results of a risk assessment. The software 'environmental/economic evaluation and the optimising of contaminated site remediation' analyses 'environmental costs' and 'environmental benefits' with an life cycle assessment approach.

The main innovative part in the three software products is the calculation of potential environmental burdens (screening life cycle assessments) of soil remediation measures. The degree of transparency of the three different life cycle assessment approaches is discussed in this chapter.

LIFE CYCLE ASSESSMENT IN SOIL REMEDIATION PLANNING

Remediation of contaminated sites is done to improve the environment. This improvement can be diminished by the possible environmental impacts of the technical measures. The planning of soil remediation concepts requires often the use of many tools. Such tools can be financial assessments, legal assessments or risk assessments. All useful tools together form a toolbox for the remediation of contaminated sites. This toolbox should include tools to evaluate the environmental burdens caused by the remediation (itself). Several governmental organisations promote the use of such tools. In the Netherlands (REC method), in Denmark (environmental/economic evaluation and optimising of contaminated sites remediation) and in Germany (environmental balancing of soil remediation measures), software tools have been developed for the consideration of the environmental burdens of the remediation (itself).

The evaluation of the overall environmental performance of a specific soil remediation option requires the knowledge of the environmental burdens caused by the remediation (itself). The life cycle assessment (LCA) method is a suitable tool to assess the potential environmental impacts of remediation. The life cycle assessment method is still under development, but practitioners can refer to four international standards (ISO 14040:1997, ISO 14041:1998, ISO 14042:2000, ISO 14043:2000). Due to the data uncertainty in the soil remediation-planning phase the requirements for the use of life cycle inventory data are relatively low. According to the ISO standards, every life cycle assessment consists of four parts as shown in Fig. 11.1.

1. Goal and scope definition.
2. Life cycle inventory.
3. Life cycle impact assessment.
4. Life cycle interpretation.

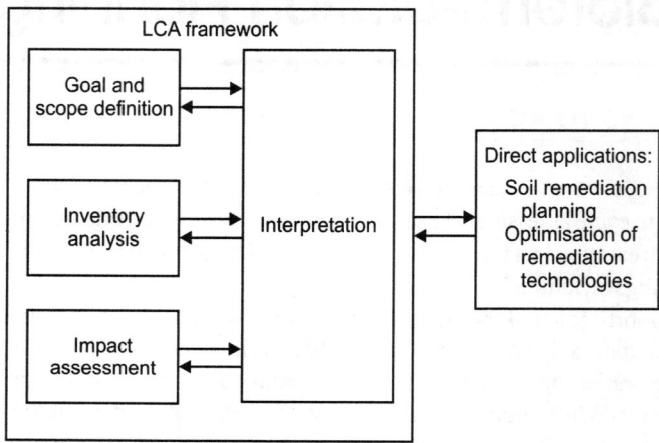

Fig. 11.1. Life cycle assessment (LCA) framework adapted from ISO 14040:1997 with special direct applications for soil remediation planning.

ENVIRONMENTAL BALANCING OF SOIL REMEDIATION MEASURES METHOD

The method is also called 'environmental balancing of soil remediation' or simply 'environmental balancing'. The software calculates a life cycle inventory. In the life cycle impact assessment, the life cycle inventory is transformed into indicator results. A rough data quality analysis is performed. In the life cycle interpretation, disadvantage factors for selected life cycle inventory entries and impact indicator results are calculated. A preliminary ranking of two soil remediation options compared can be made by the software user based on the table of disadvantage factors. Outside of the life cycle assessment framework, guidance for the improvement of remediation options is given. Also the table of disadvantage factors can be compared with the results of a separate risk assessment (area, volume) of contaminated soil and groundwater of the site before and after the remediation (Fig. 11.2).

REC METHOD

Beinat developed the decision support tool REC. REC is based on assessments of risk reduction, environmental merit and costs. REC can help in comparing soil remediation options.

The REC method provides three indices (risk reduction, environmental merit and costs), (Fig. 11.3). The environmental merit index is based on nine indices. Three of these indices (energy demand, air emission score, waste) are derived from a life cycle assessment of the remediation measures.

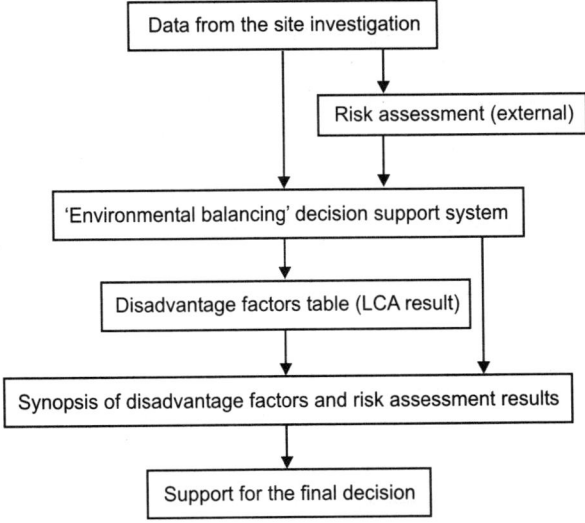

Fig. 11.2. Environmental balancing of soil remediation measures method.

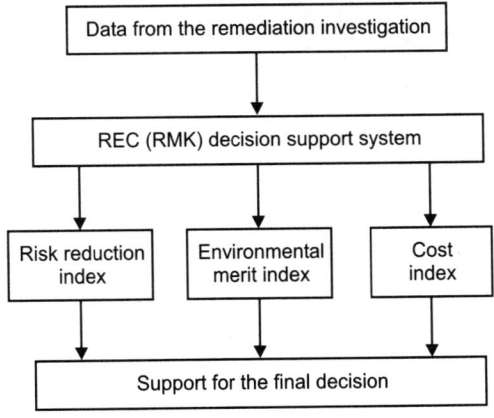

Fig. 11.3. REC method in a decision making process.

ENVIRONMENTAL/ECONOMIC EVALUATION AND OPTIMISING OF CONTAMINATED SITES REMEDIATION METHOD

A consortium of companies lead by the company ScanRail Consult developed the life cycle assessment based software tool 'environmental/economic evaluation and optimising of contaminated sites remediation'. The Excel ® based software is available in Danish and English. The software does not include the economic evaluation. The life cycle assessment method is applied in two ways: the calculation of 'environmental costs' and 'environmental benefits'. The benefits are mainly expressed in terms of life cycle indicator results of the life cycle impact categories human toxicity and ecotoxicity. Some data can be estimated as qualitative data. The single results are not aggregated to one overall score. Therefore, a synopsis is the key decision making process (Fig. 11.4).

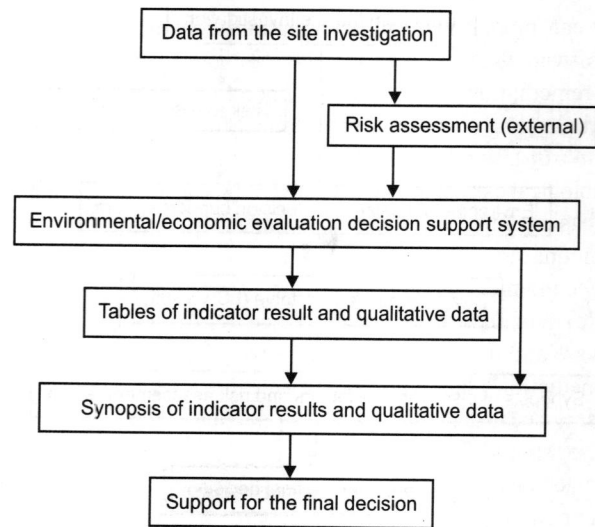

Fig. 11.4. Environmental/economic evaluation and optimising of contaminated sites remediation.

GENERAL COMPARISON OF THE THREE SOFTWARE TOOLS

The RMK (REC) software and the environmental/economic evaluation software are based on the spreadsheet programme Excel®. The Environmental balancing software works with the database programme Access®.

Allowed input data are listed in Table 11.1. With several input data in all three software tools a wide variety of bioremediation options can be modelled.

Table 11.1. Type of input data from site investigation (no costs).

Type of input data	Environmental balancing	Environmental/Economic evaluation	REC
Mass of polluted soil (water)	X	X	X
Pollutant	X	X	X
Remediation technology	X	X	X
Time of remediation	X	X	X
Transport: mass and distance	X	X	X
Type of land use	X	X	X
Amount of materials (plastics, etc.)	X	X	–
Pollutant concentration	–	–	X

The three software tools include predefined bioremediation processes. These pre-defined processes can consist of several other processes (ventilation, stirring, etc.).

The REC software and the environmental/economic evaluation include one soil bioremediation technology. Detailed descriptions of the applied technologies are not in the documentation of the two software tools and their documentation. If the software user knows the amount of electricity (REC), the amount of diesel (REC), the time of the usage of specific machines (environmental/economic evaluation) then the software user can model many bioremediation technologies. In case of the environmental/economic evaluation software the software user has to enter these data in several different sheets for the different phases of the remediation (establishment, operation, dismantling).

The environmental balancing software covers four different biotechnological technologies for the soil treatment (*in situ*, *ex situ*), two bioremediation technologies (*in situ* including reactive walls) and one technology of the biological cleansing of discharge air. It is also possible to model other bioremediation measures by using the basic technologies of civil engineering (well construction, etc.). The key data of the technology (like amount of the soil) can be entered on one screen.

The environmental/economic evaluation software offers the possibility to enter data of the usage several dozens of (single) machines. In this respect, the environmental/economic evaluation software is the most detailed software and the REC software the least detailed one of the three analysed software tools. For many soil remediation-planning studies the detailed approach of the environmental/economic evaluation is not necessary because the uncertainty in the planning phase is often very high. In the REC software the software user should have some knowledge about the calculation of the electricity amount or diesel amount of the machines used. If the software user does not has this knowledge, the environmental balancing software can be more suitable.

COMPARISON OF THE LIFE CYCLE ASSESSMENT APPROACHES

The REC method considers mainly diesel machine and electrical machine applications. These energy data are transformed directly into aggregated scores for air emissions. For example:

Input data	1 Gigagram contaminated soil in thermal soil treatment
Intermediate data	600 Gigajoule electricity
Output data	3 yearly Dutch inhabitant energy demand equivalents
	13 yearly Dutch inhabitant air emission equivalents

The assumptions and sources (literature) for the generic life cycle inventory data used are not documented.

In the environmental balancing method, the result of the life cycle assessment approach is a table with up to 19 disadvantage factors. The environmental/economic evaluation gives tables with eleven traditional life cycle indicator results and 15 common inventory results (mainly resources and wastes). Eight of the eleven indicator results are associated with the environmental 'costs' and three with the environmental 'benefits'. Most of these factors can be traced back to the indicator results (impact categories) and the single emissions (differentiated for the different processes like transportation by truck) or other inventory entries. The environmental balancing and the environmental/economic evaluation use mainly published generic life cycle inventory data. Some technologies (like the soil bioremediation) in the environmental/economic evaluation software are described with the emission data but not with the process data.

Table 11.2 shows output data concerning the three life cycle assessment approaches. Due to a missing of a clear separation between LCA data and non-LCA data in the three software tools, the definition of what can be interpreted as LCA data is taken by the distinctions made in the description about the environmental balancing method. To sum up all three-software products include the evaluation of the environmental burdens of the remediation processes. All three software products help soil remediation planners to estimate the overall environmental performance of different remediation concepts. This is a major contribution for the inclusion of the sustainability concept in soil remediation planning.

Table 11.2. LCA output data of the three software products.

Type of quantitative output data	Environmental balancing	Environmental/Economic evaluation	REC
Waste amount	X	X	X
Aggregated score for cumulated energy demand in Joule	X	–	–
Up to 19 disadvantage factors for single impact indicator results (inventory entries) for comparison of two remediation options	X	–	–
Land use (only remediation measures)	X	–	–
Water consumption (only remediation)	X	–	–
Non-renewable resources indicator result	X	–	–
Global warming indicator result	X	X	–
Acidification indicator result	X	X	–
Summer smog indicator result	X	X	–
Toxicity indicator results (air, water, soil; human or ecosystem; persistent)	X	X	–
Odour indicator results (near/remote emissions)	X	–	–
Noise indicator results (different levels)	X	–	–
Ozone depletion indicator result	–	X	–
Nutrification indicator result	–	X	–
Aggregated score for air emissions	–	–	X
Aggregated score for cumulated energy demand in yearly inhabitant equivalents	–	–	X

All three software products are useful decision support tools complementing the soil remediation planning toolbox. They require only data, which are usually available after a site investigation and a preliminary remediation concept making. All three are designed for soil remediation planners who have no (or little) experience in life cycle assessment.

The environmental balancing software contains only calculation procedures for a life cycle assessment approach. The REC software includes additional calculation procedures for risk (reduction) assessments and cost assessments. Therefore, only the life cycle assessment approach can be compared between the three software products. The transparency of the generic data used (life cycle inventory) and assumptions and the transparency of the output data (life cycle impact assessment) are higher in the environmental/economic evaluation and environmental balancing than in the REC software.

The environmental/economic evaluation software allows detailed data inputs for specific machines. By avoiding these detailed information the environmental balancing helps the planner to focus on the important issues of the remediation options.

Chapter 12

Slurry Decontamination Process

INTRODUCTION

Within the broad spectrum of technologies, focusing on the treatment and recycling of contaminated soils, sediments and sludge four types of *ex situ* bioprocessing can be identified: (i) landfarming, (ii) composting (biopiles), (iii) solid state fermentation (rotating reactors), and (iv) slurry processing.

To the latter category belongs the slurry decontamination process (SDP), the SDP is an *ex situ* continuous plug flow system based on tapered airlift slurry bioreactors. The process consists out of four major unit operations in which separation technology and biotechnology are integrate . The system has been studied at scales of 400 1,800 l and 4 m³.

The integral process was operated at pilot scale (3 m³ reactor volume) to test various solids waste streams. It was operated semi-continuously over a period of two and a half years. In the SDP efficient sand removal was combined with steady state microbial breakdown of organic pollutants such as mineral oils, PAH, BTEX and to a lesser extent PCB's. Recycling targets were reached. Major process parameters are the type and level of the contaminants, the power input, the solids hold-up, the power, capital and labour costs. The solids residence time is the key design parameter. Model calculations were made for a 1200 cubic metre scaled-up SDP-installation. For residences times ranging from 2 days up to 12 days, the costs were estimated. For the short residence times the cost level was within the market range (roughly be in between 20 and 60 euro/tonne), longer residence times were not feasible.

In terms of scale up economics, the solids residence time in the reactors of the SDP should not be longer than strictly necessary (few days). Therefore, reactor treatment (together with sand removal and flotation, if required) is to be combined with low cost, extensive, after treatment such as ripening fields, landfarming, phytoremediation or biopiles (the so-called 'constructed natural systems'). Due to the integration of intensive reactor treatment and extensive after treatment, not only recycling can take place within economic restrictions, but also flexibility is introduced to treat cocktails and solids waste streams having various compositions.

RECYCLING OF CONTAMINATED SOLID WASTE

Waste recycling plays a key role in the development of a sustainable economy. The classical approach, remediation without the production of recycled materials, does not contribute to durable material flows. Moreover, the production of reusable materials is a necessity to make waste treatment an attractive economic solution. For sustainable solutions the overall environmental efficiency should be positive and fit within the local economic and legal framework. The benefits of the treatment (decontamination and recycling) thus have to be compared to the disadvantages (power use, emissions, hindrance). Since recycling cannot take place regardless the effort and costs needed, the environmental benefits finally are to be judged by their economic merits (Fig. 12.1).

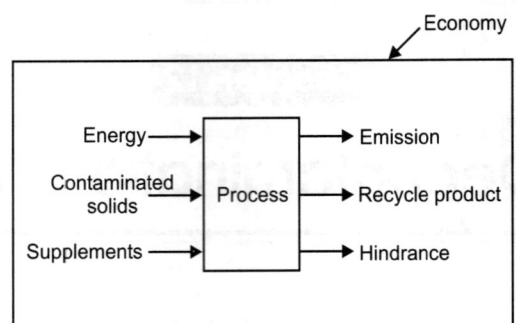

Fig. 12.1. Elements of the environmental process balance.

Solids waste streams (contaminated soils, sediments and sludge) can be recycled. The solids have to be recycled into usable products while the contaminants are removed or destroyed. In the Netherlands legal targets for recycled materials were set in the Dutch Building Material Decree. Depending on the content and the leaching of components, two different ways for using recycled materials in works are defined:

1. Category 1 products, needing no further isolation.
2. Category 2 products, needing further isolation and monitoring.

In the Dutch practice solids treatment is now-a-days mainly aiming at the production of Category 1 recycle products. Although each country still has its own standards, and standardisation is far away, it is beyond discussion that both recycling targets and environmental efficiency analyses are needed to support the development of sustainable technologies.

CHARACTERISTICS OF CONTAMINATED SOIL, SEDIMENTS AND SLUDGES

A complex solid matrix contaminated with one or more pollutants is the core of polluted soils, sediments and sludge (industrial or municipal). In soils the solid matrix is frequently dominated by sand, while the water content may be less than 25 per cent levels of debris can be found depending on the history of the site but rarely exceed the 10 per cent. River, harbour and canal sediments contain a majority of water (frequently above 60/70 per cent) while the fine fraction (below 63 micrometre) may dominates the solids. Industrial and municipal sludge mostly are very humid (more then 95 per cent water) and have a large content of organics (above 60 per cent). In industrial sludge the contaminant mostly originating directly from corrosion or wear (e.g. spent catalyst) of the installation on the site. Disregarding the heterogeneous nature of the waste, the contaminant behaviour largely is determined by the fines. This is due to the fact that submicron particles such as humic-clay structures and clay agglomerates have extreme high adsorption capacity. The solid waste, therefore, basically contains a contaminated fine fraction, a less contaminated sand/gravel fraction, cleaner debris and a contaminated water phase. Corresponding to this broad spectrum of waste streams with their contaminants, there is a variety of treatment options.

CLASSIFICATION OF TREATMENT TECHNOLOGIES

Basically solids waste treatment can be classified in three groups: *in situ* remediation, constructed natural systems (simple technology) and *ex situ* technology (Table 12.1).

Table 12.1. Classification of solids treatments.

In situ remediation	Constructed natural technology/ simple processes systems	Ex situ remediation
No excavation	Limited power input	Excavation
No power input	Low complexity	Power input
	Use of 'natural processes'	Process operations
Soil	Soil/sediments	Soil/sediment/sludge
Pump and treat	Landfarming (soil)	Separation technology
Bioremediation	Ripening (sediment)	Thermal treatment
Soil venting	Sand removal in sedimentation basins	Chemical/physical treatment
Soil washing	Aerobic lagoon treatment	Immobilisation
	Anaerobic landfill treatment	Bioreactors

In Situ Remediation

In-site bioremediation basically is used within the urban context of contaminated soils when, site conditions does not allow for excavation. A variety of *in situ* techniques have been developed in the US and in Europe to decontaminate soil without removal of the buildings above. *In situ* treatment includes electro-chemical approaches (electrodes in the soil), soil sparging or venting, soil washing with water, or bioremediation stimulating the local biosystems. Another option is to 'pump and treat' the groundwater present on the site; this means that the contamination is treated by means of treating the groundwater.

Constructed Natural Systems/Simple Technologies

The approach notified as 'constructed natural systems' or 'simple technology' combines features of natural occurring processes and technological principles. An example is landfarming used for the treatment of contaminated soils. The contaminated soil is gathered in heaps or layers in a controlled zone in which microbial breakdown takes place; forced aeration, the recycling of percolation water, addition of nutrients are ways to enhance the degradation rate. Although theoretically landfarming might be considered as a 'bioreactor', in practice it is an open system without clear system boundaries. Landfarming, therefore, typically has the features of a 'constructed natural system'.

Closely related to landfarming is the 'ripening' of contaminated sediments. Layers of contaminated sediments are spread out in a controlled zone; under the influence of the processes such as evaporation and natural dewatering an improvement of texture and composition of the ripened material is achieved. Phytoremediation is using specific vegetation in relationship to landfarming and sediment ripening, two pathways can be followed:

1. The plants or trees are used to accumulate metal contaminants such as copper, zinc, cadmium and nickel. Species which have been used in this respect are flax, maize and miscanthus.
2. The root structure (rhizosphere) of the growing vegetation is used as a matrix, which will stimulate the microbial remediation of organic, contaminates.

After the treatment the crop can be harvested and used as a sustainable biomass fuel; after incineration the contaminants are gathered in the ash or in the off gas filtration unit.

A simple separation technology making use of the 'natural' gravity is the sedimentation basin for the treatment of sediment slurries. A sedimentation basin is a natural clarifier that provides conditions to allow suspended particles to settle out of a slurry. In this way, sand is captured at the bottom of the basin while the overflow of contaminated fine fraction may be further treated.

A more advanced 'natural system' is the treatment of contaminated sediments in waste lagoons. Using air spargers at the lagoon bottom a particle suspension can be sustained in which micro-organisms can aerobically degrade the (organic) contaminants. Closely related to lagoon treatment are the processes focusing on the anaerobic microbial breakdown in sediment disposal sites.

Ex Situ Processing

Ex situ processes are characterised by the presence of:
1. The solid waste as feedstock is pre-treated.
2. Power input.
3. Use of unit operations.

A class of frequently used *ex situ* remediation options, especially for complex contaminated waste cocktails, is thermal treatment. As a follow up of soil treatment, thermal techniques also are being developed to treat (wet) sediments and sludge. Immobilisation of the solids into end products such as recycled gravel, bricks, of larger structures such as basalt have been established.

A second class of successfully applied *ex situ* processes is based on particle separation techniques mostly originating from the field of mineral ore processing. Common operations are sieves, flotation cells, hydrocyclones, Humphrey-spirals, jigs, fluid bed systems and up flow columns. These processes typically result in the removal debris and the production of reusable sand fractions while the contaminated fines are further treated or stored.

Chemical treatments, such as solvent extraction methods (e.g. supercritical CO_2 or acetone extraction) have been investigated as *ex situ* treatment technology. Also the addition of chemicals to solidify the solids is in practice being carried out. Although applied in the US and Canada chemical solidification is no common use in Europe and other developing countries.

In case the contaminants are organic (such as mineral oil, PAHs, solvents, BTEX, PCBs) bioreactors can be used. In bioreactors populations of soil-organisms degrade the contaminants to yield harmless products.

BIOREACTORS

Defining a bioreactor as a vessel or a closed system in which under controlled conditions microbial breakdown occurs, the basic kinetics can be denoted by means of the black box model as depicted in Fig. 12.2. Under steady state condition, (no accumulation in the system), the input of pollutant, oxygen, nitrogen and soil compounds (e.g. humic substances) results into the output of carbon dioxide, water, nitrate and protons.

Although the mass balances for each of the elements involved (C, H, O and N) in theory should fit for the complete 100 per cent (elements cannot be destroyed), in practical multi-phase systems proper mass balance measurements are difficult. Besides interference with the surrounding for the gaseous components (e.g. oxygen), the dissolved components have to be followed in a complex matrix. In practice the microbial breakdown, therefore, mostly is followed by the contaminant concentration only. Having defined the major microbial features of the bioreactor, two major categories can be distinguished:
1. Bioreactors with a restricted solids hold-up: slurry reactors (typical solids hold up-below 40 wt%).
2. Bioreactors with restricted humidity: solid-state fermentation, (solids hold-up typical above 60 wt%).

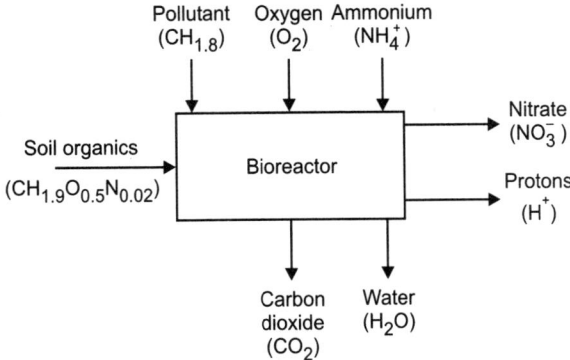

Fig. 12.2. Basics of the bioreactor conversion.

Slurry Bioreactors

Characteristic for all types of slurry bioreactors (Fig. 12.3) is the need of power input to sustain a three phase system in which the solid particles are suspended; the gravity forces acting on the solids have to be compensated by the drag forces executed by the liquid motion. In a proper designed slurry system the power input is used to maintain three phenomena:

1. Suspension.
2. Aeration.
3. Mixing.

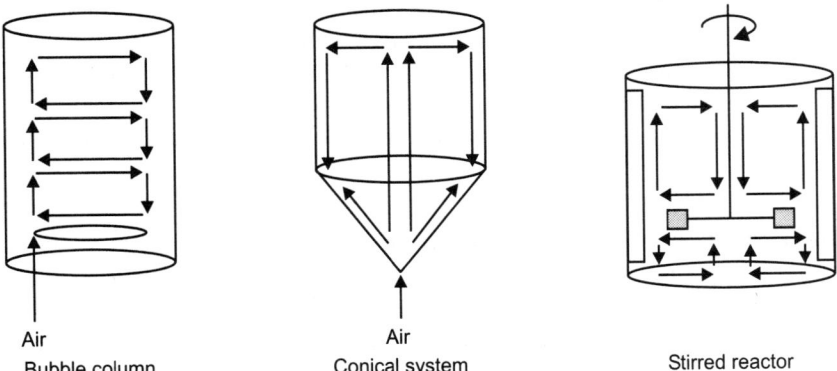

Fig. 12.3. Common configurations of slurry bioreactors.

For each reactor configuration, the appropriate balance of these three parameters depend on the reactor scale, the particle size distribution, slurry density, slurry viscosity, oxygen demand of the biomass and the solids hold-up.

Solid State Bioreactors

For solid-state fermentation there is no need to maintain a solids/liquid suspension; a compact moist solid phase determines the system. In a solid-state fermentor, process conditions are maintained by controlling the temperature, humidity and aeration. Both the fixed bed reactor as well as the rotating drum bioreactor are suited for solid-state fermentation (Fig. 12.4). In the fixed bed reactor the contaminated solids are permanently installed upon a drained bottom as a stationary phase. Forced aeration and the supply of water mostly are applied as continuous phase. A fixed bed reactor may be batch operated as a closed biopile system.

Continuous solid state processing is possible in the rotating system, here the solid phase (as a compact moist material) is 'screwed and pushed' through the reactor. In line with slurry processing power is required to maintain the transport of the solids through the system.

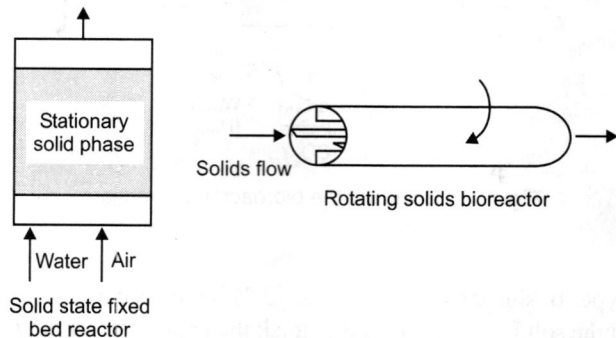

Fig. 12.4. Bioreactors for solid state processing (fixed bed and rotating drum reactor).

In line with its traditional role as a soil fertiliser, compost has been used as an additive in solid-state treatment. Basically the compost addition is used to stimulate the microbial breakdown. In experiments soil contaminated with hydrocarbons has been mixed with compost in various ratios (soil/compost ratios 2:1, 3:1 and 4:1). In 3-litre test batch reactors the hydrocarbon degradation was more than 90 per cent after a period of 44 days. Compared to the breakdown result without compost addition, the soil/compost systems showed a much faster degradation rate and a lower end concentration.

At larger scale fixed bed experiments, using 10 m³ biopiles, were carried out to investigate the degradation of chlorophenol in contaminated soil. Chalk, commercial fertiliser (NPK) and bark chips (as bulk aeration agent) were added as supplements. After two months 80 per cent of the contaminant was removed.

CONFIGURATION OF *EX SITU* BIOPROCESSES

Depending on the type of bioreactor pre- and post-treatment operations are needed. Solid-state bioreactor processing in general does not need intensive pre-treatment of the solids since the texture of the solid feedstock is not significantly changed. In contrast, slurry bioprocessing requires an extensive pre-treatment to remove large parts from the solids before the reactor is being fed. The bioreactor mostly is integrated with washing/separation operations.

Ex Situ Slurry Bioprocess

A typical set-up of an integrated *ex situ* (slurry) bioprocess is shown in Fig. 12.5. First, the feedstock is screened using a wet vibrating screen, to remove the debris (sizes above 2–6 mm). Second, sand fractions are being removed by one or more separation techniques, a typical separation diameter (the so-called cutpoint) for these separation steps is 63 microns (or 50 microns depending on the standard chosen). In the cyclone shown in Fig. 12.5 the slurry flow is split into a sand fraction (particle size above 63 microns) at the bottom and a fine fraction at the top (below 63 micrometre).

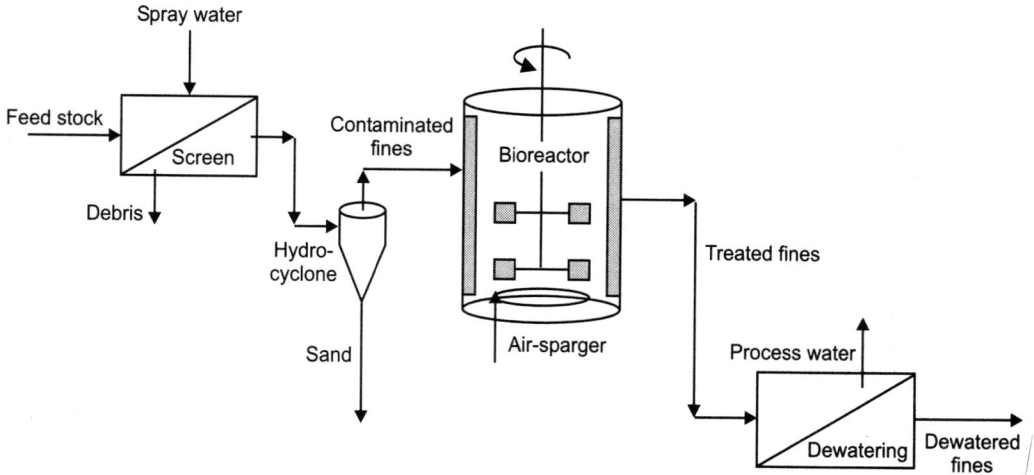

Fig. 12.5. Typical set-up of an *ex situ* (slurry) bioprocess using a batch operated aerated stirred tank reactor (typical solids hold-up is 20 wt%).

The top flow of the cyclone, containing the contaminated fines, is being fed the bioreactor (depicted is a stirred tank but any of the three types from Fig. 12.5 might be chosen). The final dewatering operation results in an end product containing the fines and process water.

1. Batch operation; no fresh material is introduced to the bioreactor during processing, the composition of the content changes continuously.
2. (Semi-) continuous operation (plug flow); fresh material is introduced and treated material removed during processing, the composition in the reactor remains unchanged with time.

Although continuous processes offer many advantages in terms of capacity, inactive periods and costs, in the treatment practice most operations are still batchwise.

Slurry Decontamination Process

The slurry decontamination process has been developed as a (semi)-continuous system (Fig. 12.6). This process contains four major unit operations:

1. The contaminated solids are mixed with (process) water into a slurry and sized over a vibrating screen. In this wet sieving step, the debris is removed and a slurry prepared having the required density (25–35 w/w%).
2. In the first reactor/separator, a tapered air lifted bioreactor: the DITS-reactor the sand fractions are removed by means of a fluidised bed. Extensive organic material is removed by fine screening of light material. In addition, the agglomerates of the contaminated fines are demolished due to the power input and therefore opened to biological breakdown (also inoculation with the active biomass takes place).
3. In a second reactor stage the fine fraction is in a cascade of air lifted tapered bioreactors which are connected (ISB-cascade).
4. A dewatering stage completes the process, the water released is partly recirculated as process water to mix up the fresh solids into a slurry.

At various scales, ranging from mini-plant level (40 litres) up to a 4-m³ parts of the system was extensively tested. A pilot plant was operated for two and a half years to test various solid waste streams at a scale of 3 m³. During several treatment periods in which various waste streams was processed, steady states degradation was measured.

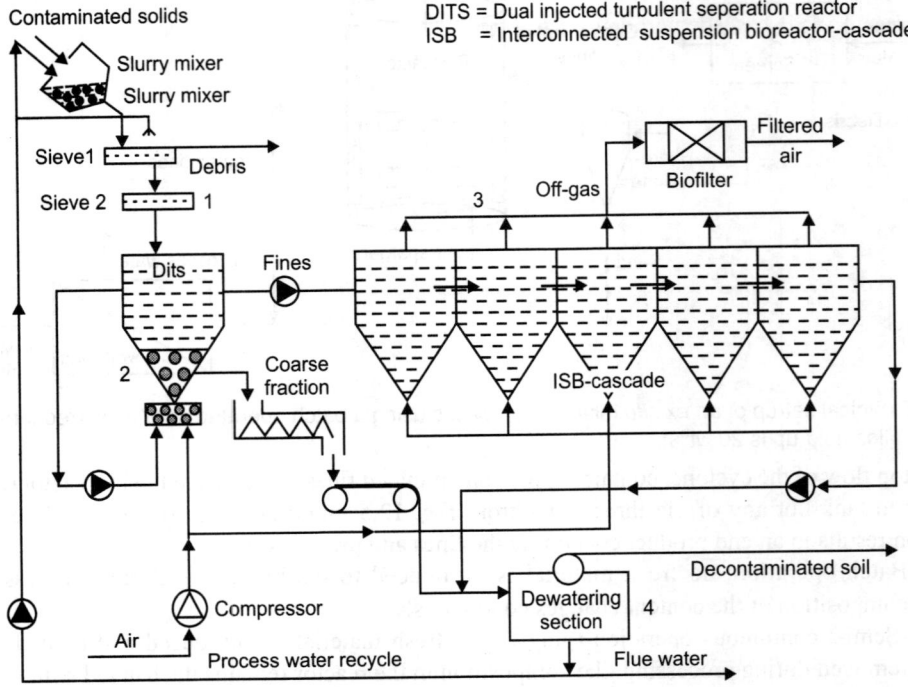

Fig. 12.6. Slurry decontamination process (SDP).

Figure 12.7 gives an artist's impression of the 3 m³ pilot plant, which was constructed by BIRD Engineering in the Netherlands. Shown is how the beginning of the process (the slurry preparation) takes place at a platform while the reactor components are at a lower level. By hydrostatic forces the slurry runs through the system. After the last treatment step, the fifth compartment of the ISB-cascade, the slurry is pumped into a chamber filter press for dewatering.

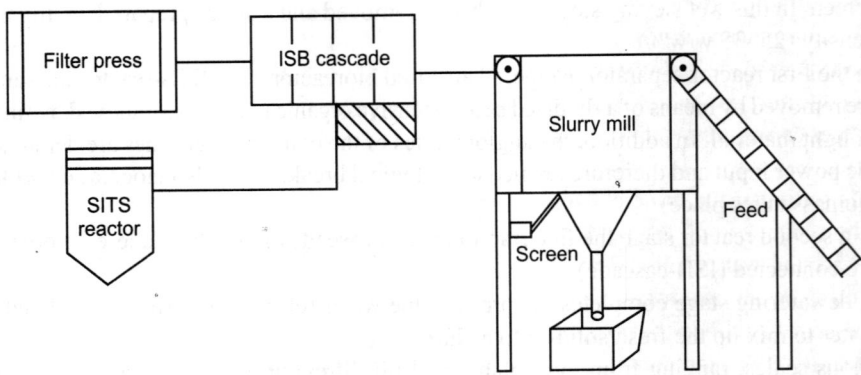

Fig. 12.7. Artist's impression of the pilot plant (units not in proper size).

Microbial Breakdown in the SDP

A contaminated soil treated in the pilot plant resulted in a steady state breakdown pattern shown in Fig. 12.8. The measure steady state concentrations (mineral oil), in each of the four units (slurry mill, DITS-reactor, ISB-cascade and dewatering stage), are depicted as a function of time. For a scattered input (black triangles for the input ranging from 600 to 1300 mg/kg), the steady state concentration further on in the process also fluctuated (+/– 350 mg/kg for the DITS-reactor and +/– 200 mg/kg for the ISB-cascade).

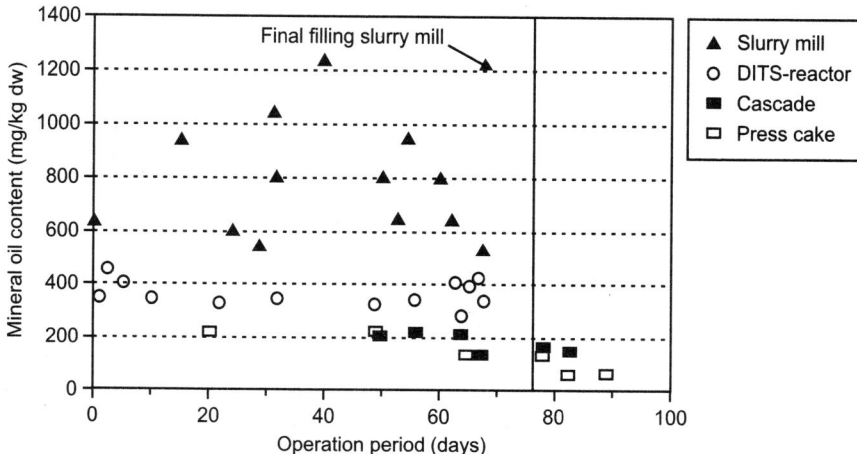

Fig. 12.8. Steady state mineral oil breakdown pattern in the SDP (soil).

After dewatering, end concentrations were reached at levels below 50 mg/kg, well below the recycling standards (residence time was 38 days). Due to scattered input, no smooth steady state breakdown pattern is observed. Each following step, however, clearly has lower steady state values.

Figure 12.9 shows the experimental results for a heavily polluted sediment (Petroleum harbour Amsterdam) over a steady state period of 6 weeks, the residence time in this experiment was 16 days. Nutrients (nitrogen, phosphorus and potassium) were added and the temperature was kept at 30 degree Celsius. The steady state PAH concentration in the solids is depicted as a function or time. The upper symbols show the feed concentration in the slurry mill with an average of about 350 mg/kg. In the DITS-reactor the steady state concentration dropped to values around 100 mg/kg (first part of the microbial breakdown).

In the ISB-cascade the average concentration dropped to values of 30/40 mg/kg. After dewatering the final concentration increased somewhat in the filter cake. The overall PAH-degradation level was about 92 per cent and recycling standards could be reached. No significant evaporation was measured in the off gas.

In this sediment the mineral oil degradation pattern showed a similar trend, however, an overall degradation level of only 65 per cent was established (16 days residence time). Final concentrations after dewatering were around 3000 mg/kg, far above the recycling target of 500 mg/kg. The load of mineral oil to be degraded thus did not match the microbial breakdown capacity generated. Therefore it was necessary to reduce the load of contaminants being fed to the system. Since the contaminants predominantly are adsorbed to the soil organics and mineral fines, froth (foam) flotation at the start of the SDP (in the DITS-reactor) was experimentally tested.

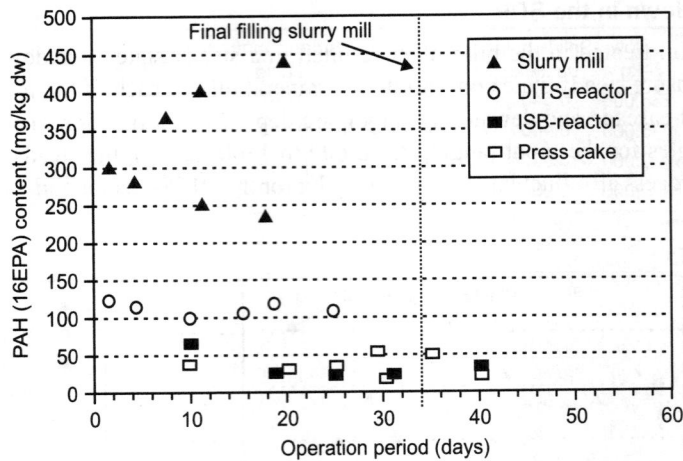

Fig. 12.9. Steady state PAH breakdown pattern in the SDP (sediment).

SDP-Improvements: Froth Flotation in the DITS-Reactor

Froth (foam) flotation is a technique used to separate particles if there is sufficient difference in their hydrophobicity. In an aerated particle suspension the hydrophobic particles tend to be collected at the air bubble/water interface; with the air bubbles these particles rise to the surface and gather in the foam on top of the slurry. If the mixture of froth and hydrophobic particles is collected from the top by means of a skimmer, a particle separation is achieved. In industry flotation is often used to separate metals from a suspension.

Flotation experiments were carried out by connecting a flotation cell to the DITS-reactor. Figure 12.10 gives the mass balances for the DITS-reactor without and with flotation for a sand free sediment. In the standard situation (no flotation) a batch of sediment was fed to the reactor (235 kg) with a solids hold-up of 54 per cent. This resulted in 126.9 kg of solids weight at the start. This load contained 12.18 kg organics (9.8 per cent) and 2.09 kg of mineral oil (at 17 gr/kg). Without flotation the only separation for this sediment took place at the debris screening, 98 per cent of the solids remained in the DITS-reactor to be treated. The mineral oil load being fed to the biomass was almost (98 per cent) equal to the input.

Using flotation the mass balance changed significantly. For a load of 126.9 kg solids an amount of 32.5 kg solids due to flotation was separated; the remaining load was 71 per cent in the input. With the flotated solids 7.47 kg of organics and 1.07 kg of mineral oil was removed. Due to flotation only 33 per cent of the organics and 45 per cent of the mineral oil remained to be treated. For PAH the flotation was less effective, 80 per cent of the PAH still were to be treated in the process.

From these experiments it was concluded that flotation is an effective way to reduce the load of contaminants in the feed flow before the bioreactors are entered. Flotation can be used as a 'safety measure' to protect the microbial population from overloading. An additional effect of flotation in the DITS-reactor is found in the capability of metal removal with the froth. For waste streams having both organic and metal contaminants, flotation opens the possibility of treating cocktails and physically removing metals without a significant change in the process.

Standard DITS

	Flow kg	Solids hold-up kg/kg	Solids flow kg	Organic matter kg/kg	Organic flow kg	Mineral oil kg/kg	Oil flow kg
Sediment input	235.000	0.540	126.900	0.096	12.182	0.017	2.094
Debris (screen)	5.000	0.480	2.400	0.149	0.358	0.017	0.040
Sand flow	0.000	0.000	0.000	0.000	0.000	0.000	0.000
Flotation flow	0.000	0.000	0.000	0.000	0.000	0.000	0.000
Amount to treat			124.500		11.825		2.054
% of input			98		97		98

DITS + flotation

	Flow kg	Solids hold-up kg/kg	Solids flow kg	Organic matter kg/kg	Organic flow kg	Mineral oil kg/kg	Oil flow kg
Sediment input	235.000	0.540	126.900	0.096	12.182	0.017	2.094
Debris (screen)	9.000	0.480	4.320	0.149	0.644	0.017	0.071
Sand flow	0.000	0.000	0.000	0.000	0.000	0.000	0.000
Flotation flow	250.000	0.130	32.500	0.230	7.475	0.033	1.073
Amount to treat			90.080		4.064		0.950
% of input			71		33		45

Fig. 12.10. Mass balances for the DITS-reactor.

SCALE-UP

Having extensively studied the major process and operational features of the SDP at pilot scale, a feasibility study for a larger demonstration plant has been made. As an example the features of plant with a working volume of 1200 m³ (average capacity of +/– 25,000 tonnes/year) were determined. At this capacity:

1. The hydrodynamics is well known, no significant scale-up problems are to be expected.
2. The kinetics are expected to be identical to the pilot plant.
3. Market demonstrations can be given.

Process Economics

For a defined SOP-plant volume the actual capacity directly is proportional to the solids residence time. The residence time in its turn defines the amount of power needed to process one tonne of solids. The costs per tonne (among costs as labour and finances) thus are a function of the solids residence time. Figure 12.11 gives the relationship between calculated cost levels per tonne input and the solids residence time. The present Dutch market range (roughly in between 20 and 60 euro/tonne) is depicted by the arrow. Shown are the upper and lower capacities at the example of a 1200 m³ plant volume. At the upper capacity (50,000 tonnes/year at 2 days residence time) costs are at the lower end of the range; at the lower capacity (10,000 tonnes/year at 12 days residence time) the costs are in the upper range.

Figure 12.11 is based on the process features shown in Fig. 12.5. This means that as much sand as possible is removed in the DITS-reactor. Flotation effects have not been incorporated in the calculations. After the DITS-reactor, the fines are treated in the ISB-cascade. For the calculations a moderately contaminated soil was taken.

Relating the design results (shown in Fig. 12.11) to the pilot experiments, it has to be concluded that the solids residence times used at pilot scale (ranging from 16 to 38 days) should not be applied. Focusing

on the shorter residence times (in between 2 and 12 days) for a scaled up system, two options are available to operate within the economic context:
1. Flotation in the DITS-reactor.
2. Combination of the SDP with extensive (low cost) treatment of the fines.

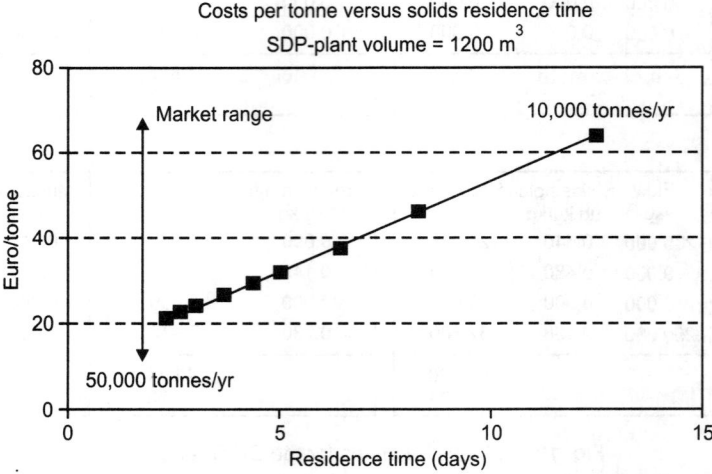

Fig. 12.11. Residence time versus estimated costs per tonne (1200 m³ SDP-installation: cost level = 2007).

Extensive (Low Cost) Treatment of the Fines

Extensive treatment of fines is possible in various ways. They all have in common that little handling is needed and that time and natural processes are allowed to improve the quality of the material. The measures to be taken depend on the nature of the contaminants concentrated in the fines. Two major groups may be distinguished being (heavy) metals and organic compounds such as mineral oil, polynuclear hydrocarbons (PAHs), chlorinated hydrocarbons and pesticides. Both groups of contaminants require a different approach.

In the case of heavy metals the environmental risk may be reduced by immobilisation or by decontamination. As a result of the treatment process in general a partial mobilisation of metals takes place. Natural ripening processes will lead to re-adsorption of metals on clay minerals and the transfer of metals from soluble into insoluble species such as the sulphides. These processes may be obtained by allowing the fines to settle and drain in a basin constructed with earthen walls. Based on the chemical composition of the fines additives may be added to increase the rate of the immobilisation processes in which micro-organisms may play an important role. These additives will specially composed on the basis of the nature of the project.

Removal of metals may take place by the use of plants (phytoremediation). Various plants can be used, which depends on the nature of the contaminants and the use, which can be made of the products (fire wood, paper, etc.). The choice of the preferred plants is depending on the way in which the plants store the contaminants. The easiest plants are those which collect the contaminants in the leaves. Harvesting, composting, incineration of the residue and collecting the ashes, is in this case the cheapest way to collect the contaminants.

Organic compounds may be removed by microbial processes. Depending on their nature these may be aerobic (mineral oil, PAHs, pesticides, etc.) or anaerobic (chlorinated hydrocarbons, pesticides, etc.).

Anaerobic processes are relatively easy to obtain, because the fines will render anaerobic conditions shortly after they settle. Additives are required to fuel, for example, dehalogenation when not present naturally in sufficient amounts and of the right source.

To obtain aerobic degradation, measures have to be taken such as the addition of additional nutrients and oxygen releasing compounds before spreading the fines to the ripening fields. A biological method is the use of plants, which have the properties to transport oxygen to their root zone such as reed (*Phragmitis communis*). In principle an aeration system may be applied, but this can very much intensify the treatment process, which sometimes is not the object. The use of appropriate plants will also improve the soil structure and will increase the rate of dewatering and, thus, decrease the period in which the area is difficult to use.

Above a number of possibilities are indicated for the use of extensive treatment of the fines in order to give these a function in land planning operations for non-food agricultural applications or as a recreational or natural environment. Based on the scale of the operation the result there of may be more or less extensively reviewed ecologically.

In the combination of the SDP and an extensive treatment the fines are ripened. In this combination after a short residence time in the SDP, the fines are further extensively treated.

Environmental Efficiency of the SDP

In order to determine the environmental efficiency of the SDP, firstly the process has to be put into a broad framework (see also Table 12.1). Being an *ex situ* treatment method, the SDP-process requires an installation using power, in addition, the feed has to be excavated, transported and stored. To operate these type of installations at full scale efficiently, clearly recycling products have to be the outcome of the SDP-treatment. Making recycling products out of waste, however, not only demands a properly designed process, also the logistics of the feed flow, the product flow and quality of the input are crucial. In addition, the economic, legal and political context should be in favour of stimulating the use of recycling products in various parts of the economy.

The overall environmental efficiency for the SDP is determined by the technical features (such as power input per tonne solids and residence time), the quality of the input and output (recycling sand and clay) and the aspects mentioned above.

Having fully explored the SDP-technology and its environmental efficiency, it was concluded that, given the present situation, the basic design of the SDP, using reactor technology only is not appropriate. Instead of focusing on reactor treatment, the combination of reactor operation (short residence times) with extensive methods is to be preferred. In this way, the benefits of both approaches are to be combined into integrated systems, resulting in environmentally efficient and flexible solid waste treatment.

Thus, from the above the following conclusions can be drawn that:

1. A transition in treatment technology from waste decontamination towards waste recycling is taking place.
2. In the broad spectrum of technologies, ranging from *in situ* soil remediation towards large-scale *ex situ* treatment installations, the category of constructed natural systems (like landfarming, phytoremediation, lagoon treatment, separation basins) fits in between.
3. The slurry decontamination process (SDP), developed and operated up to pilot level, basically was designed as an *ex situ* biotechnological reactor process.
4. In the continuously operated SDP-pilot plant mineral oil and PAH contaminated solids can be degraded down to (Dutch) recycling standards giving acceptable end products.

5. It was concluded that at the present market conditions, only short residence times (few days) in the SDP-reactors are feasible (costs). At these short reactor residence times the combination of the SDP-reactor technology with an extensive post-treatment (such as constructed natural systems in the form of phytoremediation) is aimed at. The basic SDP-set-up therefore is transformed in a combination of technologies.

6. To obtain environmentally efficient treatment the question should no longer be how a specific technology can be optimised. The major issue is how to make recycle products using any economical combination of operations, which suits the purpose.

Chapter 13

Immobilisation of Pesticides in Soil through Enzymatic Reactions

INTRODUCTION

Immobilisation phenomena occurring in soil are of great environmental importance because they may lead to a considerable reduction in the bioavailability of pesticides. Both enzymes and abiotic catalysts can mediate the immobilisation process. One of the most important catalytic reactions in soil is oxidative coupling that links naturally occurring and xenobiotic chemicals, such as pesticides, to organic matter. The reaction may be caused by oxidoreductases and may have a detoxification effect. Therefore, pesticide immobilisation through binding to soil constituents can be considered an alternative method of pollution control.

Immobilisation processes observed in soil are of great environmental significance as they may lead to a considerable reduction in the bioavailability and degradation of pesticides. The ability of soils to retain pesticides is attributed to adsorption phenomena and chemical reactions occurring on active surfaces of humus and mineral particles; pesticides can also be retained through entrapment within the soil matrix. According to the proposed models of biodegradation, pesticide molecules must be present in the aqueous phase to be available to micro-organisms. This bioavailability requirement is constantly challenged in terrestrial systems where pesticide molecules are continuously removed from the soil solution through immobilisation or diffusion into inaccessible locations.

Bound residues, by definition, cannot be removed from soil by non-destructive methods. Pesticides retained through adsorption are not considered bound as they can be desorbed by extraction with water or organic solvents. Pesticides are, in general, adsorbed faster than they are desorbed, a phenomenon known as hysteresis. According to recent observations, the rates of adsorption and desorption are subject to reduction with the length of time that the xenobiotics reside in soil or are 'aged'. As they age, chemicals show increased hysteresis. In addition, considerable amounts of aged xenobiotics become entirely resistant to desorption and thus are unable to be biodegraded.

Ageing is currently ascribed to sorption and entrapment phenomena occurring in remote micro-sites within the soil matrix. According to Alexander, xenobiotics can reach these sites by diffusion across the organic matter. Such a combination of diffusion processes with adsorption frequently is referred to as sequestration or slow sorption, because months or even years may be required to reach equilibrium. Like adsorbed chemicals, those that are sequestered can be recovered, although with difficulty, by vigorous extraction with organic solvents. From the standpoint of biodegradation, however, sequestration is practically irreversible, because the chemicals involved in diffusion and subsequent sorption do not desorb back into the soil solution.

It is well known that a large portion (20 to 70 per cent) of a particular chemical that reaches the terrestrial system becomes sequestered or bound to soil and resists extraction with water and organic solvents. Neither research in the laboratory nor practical experience has found any significant any negative or toxic impact of bound xenobiotics on the environment; consequently the immobilisation of pollutants in soil has been recognised as a promising decontamination technique.

REACTIONS BETWEEN PESTICIDES AND HUMIC MATERIAL

Binding to humus constitutes one of the major reactions by which anthropogenic compounds are transformed in nature. As discussed above, pesticides interact with soil colloids through several mechanisms; a number of reviews describe the various mechanisms. Adsorption occurs primarily as a consequence of the attraction between the solid surface of the soil and the soluble or vapour phase of the pesticide. The nature and strength of adsorption depend largely on the chemical structure of the molecule. Adsorption is reversible, and the desorbed chemicals are available to interact with the biota. However, there is abundant evidence suggesting that with longer exposure to soil, adsorbed residues become more resistant to extraction and degradation. This resistance may result from a gradual sequestration or slow incorporation of the pollutant into humus.

Covalent Binding by Soil Micro-organisms

The most persistent complexes result from the covalent binding of xenobiotics to humic material. These complexes, often referred to as the 'bound residues', are highly resistant to acid and base hydrolysis, thermal treatment, and microbial degradation. In a sense, bound residues constitute a dead-end product of microbial activity. Micro-organisms and their enzymes may, in fact, be indispensable in bound residue formation. Experiments using ^{14}C-labelled compounds demonstrated that generally only negligible amounts of bound residues are formed in sterile soils. The role of micro-organisms in these processes is to condition the xenobiotic molecules for covalent binding.

Micro-organisms also can partially degrade xenobiotics, thus converting them to more reactive derivatives that may be involved in future covalent binding. As a result of binding, however, these derivatives are resistant to further degradation or mineralisation on exposure to microbial populations.

Oxidative Coupling

Oxidative coupling is one of the most important chemical reactions occurring in soil. It leads to humification of both naturally occurring humic acid precursors and susceptible anthropogenic compounds (phenols and aromatic amines) through their incorporation into soil organic matter. The incorporation is controlled by a free radical mechanism. The resonance-stabilised free radicals, formed through the loss of an electron and a proton from a phenol molecule, couple to each other in a variety of combinations. After coupling, phenolic moieties are mostly linked through C-C and C-O bonds, whereas aromatic amines form C-N and N-N linkages.

Oxidative coupling is mediated by a number of biological and abiotic catalysts, including microbial or plant enzymes, inorganic chemicals (e.g. ferric chloride, cupric hydroxide) and clay minerals. Coupling reactions can also occur spontaneously in the presence of oxygen at neutral and alkaline pH values. Spontaneous reactions frequently lead to the incorporation of non-phenolic compounds into humic polymers.

ENZYMES AND THEIR ORIGIN

Many soil micro-organisms produce extracellular oxidoreductases capable of catalysing the coupling of aromatic compounds. These enzymes are classified as either peroxidases or polyphenol oxidases.

Peroxidases

All peroxidases contain an iron porphyrin ring and require the presence of peroxides (e.g. hydrogen peroxide) for activity. In particular horseradish peroxidase (HRP), which catalyses the polymerisation of a wide range of phenolic and aniline compounds, was tested for the detoxification of industrial waste-water.

Polyphenol Oxidases

The polyphenol oxidases are divided into two groups: laccases and tyrosinases, which require bimolecular oxygen, but no coenzyme, for activity. However, the enzymes differ in the mechanism by which they oxidise phenols. Laccases oxidise phenolic compounds to form their corresponding anionic free radicals, whereas tyrosinases form *o*-diphenols and subsequently release oxidised *o*-quinones. In an alkaline environment, the quinone products slowly polymerise through auto-oxidative processes. The laccases may prove to be the most useful of the phenoloxidases because, like the peroxidases, they produce highly reactive radicals, but unlike the latter, they do not require the presence of hydrogen peroxide.

Function of Enzymes in Binding Reactions between Pesticides and Humic Material

The main role of enzymes or minerals in oxidative coupling is to mediate the oxidation of the substrates to free radicals. Once the free radicals are generated, coupling is completed without further involvement of the catalyst. In modelling studies we investigated the catalytic effects of enzymes on pesticides or their phenolic or anionic intermediates by determining their binding to humic material, and whenever possible, we identified the resulting oxidative coupling products.

On the basis of early observations, xenobiotic anilines and phenols were assumed to form covalent linkages with soil organic matter. It was well understood that the validity of these assumptions could be verified only through direct inspection of the intact complexes. However, the intricate and heterogeneous structure of humic substances made it difficult to achieve direct insight. To overcome this problem, complex soil systems were replaced by simple models in which the xenobiotic chemicals were allowed to interact with the monomeric constituents of humic acid in the presence of enzymes. Using model substrates, the resulting products were relatively easy to isolate from the reaction mixture and could be analysed for their exact molecular configuration.

In a later study, Simmons observed only partial oxidation of 4-chloroaniline in the presence of various catalysts. The resulting free radicals first bound to each other to form a dimer that subsequently was condensed with a resonance-stabilised guaiacol anion. The aniline molecules that did not undergo oxidation were subject to Michael addition to quinone oligomers resulting from the coupling of the guaiacol free radicals. In the study of Tatsumi, free radical formation was limited exclusively to ferulic acid, and all aniline molecules were incorporated into the resulting dimers through a non-radical condensation.

In contrast to anilines, xenobiotic phenols first had to be enzymatically oxidised to aryloxy-free radicals or quinones to become bound to humic substances. For example, when Sarkar incubated 2,4-dichlorophenol with fulvic acid, no binding occurred in the absence of catalysts; however, considerable binding was observed upon the addition of oxidoreductases such as mushroom tyrosinase, horseradish peroxidase, or the laccases from *Trametes versicolor* or *Rhizoctonia praticola*.

NMR SPECTROSCOPY TO DETERMINE THE TYPE OF BINDING OF PESTICIDES IN THE SOIL

Historically, research on pesticide immobilisation was carried out using ^{14}C-labelled chemicals combined with radiation counting. Recently, labelling of pollutants with stable isotopes (^{13}C or ^{15}N) combined with nuclear magnetic resonance (NMR) spectroscopy emerged as a non-destructive technique with great identification potential. The major advantage of this approach lies in the fact that pollutant molecules enriched with the ^{13}C or ^{15}N isotope generate more intensive NMR signals than those resulting from the natural abundance of ^{13}C or ^{15}N in the studied compound and soil. The basis of the NMR approach is that any binding-related modification in the original arrangement of the labelled atoms automatically induces changes in the position of the corresponding signals in the NMR spectra. The delocalisation of the signals exhibits a high degree of specificity, indicating whether or not binding has occurred and, if so, the type of bond formed.

NMR was used successfully to determine covalent binding of pesticides and other xenobiotics. In the study of Haider, for instance, the fungicide anilazine [4,6-dichloro-N-(2-chlorophenyl)-2,3,5-triazine-2-amime] labelled with ^{14}C and ^{13}C in the triazine ring was found to be immobilised in soil through ligand exchange. The NMR spectra of humic acid extracted from soil together with the bound fungicide revealed that the chlorine substituents located at the C-4 and C-6 positions were removed from the triazine ring and replaced by the oxygen-containing functional groups of soil organic matter. This exchange resulted in the formation of strong ether and ester linkages between the dehalogenated anilazine molecule and the humic matrix.

Thorn used ^{15}N-NMR spectroscopy to demonstrate covalent binding of ^{15}N-labelled aniline to humic acid when the two components were dissolved in water and stirred for 5 days at pH 6. The changes in the chemical shifts of the ^{15}N atom indicated that binding was due to nucleophilic addition reactions of aniline with the quinone or carbonyl groups typical for humic substances. The labelled chemical was incorporated in the form of anilinohyaroquinone, anilinoquinone, anilide, imine, and heterocyclic nitrogen. The latter comprised more than 50 per cent of the bound amines.

The ^{13}C-NMR studies were carried out using two ^{13}C-labelled pollutants: 2,4-dichlorophenol, a degradation product of the herbicide 2,4-D, and cyprodinil, a new phenyl-pyrimidine amine fungicide manufactured by Ciba-Geigy. 2,4-Dichlorophenol, labelled either in the C-1 or in the C-2 and C-6 position, was incubated for 2 hours with dissolved humic acid in the presence of a peroxidase. The NMR signals generated by the ^{13}C label demonstrated bonding between the two components through carbon-carbon, ester and phenolic ether linkages.

To investigate the formation of covalent bonds under more natural conditions, cyprodinil, which was labelled either in the phenyl or pyrimidyl ring, was incubated with fresh soil for several months. After exhaustive washing with methanol, humic acid was isolated by extraction with 0.5 M NaOH. Humic acid was then purified by dialysis and/or silylated by treatment with trimethylchlorosilane to facilitate the ^{13}C-NMR analysis. The NMR signals generated by both the dialysed and silylated samples indicated cleavage of the cyprodinil molecule between the aromatic rings and covalent binding of the phenyl and pyrimidyl moieties to humic acid.

Nanny demonstrated the use of ^{13}C-NMR spectroscopy for the assessment of non-covalent complexes of xenobiotics with humic materials. The compound under investigation (^{13}C-labelled acenaphthenone) and humic material (fulvic acid) were allowed to interact directly in the NMR tube in a methanol/D_2O solution. Based on the measurements of the decreasing spin-lattice relaxation time (T_1) of the labelled atom, smith determined that the sorption of acenaphthenone to fulvic acid involved weak hydrophobic or hydrogen bonding.

The results, especially those related to binding in the soil, confirm the great potential of using ^{13}C-labelled chemicals with ^{13}C-NMR spectrometry as an analytical technique for evaluating interactions between pollutants and soil components, particularly humic substances. Establishing the physical or chemical associations between pollutants and humic substances will provide essential data for understanding principles of bioavailability.

STABILITY AND RELEASE OF BOUND PESTICIDES

Before the binding of xenobiotics to humus can be applied as a decontamination procedure, the stability of the bound complexes must be investigated. If large quantities of a bound pollutant were released at a future time, the accumulation of these complexes would pose a delayed environmental hazard. The stability of humus-bound xenobiotics has been demonstrated by several investigators. In one study, when 3,4-dichloroaniline was applied to a German soil, 46 per cent of the compound remained bound to the soil two years after treatment. In a separate study, 83 per cent of ^{14}C-labelled-atrazine remained associated with the soil after 9 years; 50 per cent of this residue presented bound material.

The activity of micro-organisms is believed to be the primary factor responsible for the release of bound residues. To study the release of bound pesticides, ^{14}C-labelled-catechol and mono-, di-, tri, and pentachlorophenols, bound to humic acid polymers, were incubated with microbial soil populations, and the release of radioactive compounds into the medium was monitored for 13 weeks. This study demonstrated that ^{14}C-labelled compounds were released in small quantities and the release was accompanied by a simultaneous mineralisation of the bound material to $^{14}CO_2$. As might be expected, the release of bound xenobiotics differs with the type of binding. A 'surface' fraction of bound residue appears to be releasable, whereas the remainder is covalently bound to a 'core' portion that is less accessible to microbial degradation.

Overall, the available data indicate that the microbial release of bound xenobiotics occurs at an extremely slow rate. Once released, the xenobiotics can be mineralised or reincorporated into humus. Consequently, released residues are not expected to accumulate and should not pose a delayed health hazard.

There is little doubt that binding interactions reduce bioavailability and considerably contribute to the recalcitrance of xenobiotics in soil. However, taking into account that a given chemical may undergo binding by several mechanisms simultaneously and that xenobiotic molecules frequently compete for binding sites with other chemicals present in soil environments, it will never be easy to determine the exact effect of bioavailability on xenobiotic recalcitrance in *in vivo* situations.

ENZYMES AS DECONTAMINATING AGENTS

The use of microbial extracellular enzymes as decontaminating agents is hindered by the fact that free enzymes are rapidly inactivated under the harsh conditions of soil. This problem may be overcome by immobilising the free enzymes on solid supports. Immobilisation has been shown to enhance the thermostability of the enzymes, to prevent their degradation by proteases, and to increase their half-life. However, the enzymatic activity retained after immobilisation depends on the method of immobilisation and the nature of the solid support.

The activity of laccase immobilised on soil supports, was investigated using radio labelled 2,4-DCP. The efficiency of laccase-kaolinite and laccase-soil complexes in removing 2,4-DCP was equivalent to that of the tree enzyme (~95 per cent). Laccases bound to montmorillonites 1 and 2 were less efficient, with removal activities of 69 per cent and 42 per cent, respectively. However, after 6 hours of incubation, the laccases, immobilised on soil particles, retained 86 to 100 per cent of their activity, whereas the tree enzyme retained only 62 per cent of its activity. Furthermore, the immobilised enzyme could be recovered from the reaction mixture and used repeatedly to transform the substrate, with minimum loss of activity.

Overall, because of their increased biochemical stability and reusability, immobilised enzymes are more cost effective than are free enzymes.

To sum up the incorporation of pesticides and their derivatives into soil organic matter occurs readily in nature. This process can be used to immobilise and detoxify hazardous compounds. The immobilisation phenomena have several important consequences: (i) the amount of compound available to interact with the biota is reduced, (ii) the complexed products are less toxic than their parent compounds, and (iii) binding restricts leaching of chemicals across the soil profile, thus preventing groundwater contamination.

The use of enzymatic coupling for detoxification raised some concerns about the ultimate fate of bound pesticides. However, all available data indicate that, once xenobiotics are incorporated into soil, they are released at a very slow rate and to a minimal extent. The gradual release should not pose a delayed health hazard because the released compounds can be mineralised to CO_2 or reimmobilised in the soil matrix. Prior to the practical application of enzymatic treatment, extensive research is required to further analyse the accumulation, bioavailability, and toxicity of bound pesticide residues under field conditions. Research should continue to focus on the development of new methods for maximising the binding process, e.g. through the use of immobilised enzymes, abiotic catalysts, or co-polymerising agents. All current evidence indicates that the enzymatic or abiotic incorporation of xenobiotics into humus provides an efficient method for detoxifying hazardous pollutants.

SECTION IV

Applications of Environmental Biotechnology

SECTION IV

Applications of Environmental Biotechnology

14. Chemical Industries

Chapter 14

Chemical Industries

INTRODUCTION

In any country, economic development and environment protection should go hand in hand. There cannot be economic development (i.e. the improvement of the standard of living of the common man) without increasing the production of goods and services. Every such activity of production has its own associated problem in the balance of ecology and environment in general. Chemical industries, in particular, are being looked at with awe and suspicion in this respect. It should be the responsibility of the chemical manufacturers to use only such technologies which contribute the least to the upsetting or downgradation of the ecology and environment. Efforts are to be made in improving the technologies to better the performance.

Technology is defined as the art of science, i.e. the mode by which irrefutable scientific data (physical, chemical or derived biological or other scientific data) are used to achieve the desired objective. Environmental friendly technologies include technologies, goods and services whose development is triggered by environmental improvement objectives. The modes initiate with research on process chemistry or changes that reduce the production and use of hazardous chemicals, research on alternative synthetic pathways to reduce or eliminate the use or generation of hazardous substances in the manufacturing process, the development of real time process sensors and controls to prevent or minimise waste generation, etc.

The environmental impact of an existing process can be reduced by using clean technologies, which will, in turn, mean higher costs. Manufacturers wanting to determine the environmental implication of their activities need to look beyond the factory fences and consider the impact of obtaining the raw materials and subsequent use of their products. This is due to the awareness created in the minds of people after major disasters like dioxin release in Italy, the isocyanate tragedy of Bhopal, etc. and the legal and third party liability suits against the manufacturers. The strategies in developing clean technologies (different than the clean-up technologies stated above) should take into account the life cycle of materials, likely changes envisaged in customer practices, environmental regulation/legislation, etc. The environmental friendly technologies or clean technologies should aim at satisfying the following basic scientific findings:

1. Handle substances (chemicals as raw material, intermediate or finished products) which are least harmful to living organisms (human, animal or plant life), i.e. which are not toxic, corrosive or flammable/explosive.

2. Reactions/processes which do not involve much of transfer of energy (neither too exothermic nor endothermic) with the transfer level of energy being not far away from environmental status, i.e. not at a very high temperature or high pressure process.

3. Suitable moderating/control mechanism at two levels, with back up system to bring the situation back to normal in the least time interval.

To further complicate the pollution control aspects of the chemical industry, the industry is constantly changing, using different raw materials and new processes, and producing new products.

In many cases, the process and its wastes are unique and pollution abatement systems must be individually engineered. However, many processes are free of wastes and many plants report no waterborne wastes. Chemical process industries over the years have developed several methodologies aimed at early detection of hazards and assessment of consequences of an untoward accidental release of hazardous materials in order to effectively attenuate residual risks. The comprehensive criteria developed for the acceptability of risks provides a satisfactory means of evaluating the technology at various stages of inplementation. Some of the polluting chemical industries are discussed in this chapter.

TREATMENT OF WASTE FROM ORGANIC CHEMICAL INDUSTRIES

The organic chemical industry, which manufactures carbon-containing chemicals, produces an enormous number of materials that are essential to the economy and to modern life. This industry obtains raw materials from the petroleum industry and converts them to intermediate materials or basic finished chemicals. Based on the type and source of chemicals, this industry is classified into three categories.

1. Gum and wood chemicals (tall oil, rosin, turpentine, pine tar, acetic acid, and methanol).
2. Cyclic organic crudes and intermediates (benzene, toluene, xylene, naphthalene, dyes, and pigments).
3. Organic chemicals not elsewhere classified (ethyl alcohol, propylene, ethylene, and butylene).

This industry is also categorised into:

1. Bulk or commodity chemicals.
2. Fine or speciality chemicals.

A wide range of chemicals are produced from common feedstock such as petrochemicals, coal, natural gas, and wood. Fossil fuels provide small (molecular size) chemicals such as benzene, ethylene, propylene, xylene, toluene, butadiene, methane, and butylene, which find end use in a large variety of industries ranging from agricultural chemicals to cosmetics (Table 14.1). Thus the organic chemicals industry forms the fulcrum for the needs of modern life.

Table 14.1. Major organic chemical products.

Category	Example chemicals	Example end uses
Aliphatic and other acyclic organic chemicals	Ethylene, butylenes and formaldehyde	Polyethylene plastic, plywood
Solvents	Butyl alcohol, ethyl acetate, ethylene glycol ether, perchloroethylene	Degreasers, dry cleaning fluids
Polyhydric alcohols	Ethylene glycol, sorbitol, synthetic glycerine	Antifreeze, soaps
Synthetic perfume and flavouring materials	Saccharin, citronellol, synthetic vanillin	Food flavouring, cleaning, product scents

(Contd ...)

Category	Example chemicals	Example end uses
Rubber processing chemicals	Thiuram, hexamethylene tetramine	Tyres, adhesives
Plasticisers	Phosphoric acid, phthalic anhydride, stearic acid	Raincoats, inflatable toys
Synthetic tanning agents	Naphthalene sulphonic acid condensates	Leather coats and shoes
Chemical warfare gases	Tear gas, phosgene	Military and law enforcement
Cyclic crudes and intermediates	Benzene, toluene, mixed xylenes, naphthalene	Eyeglasses, foams
Cyclic dyes and organic pigments	Nitrodyes, organic paint pigments	Fabric and plastic colouring
Natural gas and wood chemicals	Methanol, acetic acid, rosin	Latex, adhesives

All the same, some unavoidable problems to our environment accompany this industry — toxic wastes. Organic chemical industries are among the largest producers of toxic wastes:

1. Methanol.
2. Ammonia.
3. Nitric acid.
4. Nitrate compounds.
5. Acetonitrile.
6. Propargyl alcohol.
7. Chlorinated solvents.

Some of the chemicals released into the environment in the United States and developing countries are given in Table 14.2.

Table 14.2. Toxic releases from organic chemicals industries in the US and developing countries.

Chemical name
Ethylene
1,2-Dichloro-1,1,2-trifluoroethane
2,4-Dimethyl phenol
Acetamide
Acetonitrile
Acetophenone
Acrylamide
Acrylic acid
Acrylonitrile
Ammonia
Biphenyl
Bromine
Bromomethane
Carbonyl sulphide

(Contd ...)

Chemical name
Chlorobenzene
Chlorodifluoromethane
Cyanide compounds
Cyclohexanol
Dichlorofluoromethane
Diethyl sulphate
Ethylene glycol
Formaldehyde
Formic acid
Hydrogen cyanide
Malanonitrile
Manganese
m-Cresol
Methanol
Naphthalene
Nitrate compounds
Nitric acid
Nitrobenzene
N-Methyl-2-pyrrolidine
o-Cresol
Propargyl alcohol
Propylene
Phthalic anhydride
Pyridine
Sodium nitrite
t-Butyl alcohol
Toluene
Vinyl acetate

Oil spills are one of the major problems of present society. Humans have long exploited the volume dilution power of the sea to dispose of unwanted wastes. Although concern about waste accumulation in marine environments is increasing, especially for coastal waters, marine remediation efforts are nearly nonexistent. The notable exception to this rule is crude oil and refined petroleum product spills.

The tanker spills have remained the focus of research efforts related to remediation of marine oil contamination.

The potential for truly massive spills from modern supertankers and the readily visible direct impact on affected areas have captured the public's attention and sensitised regulatory and industry groups to the local destructive potential of such accidents. Petroleum is a complex mixture of thousands of individual compounds, and the degradation pathways of spilled oil are numerous and complex. Biodegradation, especially by microbes, is believed to be one of the primary mechanisms of ultimate removal of petroleum hydrocarbons from marine and shore environments. Acceleration of this natural process is the objective of bioremediation efforts. Bioremediation has yet to become an established spill-response technology, but some attempts to implement it have been encouraging. The inability of established nonbiological techniques to cope with recent large spills has led to increased interest in bioremediation. Special problems associated with marine oil spills include the uncontained nature of the waste, the potential size of the contaminated area, and difficulty of access for remediative and monitoring activities. As with other forms of *in situ* bioremediation, natural biodegradation of marine oil spills may be enhanced by inducing changes in either the microbial population or the availability of microbial nutrients.

Most researchers have concluded that nutrient availability is the chief limitation of natural biodegradation, and most research has been directed toward enhancing nutrient availability. Marine oil spill clean-ups represent some of the largest *in situ* remediation projects ever attempted.

Biotreatment

By and large, biodegradation is the most suitable and economic way of mineralising organic pollutants. In the case of ammonia, nitrate compounds, and cyanide compounds, biodegradation is the ideal choice because any of the chemical methods would produce a large volume of salts (sludge).

The industrial effluents in which these organic chemicals occur are frequently acidic and have elevated salinity. Activated sludge systems are usually protected from high salinity and pH by pretreatment of the waste-water entering the aeration tank; hence, these are most suited for treatment of organic wastes. However, pretreatment incurs cost; therefore, alternative methods employing organisms able to function under low pH and high salinity have to be adopted. A number of such reports have appeared in literature in recent times. Apart from the well known microbial degradations of aromatic, aliphatic, halogenated organics, PAHs, and dioxins, micro-organisms are known to degrade even hetero aromatic and hetero aliphatic compounds.

Aniline and related hetero aromatic compounds have been found to degrade under aerobic fermentative, nitrate-reducing, and sulphate-reducing conditions at a variety of salt concentrations and pH values. Sulphur heterocycles, such as the benzothiozoles and their derivatives, are degraded both by anaerobic and aerobic means (Fig. 14.1). Thermophillic aerobic processes have also been reported to clean up effluents of organic industries.

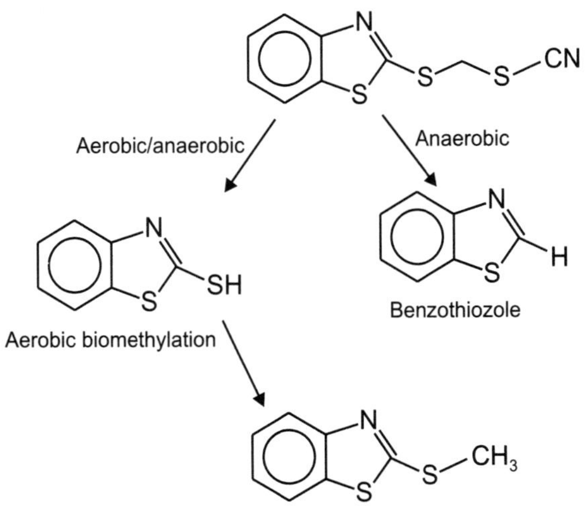

Fig. 14.1. Biodegradation of benzothiazoles.

Depending on the type of organic or inorganic pollutant, appropriate biodegradation methods (aerobic/anaerobic) can be adopted. Suitable degradation strategies for toxic releases from the organic chemicals industry are given in Table 14.3. Complete mineralisation of the pollutant is invariably brought about by a judicious combination of both processes. Anaerobic degradation usually provides intermediates that can be mineralised by subsequent aerobic processes. Excess salts and solid matter are ideally removed by pretreatment plants designed for the purpose. The effluent from the pretreatment is suitable for the biotreatment.

Table 14.3. Suitable degradation strategies for organic pollutants.

Chemical name	Aerobic degradation	Anaerobic degradation	Chemical/physical methods
Ethylene	√	√	–
1,2-Dichloro-1, 1,2-trifluoroethane	–	√	–
2,4-Dimethyl phenol	√	√	–
Acetamide	√	–	√
Acetonitrile	–	√	–
Acetophenone	√	√	–
Acrylamide	√	–	√
Acrylic acid	√	–	√
Acrylonitrile	√	√	–
Ammonia	√	–	√
Biphenyl	√	–	–
Bromine	–	–	√
Bromomethane	√	–	√
Carbon disulphide	√	–	√
Chlorobenzene	√	–	–
Chlorodifluoromethane	–	√	–
Cyanide compounds	–	√	√
Cyclohexanol	√	–	√
Dichlorofluoromethane	–	√	–
Diethyl sulphate	–	√	√
Ethylene glycol	–	–	√
Formaldehyde	–	–	√
Formic acid	–	–	√
Hydrogen cyanide	–	√	√
Malanonitrile	–	√	√
Manganese	√	–	√
m-Cresol	√	√	√
Methanol	–	√	√
Naphthalene	√	√	–
Nitrate compounds	–	√	√

(Contd ...)

Chemical name	Aerobic degradation	Anaerobic degradation	Chemical/physical methods
Nitric acid	–	√	√
Nitrobenzene	√	√	–
N-Methyl-2-pyrrolidine	√	√	–
o-Cresol	√	√	–
Propargyl alcohol	√	–	–
Propylene	√	–	√
Phthalic anhydride	√	–	√
Pyridine	√	–	√
Sodium nitrite	√	√	√
t-Butyl alcohol	√	–	√
Toluene	√	√	–
Vinyl acetate	√	√	√

Another emerging application of bioremediation, the potential of which is yet to be fully realised, is biodegradation and/or removal of environmentally undesirable compounds through biofilter technology. Naturally occurring micro-organisms are usually present in quantities adequate to handle easily biodegradable compounds like alcohols, ethers, and simple aromatics. More degradation-resistant chemicals, such as nitrogen and sulphur containing organics and especially chlorinated organics and aliphatics, may require inoculation with selected strains of microbes to achieve desired degradation efficiencies. Although every application must be evaluated individually, biofilter technology represents a volatile organic compound abatement option that is competitive in many cases on both efficiency and cost bases.

For purposes of bioremediation, aerobic microbial metabolism has traditionally been the focus of attention. Aerobic degradative pathways in microbes and in animals break down organic molecules oxidatively by using divalent oxygen or other active oxygen species, such as hydrogen peroxide, as electron acceptors. Aerobic catabolism of organics ultimately results in familiar mineral products — carbon dioxide and water. Aerobes are capable of degrading most organic wastes, provided enough oxygen is available. Some compounds, notably the organohalogens, are highly resistant to aerobic biodegradation (termed recalcitrant or persistent wastes). Resistance of most aromatic and aliphatic compounds to degradation is dramatically increased by halogenation (most commonly chlorination); further halogenation results in increased resistance.

Anaerobic microbes degrade organics reductively, eventually resulting in the mineral end product methane. In the case of carbohydrate compounds, carbon dioxide and free hydrogen also are produced. Although they are not usually utilised for routine waste degradation, some anaerobes are very adept at dechlorination of common recalcitrant organochlorine compounds, notably PCBs; organochlorine pesticides, such as DDT; and chlorinated aliphatics, such as the industrial solvent trichloroethylene (TCE). Thus anaerobic microbial catabolism (sometimes called fermentation) offers a bioremediation option to deal with persistent wastes. Complete anaerobic degradation of wastes, however, may be slow. The major problem with anaerobic digestion of organochlorine wastes is that biodegradation is often incomplete (at least on a practical time scale) and may result in toxic metabolites. The use of mixed cultures containing both aerobes and anaerobes facilitates mineralisation of many organochlorines.

In practice, a sequential bioreactor system utilising both anaerobic and aerobic reactors could be employed. For example, PCBs or chlorinated aromatics could be dechlorinated anaerobically, then fed into an aerobic bioreactor to be fully mineralised to carbon dioxide and water. Similarly, TCE and perchloro-ethylene may be reductively metabolised to vinyl chloride (a toxic chemical), which can then be subjected to aerobic biodegradation. Commercial versions of such two-stage hybrid bioreactor systems are currently under development. Isolation and characterisation of dehalogenases (dehalogenating bacterial enzymes) for possible development of immobilised enzyme reactors and biofilters are also being conducted.

Appreciation of the potential of natural systems to regulate levels of aquatic toxicants has led to the development of constructed wetlands for bioremediation of complex wastes. It has been observed that wetlands have a buffering ability on surface waters with respect to circulating nutrient and pollutant levels. Wetlands have the capacity to store excess nutrients or wastes and to release stored excesses under the right environmental conditions. A constructed wetland is an artificial habitat, most visibly made up of vascular plants and algal colonies, which also provide a structural and nutritional support for an associated, highly heterogeneous microbial community. One of the most promising applications of constructed wetlands is for *in situ* bioremediation of metal contamination. It is not always known to what extent the observed metal removal in natural wetlands is due to bacterial action and what is due to higher plant or algal activity. In any case, many of these organisms exist in a symbiotic arrangement, and multi trophic cultured systems are increasingly being viewed as an alternative to monocultures or even heterogeneous bacterial cultures. Field tests on acid mine drainage effluent have indicated that such systems are capable of removing metals via multiple pathway biological action. The use of both natural and constructed wetlands for heavy metal abatement is of great potential value, but questions remain about the eventual fates of the metals. Some means of extraction, such as removal of plant or sediment material, is necessary to prevent remobilisation of metals from dead organic material or trophic transfer to grazing animals.

Phytoremediation

Plants can adapt to a wide range of environmental conditions and are capable of modifying conditions of the environment to some extent. The unique enzyme and protein systems of some plant species appear to be beneficial for phytoremediation. Additionally, since plants lack the ability to move, many plants have developed unique biochemical systems for nutrient acquisition, detoxification, and controlling local geochemical conditions. McFarlane observed that the uptake and translocation of phenol, nitrobenzene and bromocil were directly related to transpiration rate in mature soyabean plants. Recently, the use of minced horseradish roots has been proposed for the decontamination of surface waters polluted with chlorinated phenols. Bruken and Schnoor used poplar trees for the uptake and metabolism of the pesticide atrazine. Results indicated that poplar trees can take-up, hydrolyse, and dealkylate atrazine to less toxic metabolites. Thus, plants can contribute in many ways for environmental restoration of contaminated sites.

Bioremediation is an emerging field, the full potential of which is as yet unknown, especially in the clean-up of organic contaminants. There is a tremendous need for further basic research and development, especially in the areas of environmental site and waste diagnostics, waste-technology matching, and integration of multiple remediation techniques.

There is a clear need for improved methods of environmental surveillance for the prevention of adverse environmental conditions. Continued development of new methods, including lab-bench assays and gene-probe technologies and their utilisation, may provide some of the desired information and early warning for environmental hazards. When required, bioremediative approaches need to be applied with the understanding that each local environment requires individual attention and detailed site evaluation. In bioremediation of a contaminated area, performance feedback to researchers with regard to the transport, fate, and possible toxicity of the metabolites produced is of tremendous value for method refinement. Moreover, the site evaluation processes must incorporate expertise from those knowledgeable in other remediation technologies as well as bioremediation experts. Coupled and integrated methods of containment, destruction, and biodegradation of pollutants are certain to yield more cost-effective clean-up solutions than procedures that focus on a single remediation technology. The primary limitation to the widespread use of many bioremediation approaches is often the extent to which the pollutant is available to the microbial population. The bioavailability of many chemicals diminishes with time as a result of weathering and ageing phenomena, and the time window in which appropriate bioremediation technologies can be employed requires further definition. Many organic pollutants do not readily enter the bioactive, aqueous phase of soil and sediment environments. Their bioavailability to the microbial population might be appreciably increased by the use of appropriate surfactants, dispersants, chelators, or emulsifiers. The physical matrix in which pollutants are found largely determines the rate at which the pollutants become bioavailable. Improved bioremediation of complex mixtures might take advantage of the fact that microbes can be selected to mobilise, immobilise, or fix compounds or ions in such a way that they are rendered susceptible to further treatment. The first stage of the process may require the action of a biodegrading, surfactant-producing, or bioaccumulating organism.

GASEOUS POLLUTANTS AND VOLATILE ORGANICS

Sulphur dioxide, nitrogen oxides, volatile organic compounds (VOCs), and particulates are the four major components of air pollution and are the main causes of environmental damage and many diseases, including cancer. The sulphur and nitrogen oxides and particulates are the result of burning petroleum fuels; coal, wood, etc. Printing and coating facilities and foundries, as well as the electronics, petrochemical, metal finishing, and paint industries, produce VOCs, which include solvent thinners, degreasers, cleaners, lubricants, and liquid fuels. They originate from breathing and loading losses from storage tanks, venting of process vessels, and leaks from piping and equipment, waste-water streams, and heat exchange systems.

A few common VOCs are methane, ethane, tetrachloroethane, methyl chloride, and various chlorohydrocarbons, perfluorocarbons, styrene, and naphthalenes. The European Community emissions limit is 35 grams total organic compounds (TOCs) per cubic metre of gasoline loaded (35 grams TOC/m^3); the US Environmental Protection Agency emission limit is 10 grams TOC/m^3. Particulates from air can be removed using several well established physical methods that use a gravity settler, centrifugal collector, wet spray venturi collector, electrostatic precipitator, and fabric filter.

Physical Methods

Two general methods for abatement include recovery and destruction (Fig. 14.2). The former method leads to reuse of the chemical and hence has a cost benefit. The latter method includes converting the chemical to a harmless product or into a liquid or solid pollutant that can be treated with another well established technology. Chemical, thermal, and biochemical approaches could be followed for destroying VOCs and pollutants from air, while absorption, adsorption, and cryogenic methods could be adopted for recovery and reuse of the VOCs. Chemical, catalytic, and thermal methods are very effective and well established but have several disadvantages such as high cost, conversion of one type of pollutant to another, and the possible generation of more toxic chemicals as the product. The physical methods are simple but need additional hardware for the regeneration of the absorbent or the adsorbent, and the recovery costs are high. Recovery and reuse as solvent rather than burning as fuel is more economical in all cases. Biofiltration is the cheapest and safest method, but can be slow and incomplete, and a colony of micro-organisms is needed to treat a host of VOCs. All these technologies are assumed to achieve a destruction and recovery efficiency of 90 per cent. The absorption, adsorption, and biofiltration methods are operated at ambient conditions, but the first two methods need a high temperature operation to recover the adsorbent so it can be reused. The presence of moisture leads to a decrease in the efficiency of chemical methods.

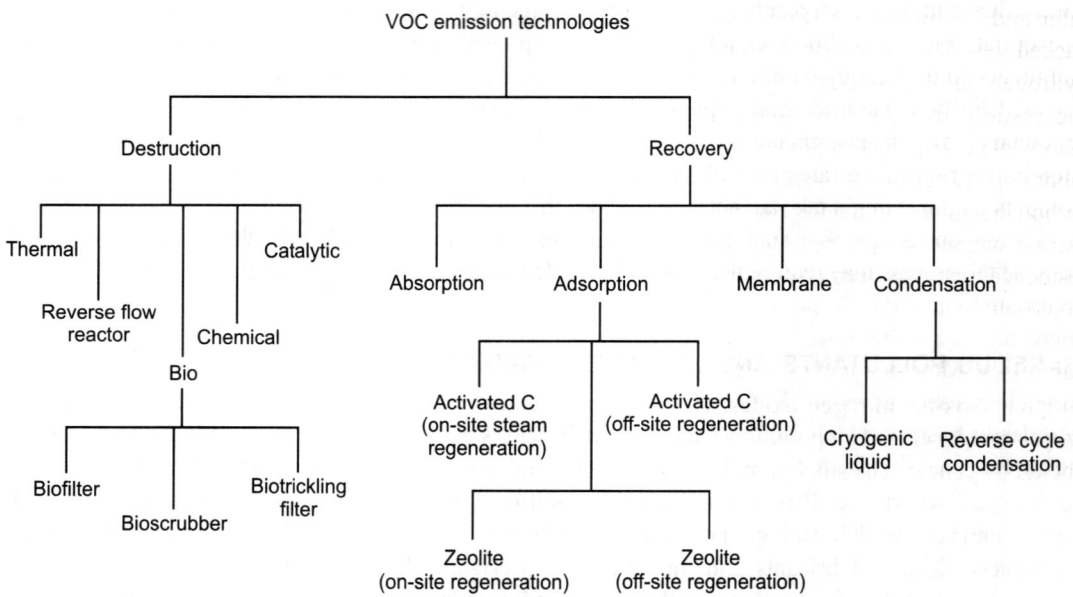

Fig. 14.2. Various recovery and treatment procedures for VOCs.

Biotreatment Processes

Three basic aerobic methods are biofilter, biotrickling filter, and bioscrubber. The type of micro-organism depends on the VOC that is being destroyed. All need 100 per cent relative humidity, long contact times, and a community of micro-organisms. The products of the process are CO_2, salts, water, and biomass. Moisture content, temperature, pH, nutrient amount, type of contaminants, presence of fine particles, and oxygen mass transfer rates play an important role in the biodegradation process. A warmer reactor can oxidise the contaminants faster, thereby increasing the destruction and the removal efficiency, but can also deactivate the sensitive micro-organisms. The reactors can work over a wide range of pH conditions (from 2 to 9). Careful thought must be given if the contaminants are sulphur or chlorine containing compounds since acid is produced on destruction of such compounds, making the biomass highly acidic. If the biomass is too dry, growth of the micro-organism stops and if too much water is present, washout of the biomass can occur. Also, shearing of the biofilm that has grown for a considerable amount of time is an issue.

Biofilter

A biofilter is a tube that is packed with material containing the micro-organism, nutrients for its growth, and support material to hold the growing colony (Fig. 14.3). A nonbioactive humidification system maintains the moisture level. The support material prevents clogging of the reactor and also keeps the pressure drop low. A pre-particulate removal system is located before the biofilter. The conditioned gas stream is introduced from the bottom or a filter bed consisting of soil, peat, compost material, ceramic, calcium alginate, activated carbon, bark chips, wood chips, yard waste, or plastic. During the process, the contaminant may be adsorbed directly on the biofilm or dissolved in the aqueous film. Biofilters can also serve as odour preventers and can be installed at the exhaust side of waste treatment plants, sewer vents, etc. Compared to the thermal oxidation process, which produces NO_x and acid rain, biofilters are safer and cheaper to run. Bed drying, short circuiting, collapse of the packing, and blocking of the packed vessel are some issues that need to be addressed. Many VOCs, including ethanol, aldehydes, hydrogen sulphide, styrene, hydrocarbon solvents, and methyl methacrylate (MMA), have been successfully treated with biofilters, achieving 85 to 95 per cent removal efficiencies. Efficiencies greater than 99.9 per cent were achieved when the H_2S inlet concentrations were in the range 5 to 2650 ppm. In laboratory experiments, removal of ethanol vapours was achieved using compost, granular activated carbon inoculated with different amounts of active biomass, and a mixture of compost and diatomaceous earth. Complete removal of H_2S from a stream containing 40 ppm in less than 30 seconds (empty bed residence time) has been reported in a biofilter packed to a height of 4 ft with synthetic inorganic media (hydrophilic mineral core) coated with hydrophobic material at 20 seconds residence time. Some of the micro-organisms that have been found to sucessfully degrade VOCs and pollutants in air are listed in Table 14.4. Most of the micro-organisms found in the biofilters were bacteria that were predominantly coryneforms and endospore formers, and occasionally pseudomonads. Yeast and fungi are less abundant. In order to achieve a high degradation efficiency, an adaptation time for the microflora is necessary; during this time the organic loading is gradually increased.

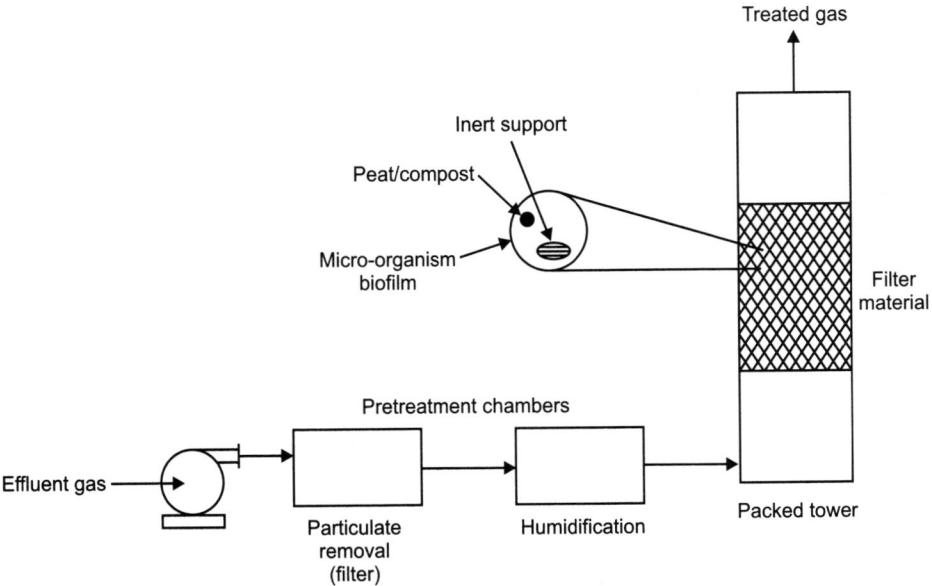

Fig. 14.3. A typical biofilter.

Table 14.3. Micro-organisms that can degrade pollutants and VOCs in air.

Organism	VOC/gas component
Pseudomonas AM1	Methanol, formaldehyde
Pseudomonas aminovorans	Dimethyl amines
Pseudomonas putida, Trichosporon cutaneum	Phenol
Pseudomonas sp.	Benzene
Pseudomonas putida	Toluene
Sphingobacterium	–
Turicella oritidis	–
Bacteria + yeast	Xylene
Exophiala yeanselmei	Styrene
Rhodococcus sp.	Methyl ethyl ketone
Thiobacillus sp.	H_2S, methyl mercaptan, CS_2
Thiobacillus thioparus	–
Pseudomonas putida	NH_3, H_2S
Arthrobacter oxydans	–
Nocardia sp.	Aniline
Hypomicrabium sp.	Dimethyl sulphide
Pseudomonas fluorescence	p-Cresol
Pseudomonas sp.	m-Cresol
Chromobacterium violaceum	Indole
Bacteria	Methyl tert butyl ether

Exhaust air from paint booths is typically of high volume and contains low concentrations of VOCs. The energy costs for biofilters to carry out destruction of such pollutants are typically one-fourth to one-tenth the energy costs of thermal oxidation technologies, and the capital costs are about two-thirds to three-fourths that of competing technologies. Chlorinated solvents may produce acid, which would affect the growth of the micro-organism. Nevertheless, biofilters are being used to treat such gases at VOC loadings of 500 to 1500 ppm, achieving more than 85 per cent reduction.

A mixture of benzene, toluene, ethyl benzene, and xylenes (BTEX) in air was effectively degraded in a biofilter packed with a mixture of compost (a mixture of yard waste and sewage sludge) and activated carbon. The micro-organisms preferentially utilised benzene, followed by toluene, ethylbenzene, and finally o-xylene. Removal efficiencies of greater than 90 per cent were achieved for inlet concentrations of 200 ppm of each of the BTEX compounds and a gas loading rate of 17.6 m³/m²·hr. The activated carbon helped in reducing the pressure drop in the bed and also acted as a buffer during shock pollutant loads. Because of the high adsorption capacity of activated carbon, the organic pollutants and oxygen got concentrated there, which in turn increased the growth of micro-organisms in the vicinity.

Biotrickling filter

A biotrickling filter also has packing material on which the micro-organisms grow, but the water is made to trickle down the packing (about 1 to 20 m³/m² day), while the gas is fed from the bottom (Fig. 14.4). The water is collected at the bottom and recycled back to the top of the column. Because of the flowing water, contaminants can be dissolved in it. The water phase is mobile here, whereas it is immobilised in the biofilter. The surface area for mass transfer is low in the latter, whereas it is high in the former. Organic bedding material has several advantages over inorganic material, which include high absorbtivity, presence of nutrients, and better porosity. The micro-organisms are immobilised on the filter packing by five different methods, including carrier binding, cross-linking, entrapment, microencapsulation, and membrane binding. Attached growth immobilisation is found to be effective for treating fluids with several different contaminants, while the entrapment methods are suitable for few contaminants. The potential release of micro-organisms to the atmosphere has been a concern for these technologies. Typical design parameters for these two filters are: a retention time in the range of 25 to 60 seconds, a typical reactor height around 0.5 to 1.5 metre, an input concentration of about 0 to 1000 ppmv VDC, waste air flow of 50 to 3,00,000 m³/hr and an inlet oxygen concentration of 11 to 21 per cent.

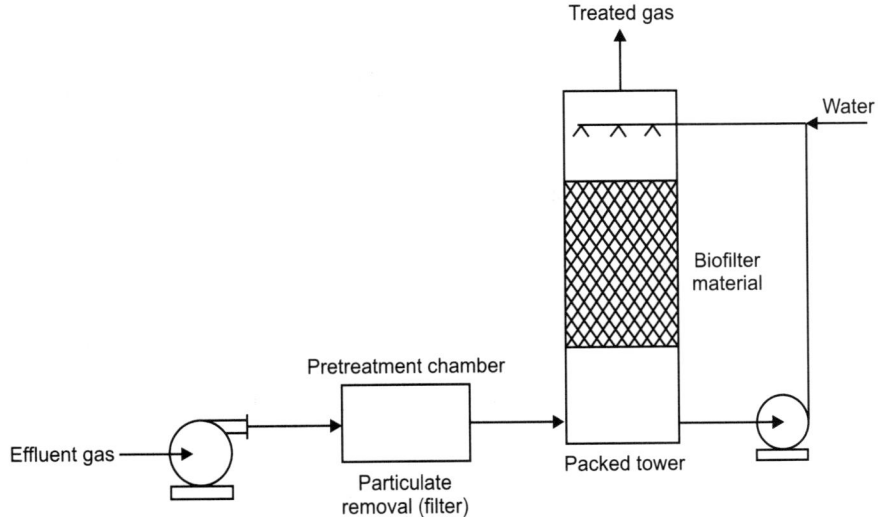

Fig. 14.4. A typical biotrickling filter.

Bioscrubber

The third biooxidation process for treating VOCs is bioscrubbing, which consists of a twin reactor system that has water scrubbing and biooxidation vessels (Fig. 14.5). The micro-organism is either suspended or attached onto a support, just like the previous cases in the biooxidation vessel. In the scrubber the VOCs and other gases get absorbed in the water medium, and are then destroyed in the second vessel by the micro-organism, which is supplied with air and nutrient solutions. The water is recycled back to the scrubber.

Membrane Bioreactor

Membrane bioreactors combine membrane technology with biotechnology, where the membrane acts as a partition that separates the liquid and the gaseous medium (Fig. 14.6). The micro-organism grows on the liquid side of the membrane, which contains water and other nutrients required for its growth. The pollutants, gases, and oxygen approach the biofilm from the gas side after diffusing through the membrane and serve as the carbon source for the growth of the microbes. The membrane does not permit the micro-organisms to pass through and contaminate the gas stream. The membrane is either hydrophobic, microporous, or dense. A hydrophobic membrane is a polymer matrix such as polypropylene or Teflon with pores of 0.01 to 1.0 μm diameter. Since the membrane material is hydrophobic, water does not enter the pores; VOCs or pollutants enter from the gaseous phase. The design generally consists of hollow fibre, spiral wound, and plate and frame modules. In the dense membrane there are no pores, but the solute dissolves and gets transported to the liquid side through diffusion. Silicone rubber (polydimethylsiloxane) has high oxygen permeability, and it is used as a dense membrane material for the aeration of waste-water.

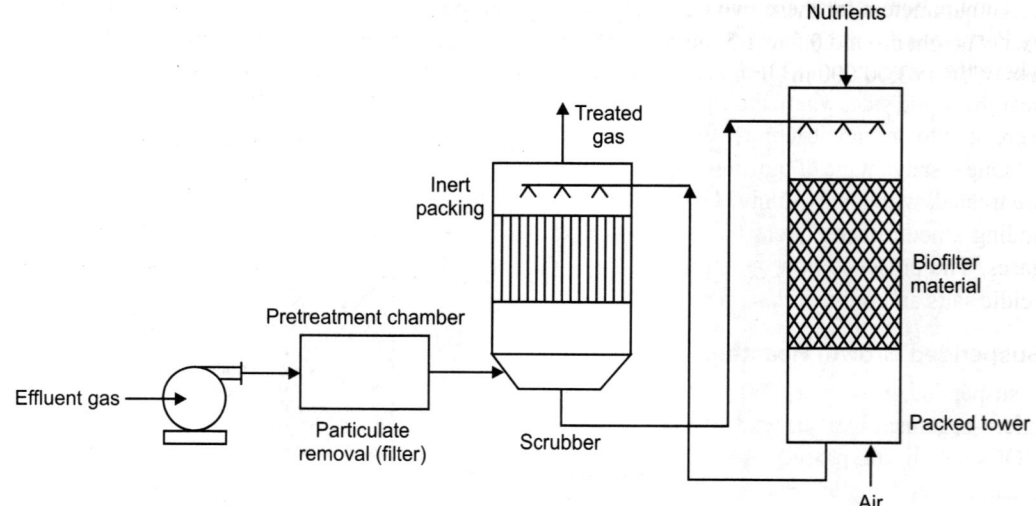

Fig. 14.5. A typical bioscrubber.

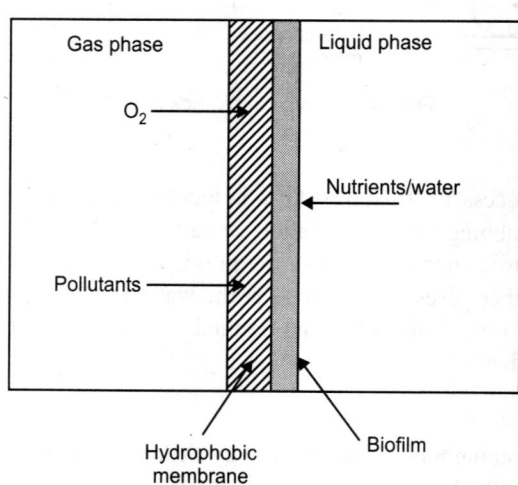

Fig. 14.6. Membrane bioreactor.

Silicone tube dense membranes have been successfully used to remove several organics, including xylenes, *n*-butanol, dichloromethane, *n*-hexane, toluene, and dichloroethane, with activated sludge as the innoculum. A porous membrane has been used to destroy organics like toluene, dichloromethane, propene, and also NO. Generally the effluent concentration is on the order of 30 to 150 ppm.

The selectivity control exhibited by membranes is demonstrated in two examples; one is related to the treatment of vehicle exhaust gases containing NO and heavy metals, and the other is the degradation of chlorinated organics in the presence of acid vapours. In the first case, the membrane could successfully prevent heavy metals from entering and poisoning the biofilm. In the second case, silicone membranes, because of their selectivity for hydrophobic components, retain acid vapours (SO_2) that could hamper biodegradation of 1,2-dichloroethane.

Having both the aerobic and the anaerobic regions in the same biomembrane reactor was considered by Parvatiyar for the treatment of trichloroethylene. On the gas side, the film near the membrane and where the oxygen concentration was high acted as the aerobic region, and the region farthest from it near the liquid side, where the oxygen concentration was zero, acted as the anaerobic zone. Both regions were able to degrade trichloroethylene completely.

One disadvantage of biofilters is that sulphates, chlorides, and nitrates accumulate when acidic gases are treated, which may inhibit the growth of micro-organisms. This is circumvented to some extent by adding a neutralising agent like lime, but it may not be possible to neutralise large amounts of acid gases. The presence of a water phase in the membrane bioreactor helps to wash out these inorganic acidic salts and prevent their accumulation.

Suspended Growth Reactors

A suspended growth reactor (SGR) is nothing but an agitated or unagitated gassed vessel containing the micro-organism in a suspended state (in a nutrient medium). In an aerobic suspended growth reactor, VOCs and air are passed through an aqueous suspension of active micro-organisms. Mass transfer of organic chemicals and oxygen from the gas to the liquid phase, where suspended active organisms biodegrade the contaminant of interest, is the crucial. In a biofilter, the micro-organism is attached to a support, whereas in this design the organism is kept suspended under agitation. Absence of plugging and better biomass and nutrient control are the advantages in this design.

SGR performance was comparable to that of a biofilter in treating gas containing toluene. The percentage removals in a biofilter and an SGR were almost similar (almost 97 per cent) for mass loadings in the range of 4 to 30 mg/l hr.

The support medium used in the biofilter was a 70:30 mixture of compost and perlite. The micro-organisms for the SGRs were cultivated from toluene degraders and compost.

Treatment of Inorganic Gases

Sulphur compounds such as hydrogen sulphide, dimethyl sulphide, dimethyl disulphide, methane thiol, carbon disulphide, and carbonyl sulphide are produced by industries like aerobic waste-water treatment plants, composting plants, and rendering plants. Generally biofilters are used for odour reduction, as they are able to clean complex waste gases, but the absence of a water phase makes it unsafe for use in areas that may produce acidic by-products. Different approaches for the degradation of dimethyl sulphide reported in the literature are shown in Table 14.4. A membrane bioreactor containing a flat-plate composite assembly made up of polydimethylsiloxane and polysulphone membranes impregnated with ZrO fillers inoculated with *Hyphomicrobium* VS, a methylotrophic micro-organism, was able to remove dimethyl sulphide from a gas stream. The removal efficiency of air contaminated with 38 mg/m^3 was found to be 99 per cent for 24 seconds residence time.

Table 14.4. Different technologies and micro-organisms used for treating H_2S.

Biofilter	Peat/night soil sludge
	Peat/*Thiobacillus thioparus* DW44
	Peat/*Hyphomicrobium* 155
	Bark/*Hyphomicrobium* MS3
	Compost/*Hyphomicrobium* M33
	Compost/dolomite/*Hyphomicrobium* MS3
Biotrickling filter	Polypropylene/*Thiobacillus thioparus* TK-m
	Polyurethane/*Hyphomicrobium* VS
	Ceramic/activated sludge from waste-water treatment plant
Membrane bioreactor	*Hyphomicrobium* VS

Gases produced during the (i) hydroteratment of oil fractions and natural gas, and (ii) synthesis gases produced by coal gasification and fuel oil partial oxidation contain highly concentrated H_2S. Scrubbing this gas using ethanoloamines at high pressures leads to recovery of H_2S, which is oxidised to produce elemental sulphur. The oxidation is performed chemically using ferric ions, which are reoxidised by air to complete the cycle. This reoxidation can be speeded up by using a micro-organism *Thiobacillus ferrooxidans* in a biological reactor, such as in the EniTecnologie process. Oxidation of a low concentration H_2S stream can also be performed biologically using *Thiobacillus thiooxidan*, as in the Shell-THIOPAQ process.

Biofilter technology has been successful for the treatment of waste gas containing H_2S at low concentrations of the contaminant and at high gas flow rates. The effect of inorganic packing material on the destruction efficiency has been studied, and the conclusion was that porous ceramic performed well. Peat as a filtering material was able to degrade H_2S without the need to inoculate the filter with oxidising microbes. Since peat was acidic (pH 4), it performed better when neutralised, removing 95 per cent of the H_2S in 1 day of operation. Sulphur is mineralised in biofilters, generating mainly sulphate ions, which remain in the biofilter. Acidification of the biofilter takes place only if the sulphur concentration is relatively high. When pellets made of pig manure and sawdust were used as the packing bed material, more than 90 per cent removal efficiency was achieved. Sulphur dioxide was reduced to H_2S biochemically by contact with sulphate-reducing micro-organisms in which *Desulfovibrio desulfuricans* was dominant. Subsequently the H_2S could be oxidised to sulphur by ferric sulphate, where ferrous ions were regenerated.

SO_2 from flue gases could be microbially oxidised to sulphate by *Thiobacillus ferrooxidans*. The sulphate-reducing bacterium *Desulfovibrio desulfuricans* used $SO_2(g)$ as a terminal electron acceptor and converted SO_2 to H_2S. The use of glucose as an electron donor in microbial SO_2 reducing cultures makes this process expensive. Heat and alkali pretreated sewage sludge was used as a carbon and energy source; it was found to reduce SO_2 completely in a continuous, anaerobic mixed culture. *Desulfotomaculum orientis* grown in batch cultures on a feed of SO_2, H_2, and CO_2 was also able to reduce SO_2 to H_2S completely at gas-liquid contact times of 1 to 2 seconds.

Treatment of NO gas poses several problems. Since the solubility of NO in water is very poor, bioprocesses that involve transfer of pollutants at low concentrations to the aqueous phase are not very efficient. One approach was to preconcentrate the gas using activated carbon and treat the desorbed, more concentrated gas using biological methods. Nitrate and nitrite ions, which are formed in this process are destroyed by a denitrificating biomass involving *Thiobacillus denitrificans* in an anoxic medium grown on a sulphur-Maerl support. The presence of oxygen during adsorption leads to the formation of NO_2, which remains on the adsorbent, whereas NO does not. This technique is also well suited for gases like NH_3 and H_2S. Two heterotrophic bacterial *Paracoccus denitrificans* and *Pseudomonas denitrificans*, have also been found in a batch culture with succinate, heat, alkali pretreated sewage sludge as carbon and energy sources, and NO as a terminal electron acceptor.

PETROLEUM REFINERY AND PETROCHEMICALS

The exploration and production sector of the petroleum business explores, develops and extracts crude oil and gas resources from natural formations beneath the earth. Exploration involves mapping geological features and drilling test wells in areas where there is a high probability of finding reserves. Proven oil fields are then developed through a well drilling programme, which leads to a producing field. The extraction techniques used depend on the geological characteristics of the area, the type and formation of the oil and/or gas deposits, and the design of the well field.

Crude oil refining operations involve extracting useful petroleum products (e.g. gasoline). Crude oil contains fractions of naphthas, jet fuel, gasoline, diesel fuel, gas oils, lubrication oils and asphalt. Refineries extract these fractions thermally or catalytically.

Crude oil is unrefined liquid petroleum; it contains predominantly carbon and hydrogen in the form of alkanes (saturated hydrocarbons), alkenes and alkynes (both unsaturated), and aromatic hydrocarbons. The other components present in oil are sulphur, nitrogen, oxygen, trace amounts of iron, silicon, and aluminium. Large amounts of hydrocarbon contaminants are spilled into the environment as a result of various human activities. Major accidental spills from oil exploration sites, oil tankers, pipelines (underwater and underground), spent marine lubricants, and storage tanks have become a common occurrence. Petroleum refineries also generate sludge and other oily effluents.

Bioremediation

Bioremediation includes stimulating the native microbial populations or introducing micro-organisms from external sources that have been known to degrade a particular contaminant, or have been engineered to do so. The environment necessary for the growth of these micro-organisms must be created. The *in situ* treatment procedures include biostimulation, bioventing, bioaugmentation, and addition of a nitrogen-phosphorous-potassium fertiliser. Bioremediation techniques have more advantages than the chemical and physical methods, including treatment cost.

Stimulation of microbial growth and activity for hydrocarbon removal is accomplished primarily through the addition of oxygen and nutrients. Several factors including temperature and pH influence this rate of growth. Biodegradation has been found to be an efficient method for the reduction of hydrocarbons. Selection of a bioremediation technology requires an understanding of the biological processes involved and the physical application methods available.

Metabolic steps in the biodegradation of hydrocarbons follow two major strategies: oxidation and/or reduction. Aerobic pathway is preferred biodegradation over anaerobic metabolism for hydrocarbon.

Aerobic

Hydrocarbon biodegradation proceeds most rapidly and efficiently under nonlimiting, aerobic conditions, where oxygen serves both as a reactant and electron acceptor, thus reflecting a greater net production of energy. Biodegradation under aerobic conditions is more complete, resulting in greater rates of mineralisation of hydrocarbons to CO_2 and water. Aerobic metabolism requires oxygenase enzymes, which incorporate molecular oxygen into reduced substrate.

The micro-organisms make use of hydrocarbons as their carbon and/or energy sources and degrade the hydrocarbons to carbon dioxide and water. Since the crude oil contains paraffinic, simple aromatic, and polyaromatic hydrocarbons (PAHs), its biodegradation involves the interaction of many different micro-organisms. The common hydrocarbon-degrading organisms in the marine environment are *Pseudomonas*, *Acinetobacter*, *Nocardia*, *Vibro*, and *Achromobacter*. Oxygen is essential for *in situ* degradation of hydrocarbons. Since injecting oxygen gas is expensive, other soluble electron acceptors such as nitrates or sulphates are also used, but these acceptors slow down the reaction.

Straight chain alkanes are easily and rapidly degraded by several micro-organisms, including *Acinetobacter* sp., *Actinomycetes*, *Arthrobacter*, *Bacillus* sp., *Candida* sp., *Micrococcus* sp., *Planococcus*, *Pseudomonas* sp., *Calcoaceticus*, and *Streptomyces*. Although micro-organisms degrade *n*-alkanes up to a chain length of 40 carbon atoms, the solubility of long chained alkanes in water is poor; therefore the availability of the alkanes decreases, leading to reduced biodegradation. The general degradation pathway is via the oxidation of the terminal methyl group to its corresponding carboxylic acid, possibly through various intermediates (Fig. 14.7), which finally get mineralised. But in some cases, the preterminal carbon is also oxidised. Anaerobic biodegradation of crude oil using seawater and sediment as inocula produced a two orders of magnitude increase in the degradation of C_{10} to C_{20} carboxylic acids in 5 days, which were further degraded, leaving behind higher (greater than C_{20}) molecular weight cyclic and branched carboxylic acids as recalcitrant material. An *Acinetobacter* sp. isolated from soil was able to mineralise long-chain *n*-paraffins(C_{16-36} chain) in car engine oil. Long chain *n*-paraffins were metabolised via the terminal oxidation pathway of *n*-alkane, which was confirmed from the products of degradation, namely *n*-hexadecane, 1-hexadecanol, and 1-hexadecanoic acid.

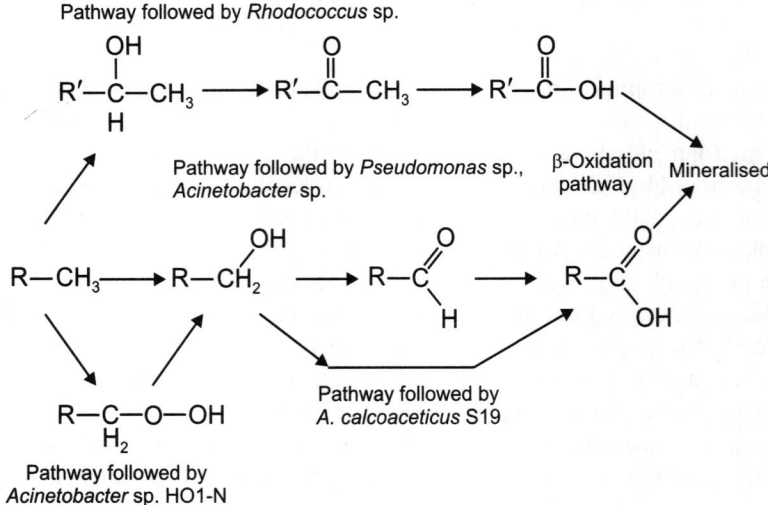

Fig. 14.7. Aerobic degradation of hydrocarbon.

Pseudomonas sp., *Ralstonia* sp., *Rhodococcus* sp., and *Sphingomonas* sp. are some of the micro-organisms that are known to oxidatively degrade monoaromatics like benzene, toluene, and xylenes (BTEX) as shown in Fig. 14.8. Toluene aerobically degrades more rapidly than other BTEX compounds in a wide variety of strains (*Pseudomonas putida* mt-2 and P., *P. mendocina, R. picketti* PKO1, etc.), either through the formation of substituent groups on the benzene ring or on the methyl group. The products could be cresols, benzyl alcohol, or dihyrol. A *Pseudomonas* sp. oxidises xylenes at the methyl group, similar to the degradation of toluene, forming several intermediates.

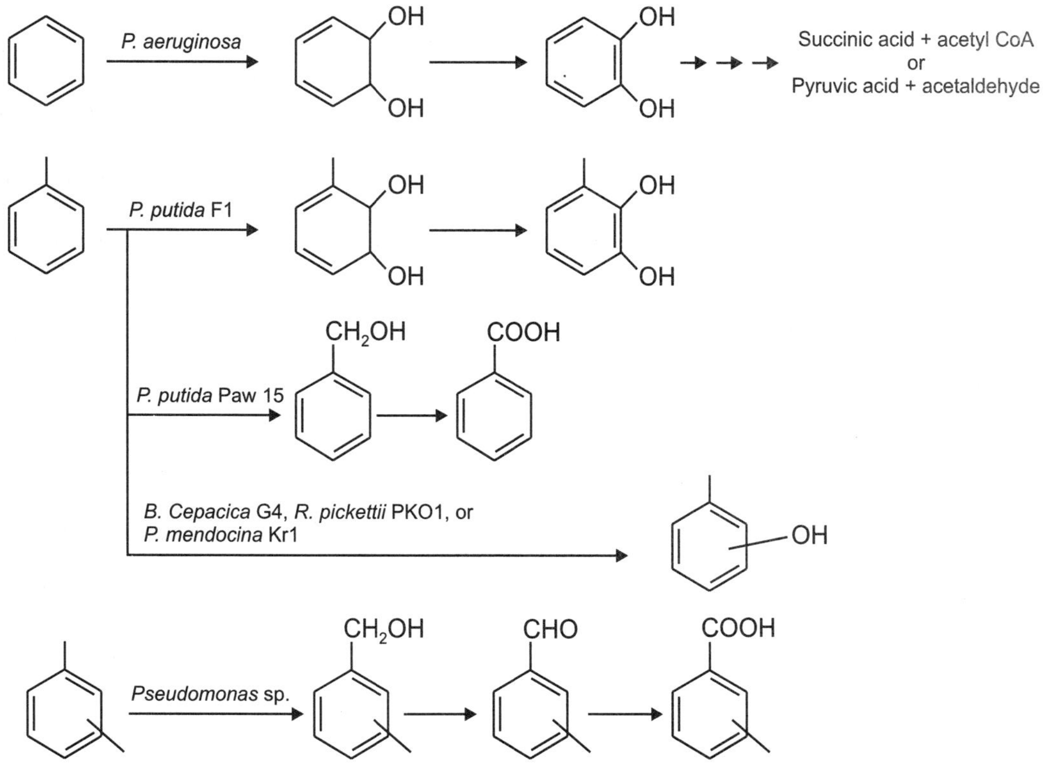

Fig. 14.8. Aerobic biodegradation pathway of aromatics.

Polyaromatic hydrocarbons (PAHs) persist in soil and sediment because of their low water solubility and high stability (because of the presence of multiple fused aromatic rings); their half-life is directly proportional to the number of fused rings. Motor vehicle exhausts, lubricating oils, paint solvents, and greases contribute to PAHs, and many of them are carcinogenic. *Burkholderia cepacia* F297 degrades a variety of polycyclic aromatic compounds, including fluorene, methyl naphthalene, phenanthrene, anthracene, and dibenzothiophene. Several micro-organisms have been reported to degrade PAHs, and they include *Rhodococcus* sp., *Alteromonas* sp., *Arthrobacter, Bacillus, Mycobacterium* sp., *Pseudomonas* sp., and *Phanaerochaete chrysporium*. Other micro-organisms, including bacteria and fungi, that are specific for a substrate include:

1. Naphthalene: *Mycobacter calcoaceticus, Pseudomonas paucimobillis, Pseudomonas putida, Pseudomonas fluorescens, Sphingomonas paucimobilis.*
2. Acenaphthene: *Beijernickia* sp., *P. putida, P. fluorescens,* and other *Pseudomonas* sp., *Burkholderia cepacia.*
3. Anthracene: *Beijernickia* sp., *Mycobacterium* sp., *Pseudomonas paucimobilis, Cycloclasticus pugeti, Ulocladium chartarum, Absidia cylindrospora.*

4. Phenanthrene: *Aeromonas* sp., *Alcaligenes faecalis*, *Achromobacter denitrificans*, *Bacillus cerus*, *A. faecalis*.
5. Fluoranthene: *Mycobacterium* sp., *P. putida, Sp. paucimobilis, P. paucinobilis*.
6. Pyrene and chrysene: *Sphingomonas* sp.
7. Pyrene: *Caenorhabditis elegans, Phanerochaete chrysosporium, Penicillium* sp., *Penicillium janthinellum*.
8. Chrysene: *P. janthinellum, Syncephalastrum racemosus, Penicillium* sp.
9. Benz[a]anthracene: *C. elegans, Trametes versicolor, Phanerochaete laevis, P. janthinellum*.
10. Dibenz[a,h]anthracene: *Trametes versicolor, P. janthinellum*.

Most degradative mechanisms reported for fungi are cometabolic, where an alternate carbon source is utilised for energy and growth, while as a consequence PAH is transformed into other products. White-rot fungus, *Phanerochaete chrysosporium*, has been reported to mineralise phenanthrene, fluorene, fluoranthene, anthracene, and pyrene in nutrient-limited cultures. Fungal metabolism of several low molecular weight PAHs has been reported in literature. They include:

1. Naphthalene: *Absida glauca, Aspergillus niger, Basidiobolus ranarum, Candida utilis, Choanephora campincta, Circinella* sp.
2. Acenaphthene by *C. elegans, T. versicolor*.
3. Phenanthrene: *C. elegans, P. chrysosporium, P. laevis, Pleurotus ostreatus, T. versicolor*.
4. Anthracene: *Bjerkandera* sp., *Bjerkandera adjusta, C. elegans, P. chrysosporium, P. laevis, Ramaria* sp., *Rhizoctonia solani, T. versicolor, Pleurotus ostreatus*.
5. Fluoranthene: *C. elegans, C. blackesleeana, C. echinulata, Bjerkandera adjusta, Pleurotus ostreatus*.
6. Pyrene: *C. elegans, P. chrysosporium, Penicillium* sp., *P. janthinellum, P. glabrum, P. ostreatus*.
7. Benz[a]anthracene: *C. elegans, T. versicolor, P. laevis*.
8. Chrysene: *P. janthinellum, Syncephalastrum racemosus, Penicillium* sp.

Algae and cyanobacteria also oxidise naphthalene (*Oscillatoria* sp., *Microcoleus chthonoplastes, Nostoc* sp.) and phenanthrene (*Oscillatoria* sp., *Agmenellum quadruplicatum*).

Sancylate, a central intermediate in the metabolism of naphthalene, undergoes oxidative decarboxylation to yield catechol; it also acts as an inducer for degradation in the presence of gram-negative bacteria like *Pseudomonas*. Whereas salicylate does not act as an inducer, it is hydroxylated to gentisate in the presence of gram-positive bacteria such as members of the *Rhodococcus* sp.

Benzo[a]pyrene (BaP), a five-ring fused compound, is known to degrade via the formation of 4,5 or 7,8 or 9, 10 dihydrols, followed by the formation of carboxylic acids in the presence of bacterial species that include *Rhodococcus* sp. strain UW1, *Burkholderia cepacia, Mycobacterium, S. maltophilia*, as well as a mixed culture containing *Pseudomonas* and *Flavobacterium*. In addition, fungal isolates that include *Phanerochaete chrysosporium, Trametes versicolor* and *Pycnoporus cinnabarinus* grown on an alternate carbon source can remove more than 90 per cent of BaP in 30 hrs, producing about 15 per cent carbon dioxide, indicating mineralisation. Fungal BaP oxidation is mediated by cytochrome P-450, leading to the formation of *trans*-dihydrol via the formation of epoxide. The green alga *Selanastum capricornutum* oxidises BaP to 4,5 or 7,8 or 9,10 or 11,12 dihydrodiols. The bioavailablity of BaP in contaminated soils could be increased by the use of surfactants, which could increase its dissolution and hence enhance the mass transfer rates. Bacterial-fungal cocultures can lead to peroxidation of BaP by fungus, which could lead to an increase in the rate of BaP mineralisation by bacteria. Similar behaviour was observed in the case of pyrene.

Naphthalene dioxygenase is induced by naphthalene, salicylate, and succinate, and is isolated in gram-negative bacteria (mainly *Pseudomonas*). The enzyme helps to incorporate molecular oxygen into the substrate to produce *cis*-dihydrodiol, which is the intermediate degradation component. *P. putida* was able to grow on naphthalene as a sole carbon source, synthesising the enzyme naphthalene-dioxygenase when activated initially on salicylate.

Operating conditions

The rate of microbial degradation depends on several operating factors that include ambient temperature, pH, salinity, oxygen availability, amount of nutrients available, chemical composition of the petroleum, its physical state and concentration in the contaminated area, and adaptation of the micro-organism to the contaminated site.

Higher temperatures lead to increased rates of degradation, as well as decreased viscosity of the oil, which in turn increases its availability for the organism in the aqueous phase. Biodegradation of petroleum has been reported in Arctic and Antarctic seawater. Strains have been known to degrade diesel oil at 0 to 10°C. Below 10°C, some of the long chain hydrocarbons also solidify, reducing their availability to the microbes. A temperature dependent diffusion barrier in the thin layer of unfrozen water limited metabolic activity. Studies carried out by Rike in winter months at an Arctic site have shown that cold-adapted micro-organisms are capable of *in situ* biodegradation. Although degradation of crude oil has been observed even at 60°C, at higher temperatures the membrane toxicity of hydrocarbons is increased, hindering biodegradation. A neutral pH is favoured by most of the strains, although degradation of hydrocarbons has been reported in acidic as well as in alkaline pH conditions. Organisms found in seawater are able to degrade oil at salt concentrations that vary from 0.1 to 2.0. *M. Pseudomonas* sp., enterobacteria, and a few gram-negative aerobes are known to work under saline conditions. Aerobic degradation requires 3.1 mg oxygen to degrade 1 mg hydrocarbon. Although the amount of oxygen dissolved in aqueous medium is good, it decreases sharply with the depth of the water. Addition of urea and ammonia-based fertilisers used for oil spills can exert an oxygen demand that results from biological oxidation of ammonia. Also on fine sediment beaches, mass transfer of oxygen may not be sufficient. Hence aerobic biodegradation is restricted to a small layer floating on top of the water layer. Oil slicks and globules of tar that sink below persist for a long time because of the absence of oxygen. Under oxygen-limited conditions, anaerobic degradation occurs in the presence of sulphate-reducing bacteria, metal-reducing bacteria, methanogens, and nitrifiers.

For sustained microbial activity, the C:N:P ratio must be maintained at 120:10:1. During oil spills, the carbon amount increases, which disturbs the nutrient balance and hence microbial growth, causing biodegradation to slow down. Organic (fertilisers) as well as inorganic sources (salts) for N and P have been added and found to be very effective. Oleophilic fertiliser was found to be very effective in degrading oil after the Exxon Valdez spill. The fertiliser preferably is added in slow-release form to have a maximum effect; it also cannot exceed the toxic concentrations of ammonia and/or nitrate so that the nutrient addition does not limit the microbial population. A field study conducted on the shoreline contaminated during the *Sea Empress* incident showed that addition of N and P led to significant decomposition of aliphatic hydrocarbons, but biodegradation of aromatics was not affected.

Petroleum has different compositions depending upon its source; hence its rate of biodegradability varies. Generally *n*-alkanes are easily susceptible, followed by branched alkanes, low molecular weight aromatics, and finally cyclic alkanes. Also biodegradation rates from highest to lowest are saturated compounds, light aromatics, heavy aromatics, and finally polar compounds, which are recalcitrant. The physical state of the oil has an effect on the degradation rate; emulsified spills degrade faster than tar balls because of the availability of the spill's large surface area. An increase in oil concentration can lead to an increase in membrane toxicity or can upset the C:N:P balance. Oxygen limitations due to the presence of a thick oil fraction can also affect the activity of the micro-organisms. Surprisingly, the percentage degradation of naphthalenes and fluorenes was greater than that of alkanes, dibenzothiophenes, and phenanthrenes in contaminated soils. There are probably two reasons for this: (i) the low molecular weight aromatic compounds have a higher solubility in water than the high molecular weight aromatics and alkanes, and (ii) the water solubility, and thus the availability, of alkanes is reduced by their high adsorption dry sand. The latter could be addressed by using suitable surfactants to solubilise the alkanes into the aqueous phase. Oil spills at sea are exposed to solar radiation, which could be hostile to microbial growth. Jezequel have observed that alkanes in oil spills that have little exposure to sunlight but that are damp degrade faster.

A mixture of *Acinetobacter* sp. and *Pseudomonas putida* PB4 degraded a light crude oil efficiently, with the degradation taking place in a sequential manner. The *Acinetobacter* sp. degraded the alkanes and other hydrocarbons and formed metabolites; the *P. putida* PB4 formed aromatic compounds by growing on the metabolites.

Anaerobic degradation

Anaerobic metabolism is a vital process with respect to petroleum hydrocarbon biodegradation and bioremediation. Because hydrocarbons are already chemically reduced stable compounds, further reduction (thermodynamically possible), is not a primary mode of degradation. Even under anaerobic conditions, it follows an oxidative strategy. In the absence of molecular oxygen, water-derived oxygen serves as a reactant, while CO_2 or sulphates serve as the electron acceptor for anaerobic degradation. Other terminal electron acceptors include manganese oxides; soil humic acids and the humic acid model compound anthraquinone-2,6-disulphonate and fumarate in a fermentative oxidation process.

Petroleum hydrocarbons can serve as electron donors and as a carbon source for bacteria under a variety of redox conditions. The *Azoarcus/Thauera* group was found to be the major bacterial group responsible for the anaerobic degradation of alkylbenzenes and *n*-alkanes, and a methanogenic consortium composed of two archaeal species related to the genera *Methanosaeta* and *Methanospirillum*, and a bacterial species related to the *Methanospirillum* was responsible for toluene degradation.

Alkanes are very inactive compounds, and during aerobic degradation, oxygen (which is absent during anaerobic degradation) is available to activate them. Sulphate-reducing and denitrifying bacteria that completely oxidise alkanes with 6 to 20 carbon atoms have been isolated. The sulphate reducers are able to produce the corrosive and toxic gas hydrogen sulphide with crude oil as a substrate. Similar to toluene, which gets added to fumarate, a common cell metabolite, via a radical mechanism, *n*-alkanes also get activated via radical mechanism and are added to fumarate. However, the *n*-alkanes were not activated at the terminal carbon but at C2, as was the case with *n*-hexane. The proposed pathway for anaerobic degradation is that fumarate reacts with the C2 of the alkane through a radical mechanism and forms (1-methyl-alkyl)-succinate. It is activated by coenzyme A (HSCoA), several rearrangements follow, and then β oxidation occurs. The final end product is CO_2 (Fig. 14.9). The metabolites formed during anaerobic biodegradation are various alkylsuccinates with alkyl chains (linked at C2) that had a carbon chain length of 4 to 8.

Under anaerobic conditions, aromatic compounds are transformed into a few intermediates [namely, to benzoate (or benzoyl-CoA) and, to a lesser extent, resorcinol and phloroglucinol], followed by the cleavage of the rings by hydrolysis, resulting in the formation of noncyclic compounds, which are then converted into metabolites by β oxidation. Two examples of activation reactions are:

1. Hydroxylation of benzene ring to form phenol.
2. Methyl hydroxylation of toluene to form benzyl alcohol.

Two examples of ring cleavage reactions are:

1. Hydrolytic cleavage.
2. Reduction of an aromatic ring to an alicyclic ring.

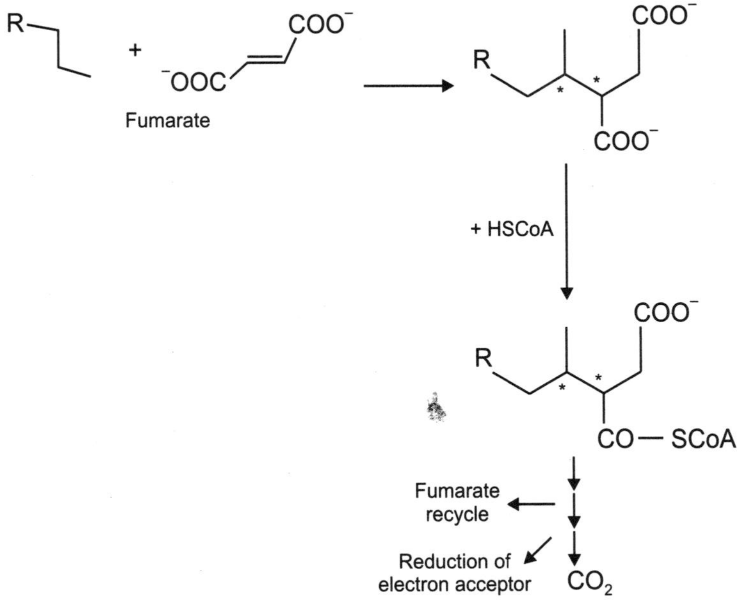

Fig. 14.9. Anaerobic biodegradation.

Benzene is transformed to phenol in the presence of methanogenic cultures and to *p*-hydroxybenzoate in the presence of denitrifying bacteria and finally to the central intermediate benzoate. Pure cultures of denitrifying, iron-reducing, and sulphate-reducing bacteria (under the genera *Thauera* and *Azoarcus*) utilise toluene as a carbon and energy source. A sulphate-reducing bacterium that oxidises toluene has been isolated and found to belong to the *Desulfobacula toluolica* genus/species. Toluene degrades via benzoyl-CoA. The oxidation of the methyl group occurs by the formation of benzyl alcohol, going to benzaldehyde, and finally to benzoate. Ethyl benzene is stable under anaerobic conditions. Denitrifying and methanogenic bacteria degrade the three isomers of xylene. Except for naphthalene, none of the PAHs have been known to degrade under anaerobic conditions.

Factors affecting bioremediation

The rate of microbial degradation of crude oil or oil waste depends on a variety of factors, including the physical conditions and the nature, concentration, and ratio of various structural classes of hydrocarbons present, the bioavailability of the substrate, and the properties of the biological system involved. Biodegradation and bioremediation processes are non-homogeneous and unpredictable in nature. A majority of HCs contaminants are degraded by cometabolism and early elimination of the cosubstrates which halt the degradation processes. Nutrient availability, especially of nitrogen and phosphorus, appears to be the most common limiting factor.

While hydrocarbon-degrading microbes must come into contact with their substrate for hydrocarbon uptake to occur (immobilisation), the insoluble nature of the majority of petroleum hydrocarbon molecules limits this contact. The most widely recognised modes of hydrocarbon accession are direct microbial adherence to large oil droplets and interaction with emulsified oil. Hydrocarbon-degrading microbes produce a variety of biosurfactants as part of their cell surface or as molecules released extracellularly. Surface have the ability to emulsify or pseudosolubilise poorly water-soluble compounds, thus influencing their efficacy including charge (non-ionic, anionic or cationic), hydrophilic-lipophilic balance, and critical micellar concentration (the concentration at which surface tension reaches a minimum and surfactant monomers aggregate into micelles). These biosurfactants and added chemical surfactants can both enhance and inhibit the biodegradation of hydrocarbons. Suppression of their production, by use of inhibitors or mutagens, retards the ability to degrade oil. Whereas the low-molecular-weight biosurfactants (glycolipids, lipopeptides) is more effective in lowering the interfacial and surface tensions, the high-molecular-weight biosurfactants (amphipathic polysaccharides, proteins, lipopolysaccharides, and lipoproteins) are effective stabilisers of oil-in-water emulsions.

Petroleum constituents cause membrane toxicity due to its lipophilic nature, as they tend to reside in the hydrophobic area between membrane monolayers in the acyl chains of phospholipids in the cytoplasmic membrane. Inside the membrane, they alter membrane structure by changing fluidity and protein conformations and result in the disruption of the barrier and energy transduction functions, while affecting membrane-bound and embedded enzyme activity. In stress response, bacteria may form biofilms, alter their cell surface hydrophobicity to regulate their partitioning with respect to hydrocarbon-water interfaces or, in gram-negative bacteria, gain protection from hydrophilic lipopolysaccharide components that offer high transfer resistance to lipophilic compounds.

Hence, attempts to optimise or accelerate processes for the degradation of hydrocarbons need to analyse microbial abundance and distribution in natural environments in the hope of evaluating the long-term effects of petroleum, developing and evaluating waste remediation approaches, tracking the enrichment of pathogenic micro-organisms during remediation, controlling deleterious community structures with ecosystem functions.

Microbial recovery and upgradation of petroleum

Petroleum processing, including exploration, refining and transportation are the major activities in the petroleum sector. At each step, chances of petroleum products getting released into environment are high, especially during transportation, i.e. oil spill. Microbial system has the capacity to process these contaminations and also upgrade the petroleum products.

Microbial oil recovery

Microbial technology is exploited in oil reservoirs to improve the recovery of oil. Injected nutrients, together with indigenous or added microbes, promote *in situ* microbial growth and/or generation of products, which mobilise additional oil and move it to producing wells. Among other microbes only bacteria are promising candidates for microbial enhanced oil recovery. On the other hand, thermophilies are potentially useful for microbial enhanced oil recovery. Five requirements, including oil, bacteria, water, nutrients, and metabolites, with adsoprtion, diffusion, chemotaxis, growth and decay of bacteria, nutrient consumption, permeability damage, and porosity reduction effects, are factors associated with microbial oil recovery.

Microbial de-emulsification

Oil emulsions are formed at various stages of oil production, recovery and refining processes, and they represent both a serious environmental and disposal problem for the oil industry and potential loss of valuable oil-products. Microbial systems have the ability to de-emulsify oil emulsion. Centrifugation, heat, electrical and other physio-chemical methods are used for it.

Microbial desulphurisation

Sulphur is the third most abundant organically found element in crude oil, normally accounting for 0.05 to 5 per cent and organically bound, mainly in the form of condensed thiopenes. It is very expensive to remove it, via physio-chemical process like hydrodesulphurisation. Biodesulphurisation is a cost-effective and efficient method.

Microbial denitrogenation

Crude oil contains about 0.5 to 2.1 per cent nitrogen, with 70 to 75 per cent consisting of pyrroles, indoles, and carbazole non-basic compounds. Several species of bacteria, including *Alcaligenes, Bacillus, Beijerinckia, Burkholderia, Comamonas, Mycobacterium, Pseudomonas, Serratia*, and *Xanthomonas* can utilise nitrogen containing indole, pyridine, quinoline, and carbazole and its alkyl derivatives. Pyrrole and indole are easily degradable, but carbazole is relatively resistant to microbial attack. Oxygenases play an important role in the initial attack in the transformation of nitrogen compounds.

Phytoremediation

Phytoremediation is a technique by which plants and the associated rhizosphere micro-organisms are utilised to remove, transform, or contain toxic chemicals located in soils, sediments, groundwater, surface water, and the atmosphere. Phytostimulation involves the stimulation of the micro-organisms in the location by using plants that have been tested for the destruction of PAH, BTEX, and other petroleum hydrocarbons.

Volatile organic carbons can be taken up by plants and transpired to the atmosphere without transformation, in a process known as phytovolatilisation, which is not an acceptable environmental solution. There is limited plant uptake of more hydrophobic and larger petroleum components. Phytoremediation is not a suitable method for remediation of high-volume oily wastes.

A multi process phytoremediation system (MPSS), using land-farming inoculation with contaminant degrading bacteria and growth of plants with plant growth-promoting rhizobacteria (PGPR), gives promising results by enhancing biomass accumulation and accelerating degradation kinetics. Plant growth-promoting rhizobacteria increase plant tolerance to total petroleum hydrocarbon and promote plant growth which results in high biomass accumulation. MPSS removes many more petroleum contaminants than landfarming, bioremediation and phytoremediation alone.

Phytoextraction, which involves removal of a contaminant from the site using plants, has been adopted in the decontamination of soil and groundwater affected by PAHs using alfalfa (*Medicago sativa*) and hybrid poplar trees. Rhizofiltration (use of micro-organisms around the zone near the roots to filter contaminants) and phytodegradation (use of plants for the degradation of the contaminants) using grasses and clover (*Trifolium* spp.) have been adopted for the treatment of a PAH-contaminated site.

Typha latifolia, T. angustifolia, Phragmites communis, Scirpus lacustris, Juncus spp., different algae, and microflora consisting of different heterotrophic and autotrophic micro-organisms, including different oil-degrading bacteria and fungi present in an artificially made wetland, were able to efficiently decontaminate water consisting of crude oil and heavy metals (namely cadmium, copper, iron, lead, and manganese). Paraffins and naphthenes were more easily degraded than other hydrocarbons, and low molecular weight PAHs degraded more easily than high molecular weight PAHs.

Reactors

Anaerobic bioremediation of soil contaminated with No.2 diesel fuel (550 mg petroleum hydrocarbon/kg of soil) in a slurry reactor at a pH of 6.5 led to 81, 55, 50, and 40 per cent biodegradation in 300 days, with mixed electron acceptor, sulphate-reducing, nitrate-reducing, and methanogenic conditions. A fibrous-bed bioreactor, constructed by winding a porous wire cloth, to which the cells are attached and entrapped, provides a suitable, novel cell immobilisation support. Such a bioreactor containing immobilised *Pseudomonas putida* and *P. fluorescens* degraded 10, 20, 20, and 12 per cent of benzene, toluene, ethylbenzene, and *o*-xylene, respectively, under hypoxic conditions.

Immobilised cells tolerated higher concentrations (greater than 1000 mg/l) when compared with the free cells. Cells in the bioreactor were relatively insensitive to benzene toxicity. Substrate inhibition was observed for all substrates.

A continuous stirred tank reactor (CSTR) and a soil slurry-sequencing stirred batch reactor (SS-SBR) were tested for the degradation of a diesel fuel-contaminated soil under aerobic conditions and with added nutrients (C:N:P ratios ~60:2:1). The diesel fuel removal efficiency was higher in the SS-SBR than in the CSTR (96 and 75 per cent, respectively). Microbial growth was approximately 25 per cent greater in the SS-SBR than the CSTR, probably because of the variety of environments faced by the organisms and because the induction or acclimatisation of the bacteria is favoured under dynamic conditions. Significant amounts of biosurfactant were produced in the SS-SBR, which was not observed in the CSTR.

Periodic aeration and venting strategy was found to be better in treating soil contaminated by diesel fuel in a SS-SBR. A combination of SS-SBR followed by a solid phase bioreactor (biopile) was found to be cost effective in treating soil contaminated (2.5 per cent oil) with car diesel fuel or *n*-decane (achieving 80 per cent degradation). Addition of an anionic surfactant increased the degradation rate. Improved porosity of the soil led to enhancement of the contaminant removal rate.

An effluent mixture containing brewery and petroleum wastes (1:2) was treated in a fluidised bed reactor using a mixed culture obtained from a petroleum refinery waste separation pond. The culture was supported on low density polyethylene (LDPE) particles. There were 36 and 64 per cent decreases in COD for petroleum-only and mixed wastes, respectively. Addition of extra nutrients to the mixed waste increased the reduction in COD to 90 per cent.

Thus, petroleum or crude oil contains a large number of hydrocarbons, aromatics, and fused ring structures; identifying microbes or microbial communities that could degrade all of them is a challenge. In addition, PAHs are refractive; they are hydrophobic, which decreases their water solubility, making them inaccessible to the micro-organisms. Thus they have a tendency to be adsorbed to the soil matrix. Nitrogen and sulphur compounds present in the petroleum may also be toxic to the micro-organisms. A large number of micro-organisms, fungi, and algae have been reported to degrade hydrocarbons under aerobic and anaerobic conditions. The white rot fungi *Phanerochaete chrysosporium* and *Pleurotus ostreatus* appear to be general-purpose organisms capable of degrading a wide range of hydrocarbons and PAHs.

Addition of extra nutrient helps degradation but adds to the operating cost. Bioaugmentation appears to be a good method for enhancing degradation if the micro-organism population at the contaminated site is not sufficient.

PULP AND PAPER

The paper and pulp process uses plenty of water, and the waste generated from this industry contains solvents, chlorinated compounds, resins, and most importantly lignin, which is highly resistant to degradation. Chlorinated compounds are also toxic to many micro-organisms. Conventional biological methods such as activated sludge and aerated lagoons help in reducing the COD load and toxicity, but these methods cannot effectively remove the colour from bleach plant effluents; in addition they consume energy for aeration. White rot fungus appears to be efficient in colour removal. Anaerobic degradation is affected by the presence of sulphate.

Destruction of adsorbable organic halogen is another aspect that needs to be addressed. Carrying out biodegradation at thermophilic conditions would be advantageous since the waste stream from the paper mill is generally around 50°C, but finding efficient micro-organisms that can perform well and overcome the other problems mentioned earlier is still a research challenge.

The principal waste parameters of concern to the paper and pulp industry are biochemical oxygen demand (BOD), pH and total suspended solids (TSS) in all categories of manufacturing. For groundwood, chemimechanical and thermochemical operations, the heavy metal ion zinc is of concern. For certain types of pulp manufacture (e.g. kraft, soda and neutral sulphite semichemical pulping), the colour of effluent is also of concern. The dominant pulping process currently used in the world is the Kraft process, largely because it can produce a strong pulp from a wide variety of species. The process also has an excellent chemical recovery system, which is important because of the high cost of chemicals.

The pulp and paper making industry is very water intensive (about 60 m^3 water per tonne of paper produced), and in terms of freshwater use ranks third after the primary metals and chemical industries. The major raw material used by the pulp and paper industry is wood, which is composed of cellulose fibres. The wood is broken down to separate the cellulose from the noncellulose material; the cellulose is then dissolved chemically to form a pulp. The pulp slurry is then vacuum dried on a machine to produce a paper sheet. Dyes, coating materials, and preservatives are also added at some point in the process. Lignin is a complex aromatic polymer that is an integral cell wall constituent that gives strength and rigidity to the tissues and allows vascular plants to resist microbial attack. The presence of residual lignin affects some properties of the manufactured pulp and paper products. Therefore, lignin is selectively removed during pulping without significant degradation of the cellulose fibres. The paper industry has several sectors such as packaging board, newsprint, boxes, printing and writings, and tissues.

Wood pulp is prepared either by mechanical or chemical means. The mechanical pulping process involves passing a debarked block of wood through a rotating grindstone where the fibres are stripped off and suspended in water. In chemical pulping, large amounts of chemicals are added to break down the wood in the presence of heat and pressure. In the kraft pulping process, sodium hydroxide and sodium sulphide are added to dissolve the nonfibrous material. The effluent generated (black liquor) contains high dissolved solids and alkali-lignin and polysaccharide degradation by-products, and has a high pH. A chemical mechanical pulping process is a combination of the two where the wood is first partially softened by chemicals and the mechanical methods are used. Thermomechanical pulping involves carrying out the process at 100°C. The yield of this process is about 93 per cent based on dry wood, implying that 30 to 70 kg/T is lost in water, leading to a chemical oxygen demand (COD) of 1000 to 5600 mg/l. The papermaking process produces an effluent that contains about 50 per cent cellulose. This contaminated water is referred to as 'whitewater'. It consists of 40 per cent lignin, 40 per cent carbohydrates, and the rest extractives. White paper is produced by bleaching, which involves addition of a bleaching agent such as chlorine, hydrogen peroxide, or sodium peroxide. After filtration, colouring materials are added. Coatings and preservatives are added during or after the paper making process. Recycled paper is also a source of cellulose fibre for corrugated paper and newsprint. The recycled fibre needs to be de-inked using flotation, which is followed by washing and screening. Typical paper industry operation and the type of chemicals used in each operation are listed in Table 14.5.

Table 14.5. Different operations and various chemicals used in paper and pulp manufacture.

Operation	Chemicals used
Chemical pulping	Acids, alkalies, lime, sulphurous acid, sodium hydroxide, sodium sulphide
Bleaching	Chlorine, bleaching agents, sulphates, solvents (chloroform)
Paper making	Pigments
Sizing and starching	Waxes, glue, synthetic resins, hydrocarbons
Colouring and dyeing	Inks, paints, solvents, rubbers, dyes
Cleaning and degreasing	Tetrachloroethylene, trichloroethylene, methylene chloride, carbon tetrachloride, trichloroethane

The quality of untreated effluent from pulp and paper manufacture varies, depending on the paper type as shown in Table 14.6. The COD of the effluent is as high as 11,000 mg/l. Dissolved small organic molecules in the effluent give a high biological oxygen demand (BOD), while more complex lignin molecules do not increase BOD but create a high COD and dark colour. The waste-water sludge from the de-inking operation contains heavy metals. The pulping process generates a considerable amount of waste-water (about 200 m^3 per tonne of pulp produced).

Table 14.6. Characteristics of effluents from the manufacture of pulps.

	Suspended solids, kg/tonne	BOD, kg/tonne
Bleached ground wood, textile, re-inked	20–360	11–220
Bine papers	22–45	7–18
Book and publication papers	22–45	9–22
Tissue	13–45	4–13
Coarse paper (boxboard, insulating, corrugated)	22–45	9–110
Newsprint	9–26	4–9

There are two main differences in the quality of the waste-waters from pulping and paper making operations, namely, (i) pulp waste-water contains dissolved wood-derived substances that are extracted from the wood during the pulping and bleaching processes, and (ii) pulping effluent will have some discolouration due to the dissolved lignin, more so when chemical pulping methods are employed. When coloured paper is manufactured, the effluent will have some discolouration because of the dyes used in the manufacturing process. Figure 14.10 gives a broad overview of the various treatment procedures for the effluent that is generated by the paper and pulp manufacturing industry.

Bioprocesses

Anaerobic process

The anaerobic degradation of complex organic compounds is affected by the presence of sulphate. The first steps in the anaerobic degradation process are the hydrolysis and fermentation of biopolymers like carbohydrates and proteins to intermediates such as propionate, butyrate, formate, and $H_2 + CO_2$ by fermenting bacteria. In the absence of sulphate, propionate and butyrate are degraded by acetogens to acetate, formate, and hydrogen, which are then converted by methanogens. In the presence of sulphate, the sulphate reducers will compete with these bacteria for propionate, butyrate, acetate, hydrogen, and formate by coupling the oxidation of these compounds to sulphate reduction. COD can be degraded via sulphate reduction if the COD to sulphate (g/g) ratio is below 0.66 (mol COD/mol sulphate <0.5). *Methanosaeta* spp. were the dominant acetate degraders, and *Methanobacterium* spp. the dominant hydrogen- and formate-consuming methanogens. *Desulfobulbus* spp. and *Syntrophobacter* spp. were necessary for propionate degradation. Butyrate was probably degraded by syntrophic butyrate degraders such as *Syntrophospora* and *Syntrophomonas*.

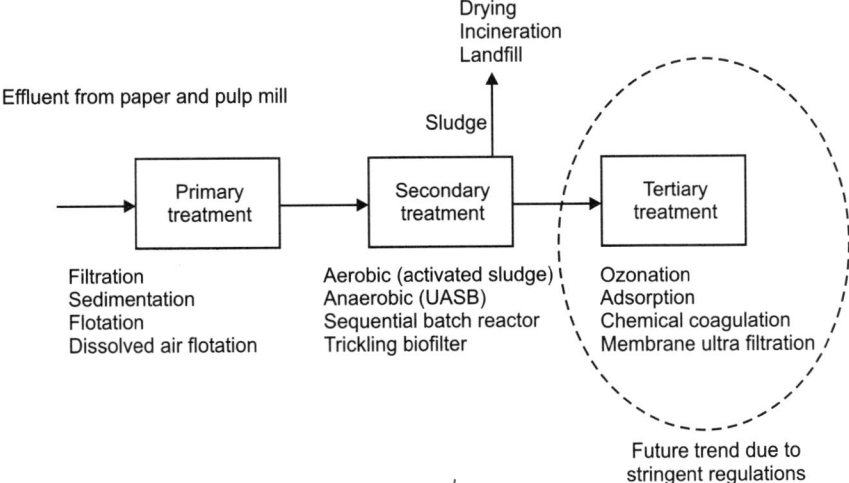

Fig. 14.10. Various treatment procedures for paper and pulp industry effluent.

Very little BOD or COD removal was observed when kraft or sulphite chlorine bleaching effluents were treated anaerobically, since they are inhibitory to methanogenic bacteria. This inhibition is attributed to organohalogens such as chlorophenols and halomethanes present in the bleaching effluents. Also methane productivity is poor unless the waste-water is not highly diluted. The alkaline steps in the bleaching process extract wood resin compounds into the effluent, which are also inhibitory to methanogens. Presently there is pressure to replace chlorine with chlorine-dioxide bleaching (elemental chlorine-free or totally replace all chlorinated bleaching agents (totally chlorine-free with ozone and hydrogen peroxide. But effluents from the chlorine and elemental chlorine-free bleaching process have similar methanogenic toxicities.

The lag phase for methane production in a batch process depends on how much of the kraft bleaching plant effluent is treated. The higher the fraction of effluent, the longer the lag phase, and once methane production starts, the rate is similar despite the differences in the length of the lag phase. This shows that the toxicity of effluent to aceticlastic methanogens is bacteriostatic rather than bacteriocidal. Aceticlastic methanogens do not easily acclimate to the toxic compounds in the effluent. We can, therefore, conclude that ethane production obtained after long lag phases in batch assays is due to a slow degradation of the toxic compounds that finally eliminates the inhibition. When the toxic compounds had been degraded to a level below the toxic threshold, methane production started.

Bioconversion of various waste paper materials by *Trichoderma viride* cellulase depends on the composition of the enzyme system, as well as the structure of cellulose. The crystalline section is difficult to hydrolyse, and the amorphous section is more susceptible to cellulase attack. Biodegradability of various paper materials tested with *Trichoderma viride* cellulase (0.2 mg/ml) incubated at 50°C for 2 hrs indicated that cardboard exhibited the highest efficiency followed by office paper and then foolscap. A decrease in hydrolytic efficiency was observed for all wastepaper materials because of the accumulation of sugar produced during biodegradation.

The solid industrial waste from the primary, secondary, and tertiary treatment stages from a pulp and paper factory contained 20 per cent solids at pH 6. When the sludge was treated with bicarbonate, a 60 per cent reduction in COD (initial COD = 1216 mg/g) and 50 per cent in extractable organic halogen (EOX) (initial EOX = 1546 mg/kg) were observed under anoxic conditions over a period of 5 months. Aerobic biological treatment by lagoons and activated sludge systems have been widely used to treat pulp and paper mill effluents to achieve BOD removal efficiencies between 65 and 99 per cent and COD reductions between 25 and 65 per cent. It is well established that fatty acids and resin acids are biodegraded aerobically, while chlorinated organic compounds are poorly degraded by these methods. Activated sludge treatment with addition of N and P to maintain a ratio of 100:5:0.3 was effective in treating *Pinus radiata* bleached kraft mill waste-water, achieving 90 per cent BOD removal and 60 per cent COD removal efficiencies in a reactor for hydraulic retention time (HRT) between 6 and 16 hrs. Generally the activated sludge processes were carried out at 35°C. Thermophilic conditions increased the effluent turbidity and decreased the sludge-settleability, leading to sludge loss. Experimental studies carried out by Vogelaar in an activated sludge tubular reactor operated at 30° and 55°C indicated that total COD removal was 58 and 48 per cent and colloidal COD removal was 86 and 70 per cent, respectively. Sludge production was the same at both temperatures.

Several thousand species of white rot fungi, most of them Basidiomycotina (which attack either hardwood or softwood) and a few Ascomycotina (which attack only hardwood) degrade lignin. Brown rot fungi extensively degrade cellulose and hemicelluloses in wood and to a very limited extent lignin. The soft rot fungi Ascomycotina or Deuteromycotina degrade both hardwood and softwood. White rot wood fungi including *Phanerochaete chrysosporium* and *Trametes versicolor* are capable of degrading wood and its constituents, such as cellulose and lignin, using the cellulose fraction as a source of carbon. Lignin peroxidases and laccase have the ability to depolymerise high molecular weight lignins and simultaneously polymerise the low molecular weight products formed. Kraft black liquor treated by the white rot fungi *Trametes elegans* showed a reduction in lignin weight (the average molecular weight decreased from 9032 to 7698) and an increase in polydispersity (from 1.6 to 3.2) after 15 days of incubation, indicating the lignin present in the effluent is degraded without the addition of extra nutrient.

Composting proceeds through three phases: (i) the mesophilic phase, (ii) the thermophilic phase (lasts from a few days to several months), and (iii) the cooling and maturation phase (lasts for several months). During composting, organic matter is transformed by micro-organisms into CO_2, biomass, heat, and a humus like end product. Aerobic conditions are prevalent in the thin topmost crust where the cellulose is oxidised to carbon dioxide; the anaerobic activity starts very close to the surface. Two thermophilic actinomycetes degrade 0.7 to 2.5 per cent of lignin in 42 days at 50°C, and a thermophilic fungus *Thermomyces lanuginosus* degrades 4.2 per cent of lignin in a compost environment.

Table 14.7 shows the results from anaerobic treatment of black liquor and bleach effluent wastes that came from a pulp and paper mill and were inoculated with sludge from a batch anaerobic reactor. There have been many reports of adsorbable organic halogen (AOX) reduction using a variety of micro-organisms; sample results are: a combination of aerobic and anaerobic treatments can achieve 65 per cent removal; treatment of bleach pulp effluents by *Phaenerochaete chrysosporium* achieves 40–60 per cent reduction; *Trametes versicolor*, 52–59 per cent; *Ceriporiopsis subvermispora*, 32 per cent; *Saccharomyces cerevisiae*, 64 per cent; and a mixture of thermophilic aerobic and anaerobic microbes, 36–56 per cent.

Bleach plant effluents from the pulp and paper industry are highly coloured and also partly toxic as a result of the presence of chloroorganics. Several micro-organisms have been used for removing colour from bleach effluent. A few promising ones are immobilised *P. chrysosporium* (50 per cent colour removal in 3 to 6 hrs) and *T. versicolor* (71 per cent colour removal in 16 hrs), and alginate-immobilised *C. versicolour* (60 per cent colour removal in 30 hrs) and *Rhizomucor pusillus* (90 per cent colour adsorbed in 3 hrs). It is reported that chlorinated phenols and adsorbable chlororganics were first adsorbed onto the fungal biomass followed by breakdown, leading to colour removal.

Table 14.7. Anaerobic treatment of waste from a pulp and paper mill.

	Black liquor	*Bleach effluent*
	Initial conditions	
COD, mg/l	24,500	2500
Total solids	31.5	3.1 g/l
	After inoculation, pH 7 at 37°C	
COD reduction, %	43	31
Methane production increase, %	33	27
	After addition of 1% w:v glucose	
COD reductions, %	71	66
Adsorbable organic halide reduction, %	73	73

Bioreactors

A moving bed biofilm reactor (MBBR) is a completely mixed, continuously operated system in which the biomass is grown on small carrier elements and circulated in the liquid. In an anaerobic or anoxic reactor, mechanical agitation is used to circulate these elements; in an aerobic reactor, aeration is used. No sludge is recycled here. Generally the carrier elements have a high biofilm growth area, are cylindrical in shape, and are made of polyethylene.

Thermophilic aerobic treatment of thermomechanical pulp white water in such a reactor led to about a 65 per cent reduction in soluble COD at a temperature of 55°C. The biodegradation was carried out with the addition of nitrogen- and phosphorous-containing nutrients. The removal rate at thermophilic conditions (55°C) was 1.1 to 1.8 kg when compared with 0.18 to 0.2 soluble COD (SCOD)/kg volatile suspended solids (VSS) day at mesophilic conditions (20° to 40°C), indicating the advantages of carrying out the reaction at thermophilic conditions. No difference in sludge yield is observed at these temperature conditions. Fibreboard manufacturing produces considerable amounts of waste-water, ranging from 3 to 15 m^3 waste-water per tonne of board produced for medium density fibreboard and wet process fibreboard, respectively, with almost 40 g COD/l, a pH of 3.0, and the presence of phenolic and tannin compounds. Such effluent has been treated in an upflow anaerobic sludge blanket (UASB) reactor at high organic loading rates (OLR), achieving COD removal efficiencies of 90 per cent and phenolics removal of 90 per cent.

A hybrid upflow sludge bed filter (USBF) anaerobic reactor consists of a UASB with a packed section located above the top of the sludge bed (Fig. 14.11). PVC corrugated rings were used as packing material in the anaerobic filter zone. Waste-water from a fibreboard manufacturing plant was treated in such a reactor, achieving COD removal efficiencies of about 90 per cent OLR, 6.5 to 8.5 kg COD/m^3 day. Eighty per cent of the COD fraction was convened into methane. The total suspended solids (TSS) removal efficiency was 54 per cent; COD and colour removal efficiencies of 10 per cent were achieved by adding 10 mg/l of neutral polyelectrolyte in the pretreatment section.

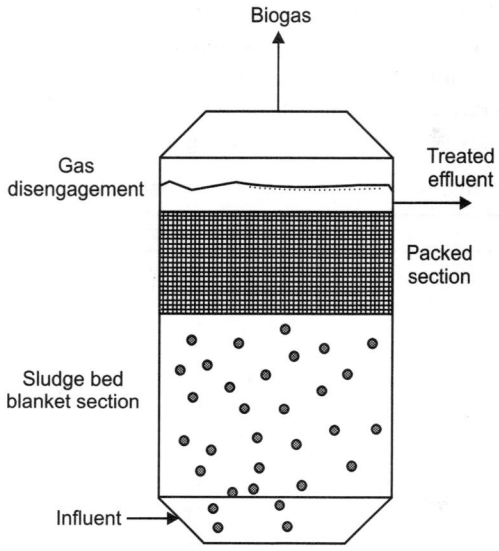

Fig. 14.11. Hybrid upflow sludge bed filter (USBF) anaerobic reactor.

Black alkaline liquor from kraft pulp mills is generally treated in activated sludge plants and aerated lagoons. Anaerobic treatment of this effluent was successfully carried out achieving a COD removal efficiency on the order of 86 per cent and a methane production efficiency of 36.9 mmol/ml at a hydraulic loading rate (HLR) of 0.60 per day. Yeast extract, ammonium chloride, and monobasic anhydrous sodium phosphate were added to supply the recommended amount of nitrogen and phosphorus, and ethanol was added as an additional carbon source. The conventional activated sludge process for the treatment of waste-water is not suitable for high organic loading and shows bulking problems during the summer months as a result of low dissolved oxygen content. Anaerobic upflow filters operated at mesophilic (35°C) and thermophilic (55°C) temperatures lead to a 75 and 90 per cent decrease in the SCOD of a simulated paper mill waste-water at an HRT of 25 hrs at an OLR of 2 g/l. The methane content of the biogas produced by the mesophilic digester was higher (85 per cent) than that produced by the thermophilic digester (81 per cent).

Effluents from a hardwood-based bleached kraft mill (BOD, COD, and adsorbable organic halogen of 200 to 300, 500 to 600, and 5 to 10 mg/l, respectively) that were treated in a sequencing batch reactor reached COD removal efficiencies of 75 per cent at 35°C, and the efficiencies decreased with increase in temperature. AOX removal decreased with increasing temperatures (from 70 to 60 per cent). The SBR was operated in four cycles of fill, aeration, settle, and withdrawal with a total cycle time of 8 hrs. BOD, COD, and AOX removal efficiencies of 99, 85, and 75 per cent, respectively, were obtained when the same effluent was treated in an activated sludge reactor operated with 38 hrs of hydraulic retention time and 10 to 15 days of solid's retention time.

An anaerobic baffled reactor (ABR) consists of a series of vertical baffles that force the waste-water to flow under and over them; therefore, the waste-water comes into contact with a large active biological mass. This reactor system has several advantages: it is simple in design, requires no gas separation system, and the over- and underflow of liquid reduces bacterial washout and enables it to retain active biological solids without the use of any fixed media. Diluted black liquor mixed with digested sewage sludge in the ratio of 3:1 (v:v) having a resultant soluble COD of 2 g/l was treated in an ABR to achieve a COD reduction of 60 per cent and a methane yield of 0.147 m^3/kg COD removed at an HRT of 2 days.

Calcium carbonate is used in the coating process, which leads to high concentrations of calcium ions in the waste-water of paper making industries. Accumulation of calcium scale in a UASB reactor can significantly decrease granule activity. Pretreatment for removal of calcium hardness includes a softening process that uses lime soda or fluidised sand-coated calcium carbonate. Another novel approach was to couple a CO_2 stripper to a UASB; the former helped in the removal of Ca ions in the form of calcium carbonate, preventing it from accumulating in the reactor and causing clogging. When a UASB and a CO_2 stripper were combined to treat a synthetic effluent containing 5000 mg/l calcium hardness and 3000 mg/l COD, 60 per cent calcium and 90 per cent COD removals were achieved. In the absence of the CO_2 stripper, the COD removal efficiency dropped down to 70 per cent.

Treatment of bleach plant effluent using *Coriolus versicolor*, a white rot fungus and *Rhizomucor pusillus* strain RM7, a mucoralean fungus in an aerobic rotating biological contactor showed 58 and 68 per cent decolourisation, respectively. Addition of glucose stimulated colour removal by *C. versicolor*, but not with *R. pusillus*. In addition, *C. versicolor* removed 55 per cent of AOX and 70 per cent COD compared with 40 and 59 per cent, respectively, by *R. pusillus*. It appeared that definite differences exist between the decolouring mechanisms of the white rot fungus and the mucoralean fungus; the former is based on adsorption and biodegradation while the latter is only adsorption.

In the Mycor process (called FPL/NCSU Mycor method), *P. chrysosporium* is immobilised on the surface of rotating disks to achieve 80 per cent colour removal and convert 70 per cent of organic-bound chlorine to chloride at an HRT of 2 days.

SUGAR AND DISTILLERY

Sugar can be produced from sugarcane or sugar beets. In Europe, sugar is extracted from sugar beets while in India, other Asian countries, South America and the Caribbean, sugar is mainly extracted from sugarcane.

The average sugar content of sugar beets is 18 per cent, but it varies greatly in sugarcane. The processing of both sugarcane and sugar beets is seasonal (campaign operation).

In recent years, the amount of waste-water of sugar beets, has been greatly reduced from 18 m^3 to approximately 0.8 m^3/T, by water-saving methods and by extensive sealing of water circuits. In modern plants, the water derives almost exclusively from the sugar beets themselves (sugar beets have approximately 0.78 m^3 of fruit water per tonne). Sugarcane processing requires still lesser amounts of water, as the water required for cleaning and pulping operations in sugar beet processing is very high.

Sugarcane is one of the most common raw materials used in sugar and ethanol production. The waste-water contains not only a high concentration of organic matter but also a large amount of dark brown pigment called melanoidin.

In sugar mills, the waste generated includes water used as splashes to extract the maximum amount of juice, and those used to cool roller bearings. As such, mill house waste contains high BOD due to the presence of sugar and oil from the machineries. The filter cloths, used for filtering the juice, need occasional cleaning. The wash water thus produced, though small in volume, contains high BOD and suspended solids.

Additional waste originates due to the leakages and spillages of juice, syrup and molasses in different sections, and also due to the handling of molasses. The periodical washings of the floor also contributes a lot to the pollution load. Though these wastes are small in volume and are discharged intermittently, they have a very high BOD.

Alcohol Distillery Effluent

The residue of the distillation process is the spent wash, which is a strong organic effluent. The other wastes from the process include yeast sludge (which is usually mixed with spent wash), floor washes, waste cooling water, and waste from the operations of yeast recovery or by-products recovery processes. About 12 to 16 litres of waste liquid effluent is generated for 1 litre of alcohol. The distillery waste-water, known as spent wash, is characterised by its colour, high temperature, low pH, and high ash content; it contains a high percentage of dissolved organic and inorganic matter (7 to 10 per cent), of which 50 per cent may be reducing sugars and 10 to 11 per cent may be proteins. The metals present in spent wash in milligrams per litre are Fe, 34.8, Mn, 12.7, Zn, 4.61, Cu, 3.65, Cr, 0.64, Cd, 0.48, and Co, 0.08, with the electric conductivity in the range of 15–23 dsm^{-1}. Indian spent wash contains very large amounts of potassium, calcium, chloride, sulphate, and BOD (around 50,000 mg/l) compared with spent wash in other countries. Organic compounds extracted from spent wash using alkaline reagents are humic in nature, similar to those found in the soil excepting that fulvic acid predominates over humic acid. The characteristics of a typical distillery effluent are give, in Table 14.8.

Table 14.8. Typical Indian distillery effluent, pH 4 to 5.5.

Compound	Concentration, mg/l
COD	1,00,000–1,50,000
BOD	35,000–50,000
Total solids	80,000–1,20,000
Total suspended solids	8000–22,000
Total volatile suspended solids	6000–22,000
Total dissolved solids	90,000–95,000
Chloride	900–3400
Total phosphorus	30–40
Sulphate as SO$_4$	1100–18,000
Nitrogen oxide	60–90
Potassium	52–62

Normally 200 per cent oxygen must be fed into the effluent to meet the oxygen demand, or, put another way, the total oxygen input required is 93.30 kg/m^3. In practice, the best of the best conventional aeration systems gives 1 kg to a maximum of 1.2 kg of O$_2$. The total energy required for this process would be 93.30 kWh/m^3.

Distillery Waste

Biological treatment of distillery effluent

Biological treatment of distillery effleunts are:

1. Anaerobic, methanogenic digestion of slops, followed by aerobic digestion.
2. Evaporation of slops, followed by aerobic composting using a cellulosic carrier material.
3. Evaporation of slops, followed by incineration of the concentrate, with or without generation of steam, along with gas cleaning.
4. Evaporation of slops, so the concentrate can be used as an additive for cattle feed.
5. Disposal of slops into the deep sea after some treatment.

The distillery wastes comprise two streams:

1. Heavy yeast residuals from fermentation tanks are separated. The waste-waters from this tank account for about 7–10 per cent of the fermentation tank capacity. The yeast sludge from the fermentation tank is a source of strong waste in distillery.
2. This comprises distillery spentwash from the distillation column. For each one litre of alcohol produced from 3–10 kg of mollasses, 10–15 litres of spentwash is produced. After including cooling and condenser water, the total volume of spentwash is 60–100 litres for every litre of alcohol produced.

Distillery wastes are variable in strength and composition. Hence, treatability also is variable.

It requires a series of biological and other treatment to bring down the effluent BOD from 40,000 mg l^{-1} (for batch process) and 1,00,000 mg l^{-1} (for continuous process) to minimal national standards (MINAS) levels of disposal. Anaerobic treatment is adopted by many in a successful way. Composting pressmud from the sugarcane industry with spentwash without allowing percolation of spentwash is still another way followed by some distilleries. Distillery waste-water is having a high BOD/COD contents and with biodegradable matter, is suitable for biotreatment. There are various options available for treatment which are generally used in combination rather than using them alone since BOD/COD reduction required is quite high. Various biotreatment routes are:

1. By-product recovery—animal feed.
2. By-product recovery—fertiliser.
3. Aerobic treatment.
4. Anaerobic digester stage—aerated tank or lagoon.
5. Fixed film biomethanisation.
6. Anaerobic digester—aerobic stage—aquaculture.
7. Anaerobic digester—aerobic stage—aerobic composting or vermiculture or irrigation or root zone treatment.

Heavy yeast residues of the fermentation tank can be used as poultry and cattlefeed. Animal feed can also be derived from spentwash by evaporation and concentration but due to its high inorganic contents, it has a laxative effect. Production of fertiliser from spentwash by evaporation and incineration has been tried but not a field scale yet.

Aerobic treatment—Considerable difficulty has been reported in using the activated sludge process to high strength distillery wastes. Even with the careful balancing of flows and pH between 7.2 to 7.5, only 33 per cent reduction in COD could be achieved, also there is difficulty in maintaining a satisfactory sludge and in controlling foam. High rate biological filtration using plastic media is applicable to an entire range of distillery effluents but multistage filtration is necessary to achieve high removal rates.

Biological treatment, including anaerobic stage followed by aerobic stage, is often used. Anaerobic digester causing 90 per cent BOD reduction and methane collection may be used or anaerobic lagoons with same BOD reduction but no methane gas collection is used. Production of H_2S impairs anaerobic digestion but can be overcome by the addition of iron salts. The effluent after anaerobic treatment still has a high BOD, so further 90 per cent BOD reduction is achieved in aerated tanks (or lagoons) with a detention time of 20–28 days or 1:1 dilution and 15 days detention. Trickling filter, activated sludge, aerobic waste stabilisation ponds may be used for aerobic treatment of predigested wastes. Raw spentwash of BOD 45,000–50,000 mg l^{-1} and COD 90,000 to 1,10,000 mg l^{-1} after anaerobic treatment will have a BOD 6000–10,000 mg l^{-1} and COD 30,000–40,000 mg l^{-1}. It will also have a characteristic dark colour and odour (H_2S). Technically, it is possible to reduce BOD to final level of 100–250 mg l^{-1} by 2 or 3 aerobic stages.

This process takes place in an anaerobic digester packed with plastic media which provide about 230 sq.m. of surface area per cu. m., enabling compact digester design. The digester is initially seeded with suitable micro-organisms which proliferate and form fixed film on the plastic media. This fixation of micro-organisms ensures safety of operation and high degree organic loading. Treatment reduces, BOD by 90 per cent and COD by 65–70 per cent and biogas is produced. Retention time is short, i.e. 7–8 days and 530 m^3 biogas is produced for each tonne of COD reduced. Biogas can substitute fuel requirements of plant by 100 per cent.

Molasses contains appreciable amounts of calcium salts, which cause deposition and scaling of heat exchangers. Since the conventional aerobic processes for primary treatment of distillery waste are not cost effective and require large land areas, the main emphasis has been on anaerobic processes, since they have the dual advantages of pollution control and fuel production. A general estimate suggests that the cost of an anaerobic biological digester is recovered within 2 to 3 years of installation as a result of substantial savings of coal and other fuels.

It is estimated that these distilleries have the potential to generate a total of $560 \times 10^6 \, m^3$ per annum of biogas if all of them would opt for anaerobic digestion. Assuming the calorific value of biogas as 5300 kcal/m^3, this amounts to 830 Gigawatt hour/annum and translates to 158 MW of power. Anaerobic digestion also reduces by a considerable amount the sludge that is produced when compared to that produced by the aerobic process.

The anaerobic processes have a few disadvantages. The process is slow because the rates of reaction and synthesis are low, long startup periods are required, and further treatment becomes inevitable since the reduction in COD achieved is only on the order of 85 per cent. Generally industries have resorted to a subsequent aerobic digestion or biocomposting. The effluent also has a caramel colour that is found to contaminate the groundwater. A number of process packages on biomethanation of distillery spent wash have been developed by international consultants.

Indistilleries primary spent wash is generally put through an anaerobic digestion step to utilise its high COD load to produce methane. The secondary spent wash produced by the anaerobically digested primary molasses spent wash (DMSW) effluent is darker in colour and needs huge volumes of water to dilute it; currently its use as irrigation water is causing gradual soil darkening (Fig. 14.12). Its disposal into natural bodies of water may result in their eutrophication. The colour leads to a reduction of sunlight penetrating the rivers, lakes, or lagoons, which in turn decreases both photosynthetic activity and dissolved oxygen concentrations, causing harm to aquatic life.

Disposal on land is also hazardous, causing a reduction in soil alkalinity and manganese availability, inhibition of seed germination, and the ruin of vegetation. The decolourisation of molasses spent wash by physical or chemical methods and subsequently directly applied as a fertiliser has also been attempted and found to be unsuitable. Anaerobic treatment of distillery waste-water has been tried in pilot and full-scale operations. Some of these are hybrid, fixed film, and continuous stirred reactors. Since it is highly acidic and hot, the effluent invariably needs pretreatment for pH and temperature. Also lime scrubbing of the biogas is needed for H_2S removal before it can be used for power generation.

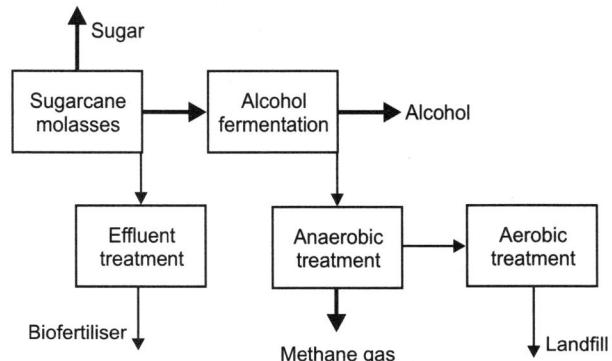

Fig. 14.12. Typical process flow for sugarcane and distillery waste.

Micro-organisms

Several micro-organisms have been reported as suitable for treating and decolourising the waste-water generated from a molasses plant. They include *Aspergillus fumigatus. Coriolus versicolor, Phanerochaete chrysospotium*, and the filamentous fungi. Anaerobic digestion studies carried out by Sirianuntapiboon with an acetogenic bacteria strain No.BP103 showed a 76 per cent decolourisation yield when cultivated at 30°C for 5 days in a molasses pigment medium. In addition, this strain could decolourise 32 and 73 per cent of molasses pigments in stillage and anaerobically treated molasses waste-water, respectively, when supplemented with nutrients.

When alcohol distillery waste-water (cane molasses vinasse) was treated in a UASB reactor under thermophilic conditions (55°C) at an influent concentration of 10 gram COD/l, the BOD removal was good (80 per cent), but the COD removal was low (39 to 67 per cent). The poor COD elimination was attributed to the low degradability of the waste itself. Phenolic compounds present in vinasse, which are produced through oxidation and cause a dark brown colour, are refractory as well as toxic for methanogens. The researchers observed more of *Methanosarcina*-like coccoids and very little of *Methanothrix*-like bamboo-shaped rods, which is more sensitive to toxic compounds. The temperature optimum for the former is 50° to 58°C and for the latter 60° to 65°C; hence operating at the elevated temperature would favour methane generation. *Methanothrix* in granular sludge is most essential for the establishment of a high performance UASB process. High concentrations of bivalent cations, such as Mg^{2+} and Ca^{2+}, induced development of single cells of the *Methanosarcina* species, which are more easily washed out from the UASB reactor than large clumps or packets. Romero reported that during anaerobic treatment of alcohol effluents COD removal is low while BOD removal is high.

Effluent from a malt whisky manufacturing plant has been treated anaerobically in different reactor configurations including UASB, upflow anaerobic filter, and batch stirred reactor. Overall COD and BOD removal efficiencies of greater than 98 per cent were achieved for effluent from a malt whisky manufacturer in a UASB reactor followed by a batch aerobic reactor. An aerobic jet loop reactor with hydraulic retention times that varied from 2.1 to 4.4 days was able to achieve about 98 per cent degradation of the effluent from a winery. *Pseudomonas*, *Saccharomyces cerevisiae*, and yeast-like fungi, such as *Trichosporon capitatum* and *Geotrichum peniculatum*, were present in the activated sludge. The white-rot fungi namely, *Coriolus versicolor* and *Phanerochaete chrysosporium* could achieve 54 and 38 per cent decolourisation efficiencies, respectively, and 60 and 49 per cent reductions in COD, respectively, in 10 days. The major shortcomings of the process were the need to add extra carbon and the effluent needed to be diluted. Smith carried out chemical decolourisation of anaerobically treated distillery effluent using chemical and biological methods. Maximum decolourisation and COD reduction of 98 and 88 per cent, respectively, were achieved by treatment with hydrogen peroxide and calcium oxide.

LEATHER AND TANNERY

Tannery waste may be classified as continuous and intermittent flow waste. Continuous flow wastes consist of wash waters after various processes and comprise a large portion of the total waste, which are relatively less polluted. Spent liquors belonging to soaking, liming, bating, pickling, tanning and finishing operations are discharged intermittently. Although these are relatively small in volume, they are highly polluted and contain varieties of soluble organic and inorganic substances.

Conversion of rawhide into leather (an unalterable and imputrescible product) requires several mechanical and chemical operations involving many chemicals in an aqueous medium, including acids, alkalies, chromium salts, tannins, solvents, auxiliaries, surfactants, acids, and metallorganic dyes; natural or synthetic tanning agents; sulphonated oils, and salts. The quantity of effluent generated is about 30 litres for every kilogram of hide or skin processed. Tannery effluents can be divided into three types based on the operations carried out in the three different sections (Fig. 14.13):

1. Unhairing and liming waste-water with high sulphide and lime content and high pH [accounts for 45 per cent of the effluent volume and contributes to 30 per cent of the overall biological oxygen demand (BOD) and chemical oxygen demand (COD)].
2. Tanning waste-water with high salinity and high chrome levels.
3. Retanning, dyeing, and fat liquoring waste-water (accounts for ~20 per cent of the total COD).

The first area of operations is the beam house in which the raw hides and skins are cleaned and prepared so that the hides are more pliable, attractive, and useful. The operations include siding, trimming, washing, soaking, fleshing, and unhairing. The last operation involves treatment with lime and sodium sulphide as the primary chemicals to dissolve the hair. These waste-waters are highly alkaline (pH of 10 to 12). Raw leather is made up of three main layers. The upper layer (epidermis) contains hair, glands, muscles, etc.

The middle layer (corium), which is useful and constitutes the leather product, is made to react with the tanning agent, while the bottom layer is removed by mechanical means. Removal of the upper layer is carried out through liming and bating processes. The skin is rehydrated by soaking and removing the globular proteins. Hair is removed from the skin by the reductive liming process. Two important processes take place during this step—hydrolysis and chemical reduction of keratin. Hydrolysis occurs in an alkaline medium, and lime acts as a buffer, maintaining the pH around 12.5. While globular proteins are easily solubilised, keratin and collagen are resistant to hydrolysis. Reduction of keratin is achieved by the use of alkali sulphide salts. Elastin, another strong fibrous protein that is not soluble under the conditions of liming, is removed using enzymes (the bating process). Pickling is another pretanning step where some globular proteins are removed with the aid of pretanning agents.

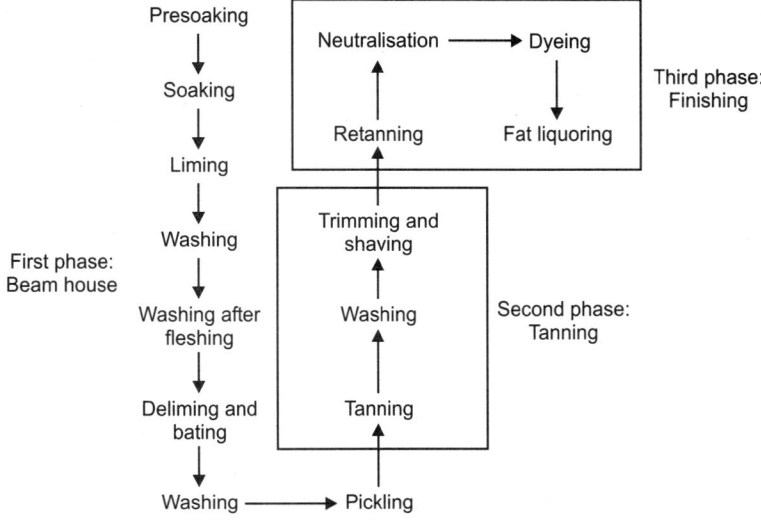

Fig. 14.13. Various steps in conversion of hide to leather.

The second area of operations is the tanyard in which a durable material is produced from the animal hides or skins. The proteinaceous matter in the hides is made to react with the tanning agent for stabilisation. This is accomplished by using synthetic tanning agents containing trivalent chromium salts, aluminium, zirconium, etc. or using vegetable tannins extracted from the bark of certain trees; 90 per cent of tanning is done using the former. These operations are carried out in an acidic medium, and the waste-water generated usually has a pH in the range of 2.5 to 3.5. The tanning process stabilises the skin structure by forming transverse bonds among its fibres.

In the case of mineral tanning agents, the tanning agent blocks the carboxylic groups (or in the case of vegetable tanning agents, the amine groups) and joins the proteinaceous colloid, thus increasing the cross-linking of the collagen fibres. The resulting stabilised leather material cannot be degraded by physical or biological means. Of the tanning agents added, 15 per cent does not get fixed to the leather and is discharged with the effluent.

The third set of process operations involve retanning and wet finishing, which gives the tanned hides special or desired features such as bleached appearance, added colouring, lubrication, or further tanning for finished leather properties. These operations usually do not alter the pH of the waste-waters. Solid waste is generated, including trimmings, degraded hide, and hair from the beam house, amounting to 70 per cent of the wet weight of the original hide.

The tannery waste-water has a very high salinity. The main contributors are 30 per cent chlorides from the pickling bath (where skins are prepared with salts and acids prior to adding tanning agent) and 60 per cent sulphates from the tanning bath. Hydrogen sulphide is released during dehairing, and ammonia is released during deliming. Characteristics of the effluent released from a tannery producing full chrome upper leather from dry salted bovine hides is given in Table 14.9; the effluent from an industrial district housing several tanneries is given in Table 14.10.

Nitrogen exists in leather tanning waste-waters as ammonia and organic nitrogen and is present in both particulate and soluble forms. All nitrogen originating from the bovine leather processing plant is from soaking, liming, deliming, bating, pickling, and tanning, and the washings from these processes, and the total nitrogen in the effluent is below 1 per cent. The main source of nitrogen is from the liming step (~7390 mg/l), followed by deliming, bating, washing, and pickling steps. The main source for protein in the effluent comes from the liming step (~13,660 mg/l), followed by the washing, deliming, and bating steps.

Table 14.9. Characteristics of effluent released by a tannery treating bovine hide.

pH	7.5–9.0
SS	1500–4000 mg/l
TS	29,000–45,000 mg/l
Chromium	100 mg/l
COD	5000–10,000 mg/l
BOD	1500–2000 mg/l

Table 14.10. Waste-water characteristics of tannery effluent.

Characteristic, mg/l	Raw waste-water	Clarifier effluent
Total COD	5094	2216
Soluble COD	2336	1187
BOD_5	1760	958
SS	2229	794
VSS	–	506
Total nitrogen	358	226
Organic nitrogen	223	62
NH_3–N	135	164
Total phosphorus	–	5.1
Total chromium (Cr^{3+})	116	41
Sulphur	51	27

Biochemical Treatment

Aerobic

A combination of biochemical oxidation and chemical ozonation of tannery effluent has been found to yield excellent results, with the first part performed in an upflow sequencing batch biofilm reactor provided with external recycle. COD, NH_4–N, and total suspended solids (TSS) removals were 95, 98, and 99.9 per cent, respectively. The combined process produced very low sludge, about 0.03 kg TSS/kg COD removed, which is much lower than the values reported in the literature for conventional biological systems. Ozone helped in the mineralisation of some organic substances and the partial oxidation of some others, leading to enhancement of the biodegradability of the effluent. The aerobic treatment of the beam house and tanyard waste-water substreams, followed by an oxidative treatment using ozone, and a second aerobic treatment improved the aerobic biodegradability of refractory organic compounds. Also, full nitrification was achieved during the subsequent aerobic degradation, and the remaining ammonia was completely removed.

A membrane sequencing batch reactor performed better than a sequencing batch reactor in treating beam house waste-water that was collected after the oxidation of sulphide compounds. The former reactor achieved a removal efficiency of 100 per cent for ammonium ion and 90 per cent for COD, and the latter reactor achieved low ammonium removal and 90 per cent for COD. The sequential batch reactor exhibited a washout in 90 days, whereas the membrane bioreactor was very stable for more than 120 days of operation.

A settled vegetable-tanning process effluent was treated successfully in a mixed continuous-flow laboratory-scale plant. The BOD and COD removal efficiencies were 85 to 96 per cent and 86 to 97 per cent, respectively, under steady-state conditions. Activated-sludge treatment of chrome-tanning waste mixed with sewage was able to remove 87 to 96 per cent of BOD under steady state conditions. About 84 to 92 per cent of the influent BOD was removed from a tannery effluent when it was treated in an activated sludge well mixed reactor.

A comparative study of tannery waste treatment was done using an upflow anaerobic sludge blanket reactor (UASB) and activated sludge (AS) reactor; interestingly, the latter was found to have more advantages than the former with respect to the capital and operating costs as well as the quality of performance. The treated UASB effluent had higher BOD and COD and considerable amounts of chromium and sulphide when compared with the AS reactor effluent.

Anaerobic treatment

Although the anaerobic treatment of tannery beam house waste-water looks attractive, the presence of sulphide, namely hydrogen sulphide, inhibits methanogenic bacteria. Undissociated H_2S is toxic, since it diffuses 'freely' through the cell membrane, denatures proteins and enzymes (sulphide cross-linking), and affects internal cell pH. In a continuous-flow fixed-film reactor, a concentration of 100 mg/l of undissociated sulphide inhibited the efficiency and degree of degradation, which was eliminated by incorporating a sulphide stripping system that reduced the concentration of undissociated sulphide to 30 mg/l. This modification improved the efficiency of the degradation by 15 per cent.

Acidogenic bacteria were not inhibited by hydrogen sulphide. A combined anaerobic and aerobic treatment of tannery waste-water effluent containing 900 mg/l organic carbon content (DOC) gave a removal efficiency of 85 per cent. Under anaerobic conditions, sulphate is convened by sulphate-reducing bacteria (SRB) into sulphide, which is not only a toxic compound but also a strong inhibitor of methanogenesis.

Also, SRB compete with methane producing bacteria (MPB) for substrates such as hydrogen and acetate and with syntrophic acetogenic bacteria (SAB) for intermediate substrates such as short-chain volatile fatty acids (VFA) and alcohols. This results in a reduction of organics available for conversion to methane. So it is advisable to remove the sulphide either before the anaerobic treatment or as part of the biotreatment cycle as shown in Fig. 14.14.

A combination of the sulphur recovery unit integrated with a USAB reactor for treating tannery effluent led to improved biogas production and also recovery of elemental sulphur. The sulphur removal unit consisted of a stripper column, absorber column, regeneration unit, and sulphur separator. A stripper efficiency of about 65 to 95 per cent in terms of sulphide removal was achieved.

The efficiency of degradation in a continuous flow fixed film reactor improved by 15 per cent when the concentration of undissociated sulphide was reduced from 100 to 30 mg/l with the help of a continuous sulphide removal system.

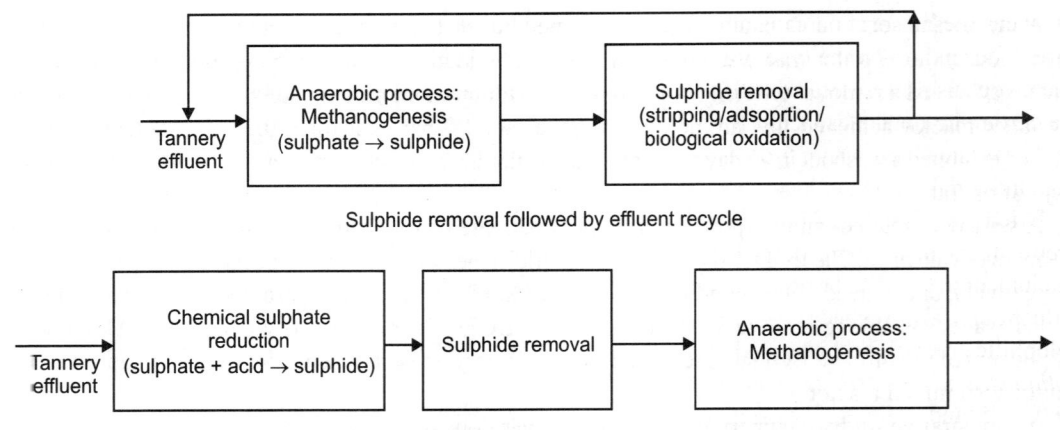

Fig. 14.14. Sulphide handling.

Chromium

Chromium is an important heavy metal used in the leather, electroplating and metallurgical industries. The moisture content of the dewatered sludge from sludge drying beds ranges from 50 to 70 per cent and the concentration of chromium as Cr ranges from 1 to 3 per cent on a dry solid weight basis. The disposal of such large quantities of hazardous solid chromium waste poses serious environmental and health problem. The earliest technique practiced for the disposal of chromium sludge consisted of solidification of the waste with cement and organic clay.

The acidic ion exchange resins Amberlite IRC 76 and Amberlite IRC 718 retained 95 per cent of the chromium at pH 5. Extraction using supported liquid membranes, chemical methods such as reduction by sodium metabisulphite, ferrous ions, zero valent iron, and a mixture of dimethyl dithiocarbamate, ferrous sulphate, and aluminium chloride have also been tested. The last method is also practiced commercially.

Several heterotrophs and coliforms were tolerant to a chromate level of greater than 50 g/ml, and many coliforms were resistant to higher levels of chromate too, whereas only a few heterotrophs were resistant to Cr^{6+} at a level of greater than 150 g/ml. A few important microbes involved in the reduction of chromium are *Pseudomonas aeruginosa*, *Enterobacter cloacae*, and *P. fluorescens*. *Desulfovibrio desulfuricans* immobilised on a polyacrylamide gel reduced 80 per cent of 0.5 M Cr (VI) with lactate or H_2 as the electron donor and Cr(VI) as the electron acceptor.

NCIM 5080 and NCIM 5109 actinomycetes strains have been found to reduce chromium levels by 99 per cent within 24 hrs and at the same time reducing 70 to 80 per cent of the COD in 74 to 96 hrs. Two strains, *Bacillus circulans* and *B. megaterium*, were able to bioaccumulate 34.5 and 32.0 mg Cr per gram of dry weight, respectively, and decrease Cr(VI) concentration from 50 mg/l to less than 0.1 mg/l in 24 hrs. Living and dead cells of *B. coagulans* biosorbed 23.8 and 39.9 mg Cr per gram of dry weight, respectively, and living and dead cells of *B. megaterium* biosorbed 15.7 and 30.7 mg Cr per gram of dry weight, respectively.

Biosorption by the dead cells was higher than that of the living cells due to pH conditioning of the dead cells. Microbes that were able to biosorb chromium include *Osciilatoria* sp., *Arthrobacter* sp.; *Agrobacterium* sp., *Pseudomonas aeruginosa* 5128, and sulphate-reducing bacteria. Pretreatment enhances the biosorption capacity as seen in the case of dead *Rhizopus nigricans*. Chromium uptake varied, depending on the type of pretreatment at pH of 2.0. Biosorbent efficiency decreased when the micro-organisms were treated with mild alkali, while treatment with acids, alcohols, and acetone improved the chromium uptake capacity.

The waste *Mucor meihi* biomass was found to be an effective biosorbent for the removal of chromium from industrial tanning effluents, reaching sorption levels of 1.15 mmol/g.

Dried and classified *Pinus sylvestris* bark was able to remove 90 per cent of trivalent chromium. Pretreatment of the bark helped to increase its chromium sorption capacity. A column packed with calcium alginate (CA) beads with humic acid could adsorb 54 per cent of the chromium from a tannery effluent and also reduce its ecotoxicity in 72 hrs of operation. *Dunaliella*, a unicellular biflagellate halophilic green algae, biosorbed 45 to 58 mg/g Cr(VI). The green algae *Carlina vulgaris*, *Scenedesmus obliquus*, *Synechocystis* sp., *Cladonia crispata*, and *Spirogyra* sp., had maximum uptakes of 33.8, 30.2, 39.0, 39.5, and 14.7 mg/g, respectively. Fungal species of *Mucor meihi*, *Rhizopus nigricans*, *R. arrhizus*, and *Aspergillus niger* biosorbed 59.8, 119.7, 58.1, and 15.6 mg Cr/g, respectively. A strain of *Streptomyces griseus* was found to grow in glucose/sodium acetate medium and reduce Cr^{6+} to Cr^{3+}.

Figure 14.15 lists the various physical, chemical, and biochemical methods that have been tried for treating tannery effluents. Several issues such as the cost of physical and chemical methods, the toxicity of chromium on biochemical methods, and the inhibitory nature of sulphides in the anaerobic degradation process have not been fully resolved. The reduction and recycle of the various streams at the source appears to be a good approach to dramatically decrease the present quality and quantity of effluent generated by this industry. Disposal of the sludge after biochemical treatment, however, has not been satisfactorily solved.

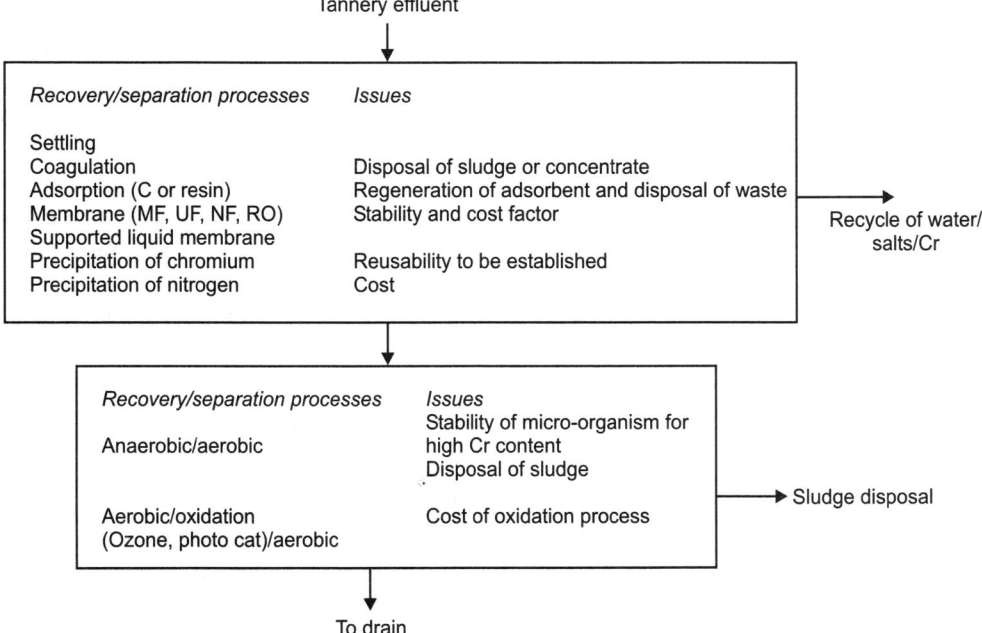

Fig. 14.15. Physical, chemical, and biochemical treatment techniques for tannery effluent.

PAINT AND DYES

Paint

A typical paint and coatings manufacturing operation involves formulation, milling, or grinding of pigments, mixing, filtering, filling, and equipment cleaning. The production process for a liquid paint starts with the dispersion of pigments, solvents, resins, and additives in a mill such as ball or bead mill, or a high-speed disperser. Diluents, resins, bactericides, fungicides, etc. are added to the dispersion mill effluent in a process known as letdown. When the formulation achieves the desired properties, mixing is stopped, the paint is filtered, and the final product is stored in cans for shipment. Paint manufacture requires several hundred raw materials, which include antifoams, defoamers, dispersants, surfactants, driers, antiskinning agents, extenders, fillers, pigments, flame or fire retardants, flatting agents, latex emulsions, oils, preservatives, bactericides, fungicides, resins, rheological and viscosity control agents, silicone additives, titanium dioxides, and colours.

The major waste generated by the paint manufacturing industry are empty raw material packages containing trace elements, equipment cleaning wastes and spills. Empty raw material packages are generated during unloading of materials to high speed mixers or mixing tanks. Water solvents are generated from equipment cleaning. Even after distillation of waste solvents for reuse, a residual paint sludge remains. The paint sludge contains solvents and residual toxic metals such as mercury, lead and chromium. Waste rinse water is generated from equipment cleaning with water and for caustic solutions. Wastes containing undispersed pigments are contained in waste filter cartridges.

The equipment cleaning wastes can be minimised by employing more efficient cleaning methods, like reduction in the frequency of equipment cleaning, use of rubber wipers to reduce the amount of paint left on the walls of a mix tank, use of teflon-lined tanks to reduce adhesion and use of plastic or foam to clean pipes to improve drainage. Pigment waste from bags and packages may be reduced by using water soluble bags. Paste pigments, which are wetted or mixed with resins, may be used in place of dry powder pigments that cause particulate or dust emissions. Bag filters or metal mesh filters may be used instead of cartridge filters. The most effective way of reducing wastes associated with bags and packages is to segregate hazardous materials from non-hazardous materials.

For example, empty bags and packages containing residual amounts of hazardous materials should be stored in plastic bags to eliminate dusting, which can cause contamination of non-hazardous materials. By installing a separate dedicated bag house for each production step, the collected pigment dust or resin dust can be recycled to the process step.

Generation of waste-water at source should also be practiced. This is to reduce the effluent load rather than finding methods to treat it. Good housekeeping can reduce generation of both waste-water and solid-wastes and spills and rejects can be reduced by increased automation. Obsolete products and rejects can also be blended into new batches of paint.

Types of pollutants

A variety of hazardous solid, liquid, and gaseous wastes is generated during the manufacturing operation. Solid waste is generated from used containers, spent filters, dried paints, pallets, and packaging materials. Equipment cleaning, spillage, and off-spec materials generate liquid waste. The various operations also lead to discharge of pollutants into the atmosphere. For example: (i) many raw materials used to manufacture paint are volatile organic compounds (VOCs) and evaporate readily in the atmosphere when the ingredients are exposed to air, (ii) pigment dust (particulate matter) is generated during the manufacturing process, and (iii) solvents used for cleaning the equipment have high evaporation rates. The industrial and home users of these paints and coatings also generate various types of waste. If these wastes are not properly treated and detoxified, they can enter the environment as shown in Fig. 14.16.

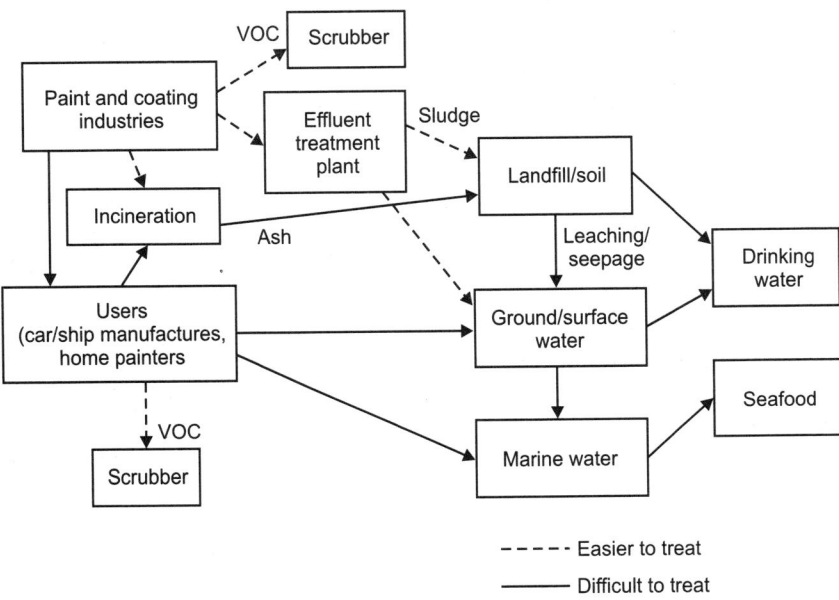

Fig. 14.16. Movement of raw materials used in paint into the environment.

Tributyltin is a herbicide used in paints as an antifouling agent to prevent marine organisms from growing, and it is known for its acute toxicity, imposex (the occurrence of induced male sex characteristics superimposed on normal female gastropods), and bioaccumulation; it causes increased shell thickness and decreases the reproductive capability of various water organisms. It is found in large harbours and dense shipping lanes, as well as in coastal areas with coral reefs and in seafood products. Its use was banned after the year 2003. Diuron and Irgarol herbicides are being used as alternatives for preventing algae growth on the surfaces of boats and ships.

Diuron has been detected in the coastal waters of the Mediterranean Sea in concentrations of more than 2 mg/l (permissible concentration 430 ng/l), and Irgarol 1051 in concentrations of up to a few hundred nanograms per litre has been detected in European, Japanese, and Australian seas. In several locations and at several times, concentrations exceeded the maximum permissible limit of 24 ng/l. The degradation products of Irgarol 1051 are known to exhibit toxicities similar to the original compound. Diuron (in the range of 3 mg/l) and Irgarol were also identified in the Japanese aquatic environment. Diuron around 1 to 40 µg/l has been detected in fresh and groundwater in many western European countries and the United States. Microgram levels of these two herbicides were also detected in the coastal waters of the United Kingdom. A reduction in *Fucus vesiculosus*, a perennial macro alga found in the Baltic Sea, has been observed in the inner parts of the archipelagos along the Swedish coast; this reduction is attributed to pollutants such as copper and Irgarol found in the antifouling paints. Copper-based antifouling paint caused toxic effects on brine shrimp nauplii. The copper released from the paint entered their cells and caused decreased enzymatic activity.

Automobiles get three layers of paint: the primer, the base coat, and the clear coat. The primer is either solvent or powder based, the base coat is waterborne, and the clear coat is also solvent or powder based. Powder based coatings generate the highest VOCs when compared with the other two, namely, 0.06 to 0.12 kg SO_x, 0.06 kg NO_x, and 0.04 kg of particulate matter per kilogram of each coating. Suspended solids (0.01 to 0.03 kg/kg of coating) and metals (about 0.004 kg/kg of coating) contribute primarily to the contamination of waste-water.

Paint solvents contribute about 45 per cent of the VOCs in Seoul, South Korea's atmosphere. Aromatics account for 95 per cent, and the remainder are alkanes. Toluene was the most abundant compound, followed by m- and p-xylene, and then o-xylene. Benzene and styrene contributed less than 1 per cent. All paints, regardless of carrier, use the same basic chemical categories, namely, resins and cross-linkers (binder system), pigments, and modifying additives. Polyurethanes are used in the manufacture of car paint. Once the paint is sprayed on the cars, thermal degradation of the polyurethane occurs, generating many new molecules of isocyanates, which are a result of secondary reactions such as chain breaking, isomerisation, and dehydrogenation. Workers in car paint shops are thus exposed to additional amounts of reacted and unreacted isocyanates contained in the paint formulation.

The lacquers or paints used in the furniture industry contain isopropanol, butanol, butyl and ethyl acetates, toluene, ethylbenzene, xylenes, and aromatic hydrocarbon solvents. The residues contain unknown complex organic mixtures, and they are found to be more toxic than the constituent basic chemicals. Latex paints generally consist of organic and inorganic pigments and dyestuffs, extenders, cellulosic and noncellulosic thickeners, latexes, emulsifying agents, antifoaming agents, preservatives, solvents, and coalescing agents. The waste-water is alkaline and contains high BOD, COD, suspended solids, toxic compounds, and colour. High-quality water with 85 per cent of the COD removed was recovered for recycling purposes from an electrocoat painting bath by reverse osmosis. A typical paint stripping facility would generate effluent consisting of methylene chloride, phenol, and other organic compounds in concentrations of about 5000, 1800 and 2200 mg/l, respectively.

Micro-organisms thrive in water-based paint by consuming oxygen. Once all the oxygen is consumed, anaerobic growth commences; during that process both bacteria and fungi produce cellulase, which breaks down long-chain cellulosic thickening agents, producing small oligomeric residual units. Fermentative bacteria break down the cellulose to glucose and the glucose to acid and carbon dioxide. Under anaerobic conditions, *Desulfovibrio desulfuricans* can use oxygen from sulphates, which generates hydrogen sulphide. Acid production by micro-organisms causes a decrease in pH.

Biochemical treatment

The general waste-water treatment facility for treating the effluent from a paint manufacturing plant consists of an equalisation basin, a primary settling tank, a pH neutralisation tank, an aeration tank, a secondary settling tank, and holding tanks. The BOD, COD, and TSS of the effluent were reduced from 588, 5632 and 2864 to 50, 100 and 100 mg/l, respectively, after the combined chemical and biochemical treatment. The concentrations of metals such as Pb, Cr, Cu, Mn, Ni, Zn, and Fe remained the same in the untreated and the treated effluent. The BOD, COD, and TSS of the effluent could be reduced to 28, 65, and 5 mg/l by coagulation-flocculation (combination alum and polyelectrolyte-anionic poly-acrylamide) and cross-flow microfiltration using a cellulose acetate membrane with pore size 0.2 μm at a pressure drop of 0.3 bar. Sulphuric acid or calcium hydroxide was added to adjust the pH of the waste-water. The microfiltration treatment procedure also removed metals and bacterial contamination from the waste stream.

Paint-stripping waste-water contaminated with phenol was treated in reactors (e.g. activated sludge and rotating biological contactor) that predominantly contained *Pseudomonas* gram-negative bacteria. Gram-positive bacteria occurred less frequently and were solely represented by the genus *Bacillus*. Other genera such as *Acinetobacter, Moraxella, Paracoccus, Acetobacter, Flavobacterium, Klebsiella, Enterobacter*, and *Vibrio* were also found but in fewer numbers. The size of the microbial communities in the continuous flow rotating biological contactor was a maximum of (10^7 bacteria/g, followed by batch and continuous flow activated-studge reactors, and least in fill and draw rotating biological contactor (10^7 bacteria/g) reactors. This difference could be explained by two factors: (i) there is higher concentration of toxic paint stripping chemicals in the batch reactor than in the continuous flow reactors (53 per cent in the former as against 20 per cent in the latter). This happened because of the dilution in the continuous reactor, (ii) continuous-flow waste-water systems favour the attachment of bacteria to surfaces instead of being washed away in the batch reactor. Both activated sludge and rotating biological contactor reactors could effectively degrade paint stripping, effluents mixed with domestic effluents.

Typical volatile compounds from paint preparation include toluene (approximately 25 per cent), methyl ethyl ketone (approximately 23 per cent), *m*- and *p*-xylene (approximately 20 per cent), and other organics such as ethylbenzene, *o*-xylene, *l*-butanol, acetone, ethane, etc. Biofilters are well suited to treating VOCs found at paint spray booths, paint manufacturing plants, or filling stations. Unlike bacterial-based biofilters, fungal-based systems function even better in slightly dry conditions and at low pH. A preadapted compost-based media bed shows good resilience to operating conditions that could easily destroy systems based on bacteria alone. Generally the VOCs are converted to carbon dioxide and water. Although steam is costly, it is effective for media wetting, moisture, and temperature control. An industrial-scale biofilter with multiple layers of compost material supported on plastic spheres with a cross-flow air and water spray humidification system degraded 75 per cent of the VOCs. In large units, maintaining wet conditions and uniform temperature are the two challenges. Capital cost is significantly less than for a thermal oxidiser, and operating costs are less than 10 per cent of a comparably sized regenerative thermal oxidiser. Biofilters neither produce toxic or hazardous products, as in the case of incomplete combustion reactions, nor create NO_x or SO_x as thermal oxidiser technologies do.

A laboratory-scale biofilter packed with cubed polyurethane foam media populated by a mixed culture of fungi was able to degrade 98 per cent of *n*-butyl acetate, methyl ethyl ketone, methyl propyl ketone, and toluene (solvent emissions from industrial painting operations) at a total VOC loading rate of 94.3 g/(m^3 hr). The mixed culture of fungal species predominantly included *Cladosporium sphaerospermum, Penicillium brevicompactum, Exophiala jenselmei, Fusarium oxysporum, F. nygamai, Talaromyces flavus*, and *Fonsecaea pedrosi*. Weekend shutdowns did not affect the performance of the biofilter, and in less than 3 hrs, the VOC removal efficiency reached its original value. The longer the shutdown, the larger the decline in removal efficiency following restart and the longer the reacclimation time required by the biofilter to recover. While removal efficiencies of acetate and ketones recovered in very short time after restart, the removal efficiency for toluene took a few days to reach its original value.

A compost-based lab-scale hybrid bioreactor could achieve more than 80 per cent removal efficiency of a paint VOC mixture consisting of toluene, xylene, methyl propyl ketone, butyl acetate, and ethyl 3-ethoxy-propionate with a total concentration of approximately 100 ppmv at a gas residence time of 46 seconds. Hydrophilic components of the gas stream were degraded completely, while minimum degradation of the hydrophobic components was observed in the bioreactor. Inoculation of a microbial solution cultivated with toluene vapour as the sole carbon source raised the degradation efficiency to 90 per cent. The hybrid bioreactor consisted of a single column divided into two sections; the first was packed with a structured plastic media and was operated as a trickling filter, and the second section was packed with a compost-based material and operated as a biofilter. A buffered solution containing phosphates was continuously recirculated and sprayed from the top of the column. Water and additional nitrogen sources were also added to the packing materials. Air was introduced from the bottom with the VOCs.

To sum up paint contains several hundred chemicals ranging from solvents to toxic chemicals and metals. These chemicals find their way into the environment through different routes. VOCs are generated during the manufacturing process as well as during usage; biofilters appear to be a promising technology for its degradation. Water-based paint industries would like to recycle their waste-water, but the major hurdle here is the microbial contamination of the recycled water and the presence of suspended matter.

Dyes

In the dye industry waste is generated due to synthesis of dye and dye intermediates; steam generation and cooling system; washing and rinsing of reaction kettles, filter press, floors, etc.; domestic and other miscellaneous activities. The water consumption pattern varies from one industry to another. In the same industry, the rate of water consumption often changes due to frequent changes of the feed material synthesis reaction and desired product. The change of product pattern needs cleaning and washing, which consumes a substantial quantity of water. The air pollutants are generated from the reaction vessel. These emissions are scrubbed by water. The other emissions are of fugitive nature and should be controlled by proper modification of plant and maintenance of equipment.

The solid wastes in the dye intermediate industry are generated from filter press from the process house, physico-chemical waste-water treatment plant and the biological waste-water treatment plant.

The treatment of wastes involves:

1. In-plant control: It is essential to have proper in-plant control measures before going for waste-water treatment.
2. Reduction of waste: The volume of waste can be reduced by proper control of fresh water consumption. The pollution load can also be reduced by recovery of chemicals and solvents as far as practicable.
3. Process modification: The production process equipment should be modified so as to generate less wastes.

Dyestuffs can be classified according to their origin, chemical and/or physical properties, or characteristics related to the application process. Another categorisation is based on the applications sector (e.g. inks, disperse dyes, pigments, or vat dyes). A systematic classification of dyes according to chemical structure is the colour index, namely, nitroso, nitro, monoazo, diazo, triazo, polyazo, azoic, stilbene, carotenoid, diphenylmethane, triarylmethane, xanthene, acridine, quinoline, methine, thiazole, indamine/indophenol, azine, oxazine, thiazine, sulphur, lactone, aminoketone, hydroxyketone, anthraquinone, indigoid, phthalocyanine, natural, oxidation base, and inorganic. Synthetic dyes are also classified according to their most predominant chemical structures, namely, polyene and polymethine, diarylmethine, triarylmethine, nitro and nitroso, anthraquinone, and diazo (Fig. 14.17).

Approximately 10,000 different dyes and pigments are manufactured worldwide. There are several structural varieties of dyes, such as acidic, reactive, basic, disperse, azo, diazo, anthraquinone-based, and metal-complex dyes. They all absorb light in the visible region. Untreated dye effluent is highly coloured and hence reduces sunlight penetration, preventing photosynthesis. Many dyes are toxic to fish and mammalian life, inhibit growth of micro-organisms, and affect flora and fauna. They are also carcinogenic in nature and hence can cause intestinal cancer and cerebral abnormalities in fetuses.

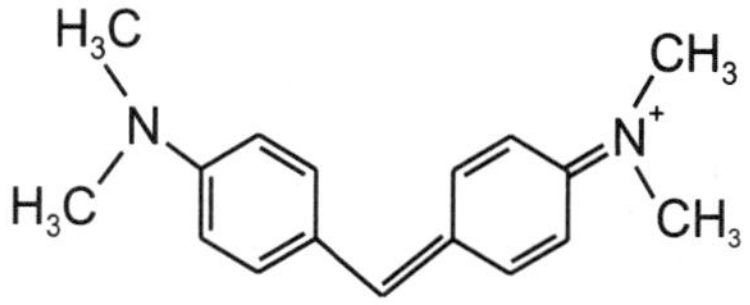

Diarylmethine dye

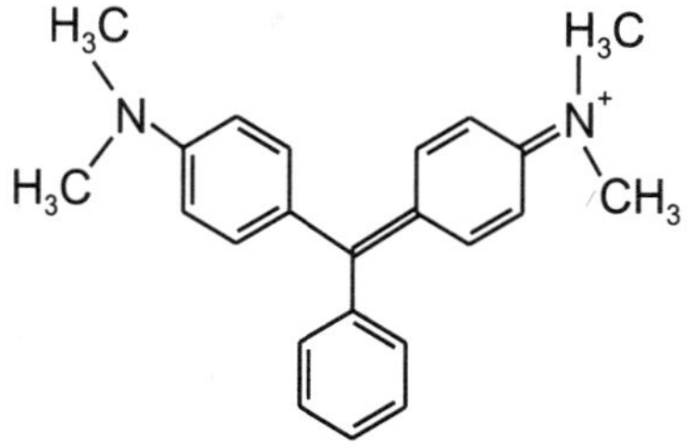

Triarylmethine dye

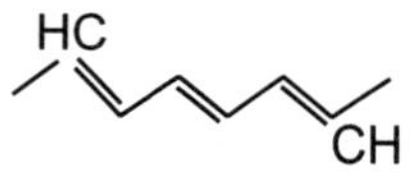

Polyene and polymethine

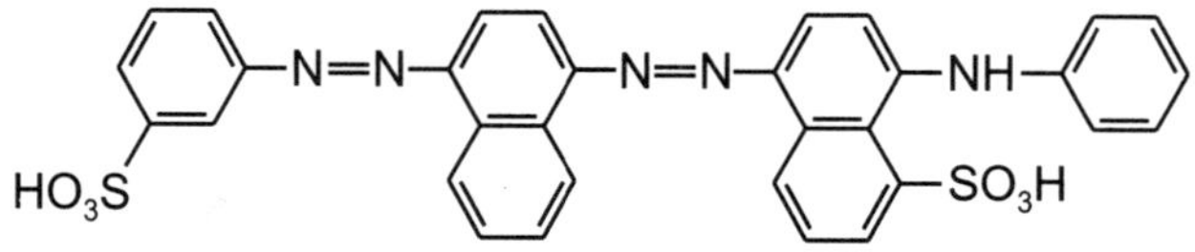

Nitro and Nitroso dyes

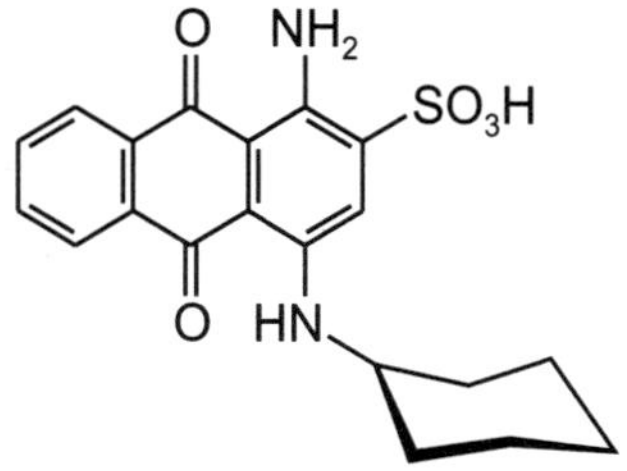

Anthraquinonic dye

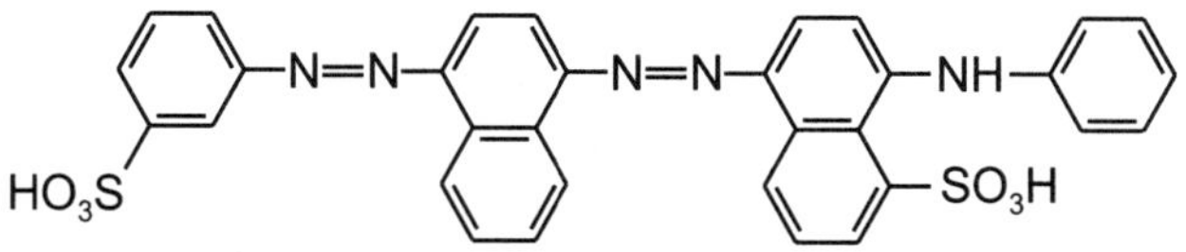

Diazo dyes

Fig. 14.17. Structure of dyes based on predominant groups.

The physical and chemical methods for the treatment of dye-containing effluent includes physico-chemical flocculation combined with flotation, electroflotation, flocculation with Fe(II)/Ca(OH)$_2$, membrane filtration, electrokinetic coagulation, electrochemical destruction, ion-exchange, irradiation, photochemical precipitation, oxidation, ozonation, adsorption with activated carbon, and the Katox treatment method, which involves the use of activated carbon and air mixtures. The chemical colour removal process leads to 60 to 70 per cent reduction in the colour, while the decrease in biological oxygen demand (BOD) is only about 30 to 40 per cent.

PESTICIDES AND INSECTICIDES

Pesticide industry has been identified as one of the highly polluting industries needing pollution control on top priority. Pesticides include insecticides, fungicides, herbicides, rodenticides, nematocides, etc. and are manufactured from chemicals.

The possible sources of pollutants are raw materials used in pesticide synthesis in excess of their stoichiometric requirements, impurities in raw materials, solvent used as a carrier medium, solvent used as an extractive medium. In view of the wide variety of process technology options, the quantity of water used and waste-water generation are widely varying from product to product and industry to industry, daily and hourly (also seasonally).

Choosing the mode of disposal for treated effluent is very important in view of the toxic nature of the effluents. The level of treatment required is to be decided based on the actual quantity of the receiving body. Recycling and reuse of waste-water within the industry will help minimise fresh water requirements and the simultaneous reduction in waste-water volume for final treatment and discharge thereby reducing related costs.

Suspended solids can be removed by screens, grift chambers, sedimentation, floatation, centrifugation and filtration. Effluents can be neutralised using acids/alkalies. Oil and grease is removed by gravity separation and air floatation. For removing heavy metals, pH is adjusted so as to precipitate these metals for removal by coagulation, settling and filtration. For the treatment of biodegradable organic effluents, biological treatment is adopted wherein micro-organisms degrade the waste in the presence of oxygen (aerobic-treatment) or in absence of oxygen (anaerobic treatment).

In addition, good housekeeping and operating practices such as waste stream segregation, employees training, better documentation, better material handling and storage and material tracking, and inventory control production runs can be scheduled to maximise efficiency. Production runs of a given formulation should be scheduled together to reduce the need for equipment cleaning between batches.

Biopesticides

After the green revolution, there has been a marked change in the pests and diseases that affect many crops. Pests like whitefly (*Bemisia tabaci*) diamondback moth (*Plutella xylostella*), mustard aphid (*Lipaphis erysimi*) and cotton bollworm/gram pod borer (*Helicoverpa armigera*), have developed resistance to chemical pesticides.

The use of synthetic organic pesticides has undoubtedly played a key role in increasing agricultural production in the world. But indiscriminate use and abuse of these compounds have led to several toxic hazards through pesticide residues in the food chain.

Most of the chemical insecticides are also highly toxic to the natural enemies of insect pests; the use of such chemicals upset the balance of life in nature, leading to large-scale outbreaks of pests. Biopesticides offer good alternative to hazardous pesticides.

The term biopesticides is usually used for all biological materials and to organisms which can be formulated for use as pesticides for the control of pests. These include material of plant origin such as neem as well as micro-organisms like bacteria, fungi, viruses, etc.

The biopesticide based on pathogens are also known as 'microbial pesticides' while those based on the plant materials as 'botanical or phytochemical' pesticides. Due to pesticide abuses, biopesticides are gaining importance for the control of pests in agriculture, horticulture, forestry and public health programme. Increased emphasis is being given by biopesticide industry and government agencies to promote their use. Neem's pest control properties have been proved beyond doubt and its role in integrated pest managment (IPM) is becoming increasingly relevant in efforts to reduce dependence on hazardous chemical pesticides.

There are number of fungi, viruses, bacteria, predators, parasites, etc. which are infectious to the insect-pests. Inclusion of these biocontrol agents, biopesticides etc. in the schedule to the insecticides act was deliberated by the central insecticides board (CIB). The board accepted to include the microbial products and biochemicals in the Schedule of the Act. The biopesticides are good pathogens of commercially important pests and highly specific to Arthropods. They are safe to mammals, plants and beneficial insects, environmentally friendly, non-polluting and leave no residues. Their large scale production is easy and offer good business prospectus for the industry and easily be manipulated to create high efficiency.

Neem (*Azadirachta indica*, Meliaceae) is a source of biopesticide of plant origin which acts as antifeedant, growth-inhibitor, nematocide and repellent. An age-old practice in India is to mix neem leaves with stored grains or to crush them on storage facility walls to prevent insect damage. Farmers have traditionally ground leaves, soaked them overnight in water and treated the planted rice crop with the extract. 'Azadiractin' is the principal and most active pesticidal compound of neem. All parts of the neem tree contain azadiractin, but is more concentrated in the seed. The content of the azadiractin per neem tree varies greatly between locations and other factors may also contribute to variability. The compound azadiraction may work as an insect growth regulator interfering with ecdysone (the key insect moulting hormone), which prevents immature insects from moulting. Neem products may also repel insects, stop their feeding, inhibit reproduction and cause other interruptions. Neem products are commercially available in the market.

The discovery of baculoviruses as eco-friendly pest-control agents came as a boon to agriculture to meet the increasing demand on food supply for the overgrowing population. Baculoviruses are promising agents for the control of insects of order Lepidoptera (butterflies and moth), Hymenoptera (sawflies) and Coleoptera (beetles). Baculoviruses do not infect vertebrates or plants. They posses a circular, covalently closed and double-stranded genome of 88–200 kb. Nuclear polyhedrosis viruses (NPV), granulosis viruses (GV) and non-occluded type viruses are the 3 subgroups baculoviruses. More than 600 species of insects are found to be infected by these viruses; and many of these insect pests are economically important like alfalfa looper, cabbage looper, armyworm, cotton bollworm and tobacco caterpillar etc. These insects are susceptible to their respective viruses while they are in the larval stage and so these viruses can be used to keep the insect population in check. This is important in view that these insects cause damage to many of our important field crops such as soyabean, cotton, tomato, pigeonpea, cabbage, tobacco.

Bacillus thuringiensis or Bt, is a member of a family of rod-shaped bacteria that are commonly found in soil in most regions of the world. Bt exhibits unique biopesticidal activity when eaten by susceptible larvae and does not have any hazards, sometimes associated with chemical insecticides. Bt provided a rather complex synergistic 'one-two punch' of enzymatic toxins and insect pathogenic bacteria. Several commercial Bt formulation are available to farmers to combat important pests like cotton bollworm (*Heliothis armigera*) and diamondback moth (*Plutella xylostella*).

Fungi can be successfully used as biopesticides against insects. They require congenial temperature and especially high relative humidity for their infection, spore germination and successful multiplication. After the first report that disease in silkworm was due to a fungus, several scientists reported entomogenous fungi controlling insects. The insect infection by fungal pathogens results in destruction of insect by physical blockage of the gut, trachea, circulatory systems, histolysis, toxin production and physiological starvation.

The use of neem and *Bacillus* based biopsecticides, NPV, GVs, antagonistic fungi and bacteria, (*Gliocladium* spp., *Pseudomonas* spp., *Bacillus subtilis*, *Trichoderma* spp.) and entomogenous fungi (*Beauverla, Metarrhizium, Nomurea, Verticilium*) is being promoted under the ambit of IPM on various crops. The neem based biopesticides, *Bacillus thuringiensis* and *Trichoderma viride* have been registered under the provision of insecticides Act. The use of *Bacillus thuringiensis* has been found to be very effective for the control of Diamondback moth on cruciferous vegetable and *Heliothis armigera* on various crops. Neem based biopesticides are being preferred for the control of mites on tea crop due to inherent problems of residues of chemical pesticides and growing demand of organically grown tea. Future is bright with biopesticides. They are potent tools of combating insect-pests and reducing pesticidal load on environment.

PROPELLANT AND EXPLOSIVES

A chemical explosive may be defined as a compound or mixture of compounds that reacts very rapidly to produce relatively large amounts of gas and heat. The rate of detonation is very high. Exothermic oxidation-reduction reactions provide the energy released during detonation. It is the nearly instantaneous formation of gases plus their rapid expansion due to pressure and heat that results in the destructive force or useful work. Large amounts of explosives are used annually, more for constructive commercial purposes than for military, combat, or terror purposes.

The discovery of explosives must be considered as one of the greatest milestones in the development of modern society. Whether it is for mining, excavation of tunnels, construction of roads and pipelines, or rock quarrying, explosives are needed. Explosives contain oxidisers and fuel. Molecular explosives contain both of these within the same molecule (2,4,6-trinitrotoluene, pentaerythritol tetranitrate, and nitroglycerine), while in composite explosives the two portions come from different molecules (ammonium nitrate and liquid fuel oil). Explosives are categorised as three groups, based on their sensitivity to detonation, as follows:

1. Primary explosives—most sensitive (get readily initiated).
2. Secondary explosives—less sensitive (less hazardous).
3. Tertiary explosives—least sensitive.

Some of the commonly used explosives are listed in Table 14.11. Of all the known explosives, the most widely known are the ones having a —N=O group. This includes nitro groups (both aromatic and aliphatic), nitrate esters, nitrate salts, nitramines, and nitrosamines. Prominent examples are nitromethane, 2,4,6-trinitrotoluene (TNT), nitroglycerine (NG), pentaerythritol tetranitrate (PETN), ethylenediamine dinitrate (EDDN), hexahydro-1,3,5-trinitro-1,3,5-triazine (RDX), cyclotetramethylene tetranitramine (HMX), and ammonium nitrate (Fig. 14.18). The synthesis and use of these explosives contaminates the environment with high amounts of nitrate compounds. The industrial effluent from these industries has low pH value and is usually high in nitrates.

Table 14.11. Commonly used explosives.

Compound name	Symbol	Composition
Primary explosives		
Mercury fulminate	–	$Hg(CNO)_2$
Lead azide	–	$Pb(N_3)_2$
Silver azide	–	AgN_3
Mannitol hexanitrate	MHN	$C_6H_8(ONO_2)_6$
Diazodinitro phenol	DDNP	$C_6H_2N_4O_5$
Secondary explosives		
Nitroglycerine	NG	$C_3H_5(ONO_2)_3$
Pentaerythritol tetranitrate	PETN	$C(CH_2ONO_2)_4$
Trinitrotoluene	TNT	$CH_3C_6H_2(NO_2)_3$
Ethyleneglycol dinitrate	EGDN	$C_2H_4(ONO_2)_2$
Cyclotrimethylene trinitramine	RDX	$C_3H_6N_3(NO_2)_3$
Cyclotetramethylene tetranitramine	HMX	$C_4H_8N_4(NO_2)_4$
Nitroguanidine	NQ	$CH_4N_3NO_2$
Nitromethane	NM	CH_3NO_2
Nitrocellulose	NC	Variable
Ethylenedinitrate	EDDN	$C_2H_{10}N_4O_6$
Prilled ammonium nitrate-fuel oil	ANFO	94/6–AN/FO
Water gels	–	Variable mixtures of oxidisers, fuels, and water
Tertiary explosives		
Mononitro toluene	MNT	$CH_3C_6H_4NO_2$
Ammonium perchlorate	AP	NC_4ClO_4
Ammonium nitrate	AN	NH_4NO_3

Toxicity and Occurrence

The toxicity of nitroorganics, inorganic nitrates, and nitrites is widely known. Some of the common symptoms are irritation of digestive tract, methemoglobinemia, disturbed heart function, kidney trouble, dysfunction of the vascular system, and severe jaundice. The nitroaromatic explosives are toxic, but their environmental transformation products, including arylamines, arylhydroxylamines, and condensed products such as azoxy- and azo- compounds, are equally or more toxic as the parent nitroaromatic. TNT is on the list of US Environmental protection agency priority pollutants. RDX is a class C possible human carcinogen and has adverse effects on the central nervous system in mammals.

Aromatic nitro compounds are resistant to chemical or biological oxidation and to hydrolysis because of the electron withdrawing nitro groups. The hydrophilic lipophilic balance (HLB) of these compounds favours lipid solubility, thereby reducing their mobility in the environment.

Thus, because of the lipophilic character and deactivated aromatic ring, these compounds accumulate in the environment. Activities associated with manufacturing, training, waste disposal, and closure of military bases have resulted in severe soil and groundwater contamination with explosives. These wastewaters are contaminated with explosives as well as the raw materials used for the production of explosives.

The nitro aromatic compound TNT is introduced into soil and water ecosystems mainly by military activities like the manufacture, loading, and disposal of explosives and propellants. This problem of contamination may increase in the future because of the demilitarisation and disposal of unwanted weapon systems.

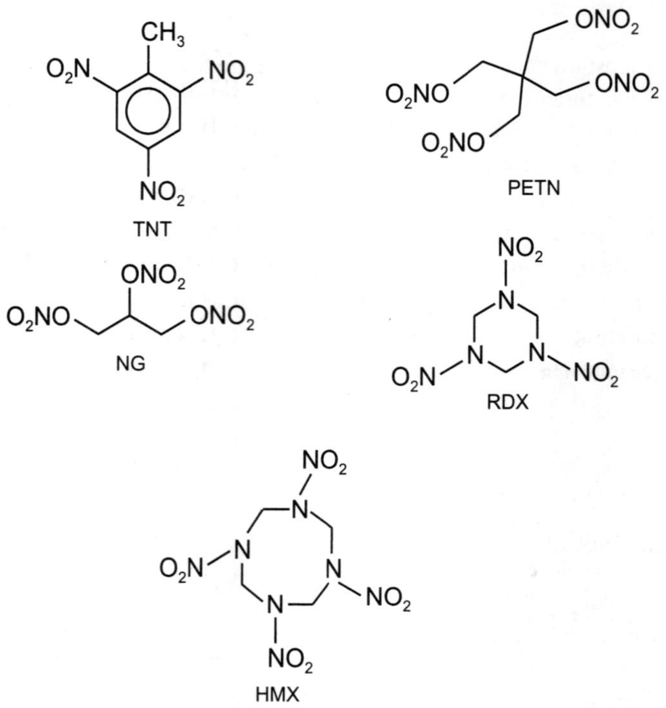

Fig. 14.18. Commonly used explosives.

The disposal of obsolete explosives is a problem for the military and associated industries because of the polluting effect of explosives in the environment.

Bioremediation

Past methods of disposing of munitions wastes have included dumping in deep sea, dumping at specified landfill areas, and incineration when quantities were small. All of these cause serious harm to the ecosystem.

For example, incineration causes air pollution, and disposal on land leads to soil and groundwater pollution. Other than these, methods such as resin adsorption, surfactant complexing, and liquid-liquid extraction have been used.

These methods only transfer the explosive from soil or water into another medium, which then needs further treatment. Chemical methods of oxidation do not yield the necessary products, and the unreacted toxic intermediates still remain. Thus, the biofriendly treatment is bioremediation.

Micro-organisms are known for their versatile metabolic activity and have evolved diverse pathways that allow them to mineralise specific nitro compounds. Despite this, relatively few micro-organisms have been described as being able to use nitro aromatic compounds as nitrogen; carbon, and energy sources because nitro groups deactivate the aromatic ring to electrophilic attack by oxygenase or other enzymes. Be that as it may, biological degradation is one of the primary routes by which nitro aromatic compounds are broken down in the environment. There has been considerable interest in the past 30 years in the microbial transformation of these compounds.

Both aerobic and anaerobic degradation of nitro aromatics has been reported. Aerobic micro-organisms use diverse biochemical reactions to initiate the degradation of nitro aromatic compounds. Reactions that attack the nitro substituent can be grouped into two general categories: oxidative or reductive. With mono- or di-nitro substituted aromatic compounds, the preferred route for their initial degradation is hydroxylation carried out by mono- or di-oxygenases.

These reactions normally result in replacement of the nitro group by a hydroxy group with nitrite release. When the number of nitro substituents on the aromatic ring is greater than two, the predominant initial reactions become reductive. These reactions reduce the nitro (NO_2) substituent first to nitroso (NO), then to hydroxylamino (NHOH), followed by an amino (NH_2) derivative prior to further processing with the release of ammonium ion. In some *Rhodococcus* and *Mycobacterium* strains, the aromatic ring, rather than the nitro group, may be reduced first to generate a hydride — Meisenheimer complex. On protonation and rearomatisation, the nitro group is replaced by a proton and nitrite is released.

Most aerobic micro-organisms reduce TNT to the corresponding amino derivatives via the formation of nitroso and hydroxylamine intermediates. However, condensation of the latter compounds yields highly recalcitrant azoxytetranitro toluenes.

Certain strains of *Pseudomonas* use TNT as the nitrogen source through the removal of nitrogen as nitrite. *Phanerochaete chrysosporium* mineralises TNT under lignolytic conditions. Because the manufacturing processes for RDX and HMX are the same, each is present as an impurity in the other. Because of the copresence of RDX and HMX in contaminated waters or at contaminated sites, degradation of both in each other's presence becomes important. *P. chrysosporium* degraded this mixture to carbon dioxide and nitrous oxide. In a study of RDX degradation by *Rhodococcus* sp., nitrite formation was observed with RDX disappearance.

Ecological observations suggest that sulphate-reducing and methanogenic bacteria might metabolise nitroaromatic compounds under anaerobic conditions if appropriate electron donors and electron acceptors are present in the environment. The successful demonstration of the degradation of RDX by sewage sludge under anaerobic conditions further indicated the usefulness of anaerobes in explosive waste treatment. Under anaerobic conditions, the sulphate-reducing bacteria *Desulfovibrio* sp. (B strain) metabolised TNT.

Of all the metabolites produced, the formation of toluene was significant. Most *Desulfovibrio* sp., have nitrite reductase enzymes that reduce nitrate to ammonia. Figure 14.19 elaborates a general pathway for the transformation of TNT that involves the initial reduction of aromatic nitro groups to aromatic amines. Boopathy and Kulpa isolated a methanogen, *Methanococcus* sp., that transformed TNT to 2,4-diaminonitro toluene.

The observations of sulphate reducers and methanogenic bacteria by many scientists suggest that these organisms could be exploited for bioremediation of explosives under anaerobic conditions by supplying proper electron donors and electron acceptors. The first step in the metabolism of nitoaromatics is reduction. This step is followed by reductive deamination, which removes all of the nitro groups present in the ring, leaving the ring intact and forming toluene and ammonia as end products. The toluene can be further degraded by toluene-degrading organisms.

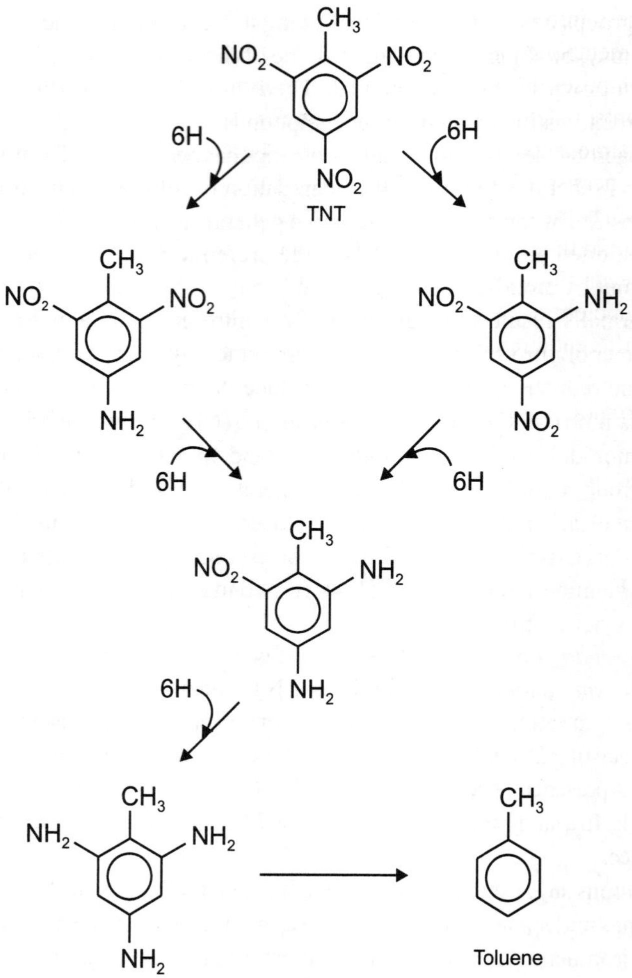

Fig. 14.19. Degradation of TNT by *Desulfovibrio* sp.

As discussed earlier, aerobic transformations of TNT have shown the production of dead-end products like amino derivatives or azoxy compounds. Therefore, the applicability of aerobes in bioremediation of sites contaminated with nitroaromatics is doubtful at present.

However, the use of anaerobes like sulphate-reducing bacteria may prove useful in decontaminating sites polluted by nitro compounds.

NUCLEAR AND RADIOACTIVE POLLUTION

Nuclear and radioactive pollution spreading into the environment has increased extensively as a result of the discovery of artificial radioactivity, particularly due to the development of the atom bomb, hydrogen bomb and of techniques of harnessing nuclear energy. Actually, this dangerous pollution enters into the environment in waste streams and stack gases from operations of power processing plants. From neutron bombardment of atomic fuel, heavy radio-nuclides are produced which are extremely toxic. Once these radio-elements find access into the environment, they enter the ecocycling processes and ultimately into the food chain and metabolic pathways.

Radioactive pollution poses a serious threat to the environment and future generation. Radioactive wastes from nuclear plants, reactors, etc. are, however, of a special kind in the sense that they do not smell bad or pollute the atmosphere like smoke, but are extremely lethal to living beings even in minute quantities. These wastes persist in the environment for a long time. Non-radiation pollutants and short half-life radio nuclides are being constantly released into the air and it is expected that they will disperse or degrade in a short span of time. Consequently, they are not regarded as a future pollution threat until their concentration exceeds the limit. They can not be disposed of into the environment like other industrial wastes. The nuclear establishments produce various types of solid and liquid radioactive wastes which contain different amounts of radioactivity and special care has to be taken for their safe disposal.

Radioactive wastes require royal disposal methods. During the phenomenon of radioactivity, some naturally unstable elements tend to become stable by emitting alpha (α), beta (β) and gamma (γ) rays. These rays can ionise the air and disarry the life activities in a cell when they pass through them.

The nuclear industry provides products that play a vital role in society. This is a unique industry that provides products both for the protection and destruction of society. They provide stable nuclides used in medicine (imaging and diagnostic) and nuclear explosives used by the military. It is one of the major energy sources for the production of electricity to meet the world's needs.

There are three types of nuclear wastes, based on their radionuclide characteristics:

1. Uranium-contaminated waste.
2. Plutonium-contaminated waste.
3. Other radionuclide-contaminated waste.

Of these types of wastes, uranium- and plutonium-contaminated wastes are potentially hazardous to human and animal health. Other nuclide wastes are low-level waste, having lower radioactivity. Although there are natural sources of radioactivity, the release of anthropogenic radionuclides into the environment is significant and a subject of intense public concern. Plutonium (Pu) contamination of soils, sediments, and/or water is an important consideration because this transuranic element can influence populations inhabiting the contaminated environment. A long half-life ($t_{1/2} = 2.41 \times 10^4$ years for ^{239}Pu and potential health effects of Pu have resulted in extensive field and laboratory studies to resolve its environmental behaviour.

Waste Management

Radioactive waste management involves the treatment, storage, and disposal of liquid, airborne, and solid effluents from the nuclear industry's operations. Four methods are employed involving chemical transformations, namely:

1. Limit generation.
2. Delay and decay.
3. Concentrate and contain.
4. Dilute and disperse.

Limiting the generation of waste is the first and most important consideration in managing radioactive wastes. Delay and decay is frequently an important strategy because much of the radioactivity in nuclear reactors and accelerators is very short lived. Concentrating and containing is the objective of treatment activities for longer-lived radioactivity. The waste is contained in corrosion resistant containers and transported to disposal sites. Leaching of heavy metals and radionuclides from these sites is a problem of growing concern. Micro-organisms corrode even the high-grade metal containers and solubilise the metal ions. Ferric sulphate formed *in situ* by the biological oxidation of pyrite (by *Thiobacillus ferroxidans*) converts uranium present in these sites to soluble uranyl sulphate (Fig. 14.20). For wastes having low radioactivity, dilution and dispersion are adopted.

Bacterial oxidation of pyrite: (*Thiobacillus ferroxidans*)
$$2FeS_2 + H_2O + 7\ 1/2O_2 \longrightarrow 2Fe_2(SO_4)_3 + H_2SO_4$$

Chemical oxidation and solubilisation of the uranium:
$$UO_2 + Fe_2(SO_4)_3 \longrightarrow UO_2SO_4 + 2FeSO_4$$

Chemical oxidation of the pyrite by ferric sulphate:
$$FeS_2 + 7Fe_2(SO_4)_3 + 8H_2O \longrightarrow 15FeSO_4 + 8H_2SO_4$$

Bacterial reoxidation of ferrous sulphate: (*Thiobacillus ferroxidans*)
$$4FeSO_4 + 2H_2SO_4 + O_2 \longrightarrow 2Fe_2(SO_4)_3 + 2H_2O$$

Fig. 14.20. Solubilisation of a radionuclide-uranium to uranyl sulphate.

Bioremediation

Chemical approaches are available for metal and radionuclide remediation but are often expensive to apply and lack the specificity required to treat target nuclides against a background of competing metal ions. In addition, such approaches are not applicable to cost-effective remediation of large-scale subsurface contamination *in situ*. Biological approaches, on the other hand, offer the potential for the highly selective removal of toxic metals and radionuclides coupled with considerable operational flexibility; they can be used both *in situ* and *ex situ* in a range of bioreactor configurations. A good degree of mineralisation is achieved during biodegradation of radioactive waste.

Reactions mediated by micro-organisms include solubilisation or volatilisation of metals ions (radionuclide ions) from organic and inorganic complexes, compounds, and minerals by production of acids or chelating agents, as well as removal from aqueous solution by a number of mechanisms that include biosorption, accumulation, and chemical precipitation. Chemical transformations such as oxidation and reduction can also be catalysed by a range of micro-organisms; these reactions can alter a number of important properties, such as speciation and water solubility, that influence biotic effects and environmental mobility of these ions. The different reactions or transformations that micro-organisms bring about on metal ions or radionuclide ions are:

1. Biosorption and accumulation.
2. Translocation.
3. Reduction and precipitation.
4. Solubilisation.

Immobilisation—biosorption and accumulation

Biosorption is microbial uptake of radionuclide species, both soluble and insoluble, by physico-chemical mechanisms, such as adsorption. Biosorption can also provide nucleation sites and stimulate the formation of extremely stable minerals. The constituent biomolecules of microbial cell walls have great affinity for radionuclides and are of greatest significance in biosorption. Once inside the cells, metals and radionuclides may be bound, precipitated, localised, or translocated. Micro-organisms can form aggregates with other colloidal materials (clay minerals) and thus help in the transport of radionuclides. Many microbial exopolymers act as polyanions under natural conditions, and negatively charged groups can interact with cationic metal and radionuclide species, thereby achieving the biosorption on the cell walls. The carboxyl groups on the peptidoglycan are the main binding site for cations in gram-positive cell walls, with phosphate groups contributing significantly in gram-negative species. Chitin is an important structural component of fungal cell walls, and this polymer is an effective biosorbent for radionuclides. Actinide accumulation by fungal biomass is one such example.

Fungi, including yeasts, have received attention in connection with metal biosorption, particularly because waste biomass arises as a by-product from several industrial fermentations, while algae have been viewed as a renewable source of metal-sorbing biomass. Both freely suspended and immobilised biomass from bacterial, cyanobacterial, algal, and fungal species have received attention. One drawback of this method of remediation is the treatment (disposal) of the radionuclide accumulated biomass. A chemical or physical treatment of the radioactivity in the biomass becomes unavoidable.

Macskie and Dean have developed a biofilter to remove and recover heavy metals from synthetic aqueous solutions. The active agent in the metal uptake is a phosphatase overproduced at the cell surface by bacteria (growing on the inner rim of a tube), a *Citrobacter* sp., originally isolated from a contaminated soil sample. The process of metal uptake relies on *in situ* cumulative deposition of insoluble metal phosphatase tightly bound to the cell surface. Soluble metals are converted to insoluble metal phosphates by a biocatalytic process that readily operates at low metal concentrations unmanageable by classical precipitation, thus overcoming the chemical constraints of the solubility product of the metal phosphate in the bulk solution. The waste-water containing the heavy metal pollutant is passed through the pipe. All the heavy metal ions get bound to the phosphatase on the cell surface. Since high loads of phosphate are produced in a localised environment, metals can be precipitated at very low metal concentrations. After the metals have been concentrated, they can be safely disposed of as metal by-products to be reused elsewhere.

Transport

The uptake and transport of radionuclides by micro-organisms is dependent on the pH and monovalent cation (K^+) concentration. Many times the entry of radionuclides into the microbial cell occurs via active transport systems for K^+ or NH_4^+. In a sense radionuclides are competitive inhibitors of the K^+ channel. For example, Cs^+ accumulation is particularly dependent on external pH and monovalent cation concentration, especially K^+.

Cyanobacteria and algae are also capable of Cs^+ accumulation. In eukaryotic micro-organisms, such as microalgae and fungi, vacuoles appear to be a preferential intracellular location for Cs^+. Metals or radionuclides may also precipitate within cells as sulphides, oxides, and phosphates. Micro-organisms are also known to produce specific biomolecules (peptides) to bind to radionuclides. The fruiting bodies of fungi are also known to have high concentrations of radionuclides. ^{137}Cs accumulation by macrofungi (mushrooms) following the Chemobyl accident in 1986 is well documented. Grazing of these fruiting bodies by animals may lead to radionuclide (cesium) transfer along the food chain.

Reduction and precipitation

Reduction is one of the most important chemical transformations catalysed by micro-organisms, affecting the solubility of radionuclides. Under anaerobic conditions, the oxidised form of the metal becomes the

TEA (terminal electron acceptor). For example, a strain of *Shewanella putrefaciens* reduced U(VI) to U(IV), giving rise to a black precipitate of U(IV) carbonate because U(IV) compounds are less soluble than U(VI) compounds. *Geobacter metallireducans* also reduces U(VI) to U(IV) species. These transformations play a significant role in the environment because they immobilise uranium.

Because many radionuclides of concern are both redox active and less soluble when reduced, bioreduction offers much promise for controlling the solubility and mobility of target radionuclides in contaminated sediments. The first demonstration of dissimilatory U(VI) reduction was by the Fe(III)-reducing bacteria *G. metallireducens* and *S. oneidensis*, which conserved energy for anaerobic growth via reduction of U(VI). It should be noted, however, that the ability to reduce U(VI) enzymatically is not restricted to Fe(III)-reducing bacteria. Other organisms, including a *Clostridium* sp., *Desulfovibrio desulfuricans*, and *D. vulgaria*, also reduce U(VI).

Although ^{238}U remains the priority pollutant in most medium- and low-level radioactive wastes, other actinides, including ^{230}Th, ^{237}Np, ^{241}Pu, and ^{241}Am, can also be present. Fe(III)-reducing bacteria have the metabolic potential to reduce Pu(V) and Np(V) enzymatically. This is significant in that the tetravalent actinides are amenable to bioremediation because of their high ligand complexing abilities and are also immobilised in sediments containing active biomass.

The most obvious applications of microbially mediated precipitation of toxic metals and radionuclides are those involving sulphide precipitation, phosphatase-mediated precipitation, and chemical reduction. Organisms capable of sulphide production (*Thiobacillus ferrooxidans*) are receiving considerable attention in bioremediation, both in reactor and *in situ* treatment systems. A promising application of biological metal reduction is uranium precipitation from nuclear effluents.

Solubilisation

Micro-organisms and plants are known to produce chelating agents that complex with metals and radionuclides. These complexes are usually soluble in water. Once in solution, they may either get converted to their corresponding hydroxides or they may be absorbed by plants. Leaching may also be brought about by autotrophic bacteria under aerobic conditions. Such processes are catalysed mainly by *thiobacilli*, such as *Thiobacillus ferrooxidans*. In fact, this organism is used on a commercial scale for the extraction of uranium from ore. Heterotrophic bacteria produce a large number of diverse chelating agents, such as dicarboxylic acids, glucuronic acids, protocatechuic acid, and salicylic acid, to complex with metals or radionuclides. Uranyl complexes with oxalic acid, citric acid, and succinic acids have been reported. Alongside these chelating agents, micro-organisms are known to excrete 'siderophores' under iron-limiting conditions. Solubilisation of Pu(IV) with siderophores has been reported and is an important means of remediation of Pu(IV).

Phytoremediation

Phytoremediation is a technology that should be considered for remediation of contaminated sites because of its cost effectiveness, aesthetic advantages, and long-term applicability. This technology can be applied for metal pollutants that are amenable to phytostabilisation, phytoextraction, phytotransformation, rhizosphere bioremediation, or phytoextraction.

Lee observed that plutonium uptake and accumulation by the Indian mustard plant (*Brassica juncea*) was higher than that by the sunflower plant (*Helianthus annuus*). They also observed that Pu uptake was dependent on the chelating agent (nitrate, citrate, etc.) present in the soil.

Composting

Composting is generally achieved by converting solid wastes into stable humus-like materials via biodegradation of putrescible organic matter. The composting process consists of microbiological treatment in which aerobic micro-organisms use organic matter as a substrate. The main products of the composting process are fully mineralised materials, such as CO_2, H_2O, NH_4^+, stabilised organic matter heavily populated with competitive microbial biomass, and ash. Compost has the potential of improving soil structure, increasing cation exchange capacity, and enhancing plant growth. Ipek showed that beta-radioactivity was greatly decreased by aerobic composting.

Bioremediation holds the key to radioactive waste management. Chemical approaches, though effective, are not economical and cannot be applied to larger field areas. A combination of phyto-remediation alongside bioremediation would certainly contain the hazardous radioactive wastes, thereby providing the much needed safety cover for the communities living near these contaminated sites.

PHARMACEUTICALS

Pharmaceutical and antibiotic residues from human and animal medical care enter the water and soil from (i) the effluent treatment plants of manufacturing facilities, (ii) the municipal sewage treatment plant, (iii) hospital waste treatment plants, and (iv) animal farms as shown in Fig. 14.21. Treating effluent from a pharmaceutical plant that manufactures drugs and antibiotics is relatively easier than treating waste from a hospital or municipal sewage plant; in the former case the substances that need to be degraded are well known. The waste from hospital or municipal sewage plants may contain low concentrations of many different pharmaceuticals and their metabolites, which makes the task very difficult.

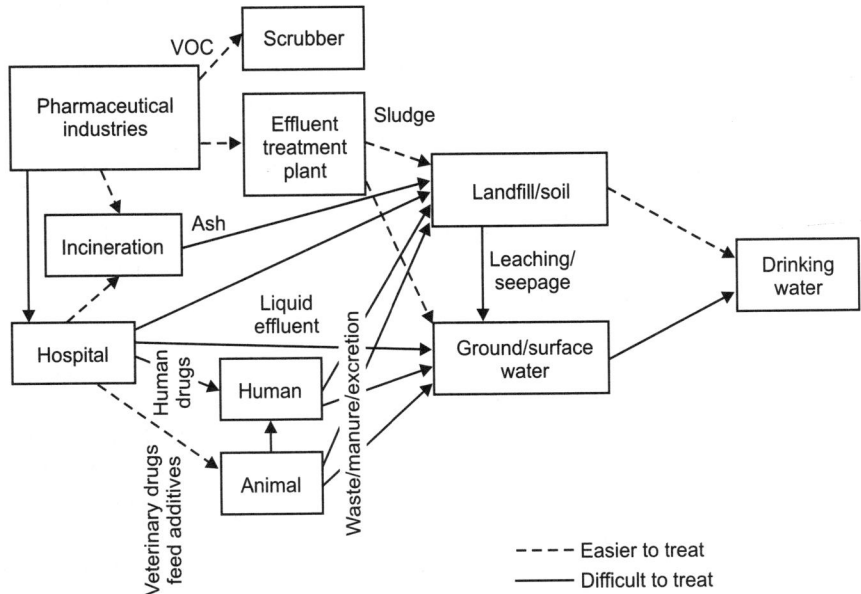

Fig. 14.21. Movement of drugs and pharmaceutical products from source to environment.

Like many other industries, the pharmaceutical industry produces a wide variety of products. This industry uses both inorganic and organic materials as raw materials, the latter being either of synthetic or of vegetable and animal origin. Some pharmaceutical plants do not discharge liquid waste at all, some discharge very small but concentrated liquid waste, while others discharge highly alkaline and toxic liquid wastes.

Therefore, it is very difficult to make any generalisation in regard to the characterisation of the pharmaceutical plant wastes. Pharmaceutical plants discharge highly alkaline and toxic liquid wastes. If crude waste from an antibiotic waste is discharged into a stream, it not only imparts an objectionable odour to it, but also adversely affects its biological population. This waste should not be allowed to be discharged into a municipal sewer, unless the sewage treatment plant is properly designed to handle a widely varying and concentrated waste from such a plant. Penicillin waste is found to have a disturbing effect on the process occurring within a sludge digestion tank.

Synthetic drugs plants utilise large number of both organic and inorganic chemicals, and usually produce a variety of drugs in different sections. The volume and composition of the liquid wastes not only vary from plant to plant, but also from section to section in a plant, producing different types of drugs from different raw materials and using varieties of processes.

Wastes containing toxic elements like cyanides and heavy metals, if discharged without any treatment, are harmful to aquatic life in the streams. These toxic elements interfere with the biological sewage treatment units very badly.

Due to the great pollution potential and the diversified characteristics of the waste from different sections of a plant, the planning for the treatment of synthetic drug wastes should be preceeded by a careful study of each waste. Segregation and equalisation very often improve the overall treatment efficiency and reduce the cost of treatment. If the wastes have high COD:BOD ratios, benchscale laboratory biological treatment studies with acclimatised seed sludge are necessary for proper planning.

The acidic wastes, wastes containing toxic elements like cyanide, and those containing offensive-odour-producing compounds are usually segregated and treated separately. Acidic wastes may be neutralised with lime. The odour-producing compounds are usually destroyed by chlorination; compounds which are resistant to chlorine may be destroyed by heating in a furnace.

Pharmaceutical plants discharge highly alkaline and toxic liquid wastes. If crude waste from an antibiotic waste is discharged into a stream, it not only imparts an objectionable odour to it, but also adversely affects its biological population. This waste should not be allowed to be discharged into a municipal sewer, unless the sewage treatment plant is properly designed to handle a widely varying and concentrated waste from such a plant. Penicillin waste is found to have a disturbing effect on the process occurring within a sludge digestion tank.

Synthetic drugs plants utilise large number of both organic and inorganic chemicals, and usually produce a variety of drugs in different sections. The volume and composition of the liquid wastes not only vary from plant to plant, but also from section to section in a plant, producing different types of drugs from different raw materials and using varieties of processes. Wastes containing toxic elements like cyanides and heavy metals, if discharged without any treatment, are harmful to aquatic life in the streams. These toxic elements interfere with the biological sewage treatment units very badly.

Due to the great pollution potential and the diversified characteristics of the waste from different sections of a plant, the planning for the treatment of synthetic drug wastes should be preceeded by a careful study of each waste. Segregation and equalisation very often improve the overall treatment efficiency and reduce the cost of treatment. If the wastes have high COD:BOD ratios, benchscale laboratory biological treatment studies with acclimatised seed sludge are necessary for proper planning.

The acidic wastes, wastes containing toxic elements like cyanide, and those containing offensive-odour-producing compounds are usually segregated and treated separately. Acidic wastes may be neutralised with lime. The odour-producing compounds are usually destroyed by chlorination; compounds which are resistant to chlorine may be destroyed by heating in a furnace.

Excess medication excreted by humans and animals, as well as unused or expired medicines, find their way into municipal sewage effluent treatment plants. Since the 1980s, pharmaceuticals like clofibrate, various analgesics, cytostatic drugs, antibiotics, and others have been reported to be present in the surface waters of many European countries. This has raised growing concern that some of these persistent products may find their way back into the drinking water. Genotoxic substances may represent a health hazard to humans and may have adverse effects on other organisms. Since antibiotics mainly interfere with bacterial metabolism, it can be assumed that bacterial communities in aquatic ecosystems feel the primary effects of antibiotic-containing effluents. One of these effects is the increase in resistance to certain antibiotics, which in turn gives rise to infections that are difficult to treat. Antibiotics are consumed by humans and are used in livestock and poultry production and fish farming. The increasing use of these drugs during the last five decades has caused genetic selection of more harmful bacteria. When animal excreta, which contain unmetabolised drugs, are applied to agricultural fields as fertiliser or manure, they contaminate the soil, and possibly the groundwater, depending upon their mobility. Terrestrial and aquatic organisms are affected as a result of leaching from the fields. Solid waste from industrial effluent treatment plants are disposed as landfill, which may lead to leaching of unmetabolised drugs into the groundwater.

Of the drugs that are administered during fish farming, 70 per cent of them are released into the environment, especially into the sediments near the fish farms. The modes of action of most pharmaceuticals in humans, animals, and fish are often poorly understood. The possible effects and side effects on nontarget receptor organisms and the synergistic effects produced as a result of mixing these drugs are also not known. The growth promoters, antibiotics, and other veterinary drugs given to poultry and cattle also end up in humans as a result of meat consumption. Natural and synthetic estrogens produce deleterious effects, such as feminisation and hermaphroditism, in aquatic organisms. The persistence of a drug in a sediment or soil depends on its photostability, its binding and adsorption capability, its degradation rate, and its solubility in water. Strongly sorbing pharmaceuticals tend to accumulate in soil of sediment; in contrast, highly mobile pharmaceuticals tend to leach into groundwater and be transported by drainage and surface runoff.

The antibiotic tetracycline and its derivatives chlortetracycline and oxytetracycline are widely used in stockbreeding and aquaculture. The average concentration of oxytetracycline in German surface waters has been estimated at 0.01 µg/l. In Germany, 0.165 mg/l of clofibric, a lipid-regulating agent, was found in river, ground, and drinking water, and of the 32 drugs that belong to the class of anti-phlogistics, lipid regulators, psychiatric drugs, antiepileptic drugs, beta-blockers and sympathomimetics, 80 per cent of them were found in the sewage treatment plant effluent with concentration levels on the order of 6 µg/l. The sewage treatment plant, which treated household effluent, consisted of three tanks: preliminary clarification, final clarification, and aerator. The concentration of tetracycline and its derivative oxytetracycline in the river Lee near London has been estimated at 9.5 µg/l and tetracycline in British surface waters at about 1 µg/l. In the United Kingdom, drugs like diazepam, methaqualone, and penicilloyl antibiotics were found in potable water and groundwater. A nationwide study carried out by the US Geological Society in 2006 found pharmaceuticals, hormones, and other organic waste-water contaminants in surface water. Apart from ceftriaxone and tilmicosin, several drugs, animal growth promoters and antibiotics, were found in nanogram levels in river sediment and river or drinking water in Italy. The concentrations found were several orders of magnitudes lower than the amount to produce any pharmacological effect, but possible effects of lifelong exposures of these pharmaceutics on humans are not known.

Effect on Plants

Erythromycin, tetracycline, and ibuprofen affect the growth of the cyanobacterium. *Synechocystis* sp. PCC6803 and the duckweed *Lemna minor* FBR006. Sulphadimethoxine alters the normal post-germinative development and growth of roots, hypocotyls, and leaves in *Panicum miliaceum*, *Pisum sativum*, and *Zea mays*. The bioaccumulation of this drug in these plants (root to stalk leaf bioaccumulation ratio is 2 to 20 µg/g) can affect other communities. *Azolla filiculoides* Lam is a water fern that can take in 58 to 2000 µg of this sulpha drug per gram for varying drug concentrations of 50 to 400 mg/l. A higher proportion of the drug was degraded in the presence of plants, between 50 and 56 per cent at a concentration of 50 to 400 mg/l, while the degradation was 5 to 30 per cent, in their absence. The drug affected the growth rate (as biomass yield per week) and nitrogen fixation.

Pharmaceutical Industry Effluent

Waste-waters from pharmaceutical manufacturing contain high levels of suspended solids and soluble recalcitrant organics. Since pharmaceutical plants operate under batch mode, changes in production schedules lead to variability in the effluent flow rate, the principal constituents, and their relative biodegradability. The pharmaceutical industry produces a wide variety of products using both inorganic and organic chemicals as raw materials. Antibiotics and vitamins are produced by fermentation of complex nutrient solutions of organic matter and inorganic salts by fungi or bacteria. Most of the wastes are toxic to biological life and have high biological oxygen demand (BOD), chemical oxygen demand (COD), and a high BOD to COD ratio; they are either highly alkaline (e.g. manufacture of sulpha drugs and vitamin B12) or acidic (e.g. manufacture of organic intermediates).

At times cyanide might also be present. But the main advantage of such effluent is that the pollutants are known; hence treatment could be exactly tailored to remove or degrade it efficiently. Common physical treatment methods include coagulation and precipitation, reverse osmosis, and ultrafiltration; biological treatment includes the activated sludge process. Typical characteristics of effluent from a pharmaceutical bulk drug manufacturing plant would be a COD of 12,500 mg/l, a BOD of 6000 mg/l, sulphate concentration of 9000 mg/l, total solids of 36,000 mg/l, a pH of 8, and dissolved solids of 29,000 mg/l.

It was believed that thermophilic treatment could lead to rapid biodegradation rates, low growth yields, and reduced cooling costs, but the operation of aerobic pharmaceutical waste-water treatment at elevated temperatures seemed to affect the performance of the process. Soluble COD removal efficiency decreased as the treatment temperature was increased from 30° to 60°C (from 62 to 38 per cent, respectively). Untreated waste-water had soluble COD and BOD of 8150 and 3800 mg/l, respectively, and a total ammonia concentration of 220 mg/l. An increase in temperature led to a reduction in the number of different bacterial populations, and probably a decrease in biodiversity. Soluble microbial product (SMP) is defined as the organic compounds released into solution from substrate metabolism and biomass decay, and has its own fraction of recalcitrant and biodegradable fractions. Thermophilic culture produced an SMP with a higher fraction of recalcitrant soluble COD than did the mesophilic culture.

Stable reactor performance requires some stability among the individual populations that comprise the microbial community in the bioreactors, even when there is variation in the influent composition. Also, flexibility is needed for the community to adapt in response to changes in the operating conditions. Flexibility with respect to bacterial community structure leads to more stable process performance. The microbial community could adapt to changing environmental conditions. This was confirmed in full-scale pharmaceutical waste-water treatment studies carried out in a series of seven reactors with the first four bioreactors operated under aerobic and thermophilic temperature conditions (T >45°C), while the last three reactors were operated at 25° to 35°C under biological nitrification and denitrification conditions. The overall treatment efficiencies were greater than 95 per cent. Short-term variability in influent waste-water composition brought about a greater community shift than did long-term operation with waste-water of consistent composition. The thermophilic reactors had similar community structures to each other; the same was true for the communities from mesophilic reactors. This study brought out the fact that during biological waste-water treatment, temperature served as a selective factor for bacterial community structure development.

Two-stage chemical and biochemical treatment of waste (with a BOD:COD ratio of 0.45 to 0.57) from a pharmaceutical bulk drug manufacturing plant produced very good results. Chemical coagulation using lime led to a reduction of 44 to 48 per cent of the sulphate. Subsequent aerobic oxidation led to COD and BOD reduction efficiencies of 86 and 80 per cent, respectively, at an MLVSS of 1500 mg/l, a temperature of 30°C, and a hydraulic retention time (HRT) of 4.5 days. The influent stream had a COD of 4000 mg/l.

Pharmaceutical waste aerobic activated sludges are normally dispersed, weak with a high solid content, and resistant to biological degradation. They have poor bacterial filament development and poor dewaterability characteristics. On the other hand, domestic waste activated sludges are usually compact and strong, with a low solid content and a thick foam.

Bioaugmentation is a technique adapted to maintain sufficient biomass in the medium when enough nutrients and carbon substrates are unavailable. Cells are grown externally (either under different operating conditions or with different substrates) and added to the main reactor from time to time to induce degradation. Manufacture of Cephradine (a main constituent of an antiosmotic drug) generates effluent containing the drug, acetic acid, and ammonia. A mixture containing this effluent and municipal sewage waste was treated in an anaerobic fluidised bed reactor to achieve 89 per cent COD reduction at an HRT of 3 to 12 hours by bioaugmentation through periodic addition of 30 to 70 grams of acclimated cells from an external enrichment reactor every 2 days.

Activated carbon was used as the carrier for the cells. The combined effluent had a COD of 12 to 15,000 mg/l, a BOD of 2000 mg/l, TSS of 6000 mg/l, dissolved solids (DS) of 11,000 to 18,500 mg/l, NH_3 of 15 to 40 mg/l, and a pH of 3 to 4. The enrichment reactor was operated as a sequencing batch reactor. A similar bioaugmentation approach was adopted for the treatment of effluent containing Cephalexin (a drug used for the treatment of bronchitis and other lung diseases) in a fluidised bed reactor to achieve an 89 per cent COD removal efficiency at an HRT of 3 to 12 days. The influent had a COD of 12 to 15,000 mg/l. Every 2 days, 30 to 70 grams of acclimated cells were added from an off-line reactor.

More than 90 per cent anaerobic degradation of waste fermentation broth from clavulanic acid production (total organic carbon, 50,000 mg/l, pH 5, N total = 3600 mg/l) was achieved in a batch mode of operation when the inoculum was waste sludge from a plant that treated a mixture of domestic and industrial waste-water. Biogas production increased from 92 to 3067 mg/l and methane content from

54 to 70 per cent when initial total organic carbon (TOC) was increased from 0.05 to 1.7 grams TOC/g volatile suspended solids (VSS). Further TOC increases inhibited the anaerobic biodegradation process.

Biodegradation of Pharmaceutical Products

The biodegradation of antibiotics and pharmaceuticals depends on the temperature, availability of organic and inorganic nutrients, concentration of the chemical, and presence of oxygen. The biodegradation rate of sulphonamides in activated sludge is identical for several of them. Nitrifying sludge degrades drugs such as chloramphenicol and oxytetracycline, but they are not mineralised. Estrogens and progestogens would be adsorbed onto sludge particles in the waste-water treatment plant and would not be biotransformed. Degradation studies carried out in artificial marine sediment under controlled laboratory conditions in a closed system indicated that oxytetracycline is highly persistent in the marine sediments (greater than 10 months), while sulphadimethoxine and ormethoprim are very short-lived (less than 21 to 62 days). Flumequine, sulphadiazine, and oxolinic acid are also not degraded and preserve their antibacterial activity for more than 180 days.

Aerobic batch biodegradation studies of veterinary and antimicrobial growth promoters such as metronidazole, oxytetracycline, olaquindox, and tylosin in the concentration range of 1 to 1000 µg/l indicated that these drugs are moderately persistent in surface water except for olaquindox, which is more biodegradable than aniline. The half-life for aerobic biodegradation is 4 to 8 days for olaquindox, 10 to 40 days for tylosine, 14 to 104 days for metronidazole, and 31 to 40 days for oxytetracycline. Addition of 1 g/l of activated sludge from a waste-water treatment plant decreased the half-life by half. Under anaerobic conditions, the biodegradation rate decreased and the lag phase increased.

A sewage treatment plant near Frankfurt, Germany, was able to eliminate through sorption on activated sludge and biodegradation more than 95 per cent of the propranolol entering the effluent stream at a rate of about 520 g/day and 90 per cent of the ibuprofen at a rate of about 250 g/day. Carbamazepine, clofibric acid, phenazone, and dimethylaminophenazone showed low biodegradation. Antibiotics such as clofibric acid and diclofenac find their way in the aquatic environment, and the former has been found even in the North Sea. In an oxic biofilm reactor, clofibric acid and diclofenac were not degraded and ibuprofen was degraded to 30 to 36 per cent of its initial concentration. When the biofilm reactor (BFR) is operated under anoxic conditions (anoxic means denitrification conditions in the absence of O_2 and presence of nitrate), ibuprofen degradation was low (only 21 per cent) and some appreciable degradation was observed for diclofenac and clofibric acid (about 30 per cent). Hydroxyibuprofen was identified as the major metabolite of ibuprofen biodegradation in the oxic BFR. The BFR used for these studies used pumice stones as support material for micro-organism growth. The biofilm was grown on the support material from activated sludge from a municipal sewage plant. Addition of acetone inhibited the degradation of ibuprofen.

The growth of *Pseudomonas putida* was inhibited by 50 per cent at a concentration of 80 and 10 µg/l in the case of ciprofloxacin and ofloxacin, respectively. These antibiotics were not biodegraded in the closed-bottle test. Metronidazole, one of the most important nitroimidazoles, is toxic to algae and daphnids in low milligram per litre concentrations and is effective against anaerobic bacteria. Strong binding to soil is one reason for the poor degradation of some of the antibiotics from contaminated terrain. For example, cyclosporine degraded very slowly after some months in moist samples of garden soils, even though several micro-organisms capable of its degradation have been isolated from soils. Sarafloxacin, a fluoroquinolone used against poultry diseases, was mineralised by less than 1 per cent in various soils in 80 days.

Virginiamycin, an antibiotic food additive for livestock, was found to biodegrade in various soils with a half-life of 87 to 173 days. Bacteriostatic sulphonamide (sulpha) drugs are used in the treatment of infections in livestock and in the treatment of human infections such as bronchitis and urinary tract infection. Eighty per cent of the drug given to livestock is excreted in urine and subsequently dispersed with the sewage on fields and can reach groundwater. Sulphamethoxazole was found in the surface waters in Germany in concentrations of 30 to 85 ng/l.

To sum up drugs, antibiotics, growth promoters, animal feed supplements, and other pharmaceutical products have been found in marine, underground, and surface waters in many developed countries around the world. Most of these drugs do not get degraded in municipal waste treatment plants. Degradation in contaminated soil is poor, since the drugs bind strongly to the earth, although microbes available for their degradation are found in the nearby proximity. Serious research should be directed toward identifying ways to degrade all these drugs, which have already contaminated the environment, as well as to prevent their entry into the environment and subsequently into the food chain.

Chapter 15

Food Processing Industries

INTRODUCTION

A number of food processing industries produce packed foods and beverages that are available in the market, in plenty. Many of these industries have no planned method of treatment and disposal of their effluents and sludge. In many instances, the direct release of untreated effluent from these industries has resulted in significant surface water pollution and reduction of the quality and productivity of the surrounding agricultural fields. The effluents and sludge released by these industries are very rich in oxidisable organic matters and contain many carbon compounds that can be substrates for various microbial processes. Recent technological developments have refined the treatment process of waste-water of food processing industries and have made the treatment procedure cost effective and environmentally acceptable. There is still scope to improve the treatment efficiency through designed microbial systems, especially for optimisation of the recovery of the resources from waste-water.

The waste-waters produced by different types of industrial units vary greatly in respect of the volume of production and waste-water characteristics. In view of the great variety of industrial processes, there is no common and comprehensive method for the treatment of waste-water of industrial origin. However, one crucial aspect is the collection and storage of the effluents for their proper purification and release into the surface water. It is often found that waste-water contains a lot of organic carbon and sometimes useful resources due to poor quality of upstream resource use and spillage of the matter at various processing steps. There is a need for the proper training of the personnel engaged in industries to substantially reduce product loss through maintenance of equipment, since these losses have a considerable impact on the concentration of pollutants in the released water. Apart from the hard statistical facts about production processes, a conscientious plant designer should, when planning the layout of the waste-water treatment units, also try to consider all operational aspects of the particular plant. Production-integrated environmental protection must be the central part of the waste-water treatment concept, with other major factors being the efficiency of the production process and prevention of product loss during the process.

The general pressure to remain cost-effective is pressing the industry to find ever new solutions, which make for ongoing optimisation. This has a considerable impact on the amount and composition of waste-water produced and thus directly on the treatment methods. Two basic tendencies have resulted from this: the first is the attempt to reduce the amount of water used, e.g. by recycling or reusing water in other processes. The result is a decreased amount of waste-water, but with a considerably high concentration of pollutants. The second tendency is to separate the fractions and to reduce the specific load (measured in terms of BOD_5 and COD), e.g. by disposing off the dried solid matter (e.g. as nutrients for agricultural use). The requirement is to separate the particulate organic and inorganic substances from the waste-water as much as possible, before leading it for chemical and/or biological purification. This is, however, not applicable for all types of industries. This chapter contains information about the procedures for treatment and disposal of waste-water of some important food processing industries.

Effluents from food and allied industries are considered to be close to domestic sewage since they mainly contain biodegradable material and suspended solids. Hence, treatment of such wastes was never felt as difficult task. A major shift in the approach as far as treatment of such wastes is concerned has been the use of anaerobic technology instead of aerobic one. Energy-saving is felt important and energy generation is possible in the treatment of such wastes. Biogas production, SCP production, by-product recovery are important aspects of treatment of food industry wastes. The large volumes of effluents, seasonal variation, high BOD, high suspended solids, presence of fats, oil and grease, solid wastes are typical of food industry wastes. Microbial processes are very much there to tackle food wastes. Since a long time improvements are towards greater efficiency in management of such wastes.

NATURE OF EFFLUENTS (WASTES) FROM FOOD PROCESSING INDUSTRIES

In general, food processing industries have wastes which fall into the category of readily degradable organics. They will be characterised by more suspended solids, high BOD/COD, no toxic matter and large volumes. Thus, treatment of these wastes is normally not considered a difficult task. However, large volumes, high BOD and suspended solids cause enough concern for their economic treatment.

Dairies operate in discontinuous manner. Many dairies may work only 8–12 hours of a day. Tank cleaning, effluent producing operations are intense only in certain hours. Conventional milk, evaporated milk, cream products, fermented milk, cheese—each process of production will have different effluent. Dairy effluents often contain milk solids. The quantity and load depend on the size of unit and the variety of products. These effluents are deficient in nitrogen and for efficient degradation, nitrogen will have to be added. Waste-water volume is part of on site management and can vary from 0.5 m^3 per m^3 of milk to 3 m^3 per m^3 of milk. Whey is a highly polluting material. 1 m^3 whey is equivalent to daily pollution production from approximately 500 people. BOD and COD of typical whey is 45,000 mg l^{-1} and 60,000 mg l^{-1} respectively.

Fruit and vegetable processing industries have a seasonal variation and a wide variety of products. Solid wastes is largely a problem here as skins, seeds, pomace, cuttings, peelings are produced to a considerable extent. Also unwanted vegetable debris is discarded to a large extent. Separation of solid wastes from effluents by screening is a must. Fruits and vegetable processing industry wastes are not soluble in cold water but are soluble in warm water. Effluents may have BOD up to 80,000 mg l^{-1} and is insoluble matter. Effluents are relatively deficient in nitrogen. The main problem with these effluents is to maintain a steady loading since pH falls with storing.

In the potato processing industry, half of potato is lost in various forms of wastes such as peel, trim, filtrable particulates, processing water, blanching water. pH of potato peeling (chemical by caustic) will be highly alkaline. While at other places, acidic pH common problem causing corrosion to plant, poor settling or primary sludges and of secondary biological processes.

Pineapple canning industry in the tropical countries like Thailand produce large quantities of liquid and solid wastes. Liquid wastes with COD 10,000 mg l^{-1} largely contain carbohydrates and have little proteins. Medium-size pineapple cannery discharges daily 150 tonnes of solid wastes. Peelings and core part are normally discarded without treatment. Similarly, banana, carrot, citrus peel, coffee pulp form large wastes during processing. Manufacturing of wheat gluten and starch from flour produces waste-waters which contain mixtures of aminoacids, proteins, carbohydrates, hemicelluloses, pentose gums, suspended starch granules, insoluble protein and bran particles. The COD ranges between 10,000 to 25,000 mg per litre. Meat processing industry is again typical in the production of high solid wastes. Bones, hair, feathers, flesh residues, paunch manure (partially digested food) are produced which have to be removed by screening the waste-waters. BOD upto 12,000 mg l^{-1} suspended solids up to 5000 mg l^{-1} and FOG (fats, oil and grease) up to 800 mg l^{-1} are common. FOG has a high BOD, more than 2000 mg BOD per gram of lipid. Blood is an essential part removed and used for separate recovery of by-products and to reduce polluting loads of effluent. Grease traps, gravity clarification, dissolved air flotation may be used to remove FOG. FOG is an insoluble but biodegradable part. FOG causes dogging.

Meat and poultry products processing industry will have slaughterhouse activities, at processing meat activities and secondary processing. High BOD, SS, NH-N FOG, extremes pH values, pathogens are common pollution problems in addition to solid wastes mentioned earlier.

BIOLOGICAL TREATMENT METHODS FOR FOOD INDUSTRY

After knowing about the nature of effluents coming about from food processing industry, it is clear that these wastes are manageable. The question is how economically we treat them to make them acceptable for discharge.

DAIRY INDUSTRY

Dairy processing (cheese, casein, butter production) effluents predominately contain milk and milk products that have been lost in the processing.

Milk lost into the effluent stream can amount to 0.5 to 2.5 per cent of the incoming milk, but can be as high as 3 to 4 per cent. Although all compounds are biodegradable, some of them, such as lactose, are readily consumed in biological treatment, whereas protein and especially fat are not easily degraded. In order to understand the environmental impact of these effluents, it is useful to briefly consider the nature of milk. Apart from water, which makes up about 87.5 per cent of its weight, raw milk typically contains 13 per cent total solids, 3.9 per cent fat, 3.4 per cent protein, 4.8 per cent lactose, and 0.8 per cent minerals. The quality control process of the raw milk prior to its use causes the generation of a particularly complex effluent that contains raw milk and a mixture of different chemicals. The liquid waste in a dairy originates from the manufacturing process, utilities, and service sections. The various sources of waste generation from dairy are spilled milk, spoiled milk, skimmed milk, whey, wash water from milk cans, equipment, bottles, and floor washing. Whey is a high-strength waste product of cheese manufacture, and it is the most difficult to degrade. It contains milk proteins, water soluble vitamins, and mineral salts. Table 15.1 shows a summary of different waste-waters from dairy factories.

Table 15.1. Characterisation of the effluents from dairy factories[a].

Origin	COD	BOD	Fats	N_t	P_t	pH	TSS	VSS
Dairy factory	4000	2600	400	55	35	8-11	675	635
Whey	61,250	–	–	2500	533	4.6	5077	4900
Cheese factory	4430	3000	754	18	14	7.32	1100	–
Yogurt and buttermilk	1500	1000	–	63		7.2	–	191	–

[a] COD—chemical oxygen demand (mg O_2/l); BOD—biological oxygen demand (mg/l); N_t—total nitrogen (mg/l); P_t—total phosphorus (mg/l); TSS—total suspended solids (mg/l); VSS—volatile suspended solids (mg/l).

Both aerobic and anaerobic processes are employed for the treatment of these wastes. Aerobic treatment is characterised by relatively high energy consumption, and biomass production is not preferred. Anaerobic processes, on the other hand, prove most suitable for the treatment of dairy wastes. The steps for treatment of waste-water generated from dairy and milk processing industries are given in Fig. 15.1.

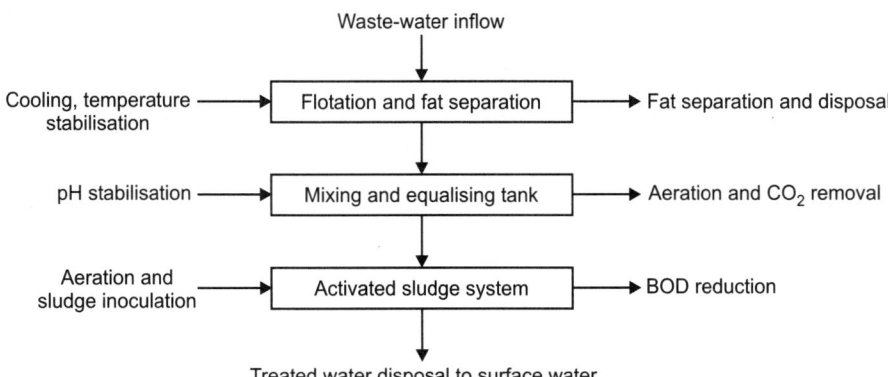

Fig. 15.1. The steps for treatment of waste-water generated from dairy and milk processing industries.

Milk fat is quite difficult to degrade biologically because of the potential toxic effects exerted by the fatty acids that result from the breakdown of fat molecules. This necessarily calls for a suitable bioreactor design to avoid undesirable fat accumulation. The treatment of cheese whey waste-waters by anaerobic degradation is constrained by the drop in pH that inhibits further conversion of acids to methane. This can be taken care of by buffering the solution in a hybrid reactor.

It is clear that buffering action is needed initially for maintaining the pH, but at a later stage, a mature microbial population improves the stability. Apart from the hybrid reactor, other, alternate reactor types have also been tried for the treatment of dairy-based waste-waters. In the study carried out by Guitonas, a fixed bed reactor with cells immobilised on rice straw was used for the treatment of milk-based synthetic organic waste. The advantage of this system was a lower adaptation time with change in the organic loading rate.

Dairy effluents were being treated for a long time by different methods. Pretreatment of dairy effluent involves: (i) flow balancing for adjustment of nutrients, (ii) adjustment of pH, (iii) removal of fat. Further treatments differ:

1. Newzealand: Dominant technique is spary irrigation.
2. Europe: Extended aeration preferred.
3. UK: Use of biofiltration either ADF or with plastic media.

Irrigation of agricultural land with the dairy effluents induces microbial action, increases earthworm activity and adds trace elements to soil. Irrigation rate does not exceed the infiltration rate of soil.

In other treatment methods for dairy effluents activated sludge process can be operated only in extended aeration mode. This is due to the fact that filamentous bacteria may dominate the sludge flora and can cause severe sludge settlement problem inspite of all other controls. Extended aeration with oxidation ditch is preferred in Europe. Here low organic loading rate (<0.1 kg BOD kg^{-1} MLSS), coupled with aeration phase, ensures environment more suitable for non-filamentous bacteria.

Biological filters are more stable but ponding problem is faced. It is overcome by using popular ADF mode of biofiltration. High rate filtration with plastic media is preferred.

Aerobic, aerated, facultative, anaerobic are the 4 main types of lagoons which may be used for dairy effluents where land costs are low. Flies, odour, insects cause nuisance. Since all the above said options are either costly due to aeration or are problematic due to other reasons, anaerobic digestion is preferred for whey (dairy effluents). Following the digester treatment and methane generation, nitrogen in wastes (1000 mg l^{-1} total nitrogen and 750 mg l^{-1} ammonia nitrogen) may be removed by aerobic nitrification/ denitrification stage and then effluents can reach to a level of discharge.

A new digester similar to 'Clarigester' has been developed which takes up to 15 kg COD/m^3/day load and has less retention time (5 days instead of 15). This is possible due to an increase in microbial mass. For the UASB reactor with two-stage system (first, primary liquifaction and acidification and second, methane production), loading rates of 25–30 kg COD/m^3/day are possible. COD, removal efficiency is 85 per cent.

Anaerobic digestion of whey is more economical than aerobic digestion. Biogas has 60 per cent methane and 40 per cent CO$_2$. With maximum whey feed of 110 m^3 per 24 hours, biogas yield of 4180 m^3 per 24 hours can be expected (38 m^3 biogas/m^3 whey).

Trickling filter and activated sludge processes have their own disadvantages and a combination technology which is known as biofilter activated sludge process is used by many fruit and vegetable processing industries. It has both trickling filter tower and activated sludge aeration basin and clarifier. Return sludge from the clarifier and secondary influent is recycled over the filter. There are over 50 biofilter activated sludge plants in the USA treating food processing wastes. Several times, high organic loading is possible in the activated sludge part of the biofilter activated sludge plant than for conventional activated sludge process.

Pure oxygen activated sludge systems are expensive and hence less used but they have smaller aeration basins. RBCs were introduced in the 1970s and are used to some extent. Land disposal is possible and an acceptable option in rural areas.

STARCH INDUSTRIES

Starch is produced from potatoes, corn and wheat. Depending on the original raw material, the wastewater fractions, amounts, and loads emerging during starch production vary considerably.

Corn Starch

The fractional flow sources during corn starch processing are: maceration station, germ washing, starch milk dewatering, gluten, thickener, glue of gluten dewatering, and chaff dehydration. The various fractions of waste-water are mainly recycled and used as processing water. The waste-water fractions that have to be treated are: (i) processing water, and (ii) the condensates resulting from evaporation of the maceration water.

Wheat Starch

During wheat starch production, waste-water is derived from the separation step and from the thickening of secondary starch. All other flow fractions are returned into the process water. The waste-water flow fraction that has to be treated is referred to as process water.

Potato Starch

During potato starch production, washing water (flume and transport water), fruit water (sometimes also condensates from a fruit water evaporation plant), and production waste-water are produced. By recycling, it has been possible to reduce the washing water demand from 5–9 m³/T to 0.3–0.6 m³/T. Fruit water separated from potatoes is usually fed into the protein recovery unit. Approximately 50 per cent of the proteins contained in the fruit water are coagulated and separated subsequently. Protein production from fruit water is always economically viable, since the price for the protein produced is comparatively low, whereas biological treatment, particularly for the elimination of nitrogen (10 g of protein contains 1.7 g N), is quite expensive (about 5–10 times the cost for protein production).

Waste-water from starch factories has a high organic load and usually consists of easily degradable matters. The undissolved organic contents are mainly carbohydrates and proteins. The fat content is normally 10 per cent. Usually, this kind of waste-water does not contain any toxic substance. The substrate ratio COD: N: P is satisfactory; actually, there may even occur an excess of N and P, so that it is not necessary to add nutrient salts. Like in the case of sugar industries, the waste-water from the starch industries are also treated in the same three distinct processes, viz. (i) soil treatment, (ii) pond processing, and (iii) small-scale technical processes (anaerobic, aerobic, evaporation).

Anaerobic waste-water treatment has become established, alongside conventional activated sludge processes, to remove organic matters and to reduce the BOD load. Fixed-film reactors and UASB reactors are mainly used, which at loads between 7–30 kg COD/m³·day, can achieve a degradation rate of 70–90 per cent to maintain operational stability. A separator for solids is usually placed upstream of the reactor. Furthermore, a separate pre-acidification stage, with a sludge removal system, is recommended. The amounts of available phosphorus and nitrogen are sufficient for the anaerobic treatment. Sometimes, trace amounts of cobalt and nickel need to be added. The pH should not exceed 7.0, since at higher pH values MAP (magnesium ammonium phosphate) might precipitate (Fig. 15.2).

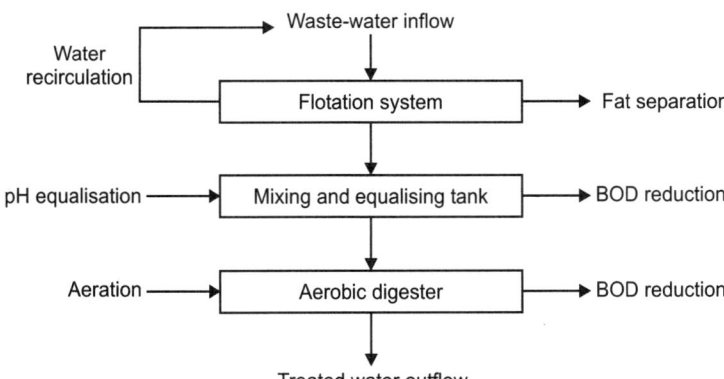

Fig. 15.2. The schematic diagram of treatment steps of waste-water from vegetable oil industries.

In the potato starch industry, a further possibility for fruit water treatment is the reduction of the waste-water by evaporation to a solid content of 70 per cent. The dried solids can then be utilised, e.g. as fertilisers. To save evaporation energy, a membrane process can be used to increase the concentration, prior to evaporation, which would be done as a cascade operation under vacuum conditions. Aerobic secondary treatment is always required if the industry intends to discharge its waste-water directly into surface water.

VEGETABLE OIL INDUSTRIES

In the vegetable oil industry one differentiates between the branches producing oils and shortening. They are: (i) extraction plants for the extraction of raw fat and oil, (ii) refining plants for refining raw fat and oil, and (iii) plants for further processing of the nutrient fats, e.g. into margarine, which consists of approximately 80 per cent fat, 20 per cent water, plus some other ingredients. The process technology for nutrient fat and oil production largely depends on the raw materials, depending on whether oil is extracted from seeds (soyabean, sunflower, coconut, rapeseed, etc.), animal fats from tallow and fat liquefiers (tallow or lard) and fruit flesh fats (palm oil, olive oil, which due to its poor storage stability, is usually extracted near the site of production), and fats from marine animals.

The processing of seed oils consists of the following stages: (i) cleaning, peeling/ shelling if required, (ii) masticating, (iii) conditioning (heating and moistening), and (iv) prepressing with ensuing extraction or direct extraction without prepressing. Extraction is accomplished by means of a solvent-oil mixture (emulsion), followed by removal of the solvent (usually hexane) by steam. The vapours are condensed and the hexane is separated from the water in static separators. In a further distillation step, the remaining hexane is removed from the waste-water. The waste-water amount produced in seed oil extraction processes is less than 10 m^3/T of seeds. Data for the waste-water pollutant concentrations is presented in Table 15.2.

Extraction of animal fats is accomplished by masticating fatty tissues and heating the macerate, followed by a separation process. Wet and dry melting processes are distinguished. The dry melting process does not produce any waste-water, whereas the wet process produces approx. 0.35 m^3/T raw material, which mainly consists of glue water and pump sealing water from the separators. Depending on the extraction method and the cleaning procedures used in the production plant, the concentration of pollutants in the waste-water from tallow melting plants can vary considerably. For waste-water that has passed the fat separators with topped sludge catcher implements, the concentration of lipophilic substances remains >100 mg/l (Table 15.2) and the COD/BOD ratio remains at about 2.5 (the ratio of emulsified fats, however, may be dramatically higher).

Table 15.2. The physico-chemical characteristics of waste-water from vegetable oil industries.

Waste-water type	pH	BOD$_5$ (g/l)	COD (g/l)	Lipophilic substances (mg/l)
Fat processing	6–7	2.0–4.0	5–10	<100
Oil refining	5–9	0.3–0.4	0.6–1.0	<600
Margarine production	5–9	0.6–1.0	1.0–2.0	<250

In refining plants, the raw oil is purified (refined) by removing undesired ingredients. The basic process steps consist of desliming, neutralising, bleaching, and dedourising (steaming). Depending on the raw material and the desired end product, further processes such as winterising, fractionating, transesterification, or hydrogenation may be carried out. In addition to this, other waste products such as saponification-water (soapstock) are processed. Waste-water fractions occur during desliming/ neutralising, oil drying and cooling, steaming (condensates), as well as during soap cracking (acidic water). The amount and composition of the waste-water depends mainly on the characteristics of the fresh water, with regard to temperature and degree of hardness, the mode of process operation (continuous or discontinuous methods, process temperature and pressure), the type and quality of raw materials, and the frequency with which the raw materials are changed. A standard value for waste-water of a refining plant, which recirculates the falling water, is <10 m^3/T of raw material. Provided that no falling water recirculation of static fat separators is used in the wet chemical refining process, the total waste-water of a refinery has the characteristics, presented in Table 15.3.

For margarine production, waste-water results only from the cleaning circuits of the CIP plants and amounts to approximately 1–3 m^3/T margarine. After rinsing and cleaning, water passes through the fat separator. The waste-water has an average BOD load of about 0.8 g/l and a COD/BOD ratio of 2.0. The concentration of the lipophilic substances is comparatively high when compared with the waste-water of oil refining plants.

Waste-water treatment processes in vegetable oil industries usually consist of a physical-chemical pretreatment by fat separators or flotation systems to decrease the amounts of undissolved solids and lipophilic substances. Whereas installation of fat separators is only a minimal pretreatment concept, because the efficiency of these systems may be completely reduced by a hot water surge, a more expensive flotation system using additives also allows the elimination of emulsified, mainly lipophilic, substances. Particularly effective are pressure flotation systems designed for a surface load of 4–5 m^3/m^2 hr, with a recirculation flow of 10–40 per cent, operating at 4–7 bar. Often a mixing and equalising (M + E) tank is installed behind the flotation system to equalise pH value and temperature peaks and to allow a more constant loading of the subsequent biological treatment stage (Fig. 15.2). The latter is an aerobic activated sludge treatment and a sludge load of approximately 0.1 kg BOD/kg MLSS.day has been found very effective. To prevent flotation of sludge and development of scum layers, the fat contents of the waste-water should be >200 mg/l.

Vegetable Canning Wastes

Vegetable canning wastes are also treated to produce methane. The total productivity of digestion depends upon the performance of liquefaction stage. A two-stage system is used where carrot peeling wastes were able to produce 2.4 m^3 methane/m^3 digester/day at 35°C. The liquefaction stage was carried out at 60°C. One-stage system produced 1.35 m^3 methane/m^3 digester/day and latter 2.27 m^3/day. For the meat processing industry, concentration has always been towards product safety considerations, and pollution control got secondary importance. It is also true that these wastes were always thought to be manageable. In the process waste, control has proved very much important for the food industry in general and the meat and poultry industry in particular. It helps to reduce volume and strength of waste-waters that are generated. Efficient recovery of by-products and care in procedures used for blood processing, hide processing, viscera handling, on site rendering, water use reduction, waste segregation (manure sewer, blood drain tank, FOG sewer, sanitary wastes, clean water sewer are particularly important.

SLAUGHTERHOUSES

Slaughterhouses and meat processing plants can be divided into four categories, according to their different production processes: (i) slaughterhouses for hogs and cattle, (ii) slaughterhouses for poultry, (iii) meat-cutting plants, and (iv) meat-processing industry. Local butcher shops are not considered, as these are very non-point sources. However, in India the local butcher shops constitute the most part of slaughter waste, that is allowed to enter the domestic sewage system in urban areas, without being treated in anyway. In the developed world, they constitute a very small turnover volume.

In the slaughtering process, not only meat from muscle tissue, but also by-products and residues are produced. The meat and the organ meats (such as liver, etc.) are fit for human consumption and can be traded freely. The residue produced in the slaughtering process is divided into two categories: (i) residues that have commercial value and are tradable, such as fat and bones, which find use as raw materials in feed plants or in the pharmaceutical industry, and (ii) non-tradable residues, such as meat unfit for human consumption and other by-products, which need to be treated in animal carcass disposal plants. Additional waste products include primary waste (stomach and intestine contents) and secondary waste (solids from waste-water screening and flotation sludge).

The primary waste-water and waste product sources are divided into three production areas: (i) truck washing and animal sheds (green line), (ii) slaughter and cutting (red line), and (iii) stomach, intestine, and entrails cleaning (yellow line) the latter, however, is often not done on the slaughterhouse grounds. The waste occurring in trucks and animal sheds consists of bedding material, faeces, and urine, which amount to 2.0 kg per hog and 10 kg per cow, if the stabling time is kept short. These materials should be removed without the use of water and spread on agricultural land. Sparing water consumption during truck cleaning can keep the washing water down to 100 l per truck. The waste-water should be screened to remove large particles and should then be fed into the main waste-water stream.

In slaughterhouses, waste-water pretreatment is mainly done with mechanical procedures. Up to now, the number of plants, for which physico-chemical or biological operational steps have been added, is comparatively small. The main cleaning effect of mechanical and physical procedures consists of retention and separation of solids with the help of stationary strainers, rotating screening drums, separators, fine rakes, screening catchers, or fat separators with a preceding sludge catcher.

In waste-water from slaughterhouses, part of the organic matter consists of oil and fats in emulsified form. Thus, it may be wise to add a physical chemical stage to the mechanical pretreatment, which would consist of a precipitation/flocculation stage and a flotation unit. Although most of the slaughterhouses operating in different countries of the world do not have their own biological treatment stages, the waste-water from slaughterhouses is suitable for biological methods, because of its composition.

The following biological methods can be used successfully on an industrial scale to reduce the BOD load in the waste-water and to regenerate the nutrients, for the use of water for irrigation: (i) large space biological methods (oxidation ponds), (ii) various activated sludge systems (single stage, cascade, two stage), and (iii) anaerobic biological methods. For activated sludge systems, the sludge load should not exceed 0.15 kg BOD_5/kg MLSS day. Direct anaerobic treatment in contact sludge reactors or joint treatment in municipal digestion tanks is particularly suitable for fats, floating materials, stomach and gut contents, and the liquid phase from the dewatering of rumen contents.

MEAT PROCESSING INDUSTRY

The meat processing industry is large, common to many countries, and generates large volumes of waste-water that require considerable treatment before release into the environment. The effluent contains high volumes of carbohydrates, proteins, fats, and other organic materials, in addition to a high concentration of phosphate, acetic acid, butyric acid, and chloride. The concentration of pollutants in various waste-water streams from slaughterhouses or rendering plants is summarised in Table 15.3. Screening, settling, and dissolved air flotation are still widely used for the removal of suspended solids and fats, oils, and greases. Anaerobic systems are well suited to the treatment of slaughterhouse waste-water. They achieve a high degree of BOD removal at a significantly lower cost than comparable aerobic systems and generate a smaller quantity of highly stabilised, more easily dewatered sludge. Furthermore, the methane-rich gas that is generated can be captured for use as a fuel. However, anaerobic treatment suffers from the disadvantage of odour generation from the ponds, thus making the development of alternate designs very essential.

Table 15.3. Analysis of waste-water from slaughterhouses.

Parameter[a]	Waste-water
BOD, mg/l	1600–3000
COD, mg/l	4200–8500
Oil and grease, mg/l	100–200
Total suspended solids, mg/l	1300–3400
Total Kjeldahl nitrogen mg/l	114–148
NH₄-nitrogen mg/l	65–87
Total phosphorus mg/l	20–30
Volatile fatty acids, mg/l	175–400

The high-rate anaerobic treatment systems such as the upflow anerobic sludge blanket (UASB) and fixed bed reactors are less popular for slaughterhouse waste-waters because of the presence of large amounts of fat, oil, and suspended matter in the influent. The anaerobic contact reactor appears to be more suitable compared with UASB because the latter is constrained by the lack of formation of granules and there is also loss of sludge due to high fat concentrations. Hence, a pretreatment step for removal of fats and suspended solids becomes essential if an UASB is to be used. However, for a low COD load, the more efficient UASB appears to result in a high COD reduction.

Two-phase reactor systems (Fig. 15.3) are best suited for degradation of food wastes. In stage one, hydrolytic and acidogenic bacteria (anaerobic) degrade organic suspended solids to volatile fatty acids (VFAs). These VFAs are then further degraded to methane by the methanogenic (anaerobic) organisms. A two-stage system for treating high-strength waste-water from an abattoir has been tried by Rivera. The system consists of an anaerobic digester followed by an artificially constructed wetland that utilises the root zone of hydrophytes planted in a gravel substrate. The treatment efficiency was high, with COD and BOD reductions of 87.4 and 88.5 per cent, respectively.

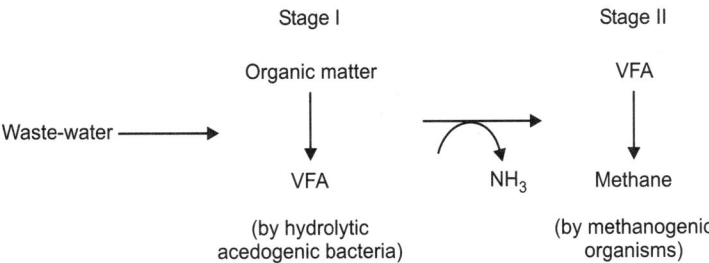

Fig. 15.3. Two-phase system for waste-waters with high concentrations of organic solids.

General Treatment Methods

The four 'Rs' of waste management (recover, reduce, reuse, and recycle) are best suited for the food industry. All the same, the waste generated from this industry (as discussed earlier) is best treated by bioremediation methods. Two-phase reactor systems are best suited for degradation. Apart from the well-known methods of bioremediation, newer methodologies have been adopted for improving the efficiency of transformation, reducing sludge formation, and aiding in the formation of sludge that can be used for farming purposes. Composting is one such option of disposal. However, odour and leaching of soluble constituents are limiting factors. Composted material is valued as a soil amendment or potting soil, but widespread use and marketability are constrained by shipping cost. Composition of the composting feedstock needs to be controlled to obtain the appropriate physical mix to allow the natural composting aerobic bioprocesses to proceed. Examples in the literature show that the full range of food processing wastes can be composted, including fruit and vegetable wastes such as peelings and skin; whole fish and fish offal; meat processing wastes such as paunch contents, blood, fats, intestines, and manure; and grain processing wastes such as chaff, hulls, pods, stems, and weeds.

Residues from extraction of oils such as cotton, olive, and palm contain tannins and phenolics that are toxic to plants and animals. Apart from the general methods, these wastes can also be detoxified by growing mushrooms (e.g. *Pleurotus* and *Lentinula* species). While actively growing, these mushrooms produce enzymes that can degrade lignins, phenolics, and tannins. Producing a crop of mushrooms while disposing of an otherwise hazardous waste has become a popular 'research model' in recent years. *Pleurotus* cultivation may even aid removal of pollutants from contaminated waste sites.

Food waste can be treated by a two-stage anaerobic process, followed by an aerobic treatment to completely mineralise the pollutants. Also, recent developments such as composting, phytoremediation, and mushroom culturing have substantial potential in clean-up of these wastes.

Chapter 16

Metal and Mining Industries

INTRODUCTION

Metallurgical industries being the largest manpower employers and the largest material handling/processing industries, contribute significantly to air, water and land pollution. Moreover, most metallurgical industries of today come into existence at a time when the concept of pollution and formulation/implementation of pollution control laws/policies were not considered very seriously. Awareness about threat to life through environmental pollution has created an urge to provide a pollution free environment for the safety of human, vegetable/plant and aquatic life, etc. Holding of education camps to discuss and develop strategies for pollution control, therefore, becomes necessary. The environmental problems associated with metallurgical and mining can be listed as under:

1. Water pollution due to wash-off of overburdened wastes.
2. Air pollution due to release of noxious gases.
3. Land degradation due to large-scale excavation, disposal of mine wastes.
4. Noise and vibration due to blasting and operation of heavy machinery.
5. Human environment problems (settlements, health, etc.)
6. Damage to sites of cultural, historical and scenic importance.
7. Problems caused by mine fires.

Metallurgical industrial activity is one of the most important examples of human ability to process, form, shape, treat and use various natural resources. Increase in metallurgical industrial activities over the last few decades has no doubt ensured national economic development but at the risk of environmental pollution. Every activity of the metallurgical industry damages the environment, posing a great challenge to life.

Public concern over environmental pollution is increasing day by day because of the awareness of its threats to health and welfare of the society. A large volume of waste-water, originating from different unit operations and containing mostly suspended solids, lubrication oils and several toxic substances are produced from an integrated steel plant.

The largest single source of waste-water from coke oven plant, having the highest pollution potential in an integrated steel plant, is the ammonia still from where the waste ammoniacal liquor comes out. The second biggest source is the benzol plant. The major pollutant of the coal washery waste is suspended solids. As such, this waste is usually treated in a clarifier with or without coagulation. However, the addition of coagulant reduces both the detention time and surface area of the tank. Several coagulants like starch, lime and indigenous coagulants like Nirmali seed (*Strychuos potatorum linn*) extracts can be used effectively for the clarification of coal washery wastes. The clarified effluent is either recycled or discharged as waste.

The biological treatment of coke oven effluents can be carried out economically in a three-stage process, with isolated or cultured bacteria, appropriate to each stage. In the first stage, phenol is oxidised, in the second, thiosulphate and thiocyanate are reduced, and in the third stage, ammonia is oxidised.

The blast furnace waste contains about 40 per cent dust coming out along with the flue gas. Iron oxide and silica comprise about 70 per cent and 12 per cent, respectively of the flue dust content. The waste can be treated in a clariflocculator even without the addition of coagulants.

Even in the most modern foundries, dust is a common problem and it is necessary to provide adequate ventilation to hold the dust concentration to acceptable levels. The air may be scrubbed before discharge to the outside in water spray type units or filtered through bag filters, in which case the collected dust must be wetted before it can be removed and hauled to a disposal area. The waste-water from air scrubbers is very high in suspended solids and must be processed for their removal for final disposal.

All these factors and environmental control activities can be achieved by good housekeeping, upgrading the existing equipment or installing new pollution control facilities. Specialised experience is required for planning and implementing a pollution abatement programme that will meet current and future needs.

The metal finishing industry uses a variety of physical, chemical and electrochemical processes to clean, etch, and plate metallic and non-metallic substrates. Chemical and electrochemical processes contribute more to the generation of hazardous waste than physical processes such as blasting, grinding and polishing. The chemical and electrochemical processes are performed in numerous chemical baths, which are followed by a rinsing operation. The most common wastes generated by the metal finishing industry are rinse water effluent and spent process bath chemicals. Typically, rinse water effluent and spent process bath chemicals are treated on-site before being discharged to a local publicly-owned treatment works (POTW). Metal finishing industry wastes are generated mostly from spent plating baths, spent process baths, rinsing/cleaning baths and degreasing.

For the metal finishing industry, available pollution prevention technologies mainly include extending the life of chemical process baths and reducing the volume of waste-water generated.

Since pollution prevention in the metal finishing industry usually involves extending the bath life and reducing the amount of waste-water generated, it is divided into two sub-sections: process baths and rinse systems. Source/waste reduction at the process-bath level can be established by material substitution, bath life extension and/or drag-out reduction. Material substitution options include modifying the chemistry of the process baths or replacing the chemicals used for a given process. Rinse water usage may be reduced by improving the rinsing efficiency and/or by controlling the water flow rate.

METAL PROCESSING, SEMICONDUCTOR AND CYANIDE

Metal Processing

Although biosorption with dead biomass appears to be very attractive, biosorption with live cells has other advantages. Metal biosorption can be combined with degradation of other organic contaminants present in the waste, and organisms can be genetically modified to improve their performance as well as survive harsh environments.

Research activities with respect to pollution control should be directed toward the following areas: (i) hastening the mobilisation of metals, (ii) designing metal-tolerant strains that can also adapt to performing biodegradation of organic pollutants, (iii) breeding natural or engineered strains, that is, design biomass with specific metal-binding properties through the expression of metal-chelating proteins and peptides, (iv) using live bacteria, (v) designing biosurfactants to assist in the solubilisation and desorption of metals from polluted soils or sediments, (vi) better understanding the cell microenvironment, (vii) studying anaerobic respiration for the *in situ* treatment of organic and metal contaminants in the subsurface, and (viii) improving process development techniques that combine biotreatment, separation, and recovery.

The semiconductor industry uses large quantities of water and a wide range of heavy metals, acids, alkalies, and toxic and hazardous organic and inorganic chemicals. Hence this industry is facing serious environmental problems. Recovery and reuse of water, acids, and other chemicals could solve many of its waste disposal problems, but the need for high purity water and chemicals makes the industry hesitant to reuse the recovered chemicals. Biofilters or biotrickling filters appear to be good technologies for treating vapours and gaseous effluents from the semiconductor plant. Coagulation followed by settling and filtration of the liquid effluent is effective and cheap for removing the hazardous material from the effluent, but the disposal of the toxic sludge generated is a serious problem that has not been solved. Bioremediation for liquid effluent appears to be very limited except for the use of biosorption for extracting metals. Phytoremediation also appears to be a good technique for treating contaminated soil and solid wastes.

Cyanide removal from waste currently relies on chemical treatment technologies, but recently biological treatment processes have been used successfully in large-scale operations. Proper closure and disposal of the spent heap leach ore that could contain adsorbed cyanide is another major problem that needs to be addressed. A combination of chemical and biological treatment technology could be highly effective and economically viable. In addition to cyanide, related compounds found in the mining effluents such as cyanate, thiocyanate, ammonia, and nitrate also must be treated and disposed of safely.

Treatment of waste from metal processing and electrochemical industries

The mining, electroplating, tannery, steel works, automobile, battery, and semiconductor industries are faced with the problem of heavy metals in their effluent streams, which harm the soil and the waterways. The metals most often encountered include lead, chromium, copper, zinc, arsenic, and cadmium. Hence treating, neutralising, and remediating these heavy-metal-polluted sites have become an utmost priority to these industries. Unlike organic contaminants that can be degraded to harmless products, metals cannot be further transmuted or mineralised to a totally innocuous form. Their oxidation state, solubility, and association with other inorganic and organic molecules can be varied so that they are made harmless. Although this does not solve the problem of pollution, it makes the environment less harmful and also aids in the recycling of the metals. Many enzymes have divalent or transition elements in their active centre. For normal cell metabolism, minute quantities of these metals are required. But when these metals are present in excess, they could be toxic to the same enzymes. Many other metals cause damage to the cells by blocking and inactivating the sulphydryl groups of proteins. Metals can be divided into three groups based on their effect on cells and micro-organisms: (i) essential and nontoxic metals such as Ca or Mg, (ii) essential but could be toxic at high concentrations like Fe, Mn, Zn, Cu, Co, Ni, and Mo, and (iii) toxic at all levels, for example, Hg or Cd.

Chemical methods for treatment of this waste-water include neutralisation, precipitation and filtration, electrochemistry, reverse osmosis, encapsulation, ion exchange, adsorption, or solvent extraction. These method are effective and well established, but require large quantities of expensive chemicals or are capital intensive, and they also generate large quantities of sludge that must be recycled or disposed of effectively. Few of these methods are very effective at high metal concentrations, and they become uneconomical under dilute conditions. Recently, biological methods have attracted interest because of their simplicity. Other advantages of biological techniques over the physical and chemical methods include their higher specificity, suitability to *in situ* methodologies, and avoidance of high energy and toxic chemical addition. Different methods have been studied for metal extraction from contaminated soil, including leaching by inorganic acids (H_2SO_4, HCl, HNO_3, etc.), leaching by organic acids (citric acid, acetic acid, etc.), bioleaching, and use of chelating agents (EDTA, ADA, DTPA, NTA, etc.), surfactants, and biosurfactants.

Mechanisms of metal-micro-organism interaction

The micro-organisms convert the metal contaminants to forms that are precipitated or volatilised from the solution, alter the redox state so that they become more soluble leading to its leaching from soil, or allow its biosorption on microbial mass, thereby preventing its migration. Different types of reactions, which take place in various parts of the cell, are given below:

1. Extracellular reactions.
   (a) Precipitation with excreted products .
   (b) Complexation and chelation.
   (c) Siderophores.
2. Cell-associated materials.
   (a) Ion-exchange.
   (b) Particulate entrapment.
   (c) Nonspecific binding.
   (d) Precipitation.
3. Cell wall.
   (a) Adsorption or ion-exchange, covalent binding.
   (b) Entrapment of particles.
   (c) Redox reactions.
   (d) Precipitation.
4. Cell membrane/periplasmic space.
   (a) Adsorption/ion-exchange.
   (b) Redox reactions/transformations.
   (c) Precipitation.
   (d) Diffusion and transport (influx and efflux).
5. Intracellular.
   (a) Metallothionein.
   (b) Metal y-glutamyl peptides.
   (c) Nonspecific binding/sequestration.
   (d) Organellar compartmentation.
   (e) Redox reactions or transformations.

Eukaryotes are more sensitive to metal toxicity than bacteria. *Cyanobacterium synechococcus* is resistant to Zn^{2+} and Cd^{2+} because of the production of the metallo thioneins (MT) gene, which is known to bind these metals. Sulphate-reducing bacteria (SRB) are anaerobes that produce sulphide and immobilise toxic ions (Cu, Fe, Zn, Ni, Cd, Pb, etc.) as metal sulphides; hence they exhibit metal tolerance as a secondary outcome of their metabolism. Hydrogen sulphide produced during the sulphate ion reduction reacts to form the precipitate. Ferric iron is also precipitated as its hydroxide. Its elimination probably occurs through two steps-the first being the reduction to ferrous iron and the second to divalent metallic sulphide as a precipitate.

Thiobacilli and *Thermophilic archaea*, iron- and sulphur-oxidising bacteria, grow at the highest metal concentrations. *Thiobacillus ferrooxidans* is dependent on Fe(II), but it is also resistant to Al, Cu, Co, Ni, Mn, and Zn at a concentration of 0.1 to 0.3 M. Reduction of Cr (VI) to insoluble Cr(III) by SRB may be due to bacterial respiration or indirect reduction by Fe^{2+} and sulphide. Under iron-limiting conditions, micro-organisms such as bacteria, fungi, cyanobacteria, and algae excrete siderophores, which are low molecular weight Fe (III) coordination compounds, to capture iron from the environment. In addition to iron, siderophores and analogous compounds can complex other metals including Ga(III), Cr(III), Sc, In, Ni, U, Th, Pu(IV), Fe (III), Pu(VI), and Th(IV).

In dissimilatory processes, the transformation of the target metal is unrelated to its intake by the microbe. The chemical species that result from the cognate biological activity generally end up in the extracellular medium. An example is Cr (VI) reduction under both aerobic and anaerobic conditions, with NADH and electron transport systems serving as the respective electron donors. *Desulfovibrio desulfuricans* couples the oxidation of a variety of electron donors to the reduction of Tc (VII) by a periplasmic hydrogenase. Membrane-bound enzymes catalyse dissimilatory metal-reducing activities.

Dissimilatory Fe^{3+}-reducers, *Geobacter metallireducens* and *Shewanella putrefaciens*, can reduce highly soluble Tc (VII) to less soluble, reduced forms of technetium and Co^{3+}-EDTA to Co^{2+}-EDTA. *Thauera selenatis* can reduce highly soluble Se (VI) to insoluble Se^0. A phosphatase-containing *Citrobacter* sp. can precipitate uranium (U^{6+}) when supplied with an organic phosphate donor. Dissimilatory iron-reducing bacteria such as *G. metallireducens* and *S. putrefaciens* couple the oxidation of H_2 or organic substrates to the reduction of ferric iron. *S. putrefaciens* could also grow by coupling the oxidation of formate or lactate to the reduction of magnetite Fe(III). *G. metallireducens* or *S. putrefaciens* has been shown to reduce uranium from its relatively mobile oxidised state U(VI) to insoluble U(IV), which precipitates as the insoluble mineral uraninite. Fe(III)-reducing *Bacillus* strains were able to solubilise up to 90 per cent of PuO_2 over a period of 6 to 7 days in the presence of nitrilotriacetic acid.

Metal ions exported from the cytoplasm will form metal-bicarbonates and carbonates around the cell surface, and at supersaturated concentration will crystallise on the cell-bound metal ions, serving as crystallisation centres. This crystallisation process leads to very high metal to biomass ratios (between 0.5 and 5.0 on a weight basis). Once the bioprecipitation process has reached a certain level, nucleation proteins and polysaccharides are released from the cells and bioprecipitation continues on these released foci.

Biosorption and bioaccumulation

Biosorbents are natural ion-exchange materials that primarily contain weakly acidic and basic groups. They have advantages over their chemical counterpart since they can remove ions at very low concentrations (on the order of 2 to 10 mg/l). Biosorbents are more specific and hence prevent the binding of alkaline earth material. Also, they have the potential of genetic modification and so can be tailored for increased specificity. Bioaccumulation of metals can take place at many locations in the cell such as the cell wall or the cell surface and periplasmically, extracellularly, or intracellularly (cytoplasmic). A few disadvantages of biosorption are: (i) its sensitivity to operating conditions such as pH and ionic strength and the presence of organic or inorganic ligands, (ii) its lack of specificity in metal binding; (iii) its requirement for large amounts of biomass if the biosorption capacity is low, (iv) reusability of the biomass after desorption is possible only if weak chemicals are used for desorption, and (v) the biomass needs to be replaced after about 5 to 10 sorption-desorption cycles.

Potamogeton lucens is an excellent biosorbent for heavy metal ions. Sorption occurs mainly by ion exchange reactions with cationic weak exchanger groups present on the plant surface. Biosorption of heavy metals using biomass has also been found to be very effective in treating mine waste as long as the heavy metal species are free in solution and do not form soluble or precipitated species with sequestering compounds. The process involves diffusion, adsorption, chelation, complexation, coordination, or microprecipitation. It has been estimated that biosorptive processes could reduce capital and operating costs by 20 and 36 per cent, respectively, and total treatment costs by 28 per cent as compared with a conventional ion exchange process. Studies done with the aquatic macrophyte *Potamogeton lucens*, which had a carboxyl functional group, indicated that copper adsorption by the biomass is not affected by equimolar concentrations of metals such as sodium, calcium, or iron, or by a nonionic surfactant like pine oil. Anionic surfactants such as sodium oleate compete with the surface groups of the biomass for the free copper ions in solution.

The root bark of the Indian sarsaparilla (*Hemidesmus indicus*) was used as a biosorbent for the successful removal of Pb, Cr, and Zn from aqueous solutions. *Spirulina* sp. (a cyanobacteria blue-green algae) was found to be an effective biosorbent and bioaccumulant of heavy metal ions such as Cr^{3+}, Cd^{2+}, and Cu^{2+}. Bioaccumulation follows the biosorption process, where metal ions that are bound to the cell wall because of ion exchange get transported into the interior of the cell (active uptake). The cell membrane is able to identify the metal species and to distinguish metal ions that are micronutrients from those that are toxins.

Cadmium is widely used in rechargeable nickel-cadmium batteries, pigments, stabilisers, coatings, alloys, and electronic components; hence waste-water from such industries may contain this metal as a pollutant. Waste-waters of dye and pigment production; film and photography processing; galvanometry and metal cleaning, plating, and electroplating; leather production; and mining operations will contain chromium (VI).

A dead biomass of *Aeromonas caviae* was reported to biosorb hexavalent chromium isolated from raw water wells. Nonliving cells of *Bacillus licheniformis* and *B. laterosporus* were able to biosorb Cd(II) and Cr. *Gloeothece magna*, a nontoxic freshwater cyanobacterium, adsorbed Cd(II) and Mn(II). Live micro-organisms *Aspergillus niger* and *Pseudomonas aeruginosa* bioaccumulated 30 to 40 per cent Cr, while several yeast, fungi, and bacteria exhibited the bioaccumulation feature for Cu ion.

Zinc is used in paints, dyes, tyres, and alloys and to prevent corrosion. Untreated and acid-treated (in HNO_3 for 24 hours) cassava waste biomass (*Manihot sculenta Cranz*) was able to biosorb Zn and Cd metal ions from the waste stream. Acid treatment inhibited desorption of the metal.

Waste-water from the electroplating, electronics, and metal cleaning industries contains high concentrations of nickel (II) ions. Batch biosorption capacities for the free biomass of *Chlorella sorokiniana* and the loofa sponge-immobilised biomass of *C. sorokiniana* were found to be 48.08 and 60.38 mg nickel (II)g, respectively. Organisms that bioaccumulated Ni include the cyanobacteria such as *Anabaena cylindrical* and *A. flosaquae*; the yeast *Candida* spp.; the fungus *Aspergillus niger*, and the bacteria *Pseudomonas* spp. Ni.

Similar to those to other fungi, the cell walls of white rot fungi consist mostly of polysaccharides, peptides, and pigments that have a good capacity for binding heavy metals; hence a broad range of metals, including Cd, Cr, Cu, Ni, Pb, Hg, alkyl-Hg, and rare earth elements U and Th are known to be biosorbed. *Phanerochaete chrysosporium* mycelia have a biosorption capacity of about 60 to 110 mg of metals ions. *Trametes versicolor* exhibited biosorption capacity in the order Pb > Ni > Cr > Cd > Cu.

The use of active, growing cells for bioremediation of metal contaminated effluent has several advantages including: (i) the ability to self-replenish, (ii) continuous metabolic uptake of metals after physical adsorption, (iii) the potential for optimisation through development of resistant species and cell-surface modification, (iv) irreversibility since metals diffuse into the cells and get bound to intracellular proteins or chelatins before being incorporated into vacuoles and other intracellular sites, (v) avoidance of a separate biomass production process such as cultivation, harvesting, drying, processing, and storage, and (vi) the possibility of developing a single stage-process. Limitations to bio-uptake by living cells are: (i) the sensitivity of the system to operating conditions like pH and metal/salt concentration, and (ii) the requirement for external metabolic energy.

Bioprocesses and reactors

Generally reactors used for metal biosorption include rotating biological contactors, fixed bed, trickle filters, fluidised beds, air lift, and biofilm reactors. The living or dead biomass has been immobilised by encapsulation, crosslinking, or supports made from agar, cellulose, or alginates. A membrane bioreactor with *Alcaligenes eutrophus* supported on a tubular membrane made of polysulphone has been successfully tested for treatment of metal-contaminated waste effluents from several industries. Zinc effluent from a plating plant was reduced from 20 to below 1.00 ppm; Zn from a zinc factory was reduced from 10 to less than 0.05 ppm; Mg from the same effluent was reduced from 28 to 20 ppm; Cu from a nonferrous industry effluent was reduced from 8 to below 0.05 ppm; and Ni from a synthetic effluent was reduced from 10 to below 0.05 ppm.

The photofilm processing industry generates effluents in the form of used film fixer solutions that contain significant amounts of silver (greater than 3000 mg/l). The effluent also contains thiosulphate, a silver complexing agent used to remove unreacted or unexposed silver from photofilms, which interferes with the silver removal process. A chemoautotrophic bacterium *Thiobacillus thioparus* was able to oxidise thiosulphate to sulphate and sulphur. This treated water was contacted with a fungal culture *Cladosporium cladosporioides* in a continuous upflow biosorbent column packed with beads of the immobilised fungus for silver recovery. *Pseudomonas maltophila*, *Staphylococcus aureus*, and a coryneform organism were reported to accumulate more than 300 mg silver per gram.

A synthetic effluent containing several metals was treated by passing it through a column packed with vermicompost. The adsorption capacities of vermicompost for Cd(II), Cu(II), Pb(II), and Zn(II) ions were 33.01, 32.63, 92.94, and 28.43 mg/g, respectively. The ability of vermicompost to bind metals was attributed to the presence of negatively charged functional groups.

A laboratory-scale up-flow algal column reactor packed with alginate—algal beads removed Cu and Ni completely from a synthetic solution. A rotating biological contactor achieved good Cu and Zn removal efficiencies. Moving-bed sand filters were used effectively with a mixed bacterial population to remove Ni from waste-water. A reactor with two strains, *Alcaligenes eutrophus* CH34 and *A. eutrophus* AE1308, removed metals such as Cd, Zn, CU, Pb, Y, Co, Ni, Pd, and Ge via bioprecipitation. Similarly, a metal accumulating strain and *Ralstonia eutropha* JMP134 together have been employed for bioaugmentation of Cd removal. When an effluent containing copper ions and nitrates was treated in a bioelectrochemical reactor in the presence of denitrifying bacterial, the reactor could remove copper by electrochemical action and it could simultaneously perform bacterial denitrification with the help of the hydrogen generated by the electrolysis of water at the anode and the nutrients added externally.

Toxic metals

Mercury

A *Pseudomonas putida* strain removed greater than 90 per cent of mercury from a 40 mg/l solution in 24 hours. An *Escherichia coli* variant containing simultaneously the merA and glutathione S-transferase genes was able to reduce mercury in the solution to Hg^0. Transgenic *Arabidopsis thaliana* plants containing a modified bacterial Hg^{2+} reductase gene converted the toxic metal to Hg^0. Organomercurials are detoxified by organomercurial lyase; the resulting Hg^{2+} then is reduced to Hg^0 by mercuric reductase.

Arsenic

The large-scale treatment of timber with chromated copper arsenate and creosote oil by the wood preserving industry leads to a significant source of arsenic in the environment. *Acinetobacter*, *Edwardsiella*, *Enterobacter*, *Pseudomonas*, *Salmonella*, and *Serratia* species are resistant to arsenic. Several bacterial and fungi species are able to methylate arsenic compounds to volatile dimethyl or trimethylarsine. Methanogenic bacteria perform methylation of inorganic arsenic under anaerobic conditions, coupling the methane biosynthetic pathway. The process consists of reduction of arsenate to arsenite followed by methylation to dimethylarsine. As(III) was oxidised to As(V) by heterotrophic bacteria such as *Alcaligenes faecalis*. Aerobic chemolithoautotrophic microbes derive metabolic energy from the oxidation of As(III). *Geospirillum anenophihs*, *G. barnseii*, and *Chysiogenes arsenatis* use As^{5+} as a terminal electron acceptor to support anaerobic growth, leading to the formation of soluble As^{3+}. This technique can be used for leaching arsenic from contaminated soil. Addition of an electron donor such as acetate can enhance arsenic reduction as well as promote the reduction of Fe^{3+} and Mn^{4+}, which bind As^{5+} to soil. *Methanobacterium* sp. in the presence of vitamin B12 as the methyl group donor is able to biomethylate AsO_3^- anaerobically to AsO_2^- followed by methylation to methylarsonic acid, dimethylarsenic acid, and finally to dimethylarsine.

Selinium

Wolinella succinogenes was able to reduce SeO_4^{2-} and SeO_3^{2-}. *Pseudomonas maltophila* O-2 was able to accumulate Se^0 both inside and outside the cells. *Thauera selenatis* is capable of anaerobically reducing SeO_4^{2-} to SeO_4^{2-} and further to Se^0 with concomitant reduction of NO_3^-. Reduction of elemental selenium to selenide (Se^{2-}) has been observed in cultures of *Thiobacillus ferrooxidans*. Reduction of SeO_3^{2-} to Se^0 has been observed with fungi such as *Fusarium* sp., *Mortierella* sp., *Saccharomyces cerevisiae*, *Candida albicans*, and *Aspergillus funiculosus*, with both extracellular and intracellular deposition of Se^0. *Aeromonas* sp., *Bacillus* sp., and *Pseudomonas* sp. micro-organisms produce dimethylselenide derivatives of SeO_4^{2-} and SeO_3^{2-}. *Alternaria alternata* fungus methylated inorganic selenium.

Tellurium

Fungus *Penicillium* sp. is reported to produce dimethyltelluride and dimethylditelluride from tellurium. TeO_3^{2-} reduction to Te^0 by *Pseudomonas maltophila* O-2, *Rhodobacter sphaeroides* (deposited at intracellular cytoplasmic membrane), and fungus such as *Schizosaccharomyces* has been reported in literature.

Acid mine water

Mine water is generally very acidic (pH < 3.0) with high concentrations of metals such as Cu, Fe, Zn, Al, Pb, As, and Cd, and a high concentration of dissolved sulphates (greater than 3000 ppm). The process to reduce the concentration of metals and sulphates that is generally adopted is addition of slaked lime to neutralise and precipitate large amounts of gypsum sludge contaminated with heavy metals. This process is expensive and labour intensive.

Bioremediation technologies include passive treatment systems (using wetlands or compost reactors under aerobic or anaerobic conditions) and active treatment methods using sulphate-reducing bacteria. In the former method, precipitated metals are retained (in the organic matrix) rather than recovered, and their long-term fate is unsure, while in the latter metals are precipitated and recovered as metal sulphides. Bioremediation using anaerobic sulphate-reducing bacteria (*Desulfibrio* sp.) has two advantages. First, sulphate can be reduced to sulphide, which reacts with dissolved metals like copper, iron, and zinc in the contaminated waters to form insoluble precipitates. Such processes have even been developed on a commercial scale to operate near mines. Second, system acidity is decreased by the reduction of sulphate to sulphide and by the carbon metabolism of the bacteria. The bacteria require an anaerobic environment. Various organic waste materials, such as straw and hay, sawdust, peat, spent mushroom compost, and whey, have been used as electron donors for the sulphate reducers in the treatment of acid mine drainage. Hydrogen has also been used as the electron source to treat mine waste to reduce sulphate and precipitate Cu and Zn in a fixed bed bioreactor.

Plants

Heavy metals have different patterns of behaviour and mobility within a tree. For example:

1. Lead, chromium, and copper tend to be immobilised and held in the roots.
2. Cd, Ni, and Zn are more easily translocated to the aerial tissues.
3. Cd moves up into the harvestable parts of a tree.

Thlaspi (Brassicaceae) can accumulate 3 per cent Zn, 0.5 per cent Pb, and 0.1 per cent Cd in their shoots; *Alyssum* (Brassicaceae) accumulate Ni; and *Thlaspi caerulescens* is known to accumulate Zn. *Salix* were found to adsorb 30 per cent heavy metals. *Salvinia minima* and *Spirodela punctata* removed 70 to 90 per cent of lead and zinc, and water hyacinth removed arsenic, cadmium, lead, and mercury. *Asellus aquaticus*, a freshwater isopod, was able to bioaccumulate Pd, Pt, and Rh. *Microspora* (a macro alga) was found to adsorb lead. *Lemna minor* (an aquatic plant) adsorbed lead and nickel. A marine algae *Chlorella* spp. NKG16014 biosorbed Cd.

Semiconductor

Semiconductor manufacturing can be grouped broadly into three categories:

1. Silicon crystal wafer growth and preparation.
2. Semiconductor or wafer fabrication.
3. Final assembly and packaging.

The semiconductor fabrication processes are always performed in a clean room and include the following steps: oxidation, lithography, etching, doping (through processes such as vapour phase deposition and ion implantation), and layering (through processes such as metallisation). Figures 16.1 to 16.3 provide a flowsheet of the entire process.

Silicon in the form of ingots is grown from seed crystals. Ingots are shaped into wafers through a series of cutting and grinding steps. The ends of the silicon ingots are removed, and individual wafers are cut from the ingot. The wafer is then polished using an aluminum oxide-glycerine solution. Further polishing is done using a slurry of silicon dioxide particles suspended in sodium hydroxide. Contaminants from the wafer are cleaned by either using a spray or immersing the wafers in acids, bases, and organic solvents.

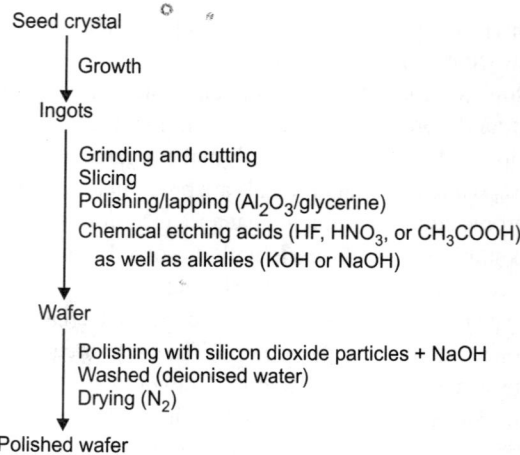

Fig. 16.1. Silicon crystal growth and wafer preparation.

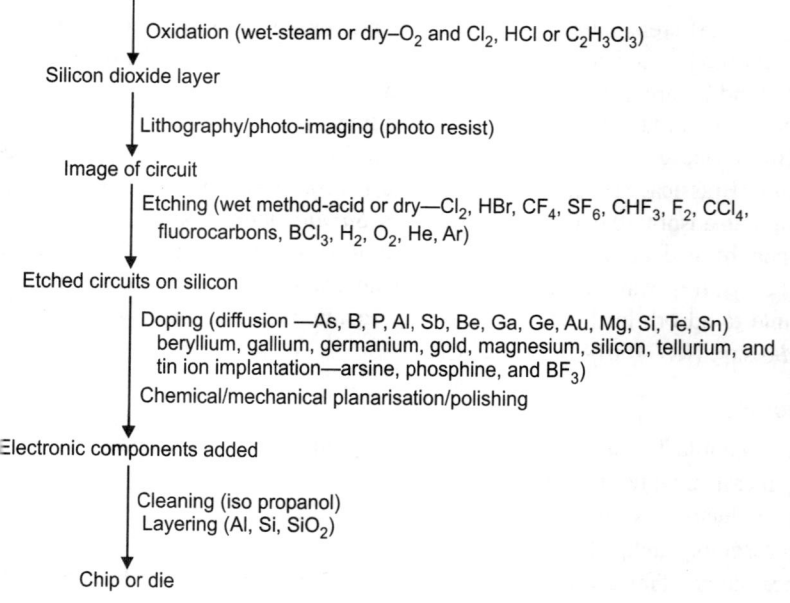

Fig. 16.2. Semiconductor fabrication.

To create the desired electronic components like transistors and resistors, impurities or dopants are introduced into the wafer to change the conductivity of the silicon. Deposition of thin films onto the silicon wafer substrate involves chemical vapour deposition, sputtering (electric deposition of a metal onto the substrate under conditions of high vacuum), and oxidation. The raw materials for deposition are in the form of gases, solid metal, and inorganic compounds. Diffusion of doping agents into the wafer layer is performed under high temperature conditions or through ion implantation, which involves bombarding the silicon wafer under high vacuum and temperature with a plasma of ionised doping agents. Photolithography is a process in which a pattern or mask is superimposed upon a photochemically coated wafer, and the etching or pattern from the mask is replicated on the underlying material. Both wet and dry etching methods are employed; the former involves a sequence of various chemicals (typically acidic), and the latter involves wafers being processed in a chamber through which gases are pumped.

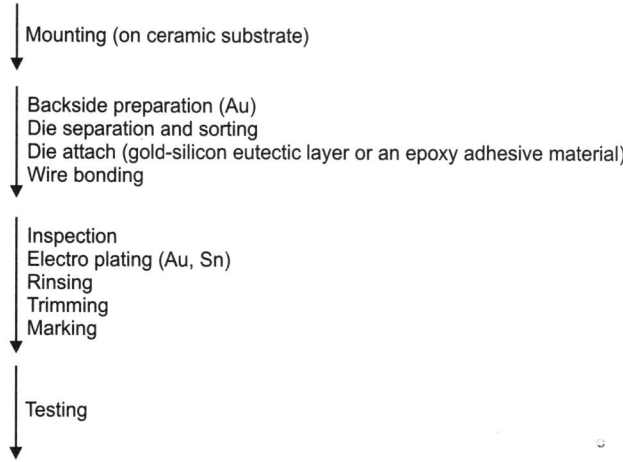

Fig. 16.3. Semiconductor assembly and packaging.

Chips or dies are mounted onto the surface of a ceramic substrate as part of a circuit, connected directly onto a printed wiring board, or incorporated into a protective package. Backside preparation involves coating with gold.

Finally the wafer is separated into individual chips by sawing. The electroplating process and the final rinse is typically the primary source of process waste-water in the semiconductor assembly and packaging process.

Waste

Water usage in integrated circuit manufacture is among the highest in any industrial sector. The process requires large quantities of deionised water. Because of the purity required, process water is not recycled, and hence waste-water discharge is a major issue. Current use of ultrapure water (UPW) is 5 to 7 l/cm^2 of silicon, and in a wet bench, it is 53 l/wafer (300 mm). This works out to 20.45 million tonnes of water for producing 2.7 billion square centimetres of wafer. The semiconductor fabricators that use chemical mechanical planarisation/polishing (CMP) consume 4.2 to 12 gallons of water per minute, which works out to more than 4.25 million gallons annually.

From Figs 16.1 to 16.3 one can see that unreacted highly toxic metals, liquids, and gases could be leaving the semiconductor manufacturing plant as waste. Hydrofluoric acid is the major inorganic acid present in the gaseous effluent stream, and calcium fluoride is also generated at 0.0018 kg per square centimetre of wafer. Fumes from lead soldering, tin plating, and other vapourised metals used in the chemical vapour deposition also escape with the effluent gases. Disposal of these hazardous effluents such as waste solvents, dissolved organic compounds, acids, alkalies, photoresistant chemicals, dissolved metals (including arsenic, copper, chromium, and selenium), waste etchants, waste aqueous developing materials, and catalyst solutions pose a major problem. Chlorofluorocarbons (CFCs), halons, carbon tetrachloride, and polychlorinated biphenyls have been banned or voluntarily phased out from the manufacturing process. Lead, cadmium, and mercury compounds used in packaging substrates, and perfluoro octyl sulphonates (PFOS), a component in some photoresists and antireflective coatings, have been grouped under the high-risk category (chemicals or materials have been targeted by a government authority for significant use restriction or potential ban). Perfluorocarbons (PFCs) and hydrofluorocarbons (HFCs), both of which have high global warming potential but shorter atmospheric lifetimes than the CFCs, have been grouped under the medium-risk chemicals (significant regulation of these compounds).

The manufacture of compound semiconductors such as gallium arsenide, indium phosphide, and indium antimonide require the use of a number of very hazardous gases, which include arsine, phosphine, trimethyl indium, trimethyl gallium, trimethyl aluminium, silane, and others.

Disposal of unconsumed process gases and the products of the deposition process pose several problems. The worst long-term environmental concern among these is arsine, which will always produce an arsenic-tainted waste stream. In addition, the presence of phosphorus and hydrogen during pumping could also lead to pyrophoric conditions.

Through process optimisation and alternative chemistries, recycling, and/or abatement, the industry must continue to diminish the emissions of by-products with high global warming potential. Restriction of use of certain hazardous substances and possible use of supercritical CO_2 for cleaning instead of water is being investigated to reduce water usage. Sulphur trioxide is being tried instead of wet chemicals as a cleaning agent for removing residual photoresist and organic polymers. This attempt could reduce the handling of large quantities of hazardous chemicals.

Physical and chemical treatment methods

Several physical and chemical methods that are being practiced for treating semiconductor waste effluent include coagulation and precipitation, ion exchange, adsorption with activated carbon, membrane filtration, and chemical oxidation. Heavy metals can be precipitated as insoluble hydroxides at high pH or sometimes as sulphides. But the disposal of this highly concentrated toxic sludge poses another problem. If the sludge is not considered hazardous, then a gravity settling system can be both economical and safe. To treat a CMP waste that contains copper, a complete system that involves removal of activated carbon oxidant, filtration of slurry particles, and ion exchange to extract copper from the effluent is necessary for its removal. Strongly complexed copper is hard to precipitate or remove, and large-scale ion exchange process is expensive. Arsenic is one of the pollutants found in the waste-water. The general method used to remove this metal is by flocculation, and other methods that have been practiced include adsorbents, such as activated carbon, amorphous aluminium hydroxide, or activated alumina. The difficulty with the removal of metal anions is the fact that they do not precipitate out as hydroxides by simple pH adjustment.

Silica and fluoride in the waste-water could be made to react with lime to form insoluble silicates and calcium fluoride salts. Coagulation and settling of these solid insoluble particles in settling tanks could be initiated by the addition of polyacrylamide. Membrane filtration for recovery of metal has several problems, which include difficulty in retaining small-sized metal particles, abrasion of the membrane, and lack of resistance to pH fluctuations.

Chemical mechanical polishing is carried out to reduce wafer topological imperfections and to improve the depth of focus of lithography processes through better planarity. CMP process effluent contains many contaminants, some of which are shown in Table 16.1.

Table 16.1. CMP process effluent contaminants.

Interconnect material	CU^{2+}, complexed Cu^{2+}, CU_2O, CuO, $Cu(OH)_2$, WO_3, Al_2O_3, $Al(OH)_3$, and Fe^{2+}/Fe^{3+}
Barrier or liner material	Tantalum, titanium oxides, and oxynitrides
Abrasives	SiO_2, Al_2O_3, MnO_2, and CeO_2
Oxidisers	Hydroxylamine, $KMnO_4$, KIO_4, H_2O_2, NO_3^-
Strong acids and weak buffering acids	HF, HNO_3 H_3BO_3, NH_4^+, and citric acid
Strong bases	NH_3, OH
Organic materials dispersants/surfactants	Poly(acrylic acid), quaternary ammonium salts, and alkyl sulphates
Corrosion inhibitors	Benzotriazole, alkyl amines
Metal complexing agents	EDTA, ethanol amines
Acids	Poly(acrylic), oxalic, citric, acetic, and peroxy acetic

CMP waste-water treatment involves neutralisation of ion and particle surface charge by oppositely charged inorganic and organic materials. When excess coagulant is added, the particles and some ions are trapped within a gel-like matrix and agglomerate. This process is known as 'sweep coagulation.' Typical inorganic coagulants used for this purpose are aluminium sulphate and ferric chloride, both of which form insoluble hydrated hydroxide gels at pH 5 to 8. Addition of organic flocculants such as polyacrylamide further destabilises the coagulated agglomerate for gravity settling or active filtration. A new technique that is being researched is called electrocoagulation and electrodecantation, which uses electric fields to agglomerate charged silica particles instead of adding polymers. Commonly used techniques to separate the floc from the clarified water include gravity settling, cross-flow filtration, and single-pass low-pressure filtration. Removal of copper from the waste-water to a 50 ppb level was achieved using polymeric metal removal agents (a polymer containing sulphide functionality) even in the presence of ammonia and other competing materials. Copper removal has also been achieved by pH adjustment followed by ion exchange. The drawbacks of this approach include the large amounts of acid and base needed in the pH adjustment steps, the need for frequent ion bed regeneration, and the bed damage due to the presence of suspended solids.

Adsorption of metals from liquid streams using treated sawdust is found to be very effective. Hg (II) is effectively removed using polymerised sawdust or peanut hulls treated with bicarbonate. Divalent Cu, Pb, Hg, Fe, Zn, and Ni and trivalent Fe are removed using untreated sawdust as well as sawdust treated with a reactive monochlorotriazine type dye. The treated sawdust showed better adsorption efficiency than the untreated sawdust. A column packed with a resin of sawdust, onion skin, and polymerised corncob could remove 86 per cent of Pb, 79 per cent of Ca, 77 per cent of Ni, 75 per cent of Zn, 71 per cent Mg, 65 per cent Mn, and 60 per cent Cu divalent ions. Sawdust modified with iron hexamine gel efficiently removed very toxic metals like Hg, Cr, and Cd. Heavy metal cations are capable of forming complexes with O^-, N^-, S^-, and P^- containing functional groups. The cell walls of sawdust consist of cellulose, lignin, and many hydroxyl groups, which are present as part of tannins or other phenolic compounds. It is speculated that ion exchange or hydrogen bonding may be the principal mechanisms for the binding of these metals to sawdust. Polyacrylamide-treated sawdust was very effective in removing Cd and Hg(II), while rubber wood sawdust could effectively adsorb Co(II), Cr(II), and Cr(VI). Treatment of exposed sawdust with nitric acid completely removes the metal ions. The binding capacity of various ion exchange resins for Cu (II) varies between 0.01 and 0.1 gram per gram of the resin.

Dimethyl sulphoxide (DMSO) is a widely used organic solvent in the semiconductor industry; hence finds it way into the effluent and requires costly treatment. Fenton treatment was also investigated using H_2O_2: Fe^{2+} at the ratio of 1000:1000 mg/l for waste-water containing 800 mg DMSO/l. Such a treatment achieved a total organic carbon (TOC) removal efficiency of 26 per cent, and the biological oxygen demand/chemical oxygen demand (BOD:COD) ratio of the waste-water was increased from 0.035 to 0.87 when the reaction was carried out at pH 3 and the coagulation at pH 7. An increase in BOD:COD ratio makes this process an attractive pretreatment step before biological treatment. Sulphuric acid is used for wafer cleaning, and its disposal involves neutralisation; the quantity of waste, therefore, exceeds the quantity of the used sulphuric acid. Generally, sulphuric acid makes up about 17 per cent of the entire quantity of waste acid in semiconductor industrial waste. Atmospheric and vacuum distillation and recovery of sulphuric acid has been attempted successfully.

Biochemical methods

Isopropyl alcohol and acetone are common solvents in the cleaning steps, and large quantities of their vapours are released into the atmosphere. A trickle bed air biofilter packed with about 7.8 litres of coal (voidage=0.44) achieved a 90 per cent removal efficiency for this vapour mixture with influent carbon loadings of the alcohol and acetone below 80 and 53 $g/m^3/hr.$, respectively, at a temperature of 30°C, relative humidity of 90 per cent, and an empty-bed residence time of 25 seconds. The biofilter was seeded with activated sludge from a waste-water treatment plant. The nutrient to the trickle biofilter feed contained inorganic salts (Mg, Na, K, Mn, and ammonium sulphates, chlorides, and phosphates) and $NaHCO_3$ as a buffer. The carbon mass ratio of the influent air stream to nitrogen, phosphorus, sulphur, and iron of the nutrient solution was equal to 100:10:1:1:0.5, respectively.

Complex effluents having a COD of 80000 mg/l and isopropyl alcohol (ipa) of 35,000 mg/l cannot be treated effectively with one technique alone but can be successfully treated using a process that combines physical, chemical and biological methods (Fig. 16.4). The initial treatment consisted of air stripping the effluent using a packed column at a temperature of 70°C to recover 95 per cent of the ipa at 9 per cent purity. Fenton oxidation of this stripped stream was carried out after diluting it with other effluents. The use of 5 g/l of $FeSO_4$ and 45 g/l of H_2O_2 for the oxidation achieved a 95 per cent reduction in COD and a 99 per cent reduction in the colour of the effluent.

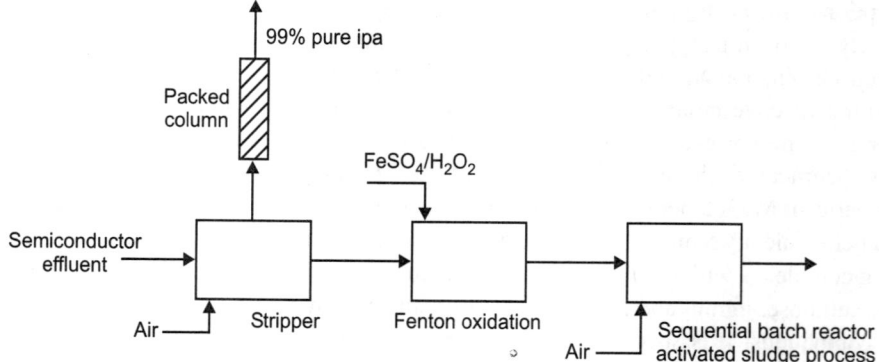

Fig. 16.4. Combined physical, chemical, and biological treatment.

Using sludge from a municipal waste-water treatment plant, an aerobic sequencing batch reactor with a 12-hour cycle, and mixed liquor suspended solids (MLSS) of 3000 mg/l was able to achieve an

85 per cent reduction in COD. The combined treatment was capable of lowering the waste-water COD concentration from 80,000 mg/l to below 100 mg/l and completely eliminated the waste-water colour. Activated sludge entrapped in polyethylene glycol prepolymer pellets was applied to the continuous treatment of organic waste-water discharged from a semiconductor plant that had a BOD of 150 to 200 mg/l at a loading rate of 5.21 kg BOD/m^3/day achieving BOD removal efficiencies of 95 to 97 per cent.

Biological breakdown of DMSO produces dimethylsulphide (DMS), which ultimately produces 2 mol of formaldehyde and 1 mol of sulphide. Formaldehyde is converted to CO_2 or used for cell synthesis, and sulphide is oxidised to sulphate. Enzyme systems such as methionine sulphoxide reductase, methionine sulphoxide-peptide-reductase, biotin sulphoxide reductase, anaerobic DMSO reductase, anaerobic trimethylamine reductase, and aerobic DMSO reductase are reported to mediate DMSO reduction to DMS. Micro-organisms that use DMSO as a terminal electron acceptor are anaerobically grown *Escherichia coli* HB101, anaerobic rumen bacterium *Wolinella succinogenes*, *Rhodopseudomonas capsulata*, and *Escherichia coli*.

Waste-water containing 800 mg/l of DMSO was treated successfully in an activated sludge process to achieve TOC, soluble COD (SCOD), and soluble BOD (SBOD) removal efficiencies of 90, 87, and 63 per cent, respectively, at a hydraulic retention time (HRT) of 24 hours at a loading rate of 0.8 kg DMSO/m^3/day. Most of the sulphur in DMSO was oxidised to sulphate.

Biosorption

Metal recovery can be achieved with the use of plant, algal, or microbial biomass; this adsorption process is termed 'biosorption'. Pretreatment enhances the metal-binding ability. Dead micro-organisms or their derivatives (bacteria, fungi, yeast, algae, and higher plants) can complex metal ions through the action of ligands or functional groups located on the outer surface of the cells. Biosorptive processes can reduce capital costs by 20 per cent, operational costs by 36 per cent, and total treatment costs by 28 per cent when compared with conventional approaches. *Mucor rouxii*, a soil fungus, can biosorb copper and silver found in CMP effluent.

Aspergillus oryzae and *Rhizopus oryzae* are able to biosorb copper (II) very effectively from waste-water. Acid-washed *A. oryzae* mycelia exhibited maximum biosorption capacity when compared with the other adsorbents. Acid washing can be used as a pretreatment step and also as a regeneration step in the heavy metal removal process. A column reactor packed with 2 to 3 mm diameter pellets of *A. oryzae* was also effective in removing Cu(II). Sodium alginate-immobilised Soil 5Y cells and immobilised *Pseudomonas aeruginosa* PU21could biosorb 0.14 and 0.15 gram Cu per gram of the biomass, respectively, at pH 5.

There were two distinct adsorption phases—an initial rapid uptake followed by a gradual uptake; the former was probably due to the adsorption of copper ions onto the cell walls. The immobilised Soil 5Y-biosorbed Cu (II) could be desorbed by treating it with HCl (achieving 90 per cent recovery). Other organisms that could adsorb Cu^{2+} are *Bacillus* bacteria, reaching adsorption equilibrium in 10 minutes at pH 7.2; planktonic *Thiobacillus ferrooxidans* cells, reaching adsorption equilibrium in 15 minutes, and immobilised *Zoogloea ramigera* cells, which produce an extracellular polysaccharide layer and reach their maximum copper adsorption capacity in 2 hours.

Brown seaweed *Sargassum* sp. (*Chromophyta*) harvested from the sea (northeastern coast of Brazil) could biosorb copper ions with a high biosorption capacity (1.48 mmol/g at pH 4.0). Other biosorbents reported in the literature were *Rhizopus arrhizus* (0.25 mmol/g), *Pseudomonas aeruginosa* (0.29), *Phanerochaete chrysosporium* (0.42), pretreated *Ecklonia radiata* (1.11), and *Ulothrix zonata* (2.77).

NaOH-pretreated *Mucor rouxii* biomass showed a high adsorption capacity for the removal of lead, cadmium, nickel, and zinc from aqueous solution. Recovery of these biosorbed metal ions was achieved with nitric acid treatment. Caustic regeneration of eluted biomass rehabilitated the metal ion biosorption capacity even after five cycles of reuse. Live biomass had a higher biosorption capacity than dead biomass (i.e. 35.69, 11.09, 8.46, and 7.75 mg/g at pH 5.0 for Pb^{2+}, Ni^{2+}, Cd^{2+}, and Zn^{2+}, respectively, as against 25.22, 16.62, 8.36, and 6.34 mg/g, respectively, with dead biomass). Biosorption depended on an intermediate pH; a value of 6.0 was found to be the maximum. At low pH (~2 to 4), the binding sites get protonated due to a high concentration of protons and the negative charge intensity on the sites is decreased, resulting in the reduction or inhibition of the binding of metal ions (which are positively charged). Yeast extract, peptone, and glucose medium, or yeast and malt broth medium had no effect, whereas dextrose and peptone medium decreased the biosorption capacity of the fungus. Biosorption capacity of Pb remained almost constant even in the presence of other ions. The biosorption capacity of Ni, Cd, and Zn decreased in the presence of other ions, indicating the operation of a competitive adsorption mechanism. Heavy metals such as Ni, Zn, Cd, Ag, and Pb were biosorbed by a *Rhizopus arrhizus* biomass under pH-controlled conditions. The maximum sorption capacity for Pb was observed at a pH 7.0 (200 mg/g). Dead *R. nigricans* obtained as a waste by-product from the pharmaceutical fermentation industry has been found to adsorb Pb over a range of metal ion concentrations, adsorption time, pH, and co-ions. The uptake process obeys both the Langmuir and Freundlich isotherms.

Phanerochaete chrysogenum, a waste by-product from antibiotic production, has been surface modified with surfactants and investigated for the removal of arsenic from the waste effluent. At pH 3, the removal capacities were 37.85 mg As/g for cationic surfactant hexadecyl-trimethylammonium bromide-modified biomass, 56.07 mg As/g for polyelectrolyte Magnafloc-modified biomass, and 33.31 mg As/g dodecylamine-modified biomass. The adsorption capacity of activated chitosan for arsenic is higher than any other adsorbent, such as fly ash, bauxite, or alumina (197.6 mg/g at pH 3.0, 30 mg/g at pH 2.5, 12.6 mg/g at pH 3.5, and 12.3 mg/g at pH 2.6, respectively). The metal-loaded biomass following biosorption (dodecylamine-modified biomass) was separated by dispersed-air flotation, leading to 75 per cent arsenic anion removal. Physical and chemical pretreatment processes enhance the biosorption capacity of cations. Physical methods include heat treatment, autoclaving, freeze-drying, or boiling, whereas chemical methods include contact with acids, alkalis, or organic chemicals.

Cyanide

Cyanide is used in the production of organic chemicals such as nitrile, nylon, acrylic plastics, and synthetic rubber. It is also used in the electroplating, metal processing, steel hardening, and photographic industries. The wastes from such industries not only contains cyanide but also significant amounts of heavy metals such as copper, nickel, zinc, silver, and iron. Since cyanide ions are highly reactive, metal complexes of variable stability and toxicity are readily formed. Ore processing in gold and silver mining operations uses dilute solutions of sodium cyanide (100 to 500 ppm), which is inexpensive and highly soluble in water, and under mildly oxidising conditions, dissolves the gold contained in the ore. Each year 2 to 3 million tonnes of cyanide are industrially produced. Food processing industries that handle crops such as cassava and bitter almonds also generate considerable quantities of cyanide waste because of the presence of the cyanogenic glucosides that are present in the plant material.

Physical processes

In nature, cyanide is oxidised to more stable products, which are relatively nontoxic when compared with the free cyanide. Cyanide treatment involves either a destruction-based process or a physical process of cyanide recovery. Cyanide and its related compounds such as ammonia, cyanate, nitrate, and thiocyanate can be destroyed by one of several processes. They include INCO SO_2/air (which uses SO_2 and air in the presence of a soluble copper catalyst to oxidise cyanide to the less toxic cyanate), copper-catalysed hydrogen peroxide (which uses hydrogen peroxide as the oxidising agent instead of SO_2 and air), Caro's acid, alkaline breakpoint chlorination (a two-step process in which the first step involves conversion to cyanogen chloride followed by hydrolysis of the cyanogen chloride to cyanate), and activated carbon adsorption followed by recovery of cyanide by desorption. Chemical and physical processes to degrade cyanide and its related compounds are expensive, complex to operate, and add toxic chemicals to the environment. Chlorination is not effective when cyanide species are complexed with metals such as nickel and silver because of their slow reaction rates. The process also produces sludge, which requires licensed disposal.

The selection of the technique for destroying cyanide will depend on the chemical characterisation of the untreated solution or slurry, as well as its quantity and environmental setting; the capital, equipment, and reagents available; the operating and maintenance costs; licensing fees; and review of the applicable regulations.

Bioprocess

Biological treatment involves the acclimation and enhancement of indigenous micro-organisms to fix or biotransform the toxic cyanide to less toxic derivatives. Biotreatment is less expensive and simple to operate. Thiocyanate is used in several industrial processes, including photofinishing, herbicide and insecticide production, dyeing, acrylic fibre production, thiourea manufacture, metal separation and electroplating, and in soil sterilisation and corrosion inhibition; hence it is found in waste-waters. Thiobacilli, pseudomonads, and *Arthrobacter* spp. are capable of degrading thiocyanate. Cyanate is an intermediate product in the first stage of thiocyanate hydrolysis and is further hydrolysed to ammonia and bicarbonate.

Although methanogens are inhibited by cyanide, a 90 per cent cyanide removal and simultaneous reduction of chemical oxygen demand (COD) and methane production were achieved when effluent was exposed to sludge adapted to cyanide (taken from an upflow anaerobic sludge blanket reactor). Cyanide inhibition on methanogenic activity was more pronounced for acetoclastic than for hydrogenotrophic methanogens. Two *Pseudomonas* sp., CM5 and CMN2 without acclimation, were able to degrade cyanide in a solution of whey from a concentration of 80 and 160 ppm to less than 1 ppm in batch mode. During metabolism, the micro-organisms used cyanide as a nitrogen and carbon source, converting it to ammonia and carbonate.

Burkholderia cepacia strain C-3 isolated from soil with a carbon source was able to biodegrade cyanide at a pH of 10. Cu^{2+} or Fe^{2+} at a concentration of 1 mM inhibited both the growth of the bacteria and cyanide degradation. The highest growth was observed in the presence of Mg^{2+}. Phenol inhibited the reaction, while ethanol and methanol had no effect. Fructose, glucose, and mannose were the preferred carbon sources for cyanide biodegradation.

Mechanism of actions

The cyanide oxygenase from the bacterium *P. fluorescens* NCIMB 11764 converted free cyanide to carbon dioxide and ammonia. *P. putida* followed a two-step enzymatic pathway for cyanide degradation. Cyanide hydratase transformed cyanide to formamide, and amidase degraded it further to formate and ammonia. *Alcaligenes xylosooxidans* sub sp., *A. denitrificans*, and *P. fluorescens* converted cyanide to ammonia and formate in a single step using cyanide dihydratase without producing formamide. *Stemphylium loti, Fusarium lateritium*, and *Gloeocerocospora sorghi* do not possess the amidase enzyme necessary to convert formamide to ammonia, which leads to the accumulation of formamide. *F. lateritium* and *G. sorghi* only detoxify cyanide to formamide by the action of cyanide hydratase, and none of these fungi utilised cyanide as a source of carbon or nitrogen. *Fusarium oxysporum, Gliocladium virens, Trichoderma koningii*, and *F. solani* IHEM 8026 grow on KCN as a sole nitrogen source. *Trichoderma* strains have the cyanide-degrading enzymes, cyanide hydratase and rhodanese. Cyanide hydratase activity in *G. sorghi, S. loti, Colletotrichum graminocola, F. moniliforme, F. lateritium, F. solani*, and *Helminthosporium maydis* was different in uninduced and induced mycelium. The enzyme cyanide hydratase present in fungi *F. solani* isolated from cyanide-contaminated soil specifically converted HCN to formamide but not the CN ion.

A microbial consortium composed primarily of *Pseudomonas* and *Bacillus* sp., degraded thiocyanate. *P. stutzeri* utilised potassium thiocyanate as a nitrogen and sulphur source and succinate as a carbon and energy source. Thiobacillus thioparus was able to assimilate 500 mg/l of potassium thiocyanate within 60 hours, but thiocyanate degradation was inhibited by the presence of thiosulphate. *Thiobacilli* and pseudomonads utilised thiocyanate as the nitrogen and sulphur source and tolerated thiocyanate at concentrations of up to 5.8 g/l. *Escherichia coli, Flavobacterium* sp., and *P. fluorescens* had the enzyme cyanase that was responsible for catalysing the hydrolysis of cyanate to ammonia and bicarbonate.

Metal-cyanide effluent

Several water management and treatment alternative are possible in mining operations, including land application, biological treatment, breakpoint chlorination, hydrogen peroxide, and the SO_2/air process. The treatment methods must take care of cyanide, metals, thiocyanate, ammonia, and nitrate as well as high levels of total dissolved solids and sulphate. Except for breakpoint chlorination, chemical oxidation processes involving hydrogen peroxide and sulphur dioxide do not remove thiocyanate, ammonia, and nitrate. But the former is very expensive and produces high residual total dissolved solid and chloride concentrations. Biological treatment techniques are of recent origin, and a combined biological and chemical treatment approach has been found to have several advantages (Fig. 16.5). Biological methods are environmentally friendly and cost less to operate, but capital costs are higher.

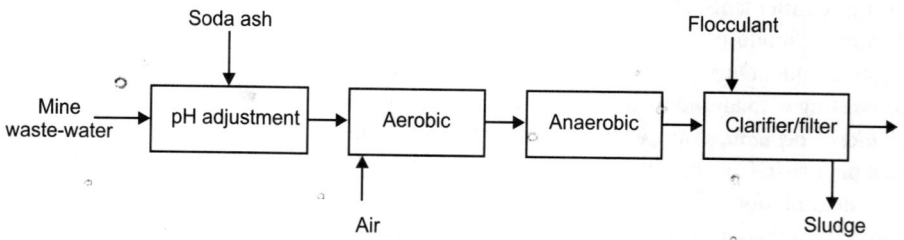

Fig. 16.5. General treatment procedure.

A typical biological and a chemical treatment procedure may involve a three-step approach.

1. A combined activated sludge treatment step for the conversion of thiocyanate to ammonia and its mediation to nitrate.
2. A denitrification treatment step leading to nitrogen gas.
3. A high density sludge ferric sulphate treatment step to precipitate arsenic and other metals in their sulphate forms.

The types of reactors available for aerobic operation include rotating biological contactors, packed beds, biological filters, sequencing batch reactors, facultative lagoons, and activated sludge systems. The aerobic treatment requires about 1 to 5 mg/l phosphate as the nutrient, 2 ng/l of dissolved oxygen, and a process temperature above 10°C. Commercial processes that have been operating are in-plant cyanide destruction; *in situ* cyanide destruction of spent heap leach piles; metal and sulphate removal using active (in-plant) sulphate reduction; and passive processes such as wetlands and ecological engineering for metals polishing.

To recover precious metals from ore in a heap leach operation, a dilute cyanide leaching solution is sprayed on the ore, which is heaped on an impermeable pad. As the solution percolates through the heap, precious metals are complexed, dissolved, and then recovered. A heap that has been treated several times by the cyanide solution has very little precious metal left and hence is discarded. The heap is considered closed if the leachate from a heap contains less than 0.2 mg/l of cyanide; this is accomplished by rinsing the heap to remove residual cyanide and then destroying the cyanide.

In biological treatment of cyanide effluent from metal ore mines, the bacteria convert free and metal-complexed cyanides to bicarbonate and ammonia, and the freed metals are either adsorbed within the biofilm or precipitated from solution. Free cyanide is the most readily degradable and iron cyanide the least, and the degradability of Zn, Ni, and Cu metal cyanide complexes fall in between. Iron cyanides have been shown to degrade the least. Ammonia to nitrate conversion follows a two-step aerobic process with nitrite as the intermediate. The nitrate is reduced to nitrogen gas under anoxic conditions. *Pseudomonas* sp. help in complete oxidation of cyanide, thiocyanate, and ammonia. Other gram-negative bacteria that play a crucial role in the process are *Achromobacter*, *Flavobacterium*, *Nocardia*, *Bdellovibrio*, *Mycobacterium*, and two nitrifiers, *Nitrosomonas* and *Nitrobacter*. Cyanide and thiocyanide serve as energy and food sources for the destruction stage bacteria and can be toxic to the nitrifying bacteria. Ammonia and bicarbonate serve as food and energy sources for the nitrifying bacteria.

Copper and zinc cyanide complexes are found in waste-waters originating from the electroplating and mining industries. *Citrobacter* sp. MCM B-181, *Pseudomonas* sp. MCM B-182, *Pseudomonas* sp. MCM B-183, and *Pseudomonas* sp. MCM B-184 were capable of degrading free as well as metal cyanide complexes by utilising metal cyanides as a nitrogen source and glucose or sugarcane molasses as a carbon source; ammonia and carbon dioxide were formed as degradation products. The degradation was not followed by metal biosorption onto the bacterial cells but by the precipitation from solution of copper and zinc as their respective hydroxides. A rotating biological contactor achieved 99.9 per cent removal of 0.5 mM metal cyanide and a COD removal efficiency of 85 per cent in 15 hours using a consortium containing all four micro-organisms. The biodegradation process was affected by the presence of metals such as Cr and Fe. A synthetic solution made up of sodium cyanide in water, ferrous sulphate, copper sulphate, zinc sulphate, and potassium thiocyanante mixed with sludge from a municipal activated sludge plant was successfully treated, achieving a greater than 90 per cent removal efficiency in a biofilter packed with a support media. The total metal content was approximately 36 per cent of the dry biomass, with first Zn being preferentially adsorbed, followed by Cu. Free cyanide, thiocyanate, and copper, iron, and zinc metallocyanides from a synthetic gold milling effluent mixed with sewage was treated in a stirred aerated bioreactor to achieve more than 95 per cent removal of free cyanide, thiocyanate, copper, and zinc. Iron removal was low, about 68 per cent.

Biodegradation of ferrous (II) cyanide ions was achieved using *Pseudomonas fluorescens* immobilised on calcium-alginate gel in a packed bed column reactor. *Cryptococcus humicolus* MCN2 yeast strain could degrade tetracyanonickelate (II) in batches. Seventy per cent of the degradation of cyanide occurred in the lag phase of cell growth. Ammonia was produced because most of the cyanide had disappeared, and its production rate coincided with the formamide degradation rate. Ammonia was assimilated directly into the cell biomass. CO_2 generation was also proportional to the cell growth.

TOXIC METAL RESISTANCES AND POTENTIAL FOR BIOREMEDIATION

Bacteria have evolved mechanisms to deal with toxic metal ions as a result of selection pressures exerted by metal-abundant environments. For the survival of micro-organisms in the environment, it is essential to maintain a proper homeostasis of the essential nutrient and nonessential toxic inorganic ions; nothing is left to chance. Homeostatic and resistance mechanisms exist towards the ions formed by almost all elements in the Periodic Table. Although most of the metal cation resistance systems are plasmid encoded, some resistance mechanisms are encoded by genes present on the chromosome. Resistance systems for most toxic ions have now been found, and understanding, at least in principle, is frequently known. For inorganic ions of a few environmentally-abundant elements, resistance mechanisms are not yet known. For example, there are no known genes for resistance towards Al^{3+} or for the halide anions.

The molecular basis for toxic ion resistance must be understood before attempts can be made to develop technologies for bioremediation based on these resistances. It is difficult to build a product based on ignorance. The genetics and molecular basis for resistances towards Ag^+, AsO_2^-, AsO_4^{3-}, Cd^{2+}, Co^{2+}, CrO_4^{2-}, Cu^{2+}, Hg^{2+}, Ni^{2+}, Pb^{2+}, Sb^{3+}, TeO_3^{2-}, Tl^+ and Zn^{2+} have been investigated. There are four basic mechanisms by which micro-organisms resist toxic metal ions. The metal ion can be prevented from entering the cell (is not bioavailable), or the metal ion is first taken into the cell and then exported out by efflux pumps. Although a futile cycle of uptake and efflux seems inefficient, efflux pumps are the most frequent resistance mechanism. Alternatively, the metal cation can be bound to specific binding proteins at the surface or within the cell; or lastly the metal ion can be transformed enzymatically to a different redox state, which is then either less toxic or dealt with by one of the previously listed three mechanisms. For bioremediation, a bacterial system using a blockage in import or the active efflux of the metal ion is not readily adaptable. However, the binding of toxic cations to proteins or the enzymatic oxidation or reduction are good candidates for bioremediation processes. Despite the advanced state of understanding of some metal cation resistances, there are only a few systems where bioremediation processes based on microbes have been used. These include 'bio-accumulation' of metal ions by live cells or fixed dead biomass and microbial reduction of chromate to Cr^{3+}, that is subsequently precipitated as $Cr(OH)_3$, both as means of removing the toxic metals.

An understanding of the molecular basis for resistance to elevated concentrations of metal ions has frequently been useful in environmental and medical sciences. For example, the Cd^{2+} resistance cation efflux pump of Gram-positive bacteria is a membrane ATPase that has been studied at the biochemical and genetic level. This resistance system serves as a model for the genes defective in two human hereditary diseases of copper metabolism, Menkes syndrome and Wilson's disease, which encode similar P-type ATPases. Silver resistance is the most recent addition to understand metal cation resistance systems. Prior to this, there were no new metal cation resistance systems described in the last decade. In this section, two well characterised (Hg and As) and a third system (Ag) that is relatively new are discussed. All these systems have unexploited bioremediation potentials.

Mercury

Mercury resistance is by far the most extensively studied metal cation resistance system and is the best example for both basic science and bioremediation. Mercury resistance systems require genes that encode regulatory proteins (MerR; for control of mRNA synthesis), transport proteins (MerT and others), a cell-surface binding protein (MerP), and the enzymes (mercuric reductase, MerA, and organomercurial lyase, MerB).

Mercuric reductase is found with all mercury resistant bacteria, but organomercurial lyase is found only sometimes, with resistance to both inorganic mercury and organomercurials. The mercury resistance system of *Bacillus* (Fig. 16.6a) is unusual in that it possess two regulatory genes, one gene for the enzyme mercuric reductase and three genes for organo-mercurial lyases. Essentially the same *Bacillus* mercury resistance system has been found in the sediments below mercury-polluted Boston Harbour, USA and Minamata Bay, Japan.

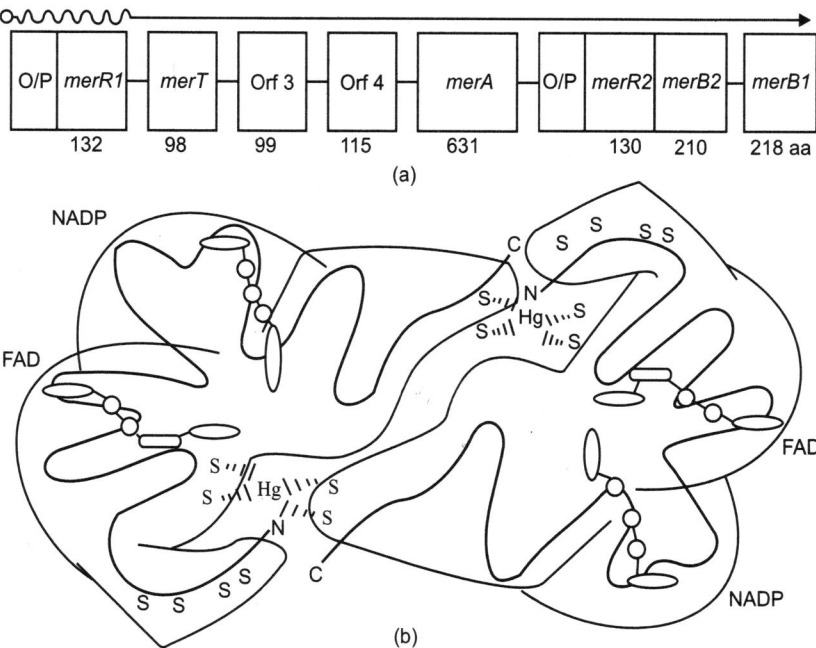

Fig. 16.6. (a) The genes for mercuric and organomercurial resistance in *Bacillus*. O/P represents the DNA MerR-binding site (Operator and the Promoter region) for initiation of mRNA synthesis; *merR1* and *merR2* the genes for the two regulatory proteins; *merT* and open reading frames ORF3 and ORF4 the presumed determinants of a Hg^{2+} uptake system; *merA* the gene for mercuric reductase; and *merB1* and *merB2* the two genes for organomercurial lysases, and (b) structure of mercuric reductase deduced from the X-ray diffraction structure of the central enzyme plus NMR structures of metal binding domains, which lack fixed positions in the *MerA* crystal.

The MerR regulatory protein is the best studied example of a larger family of such proteins found in most bacteria. MerR binds to the mRNA transcriptional start site, and upon addition of Hg^{2+}, MerR twists and bends the DNA to a conformation suitable for opening and initiation of mRNA synthesis. *merR* and its cognate DNA has been attached to genes for bioluminescence resulting in highly-specific and sensitive Hg^{2+} 'biosensors' useful for measuring low levels of Hg^{2+} in the environment. Resistance to organomercurial compounds depends on organomercurial lyase, which breaks the Hg-C bond of methylmercury and phenylmercury, converting more toxic organomercurials to less toxic inorganic

Hg^{2+}. Mercuric reductase detoxifies by converting soluble Hg^{2+} to volatile Hg^0. Thus, enzymatic detoxification results in bioremediation by bacteria in many environments. Mercuric reductase and organomercurial lyase genes have been cloned into rooted plants for phytoremediation of Hg^{2+}-contaminated soil.

The three dimensional structure of mercuric reductase from *Bacillus* was solved. The two subunits form two intra-subunit Hg^{2+} binding sites, with the active site di-thiol cysteine pair toward the amino-end of one subunit and at the carboxyl terminus of the other subunit a second cysteine pair (Fig. 16.6). The co-factors for enzymatic Hg^{2+} reduction, soluble NADPH and bound FAD, occupy positions near the active site and perpendicular to the plane shown in Fig. 16.6b.

Surprisingly, the crystal structure of Schiering starts at amino acid 160 in the sequence. The missing polypeptide in the crystal structure consists of two 'Hg^{2+}-binding domains', that are homologous to the periplasmic mercury binding protein MerP of Gram-negative mercury-resistant bacteria for which the structure has been solved by NMR. The mercury-binding domain is thought to act as a mobile 'catcher's glove' and transfers the Hg^{2+} from the inner surface of the cell membrane to the active site of mercuric reductase (Fig. 16.6b).

These Hg^{2+} binding domains (70 amino acids in length) in the two Hg^{2+} resistance proteins, MerA and MerP, are homologous in sequence and in three-dimensional structure to the copper-binding domain of the ATPase pump defective in the human copper disease Menkes syndrome. This is one example where bacterial toxic metal cation resistance studies have been useful in the understanding of cation transport in higher organisms.

Arsenic

Arsenic resistance systems are widely found with most types of bacteria. With an increasing number of microbial genome sequences becoming available, chromosomal arsenic resistance systems have been identified repeatedly, for example in *Escherichia coli*, *Bacillus subtilis* and *Mycobacterium tuberculosis*. Arsenic resistance systems include a regulatory protein (ArsR), a small soluble enzyme arsenate reductase (ArsC) that reduces intracellular arsenate [As(V)] to arsenite [As(III)], the substrate of an efflux pump (ArsB; Fig. 15.7a).

This inorganic oxyanion resistance system confers resistance to arsenate, arsenite and to antimonite [Sb(III)], a second substrate of the ArsB protein pump. The arsenate enters bacterial cells by membrane transport systems designed for phosphate uptake (Pst and Pit; Fig. 16.7a). The *arsR* gene has been used in light-emitting arsenic biosensors analogous to that for Hg^{2+} sensing.

A small number of less studied anaerobic bacteria have membrane-bound respiratory chain-linked arsenate reductase (Fig. 16.7b) or arsenite oxidase (Fig. 16.7c). The arsenate reductase shown in Fig. 16.7b is the terminal electron acceptor for an anaerobic respiratory chain that allows cell growth by oxidation of organic substrates. It seems likely that arsenate is reduced at the cell surface and arsenate and arsenite do not enter the cellular cytoplasm (Fig. 16.7b).

Aerobic arsenite oxidase found in a few Pseudomonads occurs in the periplasmic space, and arsenite (more toxic) is converted to arsenate (less toxic) by coupling with the small copper protein azurin and the electron transport chain. Recently scientists found the gene for arsenite oxidase. Bacterial enzyme activities (and therefore genes) for both oxidation and reduction of inorganic arsenic in different environments are known and form part of a global arsenic biocycle, just as there are biocycles of O and N. This means that redox state and microbial transformations must be considered in major problem areas with arsenic-polluted drinking waters, including Michigan in the USA, northeastern India and Bangladesh, that has recently received international coverage through nature and science and newspapers. Though microbial activities may exacerbate the problem; the understanding of their potential may contribute to bioremediation of ground water arsenic pollution.

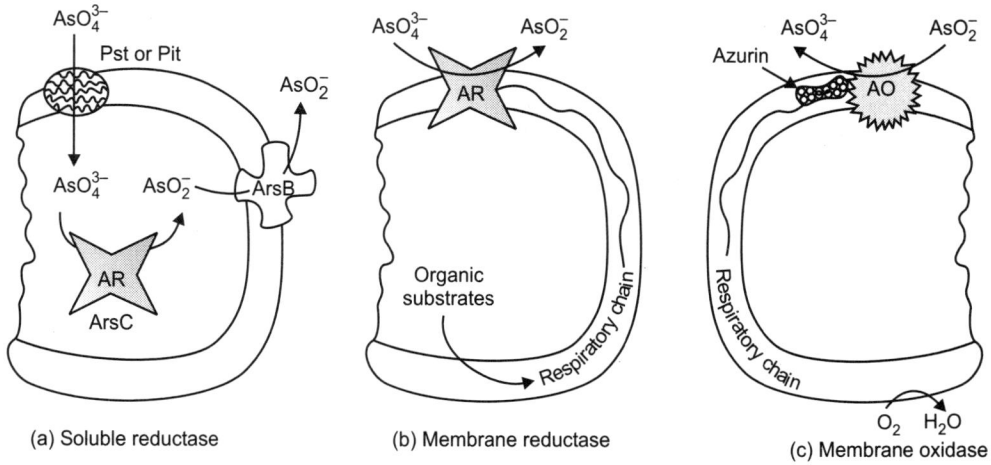

Fig. 16.7. (a) Plasmid-determined arsenate reductase. ArsC, and the ArsB arsenite efflux pump, (b) anaerobic membrane-bound arsenate reductase, AR, and (c) aerobic periplasmic arsenite oxidase, AO.

Silver

Silver resistance is a new plasmid-encoded system. Figure 16.8a shows the genetic organisation for bacterial silver resistance, with seven genes '*silPABCRSE*' (designated on the basis of their product homologies to those of other cation resistance systems) plus two open reading frames ORF105 and ORF96 (named for the lengths of the products in amino acids, for which we lack information on homologs). Three mRNAs have been identified (delineated by arrows at the top of Fig. 16.8a), with one mRNA synthesised toward the left and two towards the right, as shown.

The proposed functions of the seven gene products are diagrammed in Fig. 16.8b. These include SilE, a small periplasmic Ag^+-binding protein that has been studied in detail. SilE is described as the first protein identified to have evolved for and to be specific for binding of Ag^+. This specificity opens the possibility of using SilE for bioremediation of toxic silver-polluted waters and for recycling of silver. The other silver-resistance proteins (shown in Fig. 16.8b) include SilS (a proposed membrane bound, extracellular Ag^+-sensor that is autophosphorylated on a specific histidine residue (amino acid code H) by ATP and SilR (a responder to the sensor, that is transphosphorylated on a specific aspartic acid (amino acid code D) and regulates transcription of the three mRNAs shown in Fig. 16.8a. Finally four proteins together constitute two Ag^+ efflux pumps, one of which (SilP) is a member of the well-known metal cation-effluxing P-type ATPases and the other three (SilCBA) constitute a membrane potential-driven proton/Ag^+ exchange system. No redox chemistry of Ag^+ to Ag^0 occurs in the silver resistance system. Whereas, most metal cation resistance systems involve either an efflux mechanism or binding to small cation-binding proteins, the silver resistance system possesses both a Ag^+ specific binding protein and two efflux pumps (usually only one pump is present for any given system). This suggests that resistance to elevated concentrations of Ag^+ may be additive, with contributions separately by individual mechanisms.

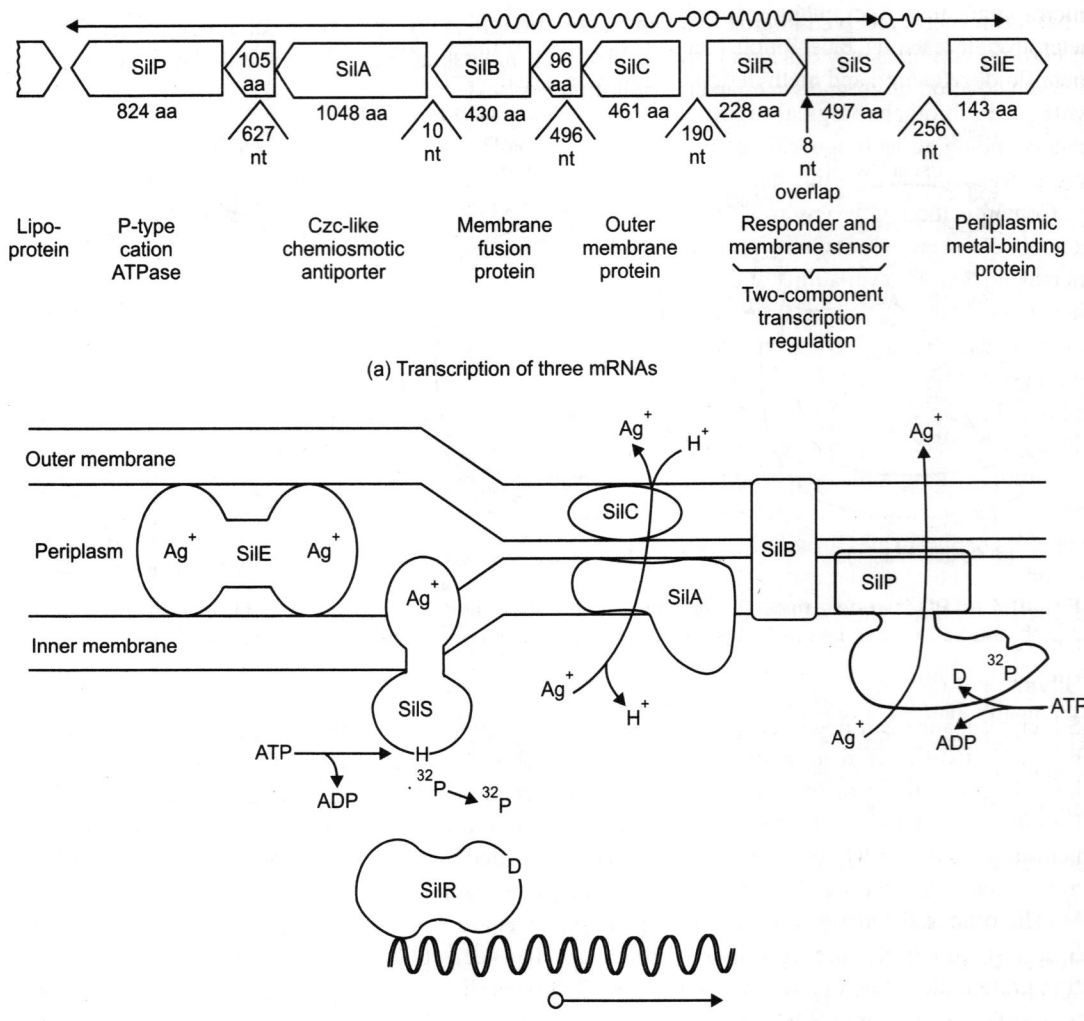

Lipo-protein | P-type cation ATPase | Czc-like chemiosmotic antiporter | Membrane fusion protein | Outer membrane protein | Responder and membrane sensor | Periplasmic metal-binding protein

(a) Transcription of three mRNAs

(b) Silver resistance proteins

Fig. 16.8. The genes and proteins of bacterial silver resistance.

MICROBIAL PROCESSES FOR IMMOBILISATION OF METALS AND THEIR POTENTIAL FOR ENVIRONMENTAL BIOREMEDIATION

Mechanisms of microbial solubilisation and immobilisation of metal(loid)s, radionuclides and related substances are of dear potential for bioremediation with some processes integral to the operation of several successful *in situ* and *ex situ* biotreatment methods. Although the biotechnological potential of most of these processes has only been explored at laboratory scale, some mechanisms, notably bioleaching, biosorption and precipitation, have been employed at a commercial scale. Autotrophic leaching is an established major process in mineral extraction and has also been applied to the treatment of contaminated land. As a process for immobilising metals, precipitation of metals as sulphides has also achieved large-scale application. This section outlines some of the main mechanisms by which micro-organisms effect changes in the speciation and mobility of metals including autotrophic and heterotrophic leaching, biosorption, metal precipitation by metal-reducing and sulphate-reducing bacteria, metal(loid) reduction and methylation, and, where possible, provides examples of field application. As well as the biotechnological significance, it should be emphasised that this work also provides understanding of the biogeochemistry of metal(loid) cycling in the environment and the central role of micro-organisms in affecting metal mobility and transfer between different biotic and abiotic locations.

Contamination of the environment by toxic metals, metalloids, organometals and radionuclides is of economic and environmental significance. Certain microbial processes can solubilise metals, thereby increasing their bioavailability and potential toxicity, where as other immobilised them and thus reduce their bioavailability. The relative balance between mobilisation and immobilisation varies depending on the organisms, their environment and physico-chemical conditions. As well as being integral component of biogeochemical cycles for metals, these processes may be exploited for the treatment of contaminated solid and liquid wastes. Metal mobilisation can be achieved by autotrophic and heterotrophic leaching, chelation by microbial metabolites and siderophores, and methylation, which can result in volatilisation.

Similarly, immobilisation can result from sorption to cell component to exopolymers, transport and intracellular sequestration or precipitation as insoluble organic and inorganic compounds, e.g. oxalates, sulphides or phosphates. In addition, and depending on the metal species, biologically-mediated reduction of higher-valency species may effect mobilisation, e.g. Mn(IV) to Mn(II), or immobilisation, e.g. Cr(VI) to Cr(III). In the contest of bioremediation, solubilisation of metal contaminants provides a route for removal of the metal from solid matrices such as soils, sediments, dumps and industrial wastes. Alternatively immobilisation processes may enable metals to be transformed *in situ* into insoluble and chemically inert forms and are particularly applicable to removing metals from mobile aqueous phases. The selected microbiological processes, which are of significance and determining metal mobility and which have actual or potential application in bioremediation of metal and metalloid pollution include autotrophic and heterotrophic leaching, reduction, precipitation and transformation.

Solubilisation

Autotrophic leaching

Most autotrophic leaching is carried out by chemolithotrophic, acidophilic bacteria which fix carbon dioxide and obtain energy from the oxidation of ferrous iron or reduced sulphur compounds which results in the production of Fe(III) and H_2SO_4. The micro-organisms involved in autotrophic leaching include sulphur oxidising bacteria, e.g. *Thiobacillus thiooxidans*, iron and sulphur oxidising bacteria, e.g. *Thiobacillus ferrooxidans* and iron-oxidising bacteria, e.g. *Leptospirillum ferrooxidans*. Both the *Thiobacillus* species are able to oxidise inorganic sulphur (Eq. 16.1) and metal sulphides such as pyrite (Eq. 16.2). *T. ferrooxidans* and *L. ferrooxidans* are able to oxidise soluble ferrous iron (Eq. 16.3) producing ferric iron, which can then indirectly solubilise metal sulphides (Eq. 16.4).

$$2S^0_{(s)} + 3O_2 + 2H_2O \longrightarrow 2H_2SO_4(aq) \qquad \text{... (16.1)}$$

$$2FeS_{2(s)} + 7O_2 + 2H_2O \longrightarrow 2FeSO_{4(aq)} + 2H_2SO_4(aq) \qquad \text{... (16.2)}$$

$$4FeSO_{4(aq)} + O_2 + 2H_2SO_{4(aq)} \longrightarrow 2Fe_2(SO_4)_{3(aq)} + 2H_2O \qquad \text{... (16.3)}$$

$$FeS_{2(s)} + 14Fe^{3+}_{(aq)} + 8H_2O \longrightarrow 15Fe^{2+} + 2SO_4^{2-}_{(aq)} + 16H^+ \qquad \text{... (16.4)}$$

As a result of sulphur and iron-oxidation, metal sulphides are solubilised, the pH of their immediate environment is decreased and solubilisation of other metal compounds takes place. While most leaching bacteria are mesophilic, moderately thermophilic iron-oxidising bacteria have also been isolated with optimum temperatures for metal sulphide solubilisation of 45°–50°C.

Autotrophic leaching of metal sulphides by acidophilic bacteria is well established in industrial scale biomining processes. Low-grade copper and uranium ores are leached to extract the metal and refractory gold ores are leached to remove arsenopyrite before conventional cyanidation and gold extraction. The bacteria used for treating gold ore are either mesophilic, operating at around 30°C (Gencor process) or moderately thermophilic operating at 45°C.

For bioremediation, production of sulphuric acid by *Thiobacillus* species has been used to solubilise metals from sewage sludge, which can then be used as a fertiliser. The elemental sulphur, which can act as an energy source for the process can be of either chemical or biological origin and it has been shown that lumps of sulphur are as effective as powder. Simultaneously sewage sludge digestion and metal leaching under acidic conditions (pH 2.0–2.5) has an advantage over conventional aerobic and anaerobic digestion in that the acidity may lead to a decrease in pathogenic micro-organisms.

Autotrophic leaching has also been used to remediate other metal-contaminated solid materials. In a two-stage process for the bioremediation of metal-contaminated soil, a mixture of sulphur-oxidising bacteria was used to acidify the soil and solubilise toxic metals before treatment of the metal contaminated leachate using sulphate reducing bacteria.

Laboratory studies have also been conducted into the bioremediation of red mud, the main waste product of Al extraction from bauxite, by autotrophic leaching. Autotrophic leaching by indigenous *Thiobacillus* spp. was found to be more efficient than heterotrophic leaching by a range of fungal strains. Although this process was developed to increase the amount of aluminium obtained from bauxite, it also decreased the toxicity of the waste product.

Heterotrophic leaching

In an industrial context, most bioleaching has been carried out using chemoautotrophic acidophilic bacteria which do not need a carbon source and have a high acidification capacity. However, their acidophilicity may make them unable to tolerate the higher pH values of many industrial wastes. Many species of fungi are able to leach metals (heterotrophic leaching) from industrial wastes and by-products, low-grade ores and metal bearing minerals and such processes may also complement the bioleaching repertoire. There may be additional advantages to using fungi for leaching purposes in that they are more amenable to bioreactor operation than *Thiobacilli* and by altering growth conditions, can be induced to produce high concentrations of organic acids.

It is known, for example, that manganese deficiency (less than 10^{-8} M) in the growth medium leads to the production of large amounts of citric acid by *A. niger*, and typical concentrations of citric acid produced industrially by this fungus can reach 600 mM. The pH of non-regulated *A. niger* cultures can fall to values between 1.5 and 2.0 due to high citric acid production. Oxalic acid production can be manipulated to yield concentrations of up to 200 mM on low cost carbon sources with the optimum pH for oxalic acid production being around neutrality. Furthermore, many species are metal tolerant and can grow over a range of pH values.

Heterotrophic leaching by fungi occurs as a result of several processes, including the efflux of protons and the production of siderophores (for iron), but in most fungal strains, leaching occurs mainly by organic acid production. Solubilisation of insoluble metal compounds results from protonation of the anion of the compound, which makes it less available to the metal cation. The production of organic acid provides both a source of protons for solubilisation and a metal-chelating anion to complex the metal cation, with complexation being dependent on the relative concentrations of the anions and metals in solution, pH and the stability constants of the various complexes.

Laboratory scale heterotrophic leaching of Ni and Co from low-grade laterite ores has been carried out using fungi. 55–60 per cent Ni was leached from the ore in the presence of *Aspergillus* and *Penicillium* strains, and 70 per cent was leached at high temperature (95°C) by application of metabolic products obtained from the cultivation of the fungal strain at 30°C in a glucose and sucrose medium. *A. niger* is able to solubilise a wide range of insoluble metal compounds, including phosphates, sulphides and mineral ores such as cuprite (CuS). There are several examples in the literature of fungal leaching of industrial wastes. *Penicillium simplicissimum* has been used successfully to leach Zn from insoluble ZnO contained in industrial filter dust and this fungus only developed the ability to produce citric acid (>100 mM) in the presence of the filter dust.

Culture filtrates from *A. niger* have also been used to leach Cu, Ni and Co from copper converter slag. A heterotrophic mixed culture has been employed for leaching manganiferous minerals. This culture was capable of reducing MnO_2, with the process being of potential for the treatment of materials not treatable by conventional processes. Cd, Zn, Cu, Pb and Al have been leached from municipal waste fly ash using *A. niger*.

A two-stage process was used, with *A. niger* being cultured and the citric acid from the culture used as a leaching agent. The environmental quality of the fly ash residue was deemed suitable for subsequent use in the construction industry.

Immobilisation

Biosorption

Biosorption can be defined as the uptake of organic and inorganic metal species, both soluble and insoluble, by physico-chemical mechanisms such as adsorption. In living cells, metabolic activity may influence biosorption because of changes in pH, E_h, organic and inorganic nutrients and metabolites in the cellular microenvironment. Biosorption can also provide nucleation sites for mineral formation. Almost all biological macromolecules have an affinity for metal species with cell walls and associated materials being of the greatest significance in biosorption. As well as by biosorption, cationic species can be accumulated by cells via transport system of varying affinity and specificity. Once inside cells, metal species may be bound, precipitated, localised within intracellular structures or organelles, or translocated to specific structures depending on the element concerned and the organisms.

Biosorption by cell walls and associated components

Microbial exopolymers can be composed of polysaccharide, glycoproteins and lipopolysaccharide, which may be associated with protein. Many exopolymers act as polyanions under natural conditions, and negatively charged groups can interact with cationic metal/radionuclide species although uncharged polymers are also capable of binding and entrapment of insoluble forms. Peptidoglycan carboxyl groups are the main cation binding sites in Gram-positive bacterial cell walls with phosphate groups contributing significantly in Gram-negative species. Chitin is an important structural component of fungal cell walls and this is an effective biosorbent for radionuclides as are chitosan, other chitin derivatives, fungal phenolic polymers and melanins.

Biosorption by free and immobilised biomass

Both freely-suspended and immobilised bacterial, cyanobacterial, algal and fungal biomass has received attention with immobilised systems having advantages which include higher mechanical strength and easier biomass/liquid separation than freely suspended biomass. Living or dead biomass of all groups has been immobilised by encapsulation or cross linking using supports which include agar, cellulose, alginates, cross-linked ethyl acrylate-ethylene glycol dimethylacrylate, polyacrylamide, silica gel and cross linking reagents such as toluene diisocyanate and glutaraldehyde.

Immobilised living biomass has mainly taken the form of bacterial biofilms on inert supports and has been used in a variety of bioreactor configurations including rotating biological contactors, fixed bed reactors, trickle filters, fluidised beds and air lift bioreactors. One problem with radionuclide-treatment using biosorption could be the disposal of radioactive biomass, although this may be amenable to conventional physical and chemical treatments and/or containment. For radionuclides, a prime consideration would be the prevention of environmental discharge, and physical destruction or elution followed by containment may be a necessary treatment step.

Metal-binding proteins, polysaccharides and other biomolecules

A diverse range of specific and non-specific metal-binding compounds are produced by micro-organisms, some of which are released into the environment. Non-specific metal-binding compounds are by-products of microbial metabolism and range in size from simple organic acids and alcohols to macromolecules such as polysaccharides; humic and fulvic acids. Humic and fulvic acids are undefined macromolecules resulting in soil and water from the microbial degradation of cellulose, lignin and other complex organic compounds, and which can bind toxic metals. Extracellular polymeric substances (EPS), a mixture of polysaccharides mucopolysaccharides and proteins are produced by bacteria, algae and fungi and also bind significant amounts of potentially toxic metals. Extracellular polysaccharides are able to both bind metals and adsorb or entrap particulate matter such as precipitated metal sulphides and oxides.

Specific metal-binding compounds include siderophores which are low molecular weight ligands (500–1000 Da) possessing a high affinity for Fe(III). Although primarily produced as a means of obtaining iron, siderophores are also able to bind other metals such as magnesium, manganese, chromium (III), gallium (III) and radionuclides such as plutonium (IV). Other metal binding molecules include low molecular weight (6000–10,000 Da) metal binding proteins, termed metallothioneins, which are produced by animals, plants and micro-organisms in response to the presence of toxic metals and phytochelatins and related peptides, which contain glutamic acid and cysteine at the amino-terminal position, and have been identified in plants, algae and several micro-organisms.

Metal Precipitation

Precipitation by metal-reducing bacteria

A taxonomically diverse range of micro-organisms are able to use oxidised metal species, e.g. Fe(III), Cr(VI) or Mn(IV) as terminal electron acceptors. Many of these organisms can utilise more than one terminal electron acceptor including several metals or other anions such as nitrate or sulphate. Most of these organisms are anaerobic; with a few being facultative anaerobes, and oxygen may also be respired. The majority of dissimilatory metal reducing bacteria are respiratory heterotrophs possessing an electron acceptor chain and can utilise a range of substrates, including organic acids, alcohols and aromatic compound. A small number of metal-reducing strains are able to reduce metals within a fermentative metabolic framework.

A significant feature of Fe(III) and Mn(IV)-reducing bacteria is the greater affinity that these organisms have for both organic substrates and hydrogen compared to sulphate-reducing bacteria and methanogens. This can lead to the total competitive inhibition of sulphate reduction and methanogenesis when these substrates are limiting.

Processes using dissimilatory metal reduction

As yet, biotechnological processes using microbial metal reduction are at the stage of laboratory demonstration. Fe(III) and Mn(IV) appear to be the most commonly utilised metals as terminal electron acceptors in the biosphere. However, Fe and Mn solubility is increased by bacterial reduction, and as neither metal is significantly toxic, other metals are potential targets in waste treatment. Molybdenum(VI) was reduced to molybdenum blue by a strain of *Enterobacter cloacae*, which was isolated from a molybdate-polluted aquatic environment. Another strain of *E. cloacae* was able to reduce Cr(VI) to Cr(III) under similar conditions, the Cr(III) precipitating from a simulated waste-water in a bioreactor. Dissimilatory Cr(VI) reduction was also carried out by a strain of *Escherichia coli* under both anaerobic and aerobic conditions, albeit at a slower rate. Metal reduction processes may be useful as pretreatments for other processes, e.g. the reduction of Cr(VI) compounds to Cr(III) may facilitate removal by biosorption or (bio)precipitation. Perhaps the most promising potential application of dissimilatory biological metal reduction is uranium precipitation, which may have potential both in waste treatment and in concentrating uranium from low-grade sources. While U(VI) compounds are soluble, U(IV) compounds such as the hydroxide or carbonate have low solubility and readily form precipitates at neutral pH. A strain of *Shewanella* (*Alteromonas*) *putrefaciens* which reduced Fe(III) and Mn (IV) also reduced U(VI) to U(IV) forming a black precipitate of U(IV) carbonate. U(IV) was also reduced by the sulphate-reducing bacterium *Desulfovibrio desulfuricans* in the presence of sulphate, utilising the electron transport chain and producing a very pure precipitate of U(IV) carbonate thus providing a potential alternative to more conventional chemical technologies. It was also reported that *Desulfovibrio vulgaris* carried out a similar enzymic reduction of uranium(VI). Bacterial uranium reduction has also been combined with chemical extraction to produce a potential process for soil bioremediation. The solubility of other radionuclides can be increased by reduction and this may favour their removal from matrices such as soils. For example, iron-reducing bacterial strains solubilised 40 per cent of the Pu present in contaminated soils within 6–7 days and both iron and sulphate reducing bacteria were able to solubilise Ra from uranium mine tailing, although solubilisation occurred largely by disruption of reducible host minerals.

Sulphate reducing bacteria

Sulphate-reducing bacteria (SRB) are strictly anaerobic heterotrophs commonly found in anaerobic environments where carbon substrates and sulphate are available. Example of such habitats are freshwater, marine and estuarine sediments and waters with a high organic content. SRB are largely mesophilic although thermophilic strains have been recovered from hydrothermal vents. Sulphate-reducing bacteria are almost entirely neutrophilic with maximum growth obtained in the range of pH 6–8. However, some isolates can grow in moderately acidic conditions such as mine and surface waters where the bulk phase pH is in the range 3–4.

In these environments, the sulphate-reducing bacteria are found in sediments and their apparent acid-tolerance results from the existence of more natural microenvironments which are maintained by buffering resulting from the low dissociation of H_2S. Sulphate-reducing bacteria utilise an energy metabolism in which the oxidation of organic compounds or hydrogen is coupled to the reduction of sulphate as the terminal electron acceptor, producing sulphide. Sulphate reducing bacteria dissimilate carbon via respiratory mechanisms. The range of carbon/energy sources used by SRB is very wide and includes alcohols, organic acids and hydrocarbons. However, individual strains are only able to metabolise a limited range of these substrates and substrate preferences have been used to divide sulphate-reducing bacteria into groups. The hydrogen-lactate group comprises mainly *Desulfovibrio* and *Desulfoto-maculum* species which utilise the organic acid lactic, pyruvic, succinic, fumaric and malic in addition to ethanol, formate and glycerol. Some organisms with this metabolic pattern can also use hydrogen as electron-donor in the presence of CO_2, acetate or another organic carbon-source. This ability has been utilised in a laboratory-scale packed-bed reactor using producer gas (synthesis gas), which contains a substantial proportion of hydrogen, as a substrate for sulphate-reducing bacteria to remove sulphate from simulated industrial waste-waters.

Bacterial sulphate reduction results in the formation of sulphide, which may reach significant concentrations in sediments or chemostat cultures. Although low concentrations (e.g. 2–5 mM) of sulphide benefit SRB growth by ensuring a low E_h, high concentrations of sulphide are inhibitory. A sulphide concentration of >16 mM was toxic to an SRB culture derived from an anaerobic treatment plant. However, such sulphide concentrations are not generally encountered due to precipitation of sulphide with metals. With the exception of the alkali and alkaline-earth metals, metal sulphides are essentially insoluble and the resultant precipitation of sulphides has been observed to protect SRB against metal toxicity: metals similarly protect the organisms against sulphide toxicity.

Metal precipitation by sulphate-reducing bacteria

The main mechanism by which sulphate-reducing bacteria remove toxic metals from solution is via the formation of insoluble metal sulphides (Fig. 16.9):

$$M^{2+} + SO_4^{2-} + 2CH_3CH_2OH \longrightarrow 2CH_3COOH + 2H_2O + MS\downarrow \qquad ...(16.5)$$

$$M^{2+} + SO_4^{2-} + 2CH_3CHOHCOOH \longrightarrow 2CH_3COOH + 2CO_2 + 2H_2O + MS\downarrow \qquad ...(16.6)$$

$$M^{2+} + SO_4^{2-} + CH_3COOH \longrightarrow 2CO_2 + 2H_2O + MS\downarrow \qquad ...(16.7)$$

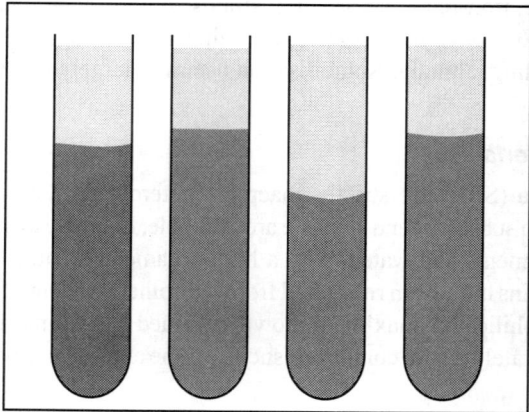

Fig. 16.9. Metal sulphide precipitates arising from bacterial sulphate-reduction. A mixed culture of sulphate-reducing bacteria was grown in a solid medium containing copper salts: the resulting black precipitate of CuS can be seen in the region where growth has occurred.

The solubility products of most toxic metal sulphides are very low, in the range of 4.65×10^{-14} (Mn) to 6.44×10^{-53} (Hg) and even a moderate output of sulphide can remove metals to levels permitted in the environment with metal removal being directly related to sulphide production. Sulphate-reducing bacteria can create extremely reducing conditions, which can reduce metals such as uranium (VI). In addition, sulphate reduction partially eliminates acidity from the system as a result of the shift in equilibrium when sulphate (dissociated) is converted to sulphide (largely protonated). This can result in the further precipitation of metals such as copper or aluminium as hydroxides as well as increasing the efficiency of sulphide precipitation.

Processes utilising metal sulphide precipitation

Acid mine drainage occurs through the activities of sulphur and iron oxidising bacteria and effluents. Laboratory studies indicate that sulphate-reduction can provide both *in situ* and *ex situ* metal removal from such waters and contribute to the removal of metals and acidity in artificial and natural wetlands. Large-scale bioreactor systems have also been developed using bacterial sulphate reduction for treating metal contaminated waters. A pilot-scale study used either 3×200 litres or using 4500 litres fixed bed vessels filled with spent mushroom compost at residence times between 9 and 17 days. Both systems raised the pH from 3.0–3 to 6–7 and removed almost all of the metals (Al, Zn, Cu, Ni) in the inflow. The most extensive use to date of sulphate reducing bacteria is in the treatment of contaminated ground water at the Budelo zinc-smelting works at Budel-Dorplein in the Netherlands. The pilot plant comprised a purpose-designed $9\ m^3$ stainless steel sludge-blanket reactor using sulphate-reducing bacteria and was developed by Shell Research Ltd., UK. This plant successfully removed toxic metals (primarily Zn) and sulphate from contaminated groundwater at the long-standing smelter site by precipitation as metal sulphides. The reactor used a selected but undefined consortium of sulphate-reducing bacteria with ethanol as the growth substrate. It was capable of tolerating a wide range of inflow pH and operating temperatures, and yielded outflow metal concentrations below the µM range. Methanogenic bacteria in the consortium also removed the acetate produced by sulphate-reducing bacteria, leaving an effluent with an acceptably low BOD. Excess gaseous H_2S was stripped out of waste gases using a $ZnSO_4$ solution. A detailed analysis of this process including mass-balance was also carried out. The process has since been expanded to commercial scale and has been in operation from October 1992. A process which integrates bacterial sulphate-reduction with bioleaching by sulphur-oxidising bacteria has been developed to remove contaminating toxic metals from soils. In this process sulphur oxidising bacteria are employed to liberate metals from soils by the breakdown of sulphide minerals and production of sulphuric acid, which liberates acid-labile forms such as hydroxides, carbonates or sorbed metals. Metals are liberated in the form of an acid sulphate solution, which enables both a large proportion of the acidity and almost the entirety of the metals to be removed by bacterial sulphate reduction (Fig. 16.10).

As the pH decreased, metals were leached in the approximate order Mn, Cr, Ni, Co, Cd, Zn, Cu, and Pb. The total amount of the metals leached corresponded closely to the amount added initially to the soil with the exceptions of Ni, Zn, and Mn where significant quantities of these were leached from soil minerals. Leaching of lead was incomplete and only occurred when the pH was below 1.5 because of the low solubility of lead sulphate. The leachate, at sulphate concentrations between 35–50 mM and pH 1.5–3.0, was fed into a bioprecipitation reactor without pretreatment. The bioreactor used for this stage was an all glass internal sedimentation feedback bioreactor (Fig. 16.11), capable of retaining a high concentration of biomass. It contained a mixed, undefined culture of sulphate-reducing bacteria produced by combining a number of metal-tolerant enrichment cultures from different environmental origins. Metals were mainly precipitated as solid sulphides and removal of the target metals by the bioreactor achieved more than 98 per cent efficiency overall with the exception of Mn and, to a lesser extent Ni and Pb. The overall process effectively removed the contaminating metal load from the soil converted it to sulphides which were concentrated 100- to 200-fold in the solid phase, while the concentrations of metals in the liquid effluent were low enough to meet environmental discharge criteria and allowed recycle of the liquor to the bioleaching stage.

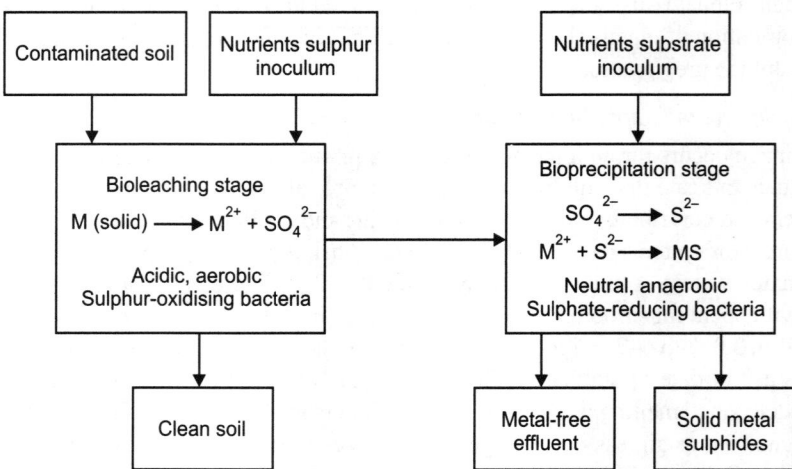

Fig. 16.10. Diagram showing the outline integrated process for bioremediation of metal-contaminated soils. The outline reactions and conditions for the bioleaching and bioprecipitation stages are shown in addition to the inputs and organisms utilised. Target metals are considered to be divalent cations and indicated as M^{2+}.

Phosphatase-mediated metal precipitation

In this process, metal or radionuclide accumulation by bacterial biomass is mediated by a phosphatase enzyme, induced during metal-free growth, which liberates inorganic phosphate from a supplied organic phosphate donor molecule, e.g. glycerol 2-phosphate. Metal/radionuclide cations are then precipitated as phosphates on the biomass to high levels. Most work has been carried out with a *Citrobacter* sp., and a range of bioreactor configurations, including those using immobilised biofilms have been described.

High gradient magnetic separation (HGMS)

This is a technique for metal ion removal from solution using bacterial rendered susceptible to magnetic fields. 'Non-magnetic' bacteria can be made magnetic by the precipitation of metal phosphates (aerobic) or sulphides (anaerobic) on their surfaces as described previously above. For those organisms producing iron sulphide, it has been found that this compound is not only magnetic but also an effective adsorbent for metallic elements.

Transformations

Metalloid transformations

Micro-organisms can transform certain metalloid and organometallic species by oxidation, reduction, methylation and dealkylation. Biomethylated derivatives are often volatile and may be eliminated from a system by evaporation. The two major transformation processes described are reduction of metalloid oxyanions to elemental forms, e.g. SeO_4^{2-} to Se^0 and methylation of metalloids, metalloid oxyanions or organometalloids to methyl derivatives, e.g. ASO_4^{3-} and methylarsonic acid to $(CH_3)_3As$ (trimethylarsine). Transformation processes modify the mobility and toxicity of metalloids, have biogeochemical significance, and are also of biotechnological potential in bioremediation.

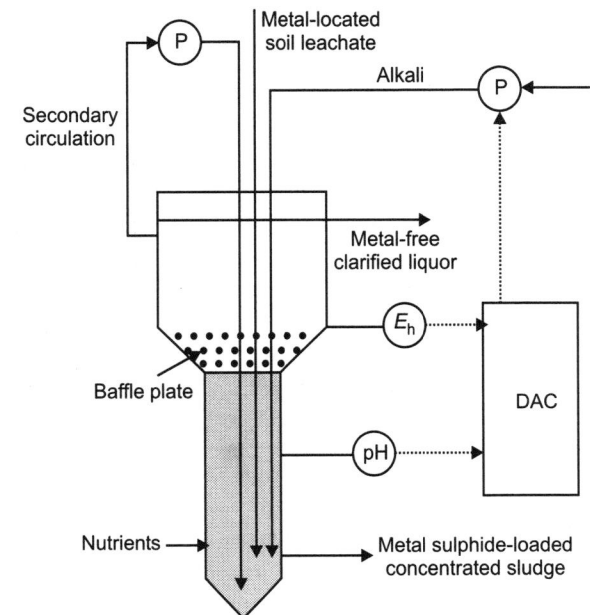

Fig. 16.11. Diagram of an internal sedimentation bioreactor for removing metals from sulphate-containing soil leachate. The upper sedimentation zone of the sulphate-reducing reactor allows extraction of clarified liquor and recirculation. It is separated from the lower, active zone containing concentrated biomass and precipitated metals by a baffle plate. Solid lines indicate material flows with arrows indicating the direction of flows: pumps are labelled P. Redox (E_h) and pH probes are labelled and the connections to a PC-based data acquisition and control (DAC) system are shown schematically as dotted lines.

Microbial reduction of metalloid oxyanions

Reduction of selenate [Se(VI)] and selenite [Se(IV)] to elemental selenium can be catalysed by numerous microbial species, which often results in a red precipitate deposited around cells colonies. Certain organisms can also use SeO_4^{2-} as an electron acceptor to support growth. *Thauera selenatis* is capable of anaerobic SeO_4^{2-} respiration to SeO_3^{2-} with contaminant reduction of NO_3^-: SeO_3^{2-} formed from this reduction was further reduced to Se^0, perhaps by means of a periplasmic nitrite reductase. It is generally believed that while SeO_4^{2-} may act as a terminal electron in some organisms, SeO_3^{2-} reduction is more likely to result in detoxification. Reduction of TeO_3^{2-} to Te^0 is also an apparent means of detoxification found in bacteria. In contrast to bacteria, fungal reduction of metalloids has received less attention although numerous filamentous and unicellular fungal species are capable of SeO_3^{2-} reduction to Se^0, deposited intra- and extracellularly, resulting in a red colouration of colonies. Fungal reduction of TeO_3^{2-} to Te^0 results in black or grey colonies.

Methylation of metalloids

Microbial methylation of metalloids to yield volatile derivatives, e.g. dimethylselenide or trimethylarsine, can be affected by a variety of bacteria, algae and fungi. Selenium methylation appears to involve transfer of methyl groups as carbonium (CH_3^+) ions via the S-adenosyl methionine system. Less work has been carried out on tellurium methylation by fungi although there is evidence of dimethyl telluride production.

Several bacterial and fungal species have been shown to methylate arsenic compounds such as arsenate [As(V), ASO_4^{3-}], arsenite [As(III), AsO_4^{3-}] and methylarsonic acid ($CH_3H_2AsO_3$) to volatile dimethyl-[$(CH_3)_2HAs$] or trimethylarsine [$(CH_3)_2As$].

Microbial metalloid transformations and bioremediation

Oremland described *in situ* removal of SeO_4^{2-}, by reduction to Se^0, by sediment bacteria in agriculture drainage regions of Nevada. Flooding of exposed sediments at Kesterson reservoir with water (to create anoxic conditions) resulted in reduction and immobilisation of large quantities of selenium that was present in sediments. Microbial methylation of selenium resulting in volatilisation, has also been used for *in situ* bioremediation of selenium-containing land and water at Kesterson Reservoir, California. The selenium-contaminated agricultural drainage water was evaporated to dryness until the sediment selenium concentration approached 100 mg Se kg^{-1} dry weight. Conditions such as carbon source, moisture, temperature and aeration were then optimised for selenium volatilisation and the process continued until selenium levels in sediments declined to acceptable levels. Some potential for *ex situ* treatment of selenium-contaminated waters has also been demonstrated.

Mercury

Mercury is briefly discussed here because as well as the physico-chemical interactions detailed previously, key microbial transformations of inorganic Hg^{2+} include reduction and methylation. The mechanism of bacterial Hg^{2+} may also arise from the action of organomercurial lyase on organomercurials. Since Hg^0 is volatile, this could provide one means of mercury removal. Methylation of inorganic Hg^{2+} leads to the formation of more toxic volatile derivatives: the bioremediation potential of this process (as for other metals and metalloids (besides selenium) capable of being methylated, e.g. As, Sn, Pb) has not been explored in detail.

Degradation of organometals

As well as organomercurials, other organometals may be degraded by micro-organisms. Organoarsenicals can be demethylated by bacteria, while organotin degradation involves sequential removal of organic groups from the tin atom, which results in a reduction in toxicity. In theory, such mechanisms and interaction with the bioremediation possibilities described previously may provide a means of detoxification. Thus, micro-organisms play important roles in the environmental fate of toxic metals and metalloids with physico-chemical and biological mechanisms effecting transformations between soluble and insoluble phases. Such mechanisms are important components of biogeochemical cycles with some processes being of potential application to the treatment of contaminated materials. Although the biotechnological potential of many processes has only been explored at the laboratory scale, some mechanisms, notably bioleaching, biosorption and precipitation, have been employed at a commercial scale. Of these, autotrophic leaching is an established major process in mineral extraction but has also been applied to the treatment of contaminated land. There have been several attempts to commercialise biosorption using microbial biomass but success has been limited, primarily due to competition with commercially-produced ion exchange media. As a process for immobilising metals, precipitation of metals as sulphides has achieved large-scale application, and this holds out promise of further commercial development.

APPLICATION OF MICRO-ORGANISMS TO THE DECONTAMINATION OF HEAVY METAL-BEARING WASTES

Metal-bearing liquid industrial wastes range from high-volume, dilute waters from mine drainages, to aggressive, concentrated or multi-component wastes from industrial processes. Simple metal cations can be removed by biosorptive or bioaccumulative processes, or by biomineralisation. Biosorption, using living or dead biomass, is essentially a simple chemical process which is governed by chemical constraints and final equilibria. Bioaccumulation usually refers to the intracellular uptake of metals by living cells.

Biomineralisation

Biomineralisation (or biocrystallisation) is a process whereby microbially-generated ligands or microbially-mediated changes in the cellular microenvironment cause precipitation of heavy metals as biomass-bound crystalline deposits (Fig. 16.12). Precipitant ligands can be hydroxide or carbonate ions, produced by localised alkalinisation (Fig. 16.12a), or microbially-generated ligands may be sulphide (Fig. 16.12b) or phosphate (Figs 16.12c,d), with corresponding metal (M) deposition to very high load as MS or $MHPO_4$, respectively. The generation of sulphides is typical of the sulphate-reducing bacteria (SRB), while production of phosphate is exemplified by *Citrobacter* or *Acinetobacter*, which produce phosphate ligand via phosphatase-mediated cleavage of suitable supplied (*Citrobacter*) or intracellular (*Acinetobacter*) phosphate substrates (Figs 16.12c,d). Most studies on phosphate-mediated biomineralisation have used *Citrobacter* (Fig. 16.12c), but it is possible to use inorganic phosphate instead of applied phosphate substrate, using the phosphate-concentrating ability of *Acinetobacter* via the polyphosphate cycle of this organism (Fig. 16.12d). These approaches overcome the problems of exceeding the solubility product of metal phosphate in a very dilute solution, providing a high localised concentration of phosphate and a nucleating surface for the initiation of formation of metal phosphate crystals.

Acinetobacter

In the case of *Acinetobacter* the requirement for an aerobic-anaerobic pulsed cycle (Fig. 16.12d) necessitates a discontinuous system, where metal is removed during anaerobic periods. In contrast the *Citrobacter* system can operate continuously. Using immobilised cells within flow-through columns continued enzymatic activity gives a steady-state metal removal, which can be described mathematically, e.g. using a metal-accumulating biofilm-bioreactor. The enzyme is held within the cellular periplasmic space and also in association with extracellular polymeric material (EPM), which provides foci for initiation and continuation of metal deposition and can also buffer the cells against adverse conditions of the bulk flow. This technique has been applied to the treatment of uranium-loaded acidic mine drainage water, where 70 per cent of the uranium was removed from a stream containing 35–40 ppm of UO_2^{2+} at a pH of 3.5–4.5. Although the enzyme is sensitive to uranyl toxicity, precipitation as HUO_2PO_4 protects the enzyme and biomass loadings of 9 grams of uranium per gram of biomass dry weight have been observed in long-term tests over several weeks.

Uranyl Phosphate Solid Waste

The uranyl phosphate solid waste from minewater remediation has a further possible use. Some metals such as Ni^{2+} are not removed readily by conventional or biotechnological methods but can be intercalated within the crystalline lattice of the crystalline HUO_2PO_4, laid down on the cells. The U-loaded biomass effectively acts as a bioinorganic ion exchanger for the remediation of 'difficult' metals and, as such, can be desorbed of the intercalating metal and reused repeatedly, with conservation of the primary HUO_2PO_4 lattice.

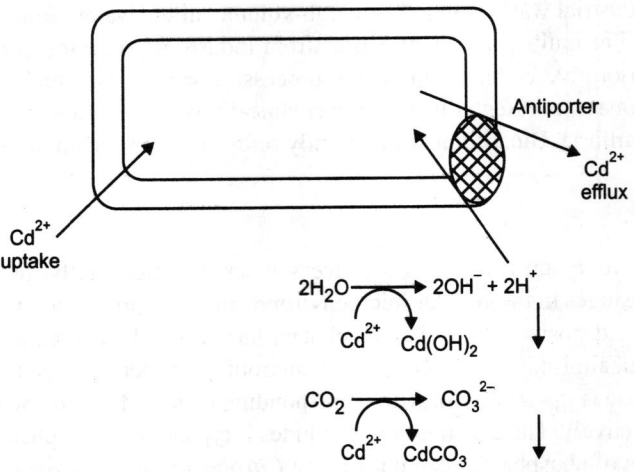

(a) Biomineralisation as hydroxides and carbonates by *Alcaligenes eutrophus*.

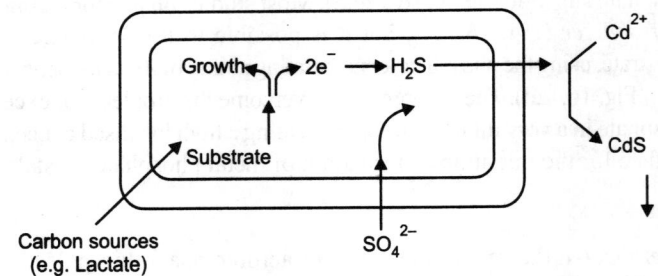

(b) Biomineralisation as sulphides by *Desulfovibrio desulfuricans*

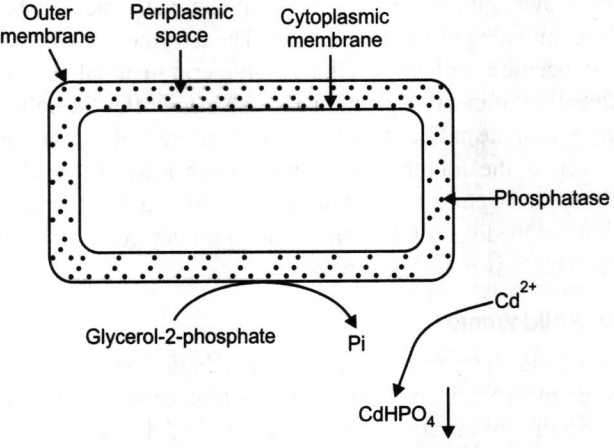

(c) Biomineralisation as phosphate by *Citrobacter* sp.   *(Contd ...)*

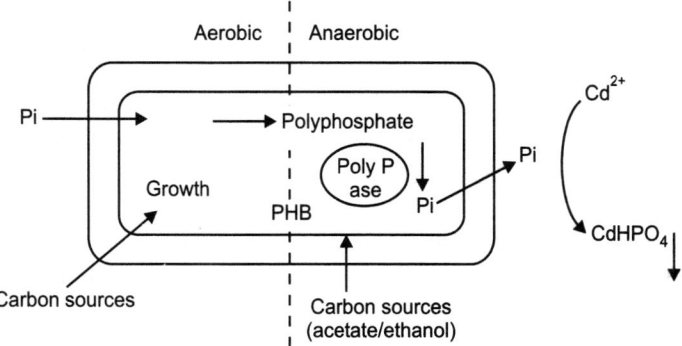

(d) Biomineralisation as phosphates by *Acinetobacter* sp.

Fig. 16.12. Examples of various mechanisms of biomineralisation: (a) in *Alcaligenes eutrophus* (now called *Ralstonia metalliducans*) metals are pumped from the cell as a resistance mechanism at the expense of metabolic energy. Metal efflux (out) is charge-counterbalanced by the uptake of two protons, causing localised alkalinisation. Metals are precipitated as hydroxides directly or as carbonates via the shift in the bicarbonate/carbonate equilibrium towards CO_3^{2-} at high pH; (b) in the sulphate-reducing bacteria, e.g. *Desulfovibrio desulfuricans* the use of sulphate as a terminal electron acceptor anaerobically *in lieu* of O_2 generates H_2S, which precipitates metals as insoluble sulphides; (c) in *Citrobacter* a cell-surface phosphatase cleaves added substrate (glycerol 2-phosphate) to form metal phosphate at the cell surface. Phosphatase was visualised using immunogold labelling to show enzyme at the surface of the cell body and also within the indistinct fuzz of the extracellular polymeric substance. Accumulated metal (in this case uranium) was visible as heavy deposits on the cells; and (d) in *Acinetobacter* the need for organic substrate is overcome by harnessing the polyphosphate cycle of this aerobic organism. Phosphate (Pi) taken up aerobically is stored as poly P, using metabolic energy from utilisation of exogenous carbon sources and breakdown of polyhydroxybutyrate (PHB) reserves. Anaerobically without cell growth poly P is hydrolysed *via* polyphosphatase to give energy, which can drive the synthesis of PHB from applied substrates; waste Pi is effluxed to form metal phosphates as with *Citrobacter*.

Formation of mixed crystals can also promote removal of other 'difficult' and highly toxic metals, such as plutonium. Pu removal, inefficient in native biomass was promoted if the cells were first allowed to accumulate $LaPO_4$. It is likely that the $LaPO_4$ acts as a nucleation focus for the deposition of $Pu(HPO_4)_2$. It is difficult to prove this using Pu because of the radiotoxicity of the large quantity needed for solid-state examination, but studies using the 'surrogate' element Th suggested the formation of a co-crystals of La and Th phosphates on the cells.

Metal Cations, Anions of High Valence

In contrast to metal cations, anions of high valence metals such as Cr(VI) and Tc(VII) (CrO_4^{2-} and TcO_4^-, respectively) do not form insoluble phosphates and the route to their bioremediation lies in the harnessing of biological reduction to the generation of low valence, insoluble forms of metal oxides and hydroxides. Bioreduction can be achieved in three ways. Normal metabolic activity generates reducing power in the form of electrons, conveyed by electron carriers and finally disposed onto molecular oxygen, reducing this to H_2O. In the absence of O_2, many bacteria can undertake 'anaerobic respiration', whereby electrons are donated to anions such as NP_3^-, SO_4^{2-}, or cationic or anionic metal species. This is called dissimilatory metal reduction and its application to metal remediation is well-described in the case of UO_2^{2+}. For example: U(VI) can be reduced to U(IV) and deposited as uranium oxide (UO_2).

Other examples, such as the use of Fe^{3+} as an electron acceptor, are well described. In these cases microbial growth occurs and biomass is a by-product, which may be undesirable as a secondary waste.

In contrast to the use of a metal as an electron acceptor, micro-organisms can also invoke specific reductive detoxification mechanisms. An example of this is the well-documented mercuric reductase system: which reduces Hg^{2+} to elemental $Hg°$. Trapping of the liberated volatile $Hg°$ is feasible but probably not economic. The reduction of Cr(VI) as the chromate ion (CrO_4^{2-}) is also well-documented. Various organisms are known to reduce Cr(VI) to Cr(III), which is removed from solution as insoluble $Cr(OH)_3$. Large-scale application of the bacterium *Bacterium dechromaticans* Romanenko has been described in a full-scale process to remove Cr(VI), but attempts to confirm the biochemical reactions using the strain were unsuccessful.

The third approach to harnessing bioreductive capabilities is the use of non-growing cells oxidising a simple electron donor. As an example, the radionuclide ^{99}Tc(VII) is problematic in wastes from the nuclear fuel cycle but TcO_4^- can be removed effectively using a reductase activity of *Escherichia coli* that was identified, by physiological studies and molecular analysis of mutants, as the hydrogenase 3 component of the formate hydrogenlyase complex. Tc(VII) can be reduced by growing cells, but metal reduction can be carried out in the absence of biomass growth by the use of formate or molecular hydrogen as electron donors. Immobilised resting cells removed Tc(VII) continuously using H_2 or formate as the electron donor. This activity extended also to the sulphate-reducing bacteria, where the extensive hydrogenase activities, e.g. of *Desulfovibrio desulfuricans*, permitted very efficient removal of Tc with a short flow residence time, and high radiotolerance of the enzyme(s). Solid-state analysis of accumulated Tc-containing precipitates confirmed that the Tc(VII) was reduced but it is not yet established whether the final valence is Tc(V) or Tc(IV). The lack of molecular and genetic information on the SRB makes confirmation of the exact mechanism of the bioreduction difficult (the metal reductase could be a cytochrome receiving electrons from H_2 via hydrogenase activity for example; uranium reductase is, nevertheless, thought to operate via cytochrome c_3 activity.

Functionally the application of growth-decoupled cells can permit application of a growth-decoupled, single step which is stable in extended use. The bioreactors accumulating Tc were run continuously for several days at a flow residence time of 2 hours with maintenance of more than 95 per cent removal of the presented Tc(VII) at an input concentration of 5.0 ppm; the experiments were terminated only because of the accumulating radiohazard.

Sulphate Reducing Bacteria

The sulphate reducing bacteria are a very versatile group of organisms, capable of removal of metal cations (e.g. Cd^{2+}) by production of H_2S, via dissimilatory reduction of SO_4^{2-} (Fig. 16.12b) and are also able to remove metal anions due to their parallel, hydrogenase-associated reductive activity. Current investigations aim to treat wastes containing both classes of metal ions (cations and anions), and also to extend these to integrated processes for the cotreatment of organic ligands which may be present, complexing the metals and reducing their availability to the remediating organisms. Examples of complexed wastes are secondary wastes from remediative soil leaching activities and nuclear decontamination operations, where the application of chelating agent (e.g. EDTA, citrate) removes metals from the solid phase but generates a secondary liquid waste which is concentrated, recalcitrant and problematic. Recent studies have developed new mixed cultures of unusual aerobic organisms, which can biodegrade EDTA to release metals in forms suitable for remediation using the biomineralisation techniques shown in Fig. 16.12.

Organophosphorus compounds such as tributyl phosphate (TBP) are commonly used as metal complexing agents in solvent extraction processes, giving TBP-metal residues. Using selective enrichments mixed cultures of Pseudomonads were developed which could grow at the expense of TBP and couple the phosphate released from TBP hydrolysis to the biomineralisation of UO_2^{2+} and removal of the latter by immobilised cells in a flow-through reactor, removing both agents in a single step.

Throughout, fundamental studies of the biochemical, physiological, and chemical processes, and the development of process models provide essential understanding for optimisation integration, and process intensification, the latter essential for economic and stable operation. These, together with the constraints or, often, absence of suitable physico-chemical treatment processes, will reinforce the future role of biotechnology in waste remediation.

SECTION V

Biodegradation and Biotransformation

Chapter 17

Biotechnology and Bioremediation

INTRODUCTION

Bioremediation can be defined as any process that uses micro-organisms, fungi, green plants or their enzymes to return the natural environment altered by contaminants to its original condition. Bioremediation may be employed to attack specific soil contaminants, such as degradation of chlorinated hydrocarbons by bacteria. An example of a more general approach is the cleanup of oil spills by the addition of nitrate and/or sulphate fertilisers to facilitate the decomposition of crude oil by indigenous or exogenous bacteria.

Naturally occurring bioremediation and phytoremediation have been used for centuries. For example, desalination of agricultural land by phytoextraction has a long tradition.

Bioremediation technologies can be generally classified as *in situ* or *ex situ*. *In situ* bioremediation involves treating the contaminated material at the site while *ex situ* involves the removal of the contaminated material to be treated elsewhere. Some examples of bioremediation technologies are bioventing, landfarming, bioreactor, composting, bioaugmentation, rhizofiltration, and biostimulation.

Not all contaminants, however, are easily treated by bioremediation using micro-organisms. For example, heavy metals such as cadmium and lead are not readily absorbed or captured by organisms. The assimilation of metals such as mercury into the food chain may worsen matters. Phytoremediation is useful in these circumstances, because natural plants or transgenic plants are able to bioaccumulate these toxins in their above-ground parts, which are then harvested for removal. The heavy metals in the harvested biomass may be further concentrated by incineration or even recycled for industrial use.

The elimination of a wide range of pollutants and wastes from the environment requires increasing our understanding of the relative importance of different pathways and regulatory networks to carbon flux in particular environments and for particular compounds and they will certainly accelerate the development of bioremediation technologies and biotransformation processes.

The use of genetic engineering to create organisms specifically designed for bioremediation has great potential. The bacterium *Deinococcus radiodurans* (the most radioresistant organism known) has been modified to consume and digest toluene and ionic mercury from highly radioactive nuclear waste.

Mycoremediation is a form of bioremediation, the process of using fungi to return an environment (usually soil) contaminated by pollutants to a less contaminated state. The term mycoremediation was coined by Paul Stamets and refers specifically to the use of fungal mycelia in bioremediation.

One of the primary roles of fungi in the ecosystem is decomposition, which is performed by the mycelium. The mycelium secretes extracellular enzymes and acids that break down lignin and cellulose, the two main building blocks of plant fiber. These are organic compounds composed of long chains of carbon and hydrogen, structurally similar to many organic pollutants. The key to mycoremediation is determining the right fungal species to target a specific pollutant. Certain strains have been reported to successfully degrade the nerve gases VX and sarin.

In an experiment conducted in conjunction with Thomas, a major contributor in the bioremediation industry, a plot of soil contaminated with diesel oil was inoculated with mycelia of oyster mushrooms; traditional bioremediation techniques (bacteria) were used on control plots. After four weeks, more than 95 per cent of many of the PAH (polycyclic aromatic hydrocarbons) had been reduced to non-toxic components in the mycelial-inoculated plots. It appears that the natural microbial community participates with the fungi to break down contaminants, eventually into carbon dioxide and water. Wood-degrading fungi are particularly effective in breaking down aromatic pollutants (toxic components of petroleum), as well as chlorinated compounds (certain persistent pesticides).

Mycofiltration is a similar or same process, using fungal mycelia to filter toxic waste and microorganisms from water in soil.

There are a number of cost/efficiency advantages to bioremediation, which can be employed in areas that are inaccessible without excavation. For example, hydrocarbon spills (specifically, petrol spills) or certain chlorinated solvents may contaminate groundwater, and introducing the appropriate electron acceptor or electron donor amendment, as appropriate, may significantly reduce contaminant concentrations after a lag time allowing for acclimation. This is typically much less expensive than excavation followed by disposal elsewhere, incineration or other *ex situ* treatment strategies, and reduces or eliminates the need for 'pump and treat', a common practice at sites where hydrocarbons have contaminated clean groundwater.

The process of bioremediation can be monitored indirectly by measuring the oxidation reduction potential or redox in soil and groundwater, together with pH, temperature, oxygen content, electron acceptor/donor concentrations, and concentration of breakdown products (e.g. carbon dioxide).

One of the newest and fastest growing applications of environmental biotechnology is bioremediation. Bioremediation most often addresses treatment of contaminated solids, such as groundwater aquifers, soils, and sediments. This focus on decontaminating solids occurs because flowing waters poorly mobilise most of the common contaminants that reach these environments.

Because the contaminants adsorb to the amply present solid surfaces or form a separate liquid phase, they are 'trapped' in the solid matrix. Clean-up strategies that rely on flushing the contaminants out with water and treating the water (i.e. so-called pump-and-treat strategies) often are unsuccessful, even after years or decades of remediation by flushing.

Bioremediation overcomes the main deficiency of conventional clean-up approaches that rely on water flushing: Dissolution or desorption of the contaminants into water is too slow, since the water's contaminant carrying capacity is very limited. With bioremediation, high densities of active microorganisms locate themselves close to the nonaqueous source of contamination. Within a short distance from its point of dissolution into the aqueous phase, the contaminant molecule is biodegraded. If the biodegradation is fast and occurs close enough to the nonaqueous source, biodegradation replenishes the water's ability to accept more dissolving or desorbing contaminant, bringing about accelerated dissolution/desorption, which decontaminates the solid phase.

Although bacteria are present in all soils, sediments, and aquifers, their naturally occurring numbers may be too small to bring about the rapid reaction needed to have enhanced dissolution/desorption. In that case, the strategy is to add to the contaminated environment the materials needed to allow growth of the bacteria active in degrading the target contaminant. These materials provide the substrates and nutrients required for the growth and maintenance of a high-density microbial population. The most commonly added materials normally are selected from among an electron-acceptor substrate (like oxygen), an electron-donor substrate (like a sugar or natural gas), inorganic nutrients (like nitrogen and phosphorus), and materials to help dissolve/desorb immobile substrates (like surfactants).

Bioremediation can be divided into three main classes: engineered *in situ*, intrinsic *in situ*, and engineered *ex situ*. The distinction between *in situ* and *ex situ* indicates whether contaminated solids remain in place (i.e. *in situ*) during the bioremediation or are excavated and transferred to an aboveground treatment system (i.e. *ex situ*). Engineered bioremediation refers to employing engineering tools to greatly increase the input rates for the stimulating materials. In contrast, intrinsic bioremediation relies on the intrinsically occurring rates of supply of substrates and nutrients, as well as the intrinsic population density of active micro-organisms. The most important factor for any type of bioremediation is ensuring that the rate of biotransformation is fast enough to meet the clean-up objectives.

Because engineered bioremediation involves using engineered measures to add the materials necessary to increase the biotransformation rates significantly, the fast-enough criterion refers to increasing the biotransformation rates well above those that would occur without the engineered additions. In this way, the time required to clean up the contamination is substantially reduced. Engineered bioremediation is a cost-effective approach when one must meet a regulated deadline, minimise exposure risk, or facilitate a property sale.

Intrinsic bioremediation, on the other hand, relies on the intrinsic (or naturally developing) biological activity to prevent the migration of contamination away from its source. While intrinsic bioremediation does not accelerate the rate of clean up, it prevents further spread of the contaminants. The natural supply of necessary materials, when coupled with the presence of appropriate micro-organisms, must be fast enough to allow biodegradation of the contaminants before they can be transported a significant distance away from the source. A monitoring plan is essential to demonstrate that these intrinsic factors remain effective for preventing contaminant migration. It cannot be emphasised too much that intrinsic bioremediation is not a 'do nothing' approach. Intrinsic bioremediation is sometimes called natural attenuation, a term that actually includes many naturally occurring mechanisms that can lead to a decrease in the concentration of a contaminant.

Prior to the design of a system for *in situ* bioremediation, several steps are required to ensure that the programme is successful. These steps are needed to characterise the site in terms of hydrology, extent and type of contamination, intrinsic microbial activity, and intrinsic supply rates of key materials.

Although bioremediation is a new and uniquely challenging application of environmental biotechnology, it is founded on the same principles as are other applications. Because of the high specific surface area of aquifers, soils, and sediments, the microbial ecology is dominated by attached growth.

This chapter focuses on the unique features of bioremediation. They are:

1. The scope and characteristics of contamination.
2. Contaminant availability for biodegradation.
3. Treatability studies.
4. Engineering strategies for bioremediation.
5. Evaluating bioremediation.

SCOPE AND CHARACTERISTICS OF CONTAMINANTS

The Office of Technology Assessment documented that over 200 substances have been detected in groundwater in the United States. The contaminants include organic chemicals, inorganic chemicals, biological organisms, and radionuclides. A summary is presented in Table 17.1.

Table 17.1. Summary of information presented on substances detected in groundwater.

Category of compounds	Examples	Prevalent uses
Aromatic hydrocarbons	Benzene	Dyestuffs
	Ethylbenzene	Solvents
	Toluene	
Oxygenated hydrocarbons	Acetone	Solvents
	1,4-Dioxane	Paints, varnishes
	Phenols	
Hydrocarbons with specific elements	2,4-D	Pesticides
(e.g. with N, P, S, Cl, Br, I, F)	Trichloroethene (TCE)	Solvents
	Trichloroethanes (1,1,1 and 1,1,2 TCA)	Munitions
Other hydrocarbons	Kerosene	Fuels
	Gasoline	
	Lignin and tannin	
Metals and cations	Iron	Alloys
	Chromium	Electrical and electronics
	Arsenic	
Non-metals and anions	Chloride	Fertilisers
	Sulphate	Food additives
Micro-organisms	Bacteria (e.g. coliforms)	–
	Viruses	
Radionuclides	Uranium 238	Tracers
	Tritium	Medical applications
	Radium 226	

Although the components listed in Table 17.1 are widely used by industry, agriculture, commerce, and households, poorly mobile contaminants trapped in the solid matrix may be under-represented when only groundwater samples are taken. The fact that the groundwater is sampled tends to accentuate compounds that are more readily mobile. In addition, detection of substances in groundwater often is biased by sampling procedures, analytical detection limits, and the circumstances that prompted the detection and reporting (e.g. was it a planned activity, such as regulatory compliance, or in response to an apparent impact, such as a public complaint).

Organic Compounds

This section focuses on organic compounds, which are most often amenable to bioremediation and are the most commonly detected contaminants in groundwater. The Council on Environmental Quality compiled a list of the 33 synthetic organic contaminants most frequently found in drinking-water wells (Table 17.2).

Table 17.2. The 33 synthetic organic contaminants reported to be most frequently found in drinking-water wells.

Trichloroethene (TCE)	Isopropyl benzene
Toluene	1,1-Dichloroethene
1,1,1-Trichloroethane	1,2-Dichloroethane
Acetone	*Bis* (2-ethylhexyl) phthalate
Methylene chloride	DBCP (Dibromochloropropane)
Dioxane	Trifluorotrichloroethane
Ethyl benzene	Dibromochloromethane
Tetrachloroethene	Vinyl chloride
Cyclohexane	Chloromethane
Chloroform	Butyl benzyl-phthalate
Di-*n*-butyl-phthalate	γ-BHC (Lindane)
Carbon tetrachloride	1,1,2-Trichloroethane
Benzene	Bromoform
1,2-Dichloroethene	1,1-Dichloroethane
Ethylene dibromide (EDB)	α-BHC
Xylene	Parathion
	δ-BHC

Organic chemicals are associated with a variety of sources, including: subsurface percolation; injection wells; land application of waste-water, waste-water by-products, and hazardous waste; landfills; open dumps; residential disposal; surface impoundments; underground and aboveground storage tanks; pipelines; materials transport and transfer operations; pesticide and fertiliser applications; urban run-off; and oil and gas production wells.

Many of the above compounds are hydrophobic, which is indicated by a relatively large octanol/water partition coefficient (i.e. log $K_{ow} > 1$) and limited water solubility (i.e. < 10,000 mg/l). Some of the compounds are highly volatile (i.e. Henry's constant $>10^{-3}$ atm-m^3/mol), which allows them to partition to a gas phase when it is present.

Chief among them is the polycyclic aromatic hydrocarbons (PAHs) derived from petroleum and the polychlorinated biphenyls (PCBs). While their hydrophobicity greatly reduces their concentrations in the water, it also accentuates their longevity as trapped sources of contamination in the soil or sediment, as well as their ability to bioconcentrate in living organisms.

Mixtures of Organic Compounds

In many situations, organic contaminants are found in mixtures. In many instances, the original contamination was a mixture of related components that co-exist normally in a commercial product. Key examples include the PCBs, various petroleum distillation fractions used for a range of fuel and lubricating purposes, and PAHs found in tars, asphalts, and petroleum sludges. One of the most widely used PCB mixtures—Arochlor 1242—has 42 per cent chlorine overall, but contains biphenyl congeners having 1 through 6 Cl substituents, with 80 per cent having 3, 4, or 5 Cl substituents. The more lightly chlorinated congeners have higher water solubilities than do the more heavily chlorinated congeners, which means the 'aged' PCB tends to gradually become enriched in more chlorinated components.

Table 17.3 lists the typical distillation fractions obtained from petroleum. Although the distillation fractions are much more homogenous than is crude petroleum, each fraction contains molecules having a substantial range of formula weights and the correlated large ranges of water solubilities and hydrophobicities.

Because of its widespread uses and improper disposal, gasoline is an excellent case to illustrate the complexity of these naturally occurring mixtures. Its chemical complexity depends on three variables: (i) the source of the crude oil from which the gasoline is refined, (ii) how the gasoline is refined, and (iii) the additives used.

The total number of distinct hydrocarbons in a gasoline fraction might be of the order of 500; however, due to the predominance of certain hydrocarbons, a smaller number of components accounts for a relatively large portion of the gasoline fraction.

Table 17.3. Typical fractions obtained by distillation of petroleum.

Boiling range of fraction	Number of carbon atoms per molecule	Use
Below 20°C	C_1–C_4	Natural gas, bottled gas, petrochemicals
20°–60°C	C_5–C_6	Petroleum ether, solvents
60°–100°C	C_6–C_7	Ligroin, solvents
40°–200°C	C_5–C_{10}	Gasoline (straight-run gasoline)
175°–325°C	C_{12}–C_{18}	Kerosene and jet fuel
250°–400°C	C_{12} and higher	Gas oil, fuel oil, and diesel oil
Non-volatile liquids	C_{20} and higher	Refined mineral oil, lubricating oil, grease
Non-volatile solids	C_{20} and higher	Paraffin wax, asphalt, and tar

Table 17.4 presents the composition of several typical straight-run gasolines (i.e. the gasoline fraction obtained by direct distillation of the crude petroleum) by class of hydrocarbon. Either alkanes or cycloalkanes dominate all of these straight-run gasolines, with those dominated by alkanes being more abundant; the aromatic hydrocarbons average below 20 per cent by volume. In general, alkenes or unsaturated hydrocarbons are absent in straight-run gasolines. Despite these general trends, Table 17.4 shows that the source of the crude oil affects the chemical composition of the gasoline mixture.

Table 17.4. Chemical composition of straight-run gasolines.

Origin and boiling range, °C	Alkanes	% by volume cycloalkanes	Aromatics
Pennsylvania, 40–200	70	22	8
Oklahoma City, 40–180	62	29	9
Ponca (Oklahoma), 55–180	50	40	10
East Texas, 45–200	50	41	9
West Texas, 80–180	47	33	20
Conroe (Texas), 50–200	35	39	26
Hastings (Texas), 50–200	27	67	6
Michigan, 45-200	74	18	8
Rodessa (Louisiana), 45–160	72	20	8
Santa Fe Springs (California), 45–150	41	50	9

(Contd ...)

Origin & boiling range, °C	Alkanes	% by volume cycloalkanes	Aromatics
Kettleman (California), 45–150	48	45	7
Huntington Beach (California), 50–210	35	54	11
Turner Valley (Canada), 45–200	51	35	14
Altamira (Mexico), 40–200	49	36	14
Portero (Mexico), 50–200	57	35	8
Bucsani (Romania), 50–150	56	32	12
Baku-Surachany, 60–200	27	64	9
Baku-Bibieibat, 60–200	29	63	8
Grozny, New Field, 45–200	64	29	7
Iran, 45–200	70	21	9
Kuwait, 40–200	72	20	8

The type of refining also plays a very important role in defining the gasoline mixture. Figure 17.1 shows that, in comparison with straight-run gasoline, thermal cracked gasoline contains alkenes, increased aromatics, and decreased alkanes and cycloalkanes; catalytically cracked gasoline has alkenes, increased aromatics, and greatly decreased n-alkanes and cycloalkanes. Further, unleaded gasolines generally have a higher aromatic hydrocarbon fraction than do leaded gasolines.

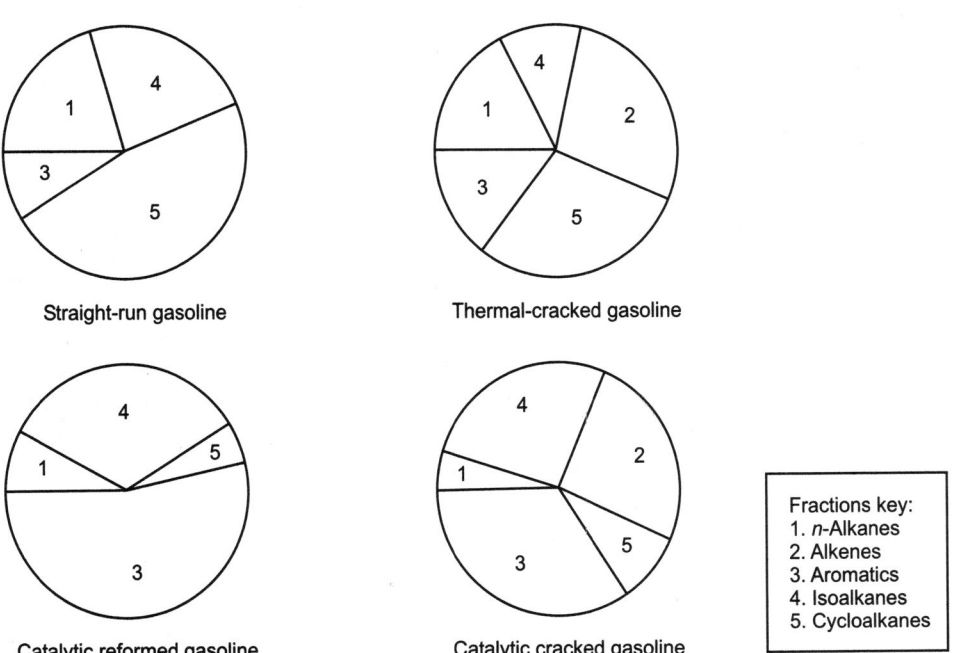

Straight-run gasoline   Thermal-cracked gasoline

Catalytic reformed gasoline   Catalytic cracked gasoline

Fractions key:
1. n-Alkanes
2. Alkenes
3. Aromatics
4. Isoalkanes
5. Cycloalkanes

Fig. 17.1. Hydrocarbon composition of gasoline components.

The most troublesome of the gasoline hydrocarbons are the single-ring aromatics: benzene, toluene, ethylbenzene, and the xylenes (BTEX). Unleaded gasoline typically contains 2–5 per cent (by volume) of benzene, 6–7 per cent of toluene, 5 per cent of ethylbenzene, and 6–7 per cent of xylenes. Compared to almost all other gasoline hydrocarbons, BTEX have by far the highest water solubility. Although the total for BTEX is roughly 20 per cent by volume, the water solubility of BTEX causes them to be the prime water pollutants.

The composition of gasoline is further complicated by additives, which are added for several purposes: (i) antiknock compounds, (ii) antioxidants, (ii) metal deactivators, (iv) antirust agents, (v) antistall agents, (vi) antipreignition agents, (vii) upper-cylinder lubricants, (viii) alcohols (e.g. ethanol), and (ix) oxygenates (e.g. MTBE). Table 17.5 summarises typical additives. With the exception of alcohols used for gasohol, antistall, or antiknock purposes and methyl-*tert*-butyl ether (MTBE) used for antiknock and oxygenate purposes, the additives are present in very low percentages and seldom affect groundwater. On the other hand, the alcohols and MTBE can be major groundwater contaminants, along with BTEX. In fact, the massive introduction of MTBE in gasoline as an oxygenate to reduce smog in California has greatly worsened the problems of groundwater contamination in that state. MTBE is being removed from gasoline in the United States in order to prevent more groundwater contamination.

Table 17.5. Additives typical in gasolines.

Additive type	Typical chemicals used	% by volume
Antiknock agents	Tetraethyl lead, tetramethyl lead	0.08
	tert-butanol, methyl *tat*-butyl ether	<3.5, <15%
Antioxidants	Aminophenols, *ortho*-alkylated phenols	< 0.06
Metal deactivators	N, N'-disalicylidene-1,2-diaminopropane	0.0004
Antirust agents	Fatty acid amines, amine phosphates	0.0005
Antistall agents	Alcohols, glycols	1–2
Antipreignition agents	Alkyl phosphates	0.02
Upper-cylinder lubricants	Light mineral oils, cyclo-paraffinic distillates	0.2–0.5
Alcohols	Ethanol	<40
Oxygenates	MTBE (methyl-*tert*-butyl ether)	<5

Mixtures Created by Codisposal

In many instances, subsurface contamination is a mixture of disparate materials whose main (or only) connection is that they were codisposed of at a single site. These codisposal mixtures can include a wide range of organic compounds that do not necessarily occur together naturally, as well as inorganic chemicals.

A common situation of codisposal is the mixture of organic and inorganic materials in sanitary landfills and in their leachates. Table 17.6 presents a list of various inorganic constituents in leachate from sanitary landfills and representative ranges of concentrations. Large numbers of inorganic contaminants can be found in leachate, some at high concentrations; many organic contaminants also can be found in leachate and cause the relatively high total dissolved organic carbon and COD values. The high concentration of inorganic ions can affect electron-acceptor availability (e.g. SO_4^{2-} and NO_3^-), precipitation potential (e.g. PO_4^{3-}, CO_3^{2-} in alkalinity), and toxicity (e.g. heavy metals, sulphides). A large fraction of the COD often is volatile acids, which tend to lower the pH, but also are good primary substrates. Biodegradation of the volatile acids removes their acidity and allows the pH to increase.

Table 17.6. Representative ranges for various inorganic constituents in leachate from sanitary landfills.

Parameter	Representative range (mg/l)
K^+	200–1000
Na^+	200–1200
Ca^{2+}	100–3000
Mg^{2+}	100–1500
Cl^-	300–3000
SO_4^{2-}	10–1000
Alkalinity	500–10,000
Fe (total)	1–1000
Mn	0.01–100
Cu	<10
Ni	0.01–1
Zn	1–100
Pb	<5
Hg	<0.2
NO_3^-	0.1–10
NH_4^+	10–1000
P as PO_4	1–100
Organic nitrogen	10–1000
Total dissolved organic carbon	10–1000
COD (chemical oxygen demand)	1000–90,000
Total dissolved solids	5000–40,000
pH	4–8

Robertson, Toussaint, and Jorque investigated the organic compounds leached into the groundwater from a landfill near Norman, Oklahoma. Refuse had been deposited below or near the water table of a sandy aquifer. They found low levels of more than 40 organic compounds in the groundwater and concluded that the source of many of these compounds was the leaching of manufactured products discarded within the landfill. In addition to constituents derived from solid wastes, many landfill leachates also contain toxic constituents emanating from liquid industrial wastes located within the landfill.

Many industrial, commercial, and military operations led to exotic mixtures of organic and inorganic contaminants. Table 17.7 shows a wide range of solvents, fuel components, and metals that resulted from wastes containing solvents, paint, fuel oil, and electroplating residues that were disposed of by landfilling and burning in pits near California, USA.

Table 17.7. Volatile and non-volatile organic compounds and trace metals found in groundwater at McClellan Air Force Base, Sacramenta, CA.

Compound	Concentration (mg/l)
1,1-Dichloroethene	60
Acetone	35
Methyl ethyl ketone	25

(Contd ...)

Compound	Concentration (mg/l)
1,1,1-Trichloroethane	12
Trichloroethene	11
Methylene chloride	5
Methyl isobutyl ketone	3.7
Vinyl chloride	2.5
Dichlorobenzene	0.17
Benzene	0.68
1,1-Dichloroethane	0.25
Toluene	0.08
Phenols	0.5
Tetrachloroethane	0.07
Trans-1,2-dichloroethene	0.2
Chromium	0.12
Nickel	0.10
Zinc	0.073
Lead	0.093
Selenium	0.049
Cadmium	0.012

Major chemical-manufacturing facilities often have disposal areas contaminated over many years with waste solvents, sludges, unacceptable products, and other residues. The whole range of common contaminants often is present. In addition, very low solubility sludges and 'bottoms' create a poorly characterised 'goop' or 'gumbo'.

The Department of Energy (DOE) has responsibility for managing the sites where nuclear weapons were produced. DOE sites are unique in that the contamination of the subsurface often involves complex mixtures of organic and inorganic chemicals, including short- and long-lived radionuclides. Important individual contaminants found at DOE sites are listed in Table 17.8. These inorganic and organic species have been found in a variety of combinations. An extremely important interaction is complexation between the heavy-metal radionuclides and the strong chelating agents, such as EDTA and NTA. The degree of complexation with the chelators controls the mobility of the radionuclides, while the biodegradation of the chelators is affected by their complexation to the heavy metals.

Table 17.8. DOE site contaminants.

Inorganic species	Organic species
Radionuclides	Organic contaminants
Plutonium 238,239	Chlorinated hydrocarbons
Americium-241	Methyl ethyl ketone
Thorium	Cyclohexanone
Uranium-232,234,238	Tetraphenyl boron
Technetium-99	Polychlorinated biphenyls (PCBs)
Strontium-90	Select polycyclic aromatic hydrocarbons (PAHs)

(Contd ...)

Inorganic species	Organic species
Cesium-134, 137	Tributyl phosphate
Cobalt-60	Toluene
Europium-152, 154, 155	Benzene
Nickel-63	Kerosene
Iodine-129	
Neptunium-237	
Radium	
Metals	Facilitators[a]
Lead	Aliphatic organic acids
Nickel	(citric, lactic, succinic, oxalic to octadecanoic)
Chromium	Chelating agents (EDTA, NTA, DTPA, HEDTA,
Copper	TTA, di-2-ethyl HPA)
Mercury	Aromatic acids (humic acids and subunits)
Silver	Solvent, diluent, and chelate radiolysis fragments
Bismuth	
Palladium	
Aluminium	
Others	
Carbon-nitrogen compounds	
Nitrite	
Nitrate	

[a] Facilitators are organic compounds that interact with and modify metal/radionuclide geochemical behaviour.

BIODEGRADABILITY

Fortunately, essentially all of the common organic contaminants found in groundwater are biodegradable, provided the proper conditions exist.

A brief summation of items most relevant to bioremediation is:

1. The aliphatic and aromatic hydrocarbons are readily biodegradable by a range of aerobic bacteria and fungi. The key is that molecular O_2 is needed to activate the molecules via initial oxygenation reactions.
2. Evidence of anaerobic biodegradation of aromatic hydrocarbons is growing. Anaerobic biodegradation rates are slower than aerobic rates, but they can be important when fast kinetics are not essential.
3. Most halogenated aliphatics can be reductively dehalogenated, although the rate appears to slow as the halogen substituents are removed.
4. Highly chlorinated aromatics, including PCBs, can be reductively dehalogenated to less halogenated species.
5. Lightly halogenated aromatics can be aerobically biodegraded via initial oxygenation reactions.
6. Many of the common organic contaminants show inhibitory effects on micro-organism growth and metabolism. Due to their strongly hydrophobic nature, many of the inhibitory responses are caused by interactions with the cell membrane. In some cases, intermediate products of metabolism can be more toxic than the original contaminant.

CONTAMINANT AVAILABILITY FOR BIODEGRADATION

A factor that frequently limits the rate of bioremediation is substrate unavailability, or when only a small fraction of all the substrate molecules is truly water soluble and, therefore, available to the micro-organisms. Two phenomena that limit substrate availability are strong sorption to surfaces and formation of a non-aqueous phase. Both factors keep aqueous-phase concentrations low. Low concentration slows degradation kinetics in general and may also prevent biomass accumulation by being lower than S_{min} or by preventing enzyme derepression or induction. However, low aqueous-phase concentrations sometimes are beneficial for biodegradation, particularly when the compound is inhibitory.

Sorption to Surfaces

The effect of sorption on biodegradation in the subsurface can be complex. In some cases, sorption of substrates stimulates biodegradation, but in many cases it retards biodegradation. In order to come to some understanding of the interactions between biodegradation and sorption, it is helpful to review sorption and how solid surfaces affect microbial physiology.

Controls of sorption

For most of the organic molecules of importance to bioremediation, their sorption to solid surfaces is controlled primarily by their hydrophobic nature. Being non-polar and of low solubility, they are thermodynamically driven out of aqueous solution by entropy effects. In other words, having these non-polar solutes dissolved in water requires a restructuring of the water molecules to a higher free-energy state. Ejecting the non-polar solutes from water solution reduces the free energy of the system. This effect is magnified when the surface to which the non-polar molecule adsorbs is itself hydrophobic.

Influences of solid surfaces on microbial physiology

Studies of the naturally occurring microbes in aquifers show that the numbers of micro-organisms attached to aquifer solids usually are 10 to 1000 times greater than those free-living in the groundwater. The ratio may be higher in soils and sediments. Although bacterial attachment to surfaces undoubtedly can affect the activity of the bacteria, what the effect will be cannot be predicted readily. Van Loosdrecht, Lyklema, Norde, and Zehnder summarised the apparently contradictory influences of solid surfaces on microbial behaviour: increased growth rate, decreased growth rate, increased assimilation and decreased respiration rates, decreased assimilation, increased respiration, increased adhesion of active cells, higher activity of attached cells, decreased substrate utilisation, lower substrate affinity, change in pH optimum, difference in fermentation pattern, increased productivity, decreased mortality, and no effect.

Some confusion can be attributed to a failure to distinguish between direct and indirect influences of solid surfaces. A direct influence results from the presence of a surface itself. An indirect influence occurs because the aggregation of micro-organisms alters their environment, such as concentrations of substrate or pH. One reason for confusion comes about because bacteria attaching to living surfaces, such as with plants and animals, often attach at and respond to specific receptors. Whereas these highly specific attachments trigger profound alterations to the physiology of the attaching microbe, as well as its host, the nonliving surfaces of soil and sediments cannot evoke the same kind of reaction. Thus, any effects on microbial physiology in environmental settings are normally the result of indirect effects via changes to the cells' local environment. These changes in local environment can include concentration gradients for substrate and pH. They also can include signalling molecules that transfer between different micro-organisms.

Biodegradation of sorbed molecules

Sorption can cause either decreased or increased biodegradation, and the observed effects depend on the characteristics of the compound, the solid phase, and the micro-organisms. One obvious way in which sorption can slow biodegradation rates is simply by decreasing the aqueous-phase concentration. Since most bacteria utilise only dissolved solutes, adsorption becomes a competing sink. In such cases, compounds having large R values see a dramatic decrease in the biodegradation rate per unit of contaminant present, since most of the solute is adsorbed to the surface and inaccessible for direct biodegradation. If equilibrium partitioning holds, only $1/R$ of the total compound present is available for biodegradation.

When sorption is important, the rate of biodegradation can, in some cases, be controlled by the rate of desorption. Irreversible sorption is an extreme case of mass-transport limitation. Adsorption of solutes inside the crystalline lattice of clay minerals can lead to irreversible adsorption if the lattice structure collapses after adsorption takes place.

Blocking of intra-aggregate pores by strongly adsorbed molecules also can lead to irreversible sorption. Polymerisation of adsorbed organic molecules, particularly phenolics, also has been implicated as a means for making adsorption essentially irreversible.

Bioremediation can be enhanced by adsorption when the compound is toxic. Sequestering the inhibitor and creating a nontoxic aqueous-phase concentration can lead to microbial growth and substrate metabolism. This beneficial sequestering is most effective when the solid has a strong intraparticle adsorption capacity. Sorption also can be beneficial when the sorbed substrate is stored and later released for biodegradation. This 'warehousing' approach allows the micro-organisms to accumulate to a high density and then modulate desorption by creating a low value of C (C is the aqueous phase concentration of solute).

Although sorption can have various positive and negative influences on biodegradation, its relevance is accentuated for soils with high organic carbon or clay content and aggregates having internal porosity. However, *in situ* bioremediation generally requires fluid-permeable deposits that encompass materials ranging from silty sands to gravel. These materials may have little organic carbon content, cation exchange capacity, or internal pores.

FORMATION OF A NONAQUEOUS PHASE

A second way in which compounds show limited availability as substrates is formation into nonaqueous phase liquids (NAPLs)—fluids that are essentially immiscible with water and migrate through the subsurface as a separate phase. This category of fluids includes petroleum, its refined fluid derivatives, and aliphatic chlorinated hydrocarbons. These fluids become trapped as residual saturation and lenses in the unsaturated and saturated zone. In the case of NAPLs less dense than water (LNAPLs, e.g. petroleum products), the pools can form at the top of the water table. Pools or residuals migrate to the aquifer bottom in the case of NAPLs more dense than water (DNAPLs, e.g. aliphatic chlorinated hydrocarbons).

This trapped NAPL serves as a long-term source of groundwater contamination via dissolution. The focus here is on petroleum-product NAPLs, although most of the subjects reviewed apply equally to other NAPLs or NAPL mixtures.

Solubility

Although NAPLs are defined as immiscible in water, they are, in general, slightly soluble in water. Table 17.9 lists selected gasoline hydrocarbons and their pure-compound water solubilities. The lowest solubilities (<1 mg/l) are associated with the normal and branched alkanes. However, aromatics have solubilities greater than 100 mg/l.

Because a gasoline NAPL is a mixture, the actual equilibrium solubilities are substantially reduced from the pure-compound solubilities shown in Table 17.9. In most cases, the water solubility for mixtures of hydrocarbons follows ideal-solution theory, which says that the equilibrium solute concentration, C_i, of the ith component in an NAPL mixture is proportional to the product of its pure-compound solubility, S_i, and its mole fraction in the mixture,

$$C_i = X_i S_i \qquad \qquad ... (17.1)$$

in which X_i is the component's mole fraction in the NAPL.

Table 17.9. Solubility of selected pure hydrocarbons in water at room temperature.

Hydrocarbon	mg/l in distilled water
n-Alkanes	
n-Propane	62
n-Pentane	39
n-Hexane	9.5
n-Octane	0.7
Branched alkanes	
2-Methylbutane	48
2,3-Dimethylhexane	0.13
Cycloalkanes	
Cyclopentane	156
Cyclohexane	55
Methylcyclopentane	42
Methylcyclohexane	14
Aromatics	
Benzene	1780
Ethylbenzene	152
Toluene	515
o-Xylene	175
p-Xylene	198

Aromatic components in gasoline, such as BTEX, have the highest S_i values, and they also are present at relatively large mole fractions. Therefore, they dissolve most rapidly into the water. Although this causes BTEX to be the most prevalent water pollutant, it also makes BTEX the most accessible for biodegradation. When combined with the fact that BTEX compounds are readily biodegradable under aerobic conditions, this relative propensity to become water-soluble has made bioremediation of BTEX by far the most widely practiced type of bioremediation.

Because the C_i values for the non-BTEX hydrocarbons in NAPLs are very low, sequential dissolution and biodegradation of the truly dissolved component is a slow means for the hydrocarbon-degrading micro-organisms to make their substrate accessible. To maximise their rate of access to hydrocarbon substrates, some bacteria and fungi able to degrade long-chain aliphatics adhere to the hydrocarbon-NAPL interface and participate in a form of 'direct uptake' of the substrates that they can metabolise. Adherent bacteria are predominant when the amount of surface area is small, a common situation when mechanical agitation cannot be provided to emulsify the NAPL. The exact mechanism by which adhesion promotes substrate accessibility is not clear. By being very close to the NAPL/water interface, adhering micro-organisms minimise the diffusion distance from the NAPL to the cell, thereby reducing the mass-transport resistance. Some believe that the hydrocarbon substrate is transferred directly into the cell without dissolving into the liquid.

When direct contact is important for increasing hydrocarbon biodegradation rates, the amount of NAPL/water surface area is critical. Emulsification or pseudo-solubilisation is a way in which the surface area can be increased. Agitation, use of synthetic surfactants, production of microbial metabolites having surface-active properties (biosurfactants), or a combination can bring them about. *Ex situ* technologies are most effective for this surface-enhancing approach. The lack of agitation and difficulties contacting the NAPL with the surfactant make *in situ* application of surface enhancement problematical.

For *in situ* bioremediation, surfactants can be used to mobilise residual NAPL. The hydrocarbons in the NAPL are extracted into surfactant micelles (i.e. colloids of nonaqueous-phase surfactant) formed when the surfactant's critical micelle concentration (CMC) is exceeded. Mobilisation of hydrocarbons by micelles may increase or decrease biodegradation. Most field experiences indicate that the application of micellular surfactants has a negative effect on biodegradation. Reduced biodegradation can be attributed to toxicity from the surfactant or to a further reduction in the dissolved concentration.

The use of surfactants to enhance biodegradation has been confused by the unfortunate use of the term 'solubilise' to refer to the partitioning of hydrocarbons into colloidal micelles of surfactant The hydrocarbon molecules are mobilised with the micelles, which often move with the water phase. However, these components are not truly soluble, because they exist inside the surfactant phase. In fact, truly soluble components often have reduced concentrations due to their partitioning into the micelles. The term 'solubilisation' is false when biodegradation of soluble components is considered. The correct term is mobilisation, and the components are mobilised in a colloidal, nonaqueous phase.

Mobilisation in micelles increases biodegradation rates when the micellular hydrocarbon is more available to the micro-organism than it would be if it remained in its original NAPL. Use of surfactants in *ex situ* bioremediation can greatly accelerate biodegradation when the nonaqueous-phase surface area is greatly increased. Most probably, the surface area is increased due to the combination of a decrease in surface tension and energy inputs, not from transfer of the hydrocarbons to surfactant micelles.

Surfactants, either biological or synthetic, could be used to mobilise hydrocarbons for the purpose of withdrawing them from the aquifer for treatment above ground. A danger concomitant with surfactant application to enhance contaminant removal in the subsurface is that the spreading of contaminants to previously uncontaminated parts of the aquifer could exacerbate the contamination problems.

TREATABILITY STUDIES

Before an *in situ* bioremediation project is attempted in the field, treatability studies may need to be performed. The overall goal of treatability studies is to verify that the *in situ* approach has a high likelihood of succeeding. The number and type of treatability studies depend upon the characteristics of the site and the contaminants. In general, the level of effort that needs to be expended on treatability studies is proportional to the uncertainty about site and contaminant characteristics. When uncertainty is low, little effort may ensure success, but extensive efforts are needed when uncertainty is high.

Table 17.10 presents a hierarchical scheme for determining what kind of treatability study is needed. Each level is used to answer different kinds of questions. A treatability study should be carried out for each level for which answers are not known from other sources. Level 1 is used to answer the fundamental question, 'Is biodegradation a feasible option with the contaminants at the site?' Level 1 tests are not needed when the biodegradabilities of the contaminants are established from the literature or from previous bioremediation experience. Level 1 is needed most often when the contaminants are unusual, are not identified (e.g. they are only peaks on a chromatogram), or occur in mixtures that may be inhibitory (e.g. with toxic organic compounds, heavy metals, or high salts) or incompatible (e.g. some contaminants are known only to be degraded aerobically, while others are degraded only anaerobically).

Table 17.10. Hierarchical approach to determining what kind of treatability studies are needed to ensure success with *in situ* bioremediation.

Level	Goals	Approach
1	Determine if biodegradation is an option	Simple laboratory microcosms, yes or no answer on biodegradability
2	Evaluate biodegradation nonidealities, such as concentration dependence of kinetics, inhibition, sorption, dissolution, mixed substrates, intermediates formation, and the need for other substrates or nutrients	Laboratory microcosms of all types, including hypovials, shake flasks, serum vials, columns, and slurries
3	Evaluate site-specific issues, such as hydrogeologic conditions and heterogeneity	Field pilot study

The techniques for Level 1 studies ought to be as simple as possible. The tube microcosms of Wilson and Noonan, serum bottles, and hypovials usually are satisfactory. The keys are to avoid complications with volatilisation and adsorption and to ensure that the reaction conditions in the microcosms are optimal for the reactions being evaluated. Usually, the disappearance of the target components, in comparison with abiotic controls, is sufficient to give the desired 'yes' or 'no' answer on the feasibility of biodegradation.

Once feasibility is established, Level 2 studies are needed to provide estimates of the rate of reaction and to identify complicating factors. Depending on the situation, Level 2 studies can address a wide range of questions. Some appropriate questions are:

1. What is the functional relationship between the concentration of contaminant and its biodegradation rate?
2. How do concentrations of other substrates, such as the primary electron donor and acceptor, affect the reaction rate?
3. What is the stoichiometry needed for addition of substrates and nutrients? In particular, the stoichiometric needs should be established with knowledge of how the added material is going to be used; for example, as a growth-supporting substrate or nutrient, as a cosubstrate, or as an electron source or sink.
4. Will environmental factors, such as low temperature, affect the rates?
5. Do intermediates form, especially hazardous ones?
6. Do the contaminants need to desorb or dissolve before they can be degraded? Can these rates be increased by addition of surface-active agents?
7. Do toxicants, including intermediates and other substrates, interfere with biodegradation?

Level 2 experiments can be performed in many types of systems, including all those used for Level 1, columns, soil beds, and slurry reactors. The design of the system should depend on the specific question being asked and on sampling requirements. Even when the experimental system is the same as for Level 1, the intensity for sampling and analysis must be much greater for Level 2. Whenever possible, Level 2 studies should be performed with actual soil, aquifer, and/or groundwater samples.

Level 2 studies should yield reasonable estimates of the rate of reaction *in situ*; limitations from inhibition, solubility, or intermediates; and needs for substrates and nutrients. This information, when combined with knowledge of the site's hydrogeology and contamination, should allow design of a field programme based on sound science and engineering.

Level 3, field pilot testing, is used to answer the question, 'Can the *in situ* bioremediation succeed under the site-specific conditions actually existing?' Real-world factors of heterogeneity and poor permeability can prevent success in the field, even though microbiological factors are positive.

Level 3 testing may not need to be performed when site characterisation shows that the site is hydrogeologically simple and highly permeable.

A Level-3 test normally is performed on a small portion of the contaminated site. The pilot location should be representative of the overall site in terms of hydrogeology and contamination. *In situ* conditions for the pilot test should simulate the proposed bioremediation scheme. The pilot site must be large enough that realistic complications are encountered. Simulation modelling of the transport and microbiological aspects of the bioremediation is recommended as part of the design and evaluation of the pilot study.

ENGINEERING STRATEGIES FOR BIOREMEDIATION

Site Characterisation

The first step in any bioremediation is site characterisation in terms of its geology, hydrology, geochemistry, type and distribution of contamination, and microbiology. Site assessments performed to meet regulatory requirements typically do not provide nearly enough or the right kind of information for evaluating the potential for bioremediation. Therefore, site characterisation needs to be tailored for bioremediation. Critical information includes:

1. The nature of the geological deposits, including the presence of fractures, thickness and extent of aquifers, location of confining units, and particle-size distribution
2. The porosity (ε), hydraulic conductivity (K_{hyd}), and the variability of these parameters for the water-transmitting units.
3. The direction and slope of the naturally occurring hydraulic gradient.
4. As much information as is possible to obtain on the location, type, and mass of the contamination source; and the extent and concentration distribution of a contaminant plume.
5. Intrinsic supply and consumption rates of electron acceptors, nutrients, alkalinity, and other geochemical species affecting biodegradation.
6. Information on microbiological activity at least at Level 1 under Treatability Studies.

ENGINEERED *IN SITU* BIOREMEDIATION

Because engineered *in situ* bioremediation is used to accelerate biologically driven removal of contaminants trapped in the solid phase, its success depends upon being able to achieve substantially increased inputs of stimulating materials.

Thus, the ideal site has these features:

1. The hydraulic conductivity is relatively homogeneous, isotropic, and large (i.e. greater than about 10^{-5} m/s).
2. Residual concentrations are not excessive; NAPL concentrations greater than about 10 g/kg reduce aquifer permeability and micro-organism access to the biodegradable contaminants.
3. The contamination is relatively shallow, in order to minimise costs of drilling and sampling.

The permeability, which controls the hydraulic conductivity, probably is the most important factor. Most successful projects have been in sandy environments having K_{hyd} values of 10^{-5} to 10^{-3} m/s. Heterogeneity is the most prevalent deviation from the ideal situation. Even when a formation has a suitably large K_{hyd}, that K_{hyd} often is an 'effective', or spatially averaged value. Heterogeneity in K_{hyd} can have a significant impact on engineered bioremediation. Contaminants trapped in regions of relatively low K_{hyd} tend to be by-passed by the fluid flows bringing stimulatory materials. Engineered *in situ* bioremediation systems can be classified according to the means by which stimulatory materials are added. Although technical details depend strongly on site-specific conditions and are advancing rapidly, these broad classifications are valuable for identifying what approaches have merit. The following methods are being applied successfully for *in situ* bioremediation (mainly) of petroleum hydrocarbons.

Bioventing

When the contaminants are trapped in the unsaturated zone (also called the vadose zone) above the water table, the easiest way to supply O_2 is by pulling air through the unsaturated soil. This technique, called bioventing, is illustrated in Fig. 17.2. Vacuum pumps create negative pressure that sweeps air through the soil and past the contaminated soil. The spacing of the vacuum points depends on the soil's permeability and the applied vacuum. Enough vacuum points are needed to ensure that O_2 is delivered to all contaminated units.

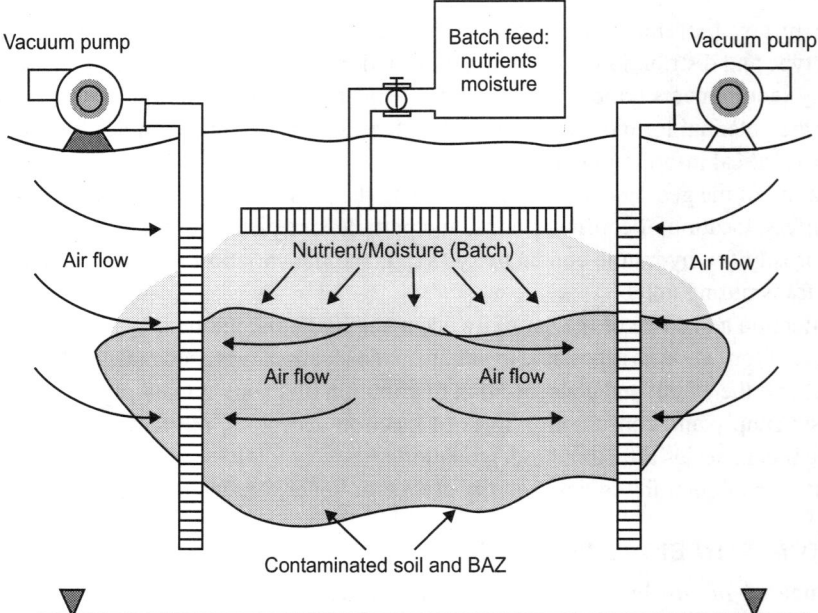

Fig. 17.2. Bioventing is used to bioremediate contaminants trapped above the water table, which is indicated by the two triangles. The BAZ occurs where the water, nutrients, and air flow coincide with the contaminated soil.

Passing air through the unsaturated zone evaporates moisture and can desiccate the soil enough that microbiological activity is slowed or even prevented. Therefore, Fig. 17.2 illustrates how water is added to the biologically active zone (BAZ) by infiltrating water. Infiltration can be accomplished by spraying or flooding the surface for permeable soils or by injection through infiltration trenches, galleries, or dry wells for less permeable soils. The infiltration rate must be carefully controlled to preclude soil 'flooding', which can decrease the soil's air permeability and leach contaminants to the water table.

When inorganic nutrients or other stimulants are required, they generally are added in soluble form (e.g. NH_4Cl, KNO_3, and NaH_2PO_4) in the infiltrating water. In some cases, nutrients can be added as gases, such as NH_3, N_2O, or triethylphosphate. Addition of methane can be employed to stimulate co-metabolic degradation of TCE. In general, gaseous additives are applied through trenches or wells located in line with the airflow routes.

Water-circulation systems

When the contamination is partly or totally within the saturated zone, stimulatory materials can be applied by water circulation. Figure 17.3 illustrates the engineered bioremediation of an LNAPL that is above and below the water table. In this case, H_2O_2 is used as a dissolved source of oxygen substantially greater than can be achieved by air saturation. The figure shows a vertical well and a horizontal infiltration gallery; in most cases, one on the other approach is used to add the circulating water and stimulants.

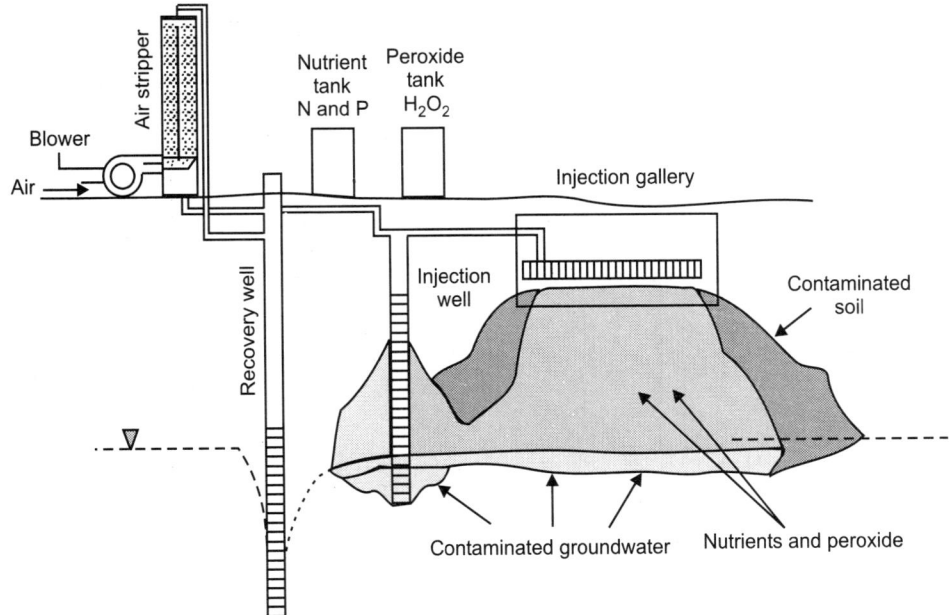

Fig. 17.3. Schematic of a water-circulation system with H_2O_2 as on O_2 source. The BAZ is present where the water, nutrients, and oxygen intersect with contaminants dissolved from the contaminated soil.

A key to using water circulation is to recover all the circulating water. Recovery systems normally involve a series of extraction wells designed to extract more water than is injected. In this way, there is no export of contaminated groundwater from the site. The extracted water commonly is treated and recycled. Above ground treatment can include air stripping (Fig. 17.3), biological treatment, activated carbon absorption, or a combination. If the extracted water is not recycled, drinking water or uncontaminated groundwater is amended and used for injection.

One problem that can occur as part of a water-circulation system is clogging near well screens and infiltration galleries. Localised growth of bacteria, sometimes coupled with chemical precipitation or gas evolution, reduces the soil's hydraulic conductivity. This can lead to decreased input rates and/or short-circuiting around clogged areas. Efforts to minimise the adverse impact of clogging include pulsing of various substrates and nutrients to 'spread out' the BAZ, reduction of substrate loading, back-flushing to dislodge accumulated solids, periodic application of disinfectants (chlorine or additional H_2O_2) or acids, and adjustment of pH and inorganic ions to preclude precipitation.

Air sparging

Originally developed in Europe, air sparging has become a popular means of engineered bioremediation in North America for strictly aerobic biodegradation. Injection of compressed air directly into the contaminated subsurface (Fig. 17.4) is an efficient way to deliver oxygen to the BAZ. In addition, air sparging can strip volatile contaminants from the saturated zone into the unsaturated zone and a vapour-capture system. Air sparging is not effective when low-permeability geological zones trap or divert the gas flow.

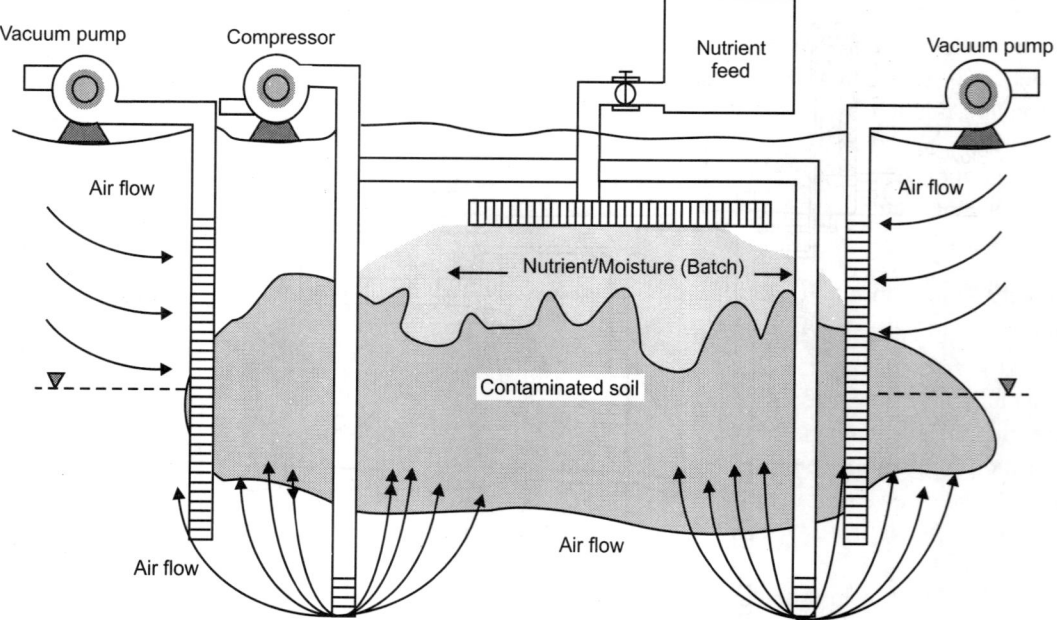

Fig. 17.4. An air-sparging system for aerobic treatment of contamination below the water table. The BAZ occurs where the air flow contacts contaminated water.

Nutrients and other amendments can be added from injection wells or an infiltration gallery, as shown in Fig. 17.4. Similar to bioventing, some nutrients can be added in a gaseous state. In most cases, a gas-recovery system is needed to capture volatile components and prevent off-site contaminant transport in the gas phase.

Intrinsic *In Situ* Bioremediation and Natural Attenuation

Intrinsic bioremediation relies on the intrinsic (i.e. naturally occurring) supplies of electron acceptors, nutrients, and other necessary materials to develop a BAZ and prevent the migration of contaminants away from the source. Although intrinsic bioremediation does notaccelerate the rate of source clean up, it can be an effective form of biological containment. Intrinsic bioremediation involves no engineered measures to increase the supply rates of oxygen, nutrients, or other stimulants. On the other hand, intrinsic bioremediation requires careful site characterisation in terms of the extent and type of contaminant source and plume, the presence of micro-organisms capable of degrading any mobile contaminants, and the intrinsic supply rates of electron acceptor and other required materials. A long-term monitoring programme is essential to ensure that the intrinsic biological activity remains effective at preventing contaminant migration. The principles of evaluating bioremediation are given later in this chapter.

Intrinsic *in situ* bioremediation is best applied in situations in which the groundwater contains naturally high concentrations of electron acceptors and adequate concentrations of nutrients, consistent groundwater levels and flow velocity, and the presence of carbonate materials to buffer pH changes. Intrinsic bioremediation can be used alone or in concert with an engineered bioremediation or other technology. Because intrinsic bioremediation depends on naturally occurring supply rates, heavy source contamination can overwhelm the intrinsic supply rates. In such a case, an engineered technology can be used to reduce the size of the contaminant source until the rate of contaminant dissolution no longer exceeds the intrinsic supply rates.

Intrinsic bioremediation sometimes is confused with natural attenuation, which is defined as the reduction of contaminant concentrations due to naturally occurring processes of biodegradation, sorption, advection, dilution, dispersion, and chemical reaction. Intrinsic bioremediation is a more stringent subset of natural attenuation in which microbial transformation reactions are responsible for the decrease in concentration. The National Research Council issued comprehensive guidance for natural attenuation. In principle, natural attenuation can minimise risks from a wide range of organic and inorganic contaminants. To date, natural attenuation has been proven to work reliably mainly for BTEX.

In Situ Biobarriers

A hybrid bioremediation technology is the *in situ* biobarrier, which is depicted schematically in Fig 17.5. Unlike the previous *in situ* methods, a biobarrier addresses mobile contaminants already being transported in a plume. The biobarrier is a containment method that prevents further transport of a plume. However, the biobarrier is an engineered system in which a BAZ is created in the path of the plume through injection of electron donor, electron acceptor, and/or nutrients. Hydraulic or physical controls on groundwater movement may be required to make certain that the plume passes through the BAZ. It seems reasonable that several different BAZs could be created sequentially by injection of different electron donors and acceptors. The Moffett Field experiment is a small-scale example of creating a specialised BAZ by injecting methane (the carbon source and electron donor) and oxygen (the electron acceptor); cometabolic biodegradation of TCE was demonstrated.

The materials needed to create a biobarrier can be injected in several ways. The most obvious way is to add them in liquid form through injection wells or trenches. An alternative to simple injection is the recirculating well, in which the injected materials and the plume water are mixed in and around wells that circulate the water between well screens placed at two different levels on the well casing. Slow-release chemical sources of O_2 and H_2 can be placed in the flow path of the plume via wells or trenches sunk to the level of the plume. Iron filings also have been used to create an *in situ* barrier. The oxidation of the elemental iron can bring about reductive dechlorination of solvents, but it also may spur microbiologically catalysed reductions.

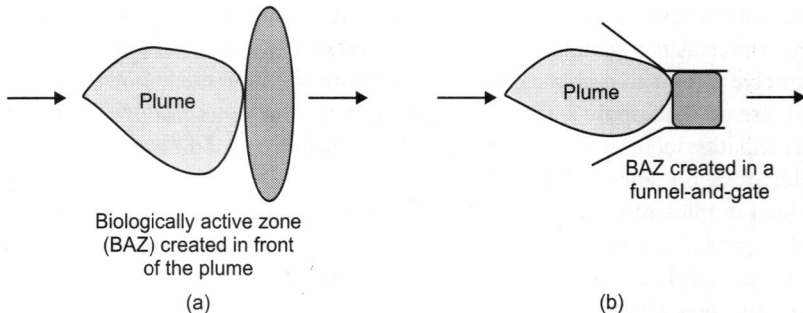

(a)

(b)

Fig. 17.5. Schematic illustration of on *in situ* biobarrier that contains a mobile contaminant plume by intercepting it with a BAZ.

Ex Situ Remediation

Contaminated soils can be excavated and treated in aboveground, or *ex situ*, treatment systems. Aboveground bioremediation for contaminated solids include slurry reactors, composting, and land farming. *Ex situ* bioremediation is most applicable for small, heavily contaminated sources and when a rapid site clean up is desired. Excavation incurs major costs and potentially increases exposure to workers and those who reside nearby.

Slurry reactors contain (typically) 5 per cent solids and are vigorously agitated for mixing and aeration. They are advantageous for maximising the rate of biodegradation. This rate increase is brought about by increased mass-transport rates due to agitation and the ease of adding oxygen, nutrients, and surface-active agents that emulsify NAPLs. The disadvantages of slurry systems are the added costs for capital, operation, and dewatering the decontaminated solids. Slurry reactors tend to be operated in a batch mode, but continuous feeding is possible.

Composting is an aerobic biodegradation scheme operated in a 'solid state' format. Solid state means that the compost material behaves as a porous solid with a moisture content of 50 to 60 per cent and through which air can be drawn to supply O_2 and to remove evaporated H_2O. Due to the high concentration of biodegradable organic material and the low moisture content of the compost mixture, the temperature rises to $60°–70°C$ during the time of peak biodegradation rates. In most cases, the air supply is determined by temperature considerations.

If the temperature is too hot, more air circulation is needed to drive evaporative cooling. In parallel to control of air circulation, the moisture content must be controlled within the optimal range, 50–60 per cent. Too much moisture prevents air circulation and slows microbial reactions.. Too little moisture initially allows the temperature to rise above the optimal range; the excess temperature and concomitant desiccation of compost materials arrest biodegradation reactions.

Land farming is a simple, 'low-tech' form of *ex situ* bioremediation. Contaminated solids are mixed into the surface layer of topsoil. Nutrients and moisture can be added initially and throughout the treatment period to optimise conditions for microbial growth. Land farming is most effective for solids contaminated by organic materials susceptible to aerobic biodegradation and where large tracts of land can be devoted to bioremediation.

Phytoremediation

Plant materials were found useful in the decontamination of water polluted with phenolic compounds. Enzymes exuded by roots of some families of Fabaceae, Gramineae, and Solanaceae release oxidoreductase, which takes part in the oxidative degradation of certain soil constituents. Horseradish-mediated removal of 2,4-dichlorophenol in a model solution was comparable with that achieved using purified horseradish peroxidase. In addition, horseradish could be reused up to 30 times. Because of the apparent ease of application, the use of plant material may present a breakthrough in the enzyme treatment of contaminated water.

Heavy metals are among the most dangerous substances in the environment because of their high level of durability and harmfulness to living organisms. Mercury has a high propensity to accumulate in organisms; the most harmful are organic compounds of Hg, especially in water. Chromium is biologically inactive in a metallic state. Organisms weakly absorb Cr (III), but Cr (VI) is more dangerous because its compounds easily penetrate physiological barriers. Phytoremediation is one of the ways to solve the problem of heavy metal pollution using plants. In the process of phytoremediation, pollutants are collected by plant roots and either decomposed to less harmful forms or accumulated in the plant tissues.

Phytoremediation is used to clean up waters, soils, slimes, and sediments from pesticides, PAHs, fuels, explosives, organic solvents, chemical manures, heavy metals, and radioactive contaminants. There are many plants that can bind heavy metals, and they are called 'hyperaccumulators'. Table 17.11 lists some of the plants that are hyperaccumulators of chromium and mercury. *Azolla caroliniana* has been tested as a biofilter to purify water and to remove nitrogen and phosphorous, elements that cause water eutrophication. It can also remove sulpha drugs and metals such as Sr, Cu, Cd, Cr, Ni, Pb, Au, and Pt and even radioactive elements as U. Bennicelli showed that *A. caroliniana* accumulates Hg (II), Cr (III), and Cr (VI).

Table 17.11. Hyperaccumulators of chromium and mercury.

Metal ions	
Cr (III)	*Hg (II)*
Dicoma niccolifera	*Arabidopsis thaliana*
Sutera fodina	*Nicotiana tobacum* (tobacco)
Pearsonia metallifera	*Liriodendro tulipifera*
Berkheya coddii	*Salix* spp.
Solanum elaeagnifolium	*Azolla caroliniana*
Azolla caroliniana	

Contaminated subsurface aquifers frequently accompany soil contamination. Bioremediation of groundwater resources presents unique problems and risks. Among the most obvious of these problems are that groundwater is mobile, whereas soil is generally stationary, and that people and livestock frequently drink untreated groundwater. Thus, there will often be an additional urgency factor associated with groundwater clean up that may justify more drastic and expensive measures.

The usual approach in remediation of contaminated aquifers is groundwater pumping and surface treatment to eliminate the water-soluble wastes. The treated water is then recharged into the aquifer via one or more injection wells at some point up gradient to the contaminated zone. Pump-and-treat operations can incorporate bioremediation in at least two ways. The most obvious method uses biological (bioreactor) surface treatment, but like any pump-and-treat approach, this method is only able to degrade wastes in the mobile, aqueous phase. It is important to recognise that many organic wastes have low water solubilities, and aquifer-associated soils will often contain larger volumes of organic wastes than the water itself. The conviction that pump-and-treat measures can be effective has led to an appreciable effort in the direction at numerous hazardous waste sites. However, the goal of remediating aquifers to drinking water standards by such techniques may be unrealistic in many, if not most, cases. Contamination levels at remediation sites are typically two to three orders of magnitude above allowable drinking water limits. Based on past experience gained in pumping and treating contaminated aquifers, treatment typically drops pollutant concentrations by a factor of 2 to 10, which then level out with no further decline. Cessation of pumping is often followed by a rebound in aquifer waste concentrations. The problem is largely that sites are typically contaminated with organic wastes that do not readily dissolve in the aqueous phase. The waste either remains adsorbed to the soil matrix, floats on the top, or sinks to the bottom of the water table. Therefore, wastes only slowly seep into the groundwater at a diffusion-limited rate and cannot be significantly changed by groundwater pumping. Pump-and-treat measures may dramatically reduce pollutant concentration in the aqueous phase of the aquifer; when the pumps are switched off, however, pollutants gradually leach out of the soil and the aqueous concentration rises again. Many leading hydrologists have concluded that hundreds to thousands of years of pumping could be required to purge some contaminated aquifers of their organic waste contaminants. The application is that although pump-and-treat measures may be useful to limit dispersal of a waste plume into the water table, massive excavation of soil is usually required to remove the source of the problem.

A more recently developed bioremediation approach to water treatment is subsurface *in situ* remediation. The treated water can be nutrient and oxygen-enriched prior to recharge, stimulating aerobic biodegradation of soil-bound, water-insoluble wastes by indigenous soil micro-organisms. The actual oxygen content of the water can be boosted by air pumps, or alternative oxygen sources such as hydrogen peroxide may be added. Surfactants and other organic waste desorbing chemicals can also be added to increase waste bioavailability. If a surface bioreactor is used, some portion of the active microbial biomass can be recharged with the water, providing continuous inoculation of the contaminated aquifer and soil. Although stimulation of aerobic metabolism is the objective of most systems, the reinjected groundwater can be enriched with nitrate to stimulate growth and enhance the biodegradative action of anaerobic denitrifying microbes. Recently, this approach has proved effective in degrading the various organic constituents of gasoline, with toxicity reductions comparable to those seen in aerobic degradation. As with *in situ* soil treatment, the success of subsurface aquifer bioremediation is largely determined by waste and soil characteristics. Soil permeability is especially important to the success of nutrient enrichment and inoculation efforts.

Over the years, a number of lakes and rivers have become seriously contaminated with various industrial wastes in many parts of the world. In some cases, the sources of pollution have been reduced or even eliminated. Public demand for remediation to a condition safe for fishing and other recreational uses is growing. Unfortunately, technologies for surface water remediation are not nearly as well developed as those for soil or even groundwater. Part of the problem lies in the size of many bodies of water. It is technically and environmentally impractical to divert a large flowing body of water from its course for treatment. Also, as with underground aquifers, the water contamination problem is largely a sediment contamination problem. Many persistent wastes become tightly bound to bottom sediments from which they slowly leach out and thus cannot readily be removed by water treatment. Conventional treatment typically involves dredging and removing bottom sediment in the most polluted areas, but such measures can themselves be environmentally devastating and there is a risk of remobilising toxicants accumulated over many years. Furthermore, the excavated sediment must still be treated and/or disposed of as toxic waste. Workers are turning to *in situ* bioremediation almost as a last resort.

Surface-water bioremediation technologies are largely being developed in place. An ongoing example is the General Electric (GE) site in Fort Edward, NY, on the upper Hudson River. For many years GE legally released PCBs into the river from a plant that manufactured capacitors. When PCBs became priority environmental pollutants in the early 1980s, at least 20 miles of the river bottom were found to be contaminated downstream of the plant. GE began looking for remediation options. In 1991, GE conducted an extensive field research programme to characterise natural degradation of PCBs at this site and discovered that the indigenous consortia of micro-organisms was exceptionally good at degrading PCBs. Presumably, since the PCBs have been present in this site for a significant period (at least 35 years), the indigenous micro-organisms have adapted to utilise the material as a food source. Both anaerobic and aerobic biodegradation have been identified as part of the natural process of remediation, which can be slow. Field tests in cylindrical caissons sunk into the river sediment at this site have identified the variables that can be manipulated to enhance *in situ* biodegradation of PCBs. The addition of inorganic nutrients, the organic cometabolite biphenyl, and oxygen significantly increased PCB degradation rates. Addition of selected PCB-degrading bacterial cultures did not dramatically improve biodegradative efficiency. No more than 60 per cent of the PCBs was degraded in any laboratory or field experiments, a finding attributed to tight sediment adsorption of the least water-soluble PCB compounds. More information on degradation rates, products, and variability under natural conditions is required for a realistic evaluation of the role that bioremediation may play in this and other surface water sites contaminated by organic waste.

Thus, groundwater, the most important source of drinking water, must be effectively and efficiently purified to ensure good health. Bioremediation is the most suitable method for the degradation of pollutants because other methods either involve elaborate expensive procedures or give rise to incompletely transformed products. Anaerobic treatment followed by aerobic treatment will ensure complete mineralisation of all pollutants. Ideally, aquifers would be inoculated with nonpathogenic bacteria that function under anoxic conditions. An aerobic treatment after pumping the groundwater will clean up the rest of the pollutants and their anaerobic transformed products.

Bioremediation of Gas-Phase VOCs

Gases contaminated with volatile organic compounds can be generated in numerous ways:

1. Bioventing and air sparging, as discussed above.
2. Vapour extraction of contaminated soils.
3. Storage tanks or production facilities for volatile organic products, such as gasoline, petroleum, and solvents.
4. Off-gases from waste-water treatment processes.
5. Off-gases from anaerobic treatment processes.
6. Off-gases from sewers or preliminary treatment of sewage.

Volatile organic compounds (VOCs) are organic chemicals that have a boiling point $\leq 100°C$ and/or a vapour pressure ≥ 1 mm Hg at $25°C$. They include alkane gases (e.g. methane), alcohols (e.g. methanol), low-molecular-weight petroleum hydrocarbons (e.g. benzene and toluene), halogenated aromatics (e.g. chlorobenzenes), and halogenated aliphatic solvents (e.g. 1,1,1-TCA and TCE). These VOCs are of particular environmental concern because they are very mobile, may affect human senses through odour, may exert a narcotic effect, and may be toxic and carcinogenic. Some VOCs also react photochemically to form ground-level ozone, a key component of smog, while others are greenhouse gases. For these reasons, emissions of VOCs to the atmosphere are becoming a greater concern to regulatory agencies, industry, and the general public.

Biodegradation of VOCs is among a suite of technologies that can be used to treat gases containing VOCs. Low capital and operating costs are the main advantages of biofiltration, the main type of biological treatment of gases. For example, Bohn found that the capital costs of a typical biofiltration system were only about 6 per cent of those for incineration, 13 per cent of those for ozone oxidation, and 40 per cent of those for activated-carbon adsorption.

Ottengraf described the biological systems commonly being used or tested in Europe, Japan, and the USA for treatment of gas-phase VOCs, as well as NH_3, H_2S, and semi-volatile odour compounds. Bioscrubbers countercurrently contact the gas stream with circulating liquid in a spray column. The bacteria are mainly dispersed in the circulating liquid. In trickling filters and biofilters, the micro-organisms are immobilised on a carrier or packing medium. In most cases, the water flow is downward by gravity, while the gas flow is countercurrent, or upward. Trickling filters are distinguished from biofilters by the amount of water applied. The trickling filter has a larger hydraulic loading so that the aqueous phase continuously flows downward. Because the hydraulic loading is less for biofilters, the water phase is essentially stationary.

Biological treatment of contaminated gas phases also can be accomplished by passing the gas through compost, peat, or soil beds. These systems are very simple, although process control may be limited. More recent developments include using three-phase fluidised-bed biofilm reactors to create highly compact biofilm systems well suited to industrial settings.

Except for bioscrubbers, all of the gas-treatment systems are of the biofilm type. The main difference is that the contaminants enter in a gas stream, which must be included in the mass balances. Because most of the contaminants are hazardous organic compounds.

EVALUATING BIOREMEDIATION

One of the factors that limit the widespread application of bioremediation is that its 'success' has been difficult to 'prove' in the field. Regulators, site owners, and the public are wary of a technology that requires a sophisticated appreciation for microbiology and how it connects to the hydrogeology and chemistry of contaminated soils. When measures for the technology's success are neither obvious nor agreed upon, the wary decision maker is likely to seek other solutions, including expensive alternatives, such as pump-and-treat or incineration.

The development and acceptance of evaluation protocols is a slow process for the following reasons:

1. The definition of success varies among the several parties involved. Regulators generally define success only in terms of meeting some compliance level for contaminant concentration in the water or soil. Buyers of bioremediation are acutely interested in cost-effectiveness. The public generally wants assurance that they are not being exposed to risk. Researchers and developers of bioremediation wish to demonstrate the cause-and-effect nature of the process. This means that agreement on evaluation protocols requires sustained communication among the many parties who are stakeholders and/or need to contribute key technical judgements: regulators, buyers, the public, engineers, microbiologists, hydrogeologists, chemists, and others.

2. Many different measures of success can be put forward, but no one measure is universally applicable for a type of contamination, soil conditions, or bioremediation approach. Expert and site-specific judgment always will play a role.

3. Contaminated soils are inherently heterogeneous. *In situ* technologies amplify the importance of heterogeneity, since sampling is difficult and expensive, while micro-organisms often are highly localised. It is well known that finding residual NAPL contamination is extremely difficult. Because the micro-organisms often accumulate on solids close to the trapped contaminants, they also are difficult to find.

Although evaluating bioremediation is challenging and not easily standardised, it can be accomplished if an evaluation programme is properly designed. The key to an evaluation programme is that the measures of 'success' must directly link microbial activity to the observed loss of contaminant. To obtain this linkage, the NRC recommends an evaluation strategy based on three kinds of evidence:

1. Documented loss of contaminants from the site.
2. Laboratory assays showing that micro-organisms at the site have the potential to transform the contaminants under the expected site conditions.
3. One or more pieces of evidence showing that the biodegradation potential is actually realised in the field.

The third type of evidence is the most crucial and the most difficult to obtain. It links the loss of contaminants in the soil and water with the potential for them to be biodegraded. A wide range of measurement approaches is available, and the NRC discusses their scientific bases. Table 17.12 briefly summarises some of the techniques and what they indicate. In all cases, the measurement techniques should be used to: (i) show that characteristics of the site's chemistry or microbial population change in ways one would predict if bioremediation were occurring, and (ii) correlate these chemical and microbial changes with documented contaminant losses.

One key distinction is between techniques that can provide principal evidence versus those that provide only confirmatory evidence. Principal evidence should be equally capable of proving the success or failure of bioremediation. Among the various techniques in Table 17.12, good examples of principal evidence include stoichiometric consumption of electron acceptors, formation of inorganic carbon that originated in organic carbon, and increased degradation rates over time. Quantification of consumption or formation rates is of great importance. The mere demonstration that a reaction occurs is not always principal evidence; instead, the rate must commensurate with the loss of contamination.

Table 17.12. Summary of techniques used to demonstrate biodegradation in the field.

Technique	Indication of
Direct measurements of field samples	
Number of bacteria	An increase in the population of contaminant degrading bacteria over background conditions
Number of protozoa	An increase in the population of predators of the contaminant-degrading bacteria
Rate of bacterial activity in laboratory microcosms	Potential rates of biodegradation
Bacterial adaptation	An increase in the rates of biodegradation since bioremediation began
Inorganic carbon concentration	Formation of inorganic carbon by oxidation of the organic contaminant
Carbon isotope ratio	Inorganic carbon originating from organic contamination
Electron-acceptor concentration	A decrease in the electron acceptors used during contaminant oxidation

(Contd ...)

Technique	Indication of
By-products of anaerobic activity	Formation of products generated when electron acceptors other than O_2 are used
Intermediary metabolites	Breakdown products of complex organic contaminants
Ratio of nondegradable to degradable components	Relative loss of biodegradable components
Experiments run in the field	
Stimulating bacteria within subsites	An increase in microbial activity with stimulation used in engineered bioremediation
Measuring electron-acceptor uptake rate	*In situ* rate of metabolism
Monitoring a conservative tracer	Contaminant losses due to abiotic mechanisms
Labelling contaminants	The fate of carbon contained in organic contaminants
Modelling experiments	
Modelling abiotic mass loss	Potential losses through abiotic mechanisms
Direct modelling	*In situ* biodegradation rates

Confirmatory evidence, on the other hand, usually only can support success, but its absence does not prove failure. Good examples of confirmatory evidence include increases in the populations of bacteria or protozoa (they are too hard to find to be principal), detection of intermediary metabolites (they can be degraded themselves), and an increase to the ratio of nondegradable to degradable components (other mechanisms also act differentially).

The complexities of the contaminated setting and the difficulties in obtaining good samples make it rare for one type of measurement to give unequivocal proof. Therefore, the three-part strategy relies upon building a consistent, logical case from convergent lines of independent evidence. A wide range of principal and confirmatory techniques is needed to create a strong case for proving (or disproving) the success of a bioremediation project. A critical evaluation of these protocols, carried out recently by a committee of the NRC, provides guidance on what should be included in an evaluation scheme. The foundation of the NRC's 2000 guidance is that the-monitoring and evaluation programme should document the presence of 'footprints', which are the products of the biological reactions capable of destroying the contaminants. Footprints include:

1. Loss of electron acceptors in proportion to loss of a contaminant that is oxidised.
2. Increases in inorganic carbon in proportion to the loss or organic contaminants that are mineralised.
3. Loss of an electron-donor substrate in parallel to the loss of a contaminant that is reduced, such as by reductive dechlorination.
4. Release of the chloride ion from organic chemicals that are dechlorinated.
5. Increases or decreases of alkalinity in proportion to reactions that release base or release acid, respectively.

In some cases, confounding reactions or high background levels make it impossible to detect all the relevant footprints. Nevertheless, the detection of several footprints at levels commensurate to the loss of contaminant is necessary to ensure that natural attenuation is reliably protecting public health and the environment. The level of effort to monitor a site depends on the likelihood that a natural-attenuation mechanism is able to destroy the contaminant in a given setting and the complexity of the setting. Reduced likelihood of destruction and/or a more complex site demands increases to the number, extent, and frequency of sampling, as well as more sophisticated evaluation of the data.

To sum up bioremediation is a cost-effective technology for the treatment of a variety of pollutants and contaminated sites. Its applicability and potential for success depend upon three factors: the properties of the pollutant (biodegradability of the specific chemical pollutants); the microbial community (enzymatic capacity to metabolise the pollutant chemicals); and the environment (properties permitting or limiting microbial growth and metabolism of the polluting chemicals). The applicability and approaches to bioremediation depend upon these three factors. In many cases bioremediation relies upon the intrinsic degradative capacity of the indigenous micro-organisms to remove the pollutant without further treatment (intrinsic bioremediation); in other cases the rates of metabolism of the indigenous microbial community are increased through environmental engineering (biostimulation); and in yet other cases the microbial community is altered through seeding with specialised cultures (bioaugmentation).

To date, most commercial applications of bioremediation depend upon naturally occurring micro-organisms and most have targeted hydrocarbon contaminated sites. Approaches to the bioremediation of chlorinated compounds and metals are more complex but have been proceeding, primarily through demonstration projects. The use of genetically engineered micro-organisms and *ex situ* treatments for remediation of additional industrial pollutants, including TCE, are likely to gain increased importance in the near future.

Chapter 18

Methods for Biocatalysis and Biotransformations

INTRODUCTION

Biotransformations are reactions of organic compounds by either enzyme or whole-cell biocatalysts. Biocatalysis is widely applied in industry for pharmaceutical, agrochemical, chemical, fragrance and flavour, nutritional, and bioremediation purposes.

Many new enzymes have been characterised from microbial cells, and methods for their isolation, stabilisation, and use have dramatically expanded. Importantly, biocatalysis has increasingly been extended to reactions in organic solvents, in which many compounds of interest are soluble and additional reactions are possible. At the same time, advances in biocatalyst improvement by recombinant technologies have provided the bases for unprecedented means of biocatalyst alteration and use. Continued advancements in the use and development of biocatalysis have drawn upon more sensitive, rapid, and informative analytical methods. Further advances in biocatalysis will be achieved from the diverse areas of organic chemistry, analytical chemistry, biochemistry, molecular biology, microbiology, and engineering. Indeed, as this chapter will make clear, the most successful practitioners of biotransformations have an appreciation and understanding of the highly interdisciplinary nature of biocatalysis development. Yet biotransformation techniques have evolved such that the synthetic chemist can utilise biocatalysts just as many other synthetic reagents are used.

Enzyme catalysts have several features that render them attractive as a class of 'reagents' for organic synthesis. Enzymes are chiral catalysts. They are proteins that have evolved into specific biocatalytic structures. They often bind substrates very specifically and display high regio-, stereo-, and enantio-selectivities. These desirable traits obviate the need to block undesirable reactions that commonly occur with other functional groups in traditional organic synthesis. Catalysis occurs under mild reaction conditions requiring no strong acids or bases, temperature extremes, rigorously controlled atmospheres, heavy metals, or other conditions commonly associated with chemical catalysts. Multistep biocatalytic processes can occur efficiently with a single micro-organism.

Enzyme reactions require little energy input because they occur very efficiently between 20° and 70°C. Most intriguingly, the maturation of genomics, molecular biology, and *in vitro* evolution techniques promise to provide highly efficient and tunable catalysts tailored for specific synthetic goals. While we realise this potential is still years off, biocatalysis is today a viable alternative for conducting many synthetic reactions.

This chapter is devoted to a consideration of biocatalysis methods applicable to the solution of problems in organic chemistry. We hope it will serve as a practical and concise guide to an enormous literature and provide a basis for simple and productive experimentation by scientists of many disciplines who may benefit from biotransformations.

CONCEPT AND GENERAL FEATURES OF BIOTRANSFORMATIONS

Organic reactions catalysed by micro-organisms are referred to as microbial transformations, bio-transformations, or bioconversions. Biotransformation reactions are catalysed by enzymes produced by microbial cells and by all living organisms. In their natural functions, enzymes catalyse, and indeed control, anabolic and catabolic reactions necessary to life processes such as bioenergetics, growth, and replication. Anabolic enzymes, involved in biosynthetic pathways, are usually substrate specific, while many catabolic enzymes, involved in digestive, defensive, and similar degradation roles in living organisms, seem to have evolved broader ranges of specificity. The substrate specificities of some enzymes are remarkably broad.

A well-known example is the reactivity of cytochromes P-450, with substrates of broadly different structures; some human hepatic forms catalyse hydroxylations or dealkylations on more than 50 diverse pharmaceutical structures. More general and convincing demonstrations are the many isolations of micro-organisms capable of degradation of synthetic organic compounds only recently introduced to the environment. Many other examples are present in the literature, and, in fact, few enzymes are specific enough to catalyse reactions with only their natural substrates. Thus, most organic compounds (excluding unstable and highly reactive compounds) can serve as substrates for enzyme-catalysed transformations.

From a synthetic perspective, as we shall summarise, it is possible to select experimental conditions that favour the production of desired enzyme catalysts that can be used to perform single and highly specific reactions.

This is done by controlling the pre-inoculation, growth, and transformation environment of the culture and the physical form of the organic substrate, and by establishing reproducible experimental protocols. Knowledge of the natural substrates of enzymes used to catalyse organic reactions, or even the identity of the enzyme itself, is not necessary.

Biotransformation enzymes may be present within (endo) or outside (exo) of the cells that produce them. Bacteria often contain soluble enzymes within the cytosol and particulate enzymes bound to membrane structures. Yeasts and fungi are more complicated; their enzymes are often compartmentalised within various organelles, including mitochondria, nuclei, vacuoles, as well as in cell membranes. A priori, there is no way to know the location of useful enzymes within the biotransforming cell. Therefore, experimental methods are designed to allow the transport of reactants to catalytic sites, wherever they might be, favouring the highest possible solubility and dispersion in the reaction medium and enhancing permeability of the cells to the reactants.

Many microbial enzymes are constitutive in nature: they are always produced by the growing cell. If enzymes are not constitutive, their formation in micro-organisms can sometimes be induced by the substrate of interest, or by related compounds.

Inducible enzymes may catalyse a variety of reactions on the inducers, substrates, and even unrelated compounds. When multienzyme pathways are induced, environmental conditions can be controlled to favour desirable single or multistep reactions.

With this basic understanding of biocatalysis, the rest of this chapter summarises methods used to conduct experiments in biocatalysis and biotransformations, particularly of organic compounds.

PROCEDURES

Huge numbers of microbes coexist in almost all natural environments, particularly soils (estimated to have 10^9 cells/g of soil), waters, and sewage. The make-up of the flora in these ecosystems is determined by the availability of oxygen and water, light exposure, temperature, and the nutrients present. Widely different mixtures of bacteria, fungi, algae, and other microscopic life can be isolated from nature by using different natural ecosystems (e.g. soils from different locations) as sources of inocula. While it may be possible to predict good candidate biocatalysts for a given transformation on a given substrate, the best catalyst most often must be identified from small-scale test reactions. This catalyst identification stage can generally be performed in two ways. The first strategy involves 'screening' large numbers of individual reactions with pure cultures for a specified transformation. The second approach involves 'selection' of a strain from mixed culture, usually using the ability to grow on the test substrate as the selective pressure.

While the 'selection' strategy is commonly used for bioremediation studies, synthetic biotransformations greatly benefit by work with pure cultures. Pure cultures are identifiable by their morphological, nutritional, and other characteristics that allow classification of organisms into taxonomic strata. Since pure cultures are definable reagents, they are easier to maintain, possible to control, and their use helps ensure experimental reproducibility. Moreover, multistep reactions can be more easily characterised with single biocatalyst strains than with microbial consortia. In essence, pure cultures are to biocatalysis as pure reagents are to chemistry. Simpler reactions are performed with straightforward and uncomplicated reagents, and the same is true with pure cultures vs. mixed cultures as specific biocatalysts.

Taxonomy

A detailed review of the science of taxonomy is beyond the scope of this chapter. Nevertheless, it is useful to consider the basic organisational framework for classification of micro-organisms commonly used as biocatalysts. Classifications are constructed from individual organisms that occur within populations of species. The species is the fundamental or most basic level of organisation in taxonomy. Species are individuals sampled from populations closely resembling each other in many different characteristics. Species that share many common characteristics are placed in a group termed the genus. Families consist of still more inclusive groups, and so on to higher organisational levels. The taxonomic classification for a given organism, *Streptomyces cretosus*, for example, is as follows: kingdom *Procaryotae*, division *Bacteria*, class *Actinomycetes*, order *Actinomycetales*, family *Streptomycetaceae*, genus *Streptomyces*, species *cretosus*.

Taxonomy can be instructive when considering biocatalysts for synthetic applications. For example, when a culture such as *Mycobacterium fortuitum* performs an interesting biotransformation reaction, but in low yield, it is logical to examine taxonomically related cultures to find other candidates that might provide higher yields or that might perform related reactions on different starting materials. To do so, other *Mycobacterium* spp., other genera of the actinomycetes, and members of closely related families such as the *Nocardiaceae* would also be examined. This approach is reasonable, since there are often similarities in enzymatic make-up among members of related genera and families. Conversely, when building and screening a library of microbial catalysts, for synthetic applications, it makes sense to sample biocatalyst diversity by including as broad a range of genera as possible.

An understanding of cell structure and morphology can be helpful when designing biocatalytic processes and equipment. Bacterial, fungal, and yeast cells all contain a variety of organelles in the cytosol, such as storage granule ribosomes, mitochondria, spores, and membranous structures. Enzymes useful for bioconversions have been found to occur in all of these structures. Importantly, cell membranes are semipermeable barriers to nutrients and waste products entering and leaving the cell. This membrane must be penetrated by organic substrates for reactions to occur with intracellular enzymes. If enzymes are located in periplasmic spaces between the membrane and the rigid cell wall, organic substrate need only to penetrate this outer wall. In addition to rigid cell walls, the shells of some micro-organisms may consist of an extra membrane (outer membrane of gram-negative bacteria), 'slime' layers, and capsules that affect mass transport into the cell.

Biocatalyst Acquisition and Preservation

Selection of the biocatalyst is the most critical of all the operations in a biotransformation experiment. Cultures with desirable properties are obtained from other investigators in the biotransformation field, from standard culture collections, or by isolation from natural habitats.

Comprehensive lists of most of the significant culture collections around the world are available on the World Wide Web (www.sv-cict.fr/bacterio/collections.html).

Well-established culture collections catalogue micro-organisms by number so that it is possible to obtain the same organism (biocatalyst) each time. The purchase of a culture (they may be expensive) by catalogue number is identical to the process whereby a specific catalyst or reagent is purchased from a chemical catalogue. In many collections, strains are maintained in lyophilised form or on agar slants suitable for mailing. Investigators usually maintain their own culture collections of 100 to 400 strains. In addition, microbiology and mycology departments on many college campuses maintain culture collections. Investigators are usually willing to share their cultures with researchers in other laboratories. Alternatively, enrichment techniques are used to isolate cultures from nature.

With access to a huge number of microbial strains, some intuition about narrowing the search for an acceptable biocatalyst can be valuable. The literature of the last 25 years provides excellent leads to available organisms with specific, desirable enzymatic capabilities. Electronic databases of this literature, allowing relational and structure-based searching, provide an excellent tool for selecting good candidate biocatalysts. Other catalogues of chemical reactions catalysed by micro-organisms have been assembled with specific attention to groups of compounds such as the alkaloids, steroids and nonsteroidal cyclic compounds, including various drugs and other xenobiotics.

Microbial strains must be handled like all complex reagents. When new cultures are procured, the following information should be recorded: culture name and number, source, acquisition and lyophilisation dates, lyophilisation medium, growth medium and temperature, literature source, reactions known to be catalysed, and unusual properties and comments. Upon receipt, it is also important to establish the purity of new cultures and to transfer them to appropriate fresh media for propagation and storage. For short-term storage and routine culturing, slants in screw-top vials should be used. After significant growth, many strains can be stored in a refrigerator. For longer-term storage, lyophilisation or ultra-low-temperature freezing is recommended.

Growth Fundamentals

Growth is the cumulative process resulting in the orderly increase of all chemical components of the living cell. Different groups of organisms behave quite differently when grown in liquid culture. As with enzyme-catalysed reactions, an approximately linear relationship exists between the amount of microbial cells (biocatalyst) present and the rate of reaction in the incubation mixture. Thus, when biotransformations are conducted with growing cultures, conditions that favour enhanced growth usually result in greater yields of reaction products. Growth rates of unicellular bacteria and yeasts are usually regular. Growth of multicellular organisms such as fungi and filamentous procaryotes (actinomycetes) such as *Streptomyces* spp. is more difficult to define.

The complement of enzymes produced by microbial cells varies greatly at five times during the life cycle of the cell. The desired enzyme activity may be present from the start of the growth cycle, or it may not appear until the late exponential phase. The changes in enzyme activities during growth reflect the changes occurring within the cell and the culture medium as the organism grows and metabolises nutrients. Thus, the optimum time for adding organic reactants or for harvesting cells must be established by experimentation. This is another motivation for using pure cultures for transformations.

Measurement of Cell Mass

For quantitative estimations of catalytic efficiency it may be necessary to estimate biomass, the amount of biocatalyst present. Wet weights of microbial cells typically reach levels of 20 to 30 g/l of culture medium. These are estimated by filtering known volumes of fungi or actinomycetes, or by centrifuging known culture volumes of bacteria and yeasts. Culture dry weights are obtained by placing aliquots of filtered or pelleted cells in a 120°C oven overnight to drive off moisture. Alternatively, optical density readings at 600 or 660 nm can be correlated to dry weights. A calibration curve between 0.1 and 1.0 absorbance units is made from a series of dilutions of the original culture. A plot of cell densities (dry weight) versus optical density should yield a usable straight line falling off somewhat in the more turbid region. A separate calibration curve needs to be constructed for each cultured strain. This procedure works well for nonfilamentous bacteria and yeasts.

Viable cell counts can be determined by plating of serial culture dilutions. A handy rule of thumb for estimating cell numbers in suspensions is that a suspension with just barely visible turbidity contains about 10^6 cells per ml. This estimate is fairly accurate for bacteria of average size such as *Escherichia coli*.

Forms of the Biocatalyst

The use of live, growing microbial cells as biocatalysts for biotransformations of organic compounds has been extensively documented. Pure cultures are grown to a point where desired enzyme activities are maximal, at which time organic chemical substrates are added to the incubation mixture in which the transformations take place. However, much experimental latitude is now possible in the use and form of the biocatalyst.

Growing Cultures

Both batch and continuous cultures are used in bioconversion experiments. In the batch culture technique, a pure culture is grown in a suitable medium. At an experimentally determined time, the substrate is added, and reaction is continued until transformation of the substrate ceases or additional reactions seriously begin to affect yields. In batch processes, the biocatalyst is used only once and then discarded. Necessary equipment is inexpensive and simple, and the procedure is straightforward for screening purposes. However, it requires the repetitive production of cells for each experiment, and the isolation of reaction products from complex fermentation media can be complicated. The physiological state of cells in batch culture varies continuously throughout the growth cycle.

This is not true of cells in continuous culture, in which cells can be maintained in a steady physiological state for long periods of time by means of continuous addition of fresh nutrient medium and simultaneous withdrawal of equal amounts of spent medium. Continuous culture has not been used widely in biotransformation screening, owing to the relative complexity of the fermentor equipment, but it may be useful for scale-up of the biotransformation.

Resting Cells

Resting cells are nongrowing, live cells retain most of the enzyme activities of growing cells. Resting cells are obtained from the culture medium at a time in the growth cycle when enzyme activities are highest, or at least present at useful levels. Mycelial growth can be removed by filtration, but yeasts and bacteria are best harvested by centrifugation. Concentrated cells are resuspended in buffers, modified culture media (usually without some required nutrient for growth), distilled water, or even nonaqueous solvent mixtures for use as biocatalysts.

As biotransformation catalysts, resting cells have several advantages versus growing cells or isolated enzymes. They are much cleaner than reactions with growing cells, resulting in easier product isolation. The cell concentration can be made higher, enhancing the sensitivity of the biocatalyst screening. Moreover, control of undesirable secondary or side reactions can be done more easily with nongrowing cells. Compared with isolated enzymes, whole resting cells can accomplish efficient multistep enzymatic reactions without the need for expensive coenzymes. For single-step reactions, the direct use of resting cells minimises loss of activity, which is unavoidable during isolation and purification of enzymes. Enzymes in intact cells usually are more stable than their isolated counterparts.

Cometabolism and enzyme induction increase the usefulness of resting-cell biocatalysis. For some reactions to occur, it is necessary to use a cosubstrate such as glucose, glycerol, succinic acid, or another oxidisable metabolite along with the organic compound to be transformed. These cosubstrates drive reactions to completion by providing the necessary energy derived during their utilisation. They also provide energy for recycling of coenzymes for the enzymatic reactions.

In some cells, desired enzyme activities are dramatically increased by cultivating the organism in the presence of the organic compound to be transformed (enzyme induction). Conversely, the use of resting cells in which enzyme activities have not been induced can result in poor yields. Many examples of the use of resting cells in biotransformations have been described.

Dried Cells

In some cases microbial cells can be dehydrated and still maintain enzyme activities. The resulting powders are convenient biocatalysts. Esterases, amidases, oxidoreductases, and dehydrogenases, among other enzyme classes, can survive cell-drying procedures. The two most common methods of drying are lyophilisation and acetone dehydration. For lyophilisation, harvested cells are suspended in distilled water or dilute buffer. The suspension is then frozen over a dry ice-acetone (or ethanol) bath in a thin shell inside a round-bottomed flask (about 5 mm thick). Water sublimes from frozen cells to form a fluffy, dry powder that may be used immediately or frozen to preserve enzyme activities for many years. When freeze-dried cells are used as biocatalysts, they must be evaluated for surviving enzyme activities before use.

Treatment of cell pastes or cakes with cold ($-20°C$) acetone is a simple method for preparing dried cells. Cells obtained by centrifugation or filtration are slurried in cold acetone and suction filtered. The drying process is repeated twice more, followed by a cold ether wash to remove residual acetone, which can be detrimental to enzyme activities. Removal of solvent from the dried cells under vacuum gives an 'acetone powder', which is most stable when stored frozen.

Dried cells offer many of the same advantages of resting cells compared to growing cultures. Both lyophilised and acetone-treated cells are easy to prepare. An adequate supply of powdered cells helps to ensure experimental reproducibility, since many experiments can be performed with one batch and it is not necessary to establish rigorous fermentation protocols for each experiment. Incubations with dried cells do not require sterile manipulations.

Permeabilised Cells

Microbial cell membranes may be made permeable to organic chemical substrates. Permeabilising agents include surfactants, solvents, and antibiotics. Permeabilising agents are usually applied after growth stops in the stationary phase, or with resting cells. Alternatively, the addition of inhibitors of cell wall synthesis during growth enhances permeability. The solvents dimethylformamide (DMF) and dimethyl sulphoxide (DMSO), commonly used to disperse steroids and other lipophilic compounds, also increase the permeability of the cells. These solvents should be used with care since at higher concentrations they may adversely affect the viability of the cells.

Isolated Enzymes and Cell-Free Preparations

Isolated enzymes are already commonly used as reagents for organic synthesis. Isolated enzymes have advantages as synthetic reagents in that they are simple, well defined, and usually catalyse a single reaction step with little side reaction. Compared with whole cells, methodology and equipment are simplified with isolated enzymes, as concerns for sterility and cell viability are minimal. A wider range of reaction environments can be used, since the stability of cellular structures is irrelevant. Removal of an enzyme from the cell also allows cleaner reactions, with greatly reduced mass transfer concerns, and no undesirable reactions catalysed by other enzymes present in the cell. Like whole-cell fermentations, isolated enzymes have been demonstrated for use on industrial scale for a number of processes. For these reasons, the use of enzymatic catalysis has expanded considerably. Several excellent general reviews on catalysis with pure enzymes are available.

The vast majority of published enzyme-catalysed reactions are acyl hydrolysis and reduction, for which the regio- and stereospecificity of enzymes allows chiral syntheses. However, a wide variety of enzymes catalysing other synthetically useful reaction chemistries, such as epoxidation, halogenation, oxidations, phosphorylation, glycosylation, condensations, nitrile hydrolysis, decarboxylation, isomerisation, and many other reactions, are available commercially. In fact, the full range of synthetic chemistries present in the structural diversity of natural products is enzyme-mediated.

However, some important enzymes, including the broad class of oxygenases that catalyse hydroxylation reactions, require multiple cofactors, multiple enzyme species, or are not sufficiently stable when purified. Other enzymes may be difficult or time-consuming to obtain in purified form. For these enzymes, catalysis with whole cells, as described above, is still very prevalent. In many cases, however, crude cell-free preparations may be a suitable alternative.

Crude enzyme preparations are obtained by breaking cells under mild conditions so that the contents are released in an active state to the buffer medium. Common techniques for the disruption of microbial cells are pressure shearing, enzymatic digestion of cell membranes, osmotic lysis, autolysis, and freezing-thawing. Ultrasonic disintegration and pressure shearing are the most widely used in exploratory bench research.

The French press is a reliable device for pressure shearing on a small scale. It consists of a solid steel cylinder containing a well that holds 5 to 40 ml of a thick cell suspension. The cylinder is fitted with a solid stainless-steel piston that can be forced into the well under high pressure (4000 to 20,000 lb/in^2). Cells are broken by the high shear forces as they are squeezed through a small release orifice in the well. Ultrasonic oscillators also break cells by shearing. Rapidly moving bubbles in the sonic field at the probe tip cause high shear forces capable of breaking the toughest cell walls. Since high-frequency sonic oscillations generate much heat, the operation must be conducted in short bursts in an ice bath. Short bursts of 15 to 20 seconds break cell suspensions of 30 to 40 grams (wet weight) per 100 ml.

Simple enzyme fractionation can be achieved by centrifugation to remove solid debris (cell membranes, unbroken cells) from crude enzyme mixtures. Centrifugation at 5000 × g for 10 minutes will produce murky supernatant mixtures containing soluble and particulate enzymes and traces of cofactors from the microbial cell. More involved and time-consuming procedures (e.g. column chromatography) are necessary to obtain pure enzymes from these crude mixtures.

Crude broken-cell suspensions and supernatant fractions with minimal purification can catalyse useful organic reactions. Appropriate volumes of these suspensions are added to reaction vessels along with organic substrates in buffer or organic solvent. If coenzymes are required, these can be added in stoichiometric amounts for small-scale reactions; otherwise, coenzyme regeneration strategies are becoming well established.

Naturally occurring, exocellular enzymes may be efficiently used with little isolation. Typical exocellular enzymes, including peroxidases (ligninases) laccases, and hydrolases are stable and can be useful biocatalysts. For convenience of use and storage, such enzymes may be concentrated by ultrafiltration, precipitation by solvents or salts, or adsorption to a carrier.

For example, *Polyporus anceps* grown in a defined medium secretes laccase (a copper oxidase). When enzyme titers are highest, cells are filtered from the fermentation broth and dry DEAE-cellulose (H$^+$ form, 3 g/l) is added to the filtrate with stirring for 30 minutes at 4°C to bind most of the enzyme activity. The resin-bound enzyme is removed by simple filtration, washed twice with distilled water, and moist resin-enzyme is stored in small portions in a freezer. Elution of DEAE-cellulose with 0.2 M phosphate buffer (pH 5.0) gives quantitative recoveries of the active enzyme that catalyses the oxidations of alkaloids.

Immobilised Systems

In developing biotransformations with an eye on practical applications, the issue of biocatalyst immobilisation will often be important. Immobilisation theoretically allows more convenient continuous processing and product isolation, improved biocatalyst stability, and reuse of the biocatalyst. The use of an immobilisation support, however, does introduce additional development costs and mass transfer considerations. In practice, interestingly, relatively few industrial biocatalytic processes have employed immobilisation.

In general, the major approaches that have resulted in successful biocatalyst immobilisation include noncovalent adsorption, covalent attachment, covalent cross-linking, physical entrapment within a porous support, and compartmentalisation within a membrane.

Although each of the general approaches has proved useful for different applications, the most common immobilisation format for whole-cell biocatalysts on small scales is gel entrapment. Empirically, this simple-to-apply procedure has generally resulted in improved biocatalyst stability and handling, while introducing moderate mass transfer barriers. In a typical laboratory-scale application, a 1 to 8 per cent sodium alginate solution is mixed with an equal amount of a concentrated resting-cell suspension in a syringe. The mixture is injected through a small-gauge needle and dropped into a 0.1 M Ca^{+2} (or other divalent cation) solution to promote gelling. After several minutes the gelled beads can be filtered off and used for transformation.

TECHNIQUES

Success in the application of micro-organisms and microbial enzymes as catalysts for organic reactions requires a working knowledge of simple microbiological laboratory techniques. Sterile or aseptic techniques, medium preparation, and the use of the light microscope are the basics.

Aseptic technique is essential to the maintenance and use of pure cultures and can be simplified to two requirements: (i) the use of sterile equipment, vessels, substrates, media, etc. and (ii) the exclusion of airborne particles containing contaminating organisms when making additions or transfers to medium. For many synthetically useful micro-organisms, practicing aseptic technique adds little to the complexity of a properly conducted reaction.

Sterilisation is the complete removal or destruction of all living entities from materials by using heat, filtration, radiation, or chemicals. The best and most convenient sterilisation method for heat-resistant materials likely to be used in bioconversion research is steam sterilisation or autoclaving with steam under pressure (15 lb/in^2, 121°C). Flasks, culture media, and pipettes are all suitably sterilised by autoclaving. Common problems that can be encountered during sterilisation are the precipitation of inorganic or organic salts and the destruction of sugars when heated in the presence of nitrogenous organic nutrients. Ovens heated to 180°C can be used to dry-sterilise glassware, pipettes, and other utensils in 1 hour. Slow cooling for about 2 hours minimises breakage of glassware. Filtration through 0.1- to 0.2-μm membranes is a reliable method for obtaining sterile solutions of heat-labile materials or of materials dissolved in nonaqueous solvents. Flame sterilisation or chemical sterilisation with ethanol is usually the method of choice for small-scale sterilisation of hands and utensils used during the course of an experiment.

The maintenance of aseptic conditions while working with sterilised equipment commonly requires the use of a laminar flow hood and common sense. The laminar flow hood provides a positive pressure of filtered air over the work area to prevent airborne particles from contaminating a culture. Common sense dictates that hands, tools, and other objects that are brought into the laminar flow hood, or contact cultures within the hood, must be sterilised before use with another culture. Proper use of aseptic techniques and equipment will ensure maximum reliability and reproducibility of cultures and the biotransformations they catalyse.

MEDIA

Catalytically active microbial cells are obtained by growth in balanced nutrient media, especially those containing inducers of the desired enzyme activities. Different micro-organisms have special requirements for optimal growth. In addition to environmental factors (temperature and pH), the ratios and amounts of carbon, nitrogen, phosphorus, trace minerals, and special growth factors are important in proper nutrition. The elemental composition of a dried cell provides insight into the nutritional requirements of that cell. Water makes up 80 to 90 per cent of the cell weight. For dried *E. coli* cells, the relative concentrations of the various elements are as follows: carbon (50 per cent), nitrogen (15 per cent), phosphorus (3.2 per cent), sulphur (1.1 per cent), sodium (1.3 per cent), potassium (1.5 per cent), magnesium (0.5 per cent), calcium (1 per cent), and iron (0.24 per cent), with trace amounts of manganese and copper. Hydrogen and oxygen account for the balance. Conversely, cell composition reflects the growth medium used. For instance, the high amount of sodium in this particular analysis reflects the fact that the *E. coli* was grown in nutrient medium containing sodium chloride, which is customarily added even though there may be no requirements for it. Several different types of culture media have been used to accommodate these nutritional principles for the growth of micro-organisms used in biotransformations.

Chemically Defined Media

Chemically defined media are made by the addition of specified ingredients to distilled water. Although more expensive, these media offer the very important advantages of reproducibility and greater simplicity in the analysis of biotransformation end products. A variety of carbohydrates, organic acids, alcohols, hydrocarbons, and lipids can serve as carbon sources. Nitrogen sources can be salts other than ammonium sulphate, such as sodium or ammonium nitrate. Urea is another good nitrogen source, as are certain amino acids (e.g. asparagine). Vitamins, purines and pyrmidines, and amino acids are added to the defined media to stimulate growth of more fastidious organisms.

Semidefined Media

Small amounts (from 0.05 to 0.5 per cent) of single vegetable or meat extracts or preparations added to chemically defined media result in semidefined culture media. For growth and screening of a large number of micro-organisms, semirefined media can serve as more generally applicable standard media. Yeast extract, meat peptones, soya peptones, malt extract, casein hydrolysates, and corn steep liquor are some of the most common and useful additives.

Small amounts of these organic nutrients supply growth factors and vitamins that often enhance growth for a variety of micro-organisms quite significantly compared to the completely defined medium, without greatly complicating reaction analysis.

Complex Media

Most of the nutrients in complex media are provided by extracts or enzyme digests of plant and animal products. The importance of reproducibility and ease of analysis and interpretation make complex media rarely the best choice for biotransformation. Of course, the use of pregrown resting-cell or dried-cell preparations in simple aqueous or nonaqueous reaction media largely alleviates these concerns.

A list of culture media used in biotransformations has been compiled. Representative recipes are given below for convenience.

Defined medium

1. Carbon source, 2 grams; ammonium sulphate, 1 gram; dipotassium phosphate, 1 gram; salt solution A, 10 ml; distilled H_2O_2, 990 ml. Adjust medium to pH 7.0 before autoclaving.
2. Salts solution A: magnesium sulphate·$7H_2O$, 25 grams; ferrous sulphate·$7H_2O$, 2.8 grams; manganous sulphate·H_2O, 1.7 gram; sodium chloride, 0.6 gram; calcium chloride·$2H_2O$, 0.1 gram; sodium molybdate $2H_2O$, 0.1 gram; zinc sulphate·$7H_2O$, 0.06 gram; HCl (0.1 M), 1 litre.

Complex biotransformation or maintenance media

1. Nutrient broth: beef extract, 3.0 grams; peptone, 5.0 grams; distilled H_2O, 1.0 litre; pH 6.8 after autoclaving.
2. Sabouraud dextrose (or maltose) broth/agar: neopeptone, 10 grams; glucose (or maltose), 40 grams; distilled H_2O, 1 litre; pH 5.7 before autoclaving.

3. Glucose, 20 grams; soyabean meal (or soya flour), 5 grams; yeast extract, 5 grams; sodium chloride, 5 grams; potassium phosphate, dibasic, 5 grams; distilled H_2O, 1 litre. Adjust to pH 7 with 6 N HCl.

4. Corn steep liquor (60 per cent solids), 20 grams; glucose, 10 grams; tap H_2O, 1 litre. Adjust to pH 4.9.

REACTIONS IN SOLVENT MIXTURES

The use of organic solvents or aqueous/organic solvent mixtures as media for biocatalytic reactions using enzymes or suspended cells is a powerful and often necessary modification. From a practical, synthetic perspective, reactions in nonaqueous media provide three primary advantages: the ability to shift the thermodynamic equilibrium of hydrolytic reaction toward synthesis, the ability to solubilise a broad range of organic molecules at synthetically useful concentrations, and the ability to rapidly separate soluble reaction products from the insoluble biocatalyst. The inclusion of organic solvents may also minimise certain side reactions and permit continuous extraction and recovery of reaction products. Much has been presented in the literature about other advantages of nonaqueous solvents, including improved thermostability, altered specificity, or decreased chance of contamination, which are of more limited applicability.

The primary difficulty with conducting biotransformations in the presence of organic solvents is lower catalytic activity and catalyst stability. Substantial literature is devoted to determining reasons for loss of catalytic activity and methods for preventing it. A complete description is well beyond the scope of the present work but is available from many excellent reviews. In many cases, the practice of nonaqueous biocatalysis, widely regarded as untenable less than 20 years ago, is today a successful reality. Practical guidelines for conducting biocatalytic reactions in the presence of organic solvents will be the focus here.

The behaviour of whole-cell biocatalysts in the presence of organic solvents is somewhat distinct from that of isolated enzyme catalysts and will be treated separately. Salter and Kell offer an excellent review of activity preservation and solvent toxicity of whole-cell-catalysed reactions in organic solvents. Much is still unknown about mechanisms for whole-cell solvent tolerance, owing to the complex nature of the living cell, and some individual strains exhibit large deviations from general trends. Empirically, however, several general recommendations can be made.

First, although no single solvent property has been definitively correlated to solvent tolerance, cell biocatalysts (both growing and resting) tend to maintain higher activity for a longer period with solvents of high hydrophobicity (normally expressed as solvent octanol/water partition coefficient, $\log P$). Solvents with $\log P > +4 - 5$ tend to make the most compatible media, while solvents of intermediate hydrophobicity ($\log P = 0$ to 4) are often most toxic. Water-immiscible solvents are much better choices for bulk organic phase than are water-miscible ones. In general, cell immobilisation, usually by entrapment or encapsulation, significantly improves organic solvent tolerance while permitting substrate access to the catalyst. In contrast to the behaviour of isolated enzymes in predominantly nonaqueous environments, whole cells often exhibit decreased thermotolerance, and reactions are often more favourably run at lower temperatures than usual for a given strain.

While hydrophobic solvents are biocompatible media for reactions with hydrophobic substrates, such as steroids, many organic molecules of interest are of intermediate polarity and are not highly soluble in either nonpolar solvents or aqueous media. In many of these cases, the use of small quantities of a 'good solvent' in either the organic or aqueous phase will provide successful reaction conditions.

The incorporation of organic 'carrier solvents', such as DMSO, DMF, or ethanol in final concentrations of <5 per cent is one very important form of this strategy. Likewise, the addition of a toxic solvent with good solvating power to a biocompatible, hydrophobic bulk solvent can provide the positive attributes of both. The biocompatible solvent extracts the toxic one away from the catalyst, yielding an organic phase capable of holding a suitable concentration of reactant molecules.

Isolated enzymes tend to exhibit much better retention of catalytic activity in the presence of organic solvents than whole cells. This is likely due to the lack of a cell membrane and other cellular substructures that are likely targets for general solvent toxicity. Like whole cells, enzymes tend generally to prefer more hydrophobic solvents with log P values >2 – 4 but tolerate a much broader range of solvents and solvent mixtures than do whole-cell catalysts. Polar solvents such as THF (tetrahydrofuran), acetonitrile, *tert*-amyl alcohol, methyl tert-butyl ether, and monglyme preserve adequate catalytic activity of many enzyme catalysts.

As mentioned previously, however, general rules for nonaqueous biocatalysis are rare; indeed, some highly tolerant whole-cell strains, such as pseudomonads may serve as excellent recombinant hosts for nonaqueous biocatalysts, while important enzyme catalysts, such as cytochromes P-450, exhibit a low tolerance even to minor levels of organic carrier solvents. Thus, the most prudent strategy at present is to screen an abbreviated list of good candidate organic solvents with each chosen biocatalyst.

In summary, to be considered general catalysts on par with other, traditional chemical catalysts for organic synthesis, biocatalysts must be functional in a fair range of organic solvents. Practically, many organic molecules of interest for transformation have limited solubility in aqueous media, or in the highly lipophilic solvents most often described in the literature for use with biocatalysts. Moreover, thermodynamic control of normally hydrolysis-favouring equilibria, ease of product recovery, and minimisation of certain side reactions are also important motivations for conducting biocatalytic reactions in organic media. Over the last 10 to 15 years, significant strides have been made toward making practical, synthetic biocatalysis feasible.

ADDITION OF ORGANIC COMPOUNDS TO REACTION MIXTURES

Most organic chemical reactions are run in nonaqueous solvents. Since microbial growth and biological reactions typically take place in aqueous environments, there is a natural tendency to restrict biotransformation reactions to aqueous media, and therefore to water-soluble organic substrates. In fact, biotransformations occur equally well with both lipophilic and hydrophilic substrates as long as an adequate concentration of reactants can be delivered to the biocatalyst. More directly, the key to success with biotransformations of lipophilic compounds is the enhancement of substrate availability to the active site of the appropriate enzyme.

It is generally assumed that access to the active site of microbial enzymes is possible only for compounds dissolved or dispersed in the reaction medium. An examination of growth rates of bacteria using poorly water-soluble hydrocarbons as their carbon source illustrates this point. Bacteria grown on naphthalene, phenanthrene, or anthracene have generation times of 1.5, 10.5, and 29 hours, respectively. These growth rates are directly proportional to the water solubilities of the hydrocarbons but independent of the total amount of solid substrate present. For whole-cell reactions, once contact with the cell occurs, substrates can penetrate the cell wall and membrane by passive or active transport. Cell surfaces and membranes, as well as enzymes themselves, have hydrophobic domains that facilitate transport, binding, and reaction with lipophilic compounds. In addition, micro-organisms produce a variety of endogenous emulsifiers that promote these reactions.

Thus, several methods have been developed to improve the solubility and dispersion of reactants in water. As we just discussed, one strategy is to conduct the biotransformation in bulk organic solvent media. Another successfully practiced approach is the delivery and dispersion of lipophilic substrates through chemical agents or physical methods that have a minimal impact on the bulk aqueous reaction medium.

Organic Carrier Solvents

The most common method for adding water-insoluble substrates to a bulk aqueous reaction medium is in water-miscible organic carrier solvents. Preferably, these solvents should have low toxicity to the biocatalyst and excellent solvation capacity. Common carriers include many of the same solvents used for organic compound transfer and storage, such as DMSO, DMF, ethanol, methanol, and acetone.

In a typical application of this strategy, the organic compound is dissolved in dry DMF (stored over molecular sieves) at a 20- to 100-fold higher concentration than desired in the reaction. Dissolution may be hastened by gentle treatment with a sonifier for a few seconds. If necessary, the substrate stock should be sterilised by filtration (with a solvent-resistant cartridge filter) before addition to the medium. Concentrated substrate solution is then added to incubation mixtures at the required level by sterile pipette. A milky precipitate forms instantly as the DMF mixes with the aqueous medium. To prevent reaggregation of the substrate and to ensure even distribution, each flask or vessel should be shaken immediately upon addition of substrate stock.

This technique works with most water-miscible solvents. Since many hygroscopic organic solvents lose solvent power as they take up water, they should be kept dry. As a case in point, a small amount of water in DMF greatly reduces the capacity of this excellent solvent. The use of these carrier agents is also exceptionally well tolerated by most microbial strains and isolated enzymes. However, there are some exceptions. For example, microsomal cytochrome P-450 enzymes tolerate only very low levels (<1 per cent) of organic carrier solvents. Thus, additional strategies for compound delivery must sometimes also be considered.

A good empirical comparison of appropriate protocols for lipophilic substrate delivery to biocatalysts is offered by Lee and coworkers. They examined in detail the aggregation and solubilisation phenomena of steroid substrates. A mixed culture of *Arthrobacter simplex* and *Curvularia lunata* catalysed the simultaneous 1-dehydrogenation and 11β-hydroxylation of 16-α-hydroxycortexolone-16,17-acetonide. Substrate was prepared: (i) as a suspension in cold solvent, (ii) in 0.1 per cent (wt/vol) aqueous Tween 80 surfactant, and (iii) as solutions in hot and cold solvents. The substrates were added to the cultures immediately after preparation and again 25 hours later. Best yields (60 to 90 per cent) were obtained with hot solvents and cold DMF. Yields were related to the particle size of the substrate. Hot solvents gave dispersions with 0.5- to 2-μm particles; those from cold solvents ranged from 10 to 100 μm. Apparently, ultrafine, amorphous particles are more accessible to enzyme active sites than crystalline forms. This may be due to improved rates of compound dissolution and improved cell permeability.

Additional vehicles can be used to solubilise substrates and improve cell permeability. For instance, Chien and Rosazza used polyvinylpyrrolidones (PVPs) to enhance the hydroxylation of ellipticine by *Aspergillus alliaceus*. This brilliant yellow alkaloid is barely soluble in water (<5 mg/l), but solutions of 30 per cent PVP (40,000 average molecular weight) gave the highest initial water solubilities of ellipticine, and the solubility increased proportionately with the concentration of PVP (60 grams of PVP per litre solubilised 100 mg of ellipticine per litre). At that concentration, yields of hydroxylated ellipticines were doubled.

PVP disperses many types of aromatic compounds in aqueous media by formation of coprecipitates. The aromatic substrate and PVP 40,000 are dissolved in chloroform-methanol (9:1), and the mixture is evaporated to dryness in a rotary evaporator. Ratios of aromatic compound to PVP of 1:5 up to 1:120 should be used. To prepare concentrated solutions or dispersions, suspend compounds in 10 to 30 per cent solutions of PVP 40,000 by grinding them together with a glass mortar and pestle. Cyclodextrins also enhance solubilities of water-insoluble substrates, and their uses in small-scale reactions have been documented.

Nakamatsu evaluated the influence of surfactants on the oxidation of sterols by *Nocardia corallina*. The bioconversions of substrates dispersed with several different surfactants were compared with the performance of substrates sonicated to reduce their particle size. Cationic, nonionic, and anionic surfactants were used at 0.01 per cent concentration. Two cationic detergents and one nonionic detergent significantly, inhibited cell growth. Most nonionic surfactants did not inhibit growth and provided good emulsification. Emal 10C, Emulbon T-83, Sorbon T-40, and Tween 80 surfactants stimulated the oxidation of soya sterols.

Inert supports may be used to adsorb or dissolve a variety of compounds within the lattices of inert materials, such as zeolites, molecular sieves, diatomaceous earth, and polymers such as divinylbenzene-polystyrene. The resulting ultrafine particle sizes and large surface areas promote a high degree of dispersion of lipophilic substrates. Adsorbed substrates are remarkably available to biocatalysts. Liquid paraffins are adsorbed to the supports from solvent solutions. After evaporation of the solvent, bound compounds are added directly to incubation mixtures.

A physical milling and wetting method has been used effectively to disperse steroids such as progesterone, as follows. USP-grade progesterone was ground with a Jet-O-Mizer model 202 grinder (Fluid Energy Processing and Equipment Co., Philadelphia, Pa.) to a fine particle size of about one-third the density of the starting material. The ground progesterone was added to 250-ml Erlenmeyer flasks wetted with suitable amounts of 0.01 per cent aqueous Tween 80 surfactant, and sterilised by exposure to steam at atmospheric pressure for about 30 minutes. By this technique, 20 to 50 grams of steroid substrate was dispersed per litre in the aqueous fermentation medium, and yields of the hydroxylated product were 60 to 90 per cent.

Gases, volatile solvents, and other compounds with high vapour pressure are relatively simple to handle in small fermentors and other types of bioreactors, except for the danger of explosions. Gases and other volatile substances can be carried into vessels along with sterile air. Air that is bubbled over the surface of a volatile solid or through a liquid, like toluene, will carry the compound into the reaction mixture. Enclosed incubator-shakers are the best way to handle volatile compounds and gases in shake-flask reactions. Extreme care must be taken to avoid the accumulation of explosive mixtures. For a small number of flasks, individual spargers or a gas manifold could be used.

Timing of Substrate Additions

When growing cells are used for biotransformations, the time of addition of the organic substrate profoundly influences the yield of product. Toxic substances, such as many antibiotics and antitumour compounds, often inhibit growth and enzyme production if they are added early in the growth cycle. In many cases, however, it is advantageous to add at least small amounts of substrate at the beginning of the growth phase to promote enzyme induction. The addition of substrate during the late logarithmic growth phase minimises toxicity effects while promoting enzyme induction. At this point in their growth cycle, cells are still capable of enzyme synthesis, while the proliferation of the biomass is less inhibitable by toxic substrates. The same reasoning applies to substrates added in toxic solvents.

The timing of substrate addition must take into account the physiological state of the micro-organism. The position of the cell in its growth cycle determines its enzyme capabilities, and, in general, enzyme levels will be determined by the competing rates of enzyme expression and degradation/inactivation. Enzymes of interest may be expressed only at specific times during the growth cycle, such as late log or stationary growth phases.

Looking for reaction when the enzyme is not present would be futile. Enzyme concentration may be subject to the presence of inducers of expression, fluctuations in the pH or temperature of the medium, the amount and kinds of carbon and nitrogen nutrients in the medium, and the degree of oxygenation of the medium. The optimal time for substrate addition is difficult to predict and is best determined experimentally.

Toxic substrates or substrates in toxic solvents may be added incrementally by 'dosing'. The addition of progesterone semicontinuously to growing *Aspergillus ochraceus* cultures minimises toxicity as well as the mechanical loss of starting material through aggregation. Unexpectedly, fewer side reactions occur. Lee used a dosing technique to obtain 38 g/litre of β-hydroxy-β-methylbutyric acid from the substrate β-methylbutyric acid, which was toxic to the *Galactomyces reesii*. Dosing techniques also sidestep the undesirable phenomenon of substrate inhibition, which almost invariably occurs when large amounts of substrate are added at a single time. The effect tends to be most prominent with water-soluble materials, but well-disposed lipids display the same phenomenon.

EQUIPMENT

Erlenmeyer flasks on shakers have been the traditional reactors for aerobic culturing. For screening, the smaller sizes (50 to 250 ml) are recommended. Larger flasks (up to 2 litres) are convenient for scaled-up experiments. At this size, 2.8 litres femback flasks are used frequently. Normally, only 10 to 20 per cent of the volume of the flask is filled with medium, since this allows for maximum agitation and aeration without splashing or excessive evaporation. Sterile closure of the flasks, while permitting gas transfer, is essential. Cotton and plastic foam plugs are widely used, but cotton-gauze filter disks are better; these are held in place by stainless-steel springs or rubber bands. Flasks with flush necks (DeLong flasks) are closed with special stainless-steel or plastic caps. Petri dishes about 100 mm in diameter and sterile, cotton-plugged pipettes are routinely used. From the standpoint of housekeeping in the laboratory, sterile, disposable labware is very convenient.

Incubators and Shakers

Bioconversion experiments require some form of temperature-controlled environment. Incubators that control temperatures from below ambient temperature to 50°C or higher are available in benchtop sizes up to full-room size.

The value of shakers in fermentation experimentation is well known. It is important to have the capability for shaking aerobic organisms, as this is an economical and practical way to screen a large number of cultures. The two common types of shakers are the rotary (or orbital) shaker and the reciprocal shaker. Shaking speeds are continuously adjustable from 0 to about 350 rotations or oscillations per minutes. Shakers range from desktop sizes to ones that can accommodate hundreds of 250-ml flasks. Reciprocal shakers are best for tube cultures, and orbital shakers are best for flasks. With either type, different platforms are available for holding various sizes of flasks. It is generally important, however, to mate the stroke length of the shaker with the diameter of the vessel.

Sterilisers (Autoclaves)

Steam sterilisers are essential for microbiological work. Culturing vessels and media must be sterilised. Automatic autoclaves with capacities for several hundred 250-ml flasks are generally used. For small-scale work, a desktop size or even a pressure cooker can be used.

Fermenters

Fermenters are useful for larger-scale biotransformations. Although the general sophistication of the devices has increased, the basic design of the vessel has not changed for many years. With a fermenter it is possible to control culture parameters in ways and degrees not possible in flasks and tubes. Stirring and air-sparging devices allow the maximum possible aeration. Many parameters (e.g. pH) can be measured and controlled continuously. Therefore, it is useful to have access to several benchtop fermenters (1 to 10 litres) for experiments that cannot be done conveniently in flasks and for scaling-up processes. Larger-scale fermenter studies (20 to 1000 litres) often involving sophisticated downstream processing will require cooperation with more specialised laboratories.

Microscale Conversions

Often, one is faced with a small quantity of precious organic compound and a large number of biocatalysts to screen for transformations. In these cases, microscale equipment should be used. Essentially, all of the protocols and guidelines mentioned above can be scaled down for individual fermentation volumes of less than 1 ml. However, several issues require additional consideration when working with small volumes in nontraditional fermentor geometries. Several considerations relate to the supply of oxygen to microfermentors. As mentioned before, the shaker stroke should also be short, consistent with the reaction vessel diameter, to ensure adequate agitation. Because of the gross morphology of some microbial strains, the small fermentor dimensions may result in significant surface effects and poor mass transfer. As a result, resting cells and immobilised or soluble isolated enzymes may be more appropriate and reproducible catalysts for microscale applications. To reduce heterogeneity in resting-cell preparations, an efficient cell homogeniser, used in short bursts on ice, is an important tool.

Microscale experiments will also require micropipettes able to handle 1- to 10-µl volumes of test compound stock or analytical aliquots. With less reaction sample available, sensitive analytical techniques providing more information per analysis should be favoured. Finally, care should be taken to prevent evaporation of the small reaction volumes by sealing the reactions or saturating the reaction headspace with reaction medium.

AUTOMATION

Biotransformations, especially involving whole cells, can be labour-intensive. The repetition involved with reproducibly preparing, inoculating, adding test compound to, monitoring, sampling, and, working-up a large number of cultures and reactions encourages the consideration of automated equipment to speed the process and reduce tedium and human error. However, sterility requirements and the vast morphological, growth rate, and medium differences between strains greatly complicates the task of automation. For these reasons, automated culturing has been applied when only one or a few strains need to be accommodated in an automated process, such as for screening large numbers of recombinant mutants, testing for specific pathogens, or processing host cell lines for genomic studies. However, commercially available automated equipment can also greatly facilitate the processing of samples from biotransformations, since sterility becomes a minor issue after the biocatalytic reaction is complete.

STANDARDISATION, QUALITY CONTROL, AND QUALITY ASSURANCE

As established earlier, screening biocatalysts typically requires the execution and evaluation of large numbers of individual reactions. Therefore, once reliable and efficient biocatalyst reaction protocols have been established, the best improvement in the frequency of identifying new biotransformations comes from improving the throughput, sensitivity, and interpretation of reaction analysis.

Prerequisite for most high-efficiency analytical methods is the development of rapid, parallel methods for the preparation of samples for analysis; catalyst removal, macromolecule (protein, polysaccharide, polynucleotide, etc.) removal, and/or solvent exchange can be important steps prior to reliable use of many analytical techniques described below. Useful in this regard are the wide variety of filtration, ultrafiltration, liquid-liquid extraction, and solid-phase adsorption products that are now commercially available. Multicartridge manifold and 96-well-plate-based techniques are particularly increasing in popularity owing to the large number of samples that can be processed simultaneously with automated liquid handlers or manually. The best analytical method may be different for different lead molecules and different objectives. However, for almost all high-throughput screening studies, thin-layer chromatography (TLC), gas chromatography (GC), and high performance liquid chromatography (HPLC) have been the proven workhorses. Improvements in laboratory scale mass spectrometry (MS) equipment, however, have made MS an important addition to the biotransformation practitioner's repertoire, either in direct flow injection mode or in tandem with other analytical techniques (e.g. LC/MS).

Thin-Layer Chromatography (TLC)

Traditionally, thin-layer chromatography has been the primary method for analysis of biotransformations. TLC is well suited for this work because it is an inexpensive method for parallel analysis and, thus, can be used to analyse a large number of reaction samples simultaneously. TLC is also simple to set up; the basic apparatus includes developing chambers, common laboratory solvents, and chromatography plates with various absorbents that can be prepared directly in the laboratory or are available commercially.

The theory and techniques of TLC are discussed in detail in several excellent texts. Silica gel, alumina, kieselguhr, and cellulose are the most commonly used absorbents and have a wide range of properties that can be altered to suit the particular need by pretreatment with acids, bases, buffers, or specific reagents (e.g. $AgNO_3$). A suitable solvent system will depend on the nature of the compounds to be separated. However, established procedures are available for a large number of organic compounds.

TLC can work very well as an initial screen if a sensitive, and preferably specific, indicator reagent is available for visualising reaction components. It may also be an excellent technique if degradation or conversion of the test substrate is the primary endpoint. However, its application to highly polar compounds can be complicated if they cannot be simply extracted from an aqueous reaction into a volatile organic solvent. Moreover, improvements in equipment and methodology for other, higher-resolution and more informative techniques, such as HPLC and MS; have made them increasingly attractive for the rapid characterisation of reaction products.

Gas Chromatography (GC)

Gas chromatography is another commonly applied tool for analysis of biotransformation mixtures. GC typically permits rapid separation of any compounds that are volatile or that can be derivatised to a volatile substance. Although, it is a serial analysis technique, separations are typically rapid (3 to 20 minutes). Sample introduction and data processing are typically automated on most modern equipment, further accelerating the analytical process. Furthermore, when these instruments are used in combination with

MS, detailed structural analyses of many samples can be obtained. Separation by GC is achieved by partitioning of the analytes between a mobile gas phase and a liquid or solid adsorbant stationed in the column. Retention times of compounds on particular columns at specified temperatures and gas flow allow characterisation of the compounds. Many stationary-phase-column chemistries are commercially available for high-resolution separations of structurally similar derivatives, and in some cases even enantiomers.

GC permits rapid analysis of microlitre quantities of sample with high resolution. The method can be quantitative or qualitative, it is highly sensitive (parts per billion), it is simple to operate, and it can be combined conveniently with MS. However, like TLC, GC usually requires extraction of the reaction mixture into a volatile organic solvent for application to the column. More important, many nonvolatile, functionalised organic compounds or thermally labile compounds are poorly analysed by GC; for analysis of unanticipated products of biotransformation screens, these limitations can be undesirable. Nonetheless, for many volatile test substrates, GC is the method of choice.

High Performance Liquid Chromatography (HPLC)

High performance liquid chromatography (HPLC) methods have the advantage of providing detailed analytical information for a very broad range of substrate molecules (and their derivatives). Analogous with GC, resolution in HPLC is achieved by partitioning of analytes between a mobile liquid and a solid adsorbant. The general versatility of HPLC methods makes them very attractive for analysis of biotransformation screens. HPLC analyses are not limited by the molecular weight, volatility, thermal stability, or organic extractability of test compounds and derivatives. Moreover, a wide variety of high-resolution separation columns with different solid-phase chemistries and analyte detection methods are commercially available. However, typical analysis times of 15 to 45 minutes per sample for a serial analytical technique have limited the use of HPLC for biotransformation screening from large biocatalyst collections. Recently, very rapid, high-throughput HPLC methods have been described for the analysis of large libraries produced by combinatorial chemistry or natural product discovery. These approaches also apply 'universal' gradients of acetonitrile (or methanol) with water to extract from a nonpolar (octyl or octyldecyl) solid phase to separate a broad diversity of compound classes. Automated instruments allow the convenient processing of many samples. Such approaches have also been adapted for general application to biotransformation screening. Several hundreds to thousands of injections a day, yielding resolution adequate for biocatalyst screening, can be performed using 1- to 10-minute run times. Proper sample preparation, however, is more critical; sharp solvent gradients at high column pressures on high-efficiency, small-particle-size packed columns result in a higher susceptibility to plugging with microbial debris or precipitated proteins.

As described below HPLC is highly compatible for both analytical and preparative work; analytical methods may be extended for the preparation of adequate quantities of products for structural determination by nuclear magnetic resonance (NMR) or for other characterisation. Recent advances in HPLC with direct NMR detection of the eluant are notable for providing the promise of immediate structural characterisation of biotransformation products, but this method is currently cost-effective for only a limited number of postscreening biotransformation analyses.

Mass Spectrometry (MS)

Traditionally, mass spectrometry (MS) has been a useful method for confirmation of a biotransformation product, most commonly used in tandem with GC separation during later stages of biotransformation product characterisation. MS provides a spectrum of molecular weights of the parent molecule, and of submolecular fragments, that help identify the nature of a transformation and its position on the test compound. Improvements in 'soft' methods for nondestructive compound ionisation from liquid samples have recently transformed MS into a more powerful tool for high-throughput direct analysis, as well as general characterisation of analytes eluting from GC or HPLC columns. In direct injection mode, MS can deliver specific molecular weight information that can identify products in less than 1 minute per sample. Information can be gleaned even from relatively crude samples from a reaction mixture, although impurities may interfere by suppressing ionisation of the desired analytes. Even more powerful is a connection of MS with GC or HPLC separations, as this allows two-dimensional resolution of complex samples (initially by chromatographic retention time, then by mass). Especially coupled with high-throughput separation methods described above, HPLC/MS yields a broadly applicable, rapid analysis (~5 minutes per sample) giving an unparalleled degree of information.

Depending upon the test compound, different ionisation interfaces may be most appropriate for introduction of a sample or chromatography column stream to MS. Typically, chemical ionisation represents a good interface for smaller, and less functionalised analytes, while electrospray offers a better ion source for more polar and functionalised organic test compounds and products.

After ionisation of the sample, there are a number of alternative designs for separation and detection of molecular species by weight. From the perspective of biotransformation analysis, commercially available quadrapole, triple quadrapole, ion trap, and time-of-flight instruments have relatively minor distinctions in analysis time, sensitivity, versatility, ruggedness, and cost that are beyond the scope of this review.

The advantages of MS analysis include broad applicability, high sensitivity, large information content, relative ease of interpretation, and very small volumes of sample required. By itself, however, MS does not provide accurate quantitative information on yields. And although equipment costs are decreasing rapidly, MS remains a very expensive and technically demanding tool, especially in comparison with techniques such as TLC.

Thus, careful consideration of analytical strategies for biotransformation analysis is very important, especially in the common case when a large number of biocatalysts and several test compounds result in a considerable number of analyses to be performed. Analysis and interpretation can easily be the most time- and labour-consuming step of the process and an important one, since undetected or unidentified products are lost, along with the work to produce them. For convenient initial screening for major transformations or degradation, TLC is a proven, cost-effective, efficient parallel technique. GC and HPLC can be more informative but are more expensive to run and will typically require more time per sample. MS and GC or HPLC/MS are very expensive but will likely give the most information per unit time and the greatest level and clarity of information. Selection of the best methods will ultimately depend on the type of test compounds and expected products, number of samples, time and resources available, stage of the biotransformation development, degree of information needed, and cost of missed information.

OPTIMISATION PROCEDURES

To obtain enough product for identification and further testing, preliminary optimisation studies may be necessary. Yields can be improved substantially by systematic studies of environmental and nutritional parameters. Such studies are of use in scaling up the process.

Environmental Parameters

Changes in temperature can drastically affect biocatalytic reactions. The temperature should be varied between 20° and 50°C for mesophilic organisms and enzymes. Large differences in yields can occur with a 1° or 2°C difference in temperature, as demonstrated with the bioconversion of isobutyric acid to L-(+)-3-hydroxybutyric acid by stationary-phase cells of *Pseudomonas putida*. The optimum temperature for growth of cells may well be different from the optimum for biocatalysis. Resting cells, stationary-phase cells, and even enzyme preparations frequently perform well at high temperatures.

It is difficult to study the effect of changes in pH in small-scale flask cultures. Systematic pH variations studies with growing cultures should be done in small fermentors where pH can be controlled automatically. With enzyme reactions or resting-cell reactions, the selection of appropriate, non-inhibitory buffers is important. A pH stat may be useful to study reactions that produce pH changes.

Aerobic organisms require oxygen for growth. It may be difficult to achieve optimum growth in shaken flasks because almost always, as cultures proliferate, oxygen becomes the growth-limiting factor. The medium is easily saturated with oxygen at the beginning of growth. However, rapid cell growth during the logarithmic phase depletes oxygen faster than it can be dissolved in the medium. As growth slows toward late log phase, oxygen levels rise. Even in highly aerated vessels, rapidly growing cultures can reduce medium dissolved oxygen concentrations to zero. In culture flasks, the efficiency of aeration is determined by the shape of the flask, the volume of liquid it contains, the type of shaking (reciprocal or orbital), the gaseous environment, culture medium composition, the type of flask closure, and ambient conditions.

Oxygen is also a substrate in many important biocatalytic reactions, such as aromatic hydroxylation, N dealkylation, O dealkylation, and sulphur oxidation. These reactions are catalysed by monooxygenases, dioxygenases, and other enzymes that activate molecular oxygen. The dynamics of medium oxygenation are important to all these types of biotransformations, whether the reactions are performed with growing cells, dried cells, or enzyme preparations.

A few simple rules can be used to obtain the best aeration in shaken flasks. Maximum aeration is attained when the liquid volume is not more than 20 per cent of total flask volume. Shaking rates should be high but adjusted so that splashing is not excessive. Rates of 100 to 250 rpm, depending on the flask size, are usually best. For larger flasks, baffles improve aeration efficiency.

Aeration rates achieved in culture media can be defined in terms of oxygen absorption rates (OAR). OAR is defined as millimoles of oxygen absorbed per litre of solution per minute. The OAR of any vessel incubated under any condition can be determined by iodometric titration, which measures the amount of sodium sulphite oxidised by molecular oxygen.

The OAR varies with the type of aeration used. By far the best aeration is achieved with stirred and sparged fermentors. Shaking is essential to achieve reasonable aeration with flasks or tubes. Typical OAR values are: (i) 0.27 for 100 ml of medium and 0.60 for 50 ml of medium in 500-ml conical flasks shaken at 250 rpm, and (ii) 2.0 in a 20-litre fermenter with a sparger operated at 250 rpm.

In modern fermentors, the measurement of dissolved oxygen is done with oxygen electrodes. When procedures are scaled up from shake-flask cultures to fermenters, it is important to increase OAR values as much as possible.

Nutritional Parameters

A discussion of the nutritional improvement of processes is given already in this chapter. Generally, the components of the culture medium should be tested for effect one at a time, if possible. Sampling times for monitoring the effect on biocatalytic reactions should be arranged to account for possible changes in growth kinetics. Variations in medium components should be checked in the order of their decreasing concentration. Concentrations and types of the carbon sources should be evaluated first by using different sources at the same concentration, then at different concentrations. Carbon sources to compare include glucose, other carbohydrates, and glycerol. Citric acid cycle intermediates are good candidates, as are pyruvate and acetate. Combinations of carbon sources can be effective for improvement of cell growth and enzyme induction and for diminishing catabolite repression of enzyme expression.

After carbon, the next most abundant nutrient is the nitrogen source. The first nitrogen compounds to compare are the simple organic salts, ammonium sulphate, ammonium nitrate, and potassium nitrate. Afterward, urea, glutamate, asparagine, and glutamine should be tested, then the various complex nitrogen sources such as yeast extracts, peptones, and tryptones. Combinations of inorganic salts may then be tried, followed by vitamins, purines and pyrimidines, amino acids, sulphur and phosphorus sources, and the various required inorganic salts and trace elements.

EXAMPLES OF TYPICAL BIOCONVERSION PROCEDURES: PULLING IT ALL TOGETHER

As should be evident, biotransformation is an interdisciplinary field involving microbiology, biochemistry, organic chemistry, analytical chemistry, and engineering. An appreciation for the contributions of all these fields is very important for the successful application of biotransformations. However, a complete understanding of all of these fields is not a prerequisite for success if the practical guidelines arising from these disciplines are recognised and followed.

To help illustrate the successful practice of biotransformation, the following examples serve as model solutions for some typical situations encountered when applying biocatalysis to organic compounds.

Aerobic Screening

Of central importance for microbial transformations is a basic, general strain-screening method for checking the activity of large numbers of micro-organisms on large numbers of compounds. For the first screening experiments, the protocol should be simple so that many samples can be processed. With a long history in the literature, the most reliable procedures involve a two- or three-stage incubation. During the first stage, the culture is grown to late logarithmic phase in a rich medium to provide a heavy inoculum for the second stage. The compounds to be screened are added to the growing second-stage culture when it has reached near-maximum growth. Alternatively, if nongrowing cells are desired, the second-stage culture is prepared by using small amounts of known inducers or substrate to raise desired enzyme activities. The fully grown second-stage cell mass is then processed (e.g. made resting, dried, permeabilised, or immobilised) for use as catalyst in a third stage, in which the compound to be transformed is added immediately. Reaction progress should be monitored occasionally from approximately 6 hours up to 1 week using work-up and analytical techniques of suitable throughput and sensitivity to indicate which catalysts convert the substrate.

For improved efficiency, the first screen can be done with few controls: the similar reaction setup for multiple biocatalysts should act as internal controls. However, to confirm presumed transformation products, initial optimisation of the most promising biocatalysts must be done with suitable controls. Controls should include cultures without substrate and substrates without micro-organisms in sterile medium and in buffers at pH 3, 6, and 8 to account for the range of pH typically observed in cultures. Following screening, biocatalysts that produce even very low yields of desired products can be optimised by using the procedures described above.

By incorporating slight variations, this general procedure can be used to screen for biotransformation reactions using different forms of microbial biocatalysts and, when appropriate, different reaction environments. Some examples of typical modifications are described below.

Microscale Screening of Resting Cells

A good example of the screening of resting cells in a microscale format is given by Semba. The objective was to identify microbial catalysts with efficient *para* hydroxylation activity on aromatic substrates. After an initial growth stage that isolated 23,400 strains from soil, colonies were regrown and induced on a solid medium. Each grown strain was transferred to separate wells of a microplate containing 50 µl of buffer, phenol as a probe substrate for the reaction, and glucose as an electron donor for the biocatalyst. A rapid dye indicator of the transformation of phenol to hydroquinone identified 1263 biocatalysts with the desired activity.

Permeabilised Cells

Cell permeabilisation procedures are a good solution if substrate transport through a cell membrane is likely to be poor and use of an isolated enzyme is impractical. As an illustration, D-malate is a rare isomer of malic acid in nature that may be produced by the conversion of the cheap bulk chemical maleic acid with maleate hydratase. Normal intact microbial cells do not catalyse the hydration reaction, and the pure enzyme is unstable. To overcome these difficulties, permeabilised cells were developed and analysed versus pure maleate hydratase. *Pseudomonas pseudoalcaligenes* was cultivated (200 litres) using a mineral salts medium containing yeast extract and 3-hydroxybenzoate. Cells harvested by centrifugation (251 grams) were suspended in 1.5 litres of 50 mM potassium phosphate buffer, pH 7, and incubated with 1 per cent Triton X-100 for 0.5 minute before being frozen at $-80°C$ for bioconversion studies. Enantiomerically pure (ee [enantiomeric excess] 99.97 per cent) D-malate could be produced using this permeabilised, nongrowing biocatalyst.

Permeabilised *Cephalosporium acremonium* cells were used to transform the antibiotic rifamycin S. A 10-ml reaction mixture containing 2.5 ml of cells, 0.5 mM rifamycin S, 0.5 mM NADH or NADPH, 1.5 mM MgCl, and 0.05 M phosphate buffer (pH 7.6) is incubated with shaking at 250 rpm and $288°C$ in an Erlenmeyer flask. The antibiotic is converted to the related rifamycins B and L by the permeabilised cells. The results compare favourably with those obtained with resting cells and cell-free preparations of *Nocardia mediterranei*.

Reductions with Yeast

Bioconversions catalysed by dried baker's yeast are some of the most commonly applied processes because of their simplicity and their utility for generating chiral centres. The asymmetric reduction of carbonyl compounds frequently occurs in good yield. The yeast powder is often rehydrated by simply mixing with a tap water reaction medium.

The only other required reagent is an ultimate electron donor, such as sugar, which serves to recycle yeast cell cofactors. Typically, a mixture containing substrate (10 grams), baker's yeast (100 grams), and sucrose (150 grams) in 800 ml of water can be incubated at room temperature for 1 to 2 days, after which it may be extracted with solvent such as ethyl acetate. Evaporation of the solvent leaves a residue that may be subjected to chromatography to obtain stereoselectively reduced product in high yields. By utilising a variety of available yeast catalysts, this general procedure can be used to reduce a broad range of carbonyl-containing compounds.

Catalysis with Dried Cells

Bioconversions with dried cells resemble the procedure for yeast cells. However, dried bacterial and fungal cells usually are not available commercially; they may be prepared as described earlier. 9α-Fluoro-16α-hydrocortisol (20 grams), acetone-dried cells of *A. simplex* (250 grams), phosphate buffer (pH 7.0, 0.1 M), and 2-methyl-1,4-naphthoquinone (3 grams) in 2.5 litres of water are agitated and aerated for 2 to 3 hours. Triamcinolone is obtained by $\Delta^{1,2}$-dehydrogenation 90 per cent yield. In this reaction, naphthoquinone serves as a hydrogen acceptor cofactor. Acetone-dried cells remain active for relatively long periods when stored in a refrigerator. These cells also may be used for nonaqueous solvent procedures.

Use of Metabolic Inhibitors

During screening experiments, micro-organisms frequently destroy compounds without the accumulation of recognisable products. Whole-cell biocatalysts contain many enzyme activities, which can result in undesirable side reactions or overmetabolism. The addition of metabolic inhibitors will stall utilisation of certain intermediates to allow for the accumulation of products.

This strategy is illustrated in the synthesis of derivatives of monensin, a structurally complex polyether antibiotic. Biosynthetic studies revealed that the compound derives from a variety of precursors and that epoxidases and hydroxylases participate in antibiotic formation. Meryrapone, a potent cytochrome P-450 inhibitor, was added (9 mM) to cultures of *Streptomyces cinnamonensis* to cause partial inhibition of monensin biosynthesis. The use of metyrapone selectively inhibited the cytochrome P-450-mediated hydroxylation of a 26-methyl group, resulting in the synthesis of a rare monensin analogue. As a result of inhibition, two new metabolites were obtained and designated 26-deoxymonensins A and B.

Another excellent example is the accumulation of a steroid intermediate in the presence of an iron chelator during the degradation of sterols by *A. simplex* and *N. corallina*. The addition of α,α'-dipyridyl (0.001 M), *o*-phenanthroline (0.0001 M), or 8-hydroxyquinoline (0.001 M) to logarithmic-growth-phase cultures with cholesterol as substrate causes the accumulation of androstadienedione by blocking the 9α-hydroxylase reaction that leads to complete destruction of the sterol. This procedure was first used to elucidate the pathway of sterol degradation in micro-organisms, but for economic reasons it is not the method of choice for large-scale androstadienedione production.

Blocked Mutants

Mutants blocked at various stages of a metabolic pathway accumulate isolable intermediates in their culture medium. Such mutants have been used for large-scale production of biotransformation products. The method can be laborious, since it involves the induction and selection of specifically blocked mutants. Coupled with enrichment culture techniques, the use of mutants is a powerful tool for producing biotransformation products of a wide variety of organic compounds. Thus, if it is possible to induce metabolic pathways for the degradation of a particular compound, it is reasonable to assume that mutants can be obtained that are blocked at points in this pathway, such that transformation products of the starting material will accumulate. Mutants have been used with great success for producing useful intermediates of sterol degradation, for example, with *Mycobacterium* species.

Solid Adsorbents

Solid adsorbents can be used when it is desired to maintain bulk substrate in a separate phase, owing to compound instability, toxicity, or for ease of handling. As an example, 3,4-methylene-dioxyphenyl acetone was stereoselectively reduced to S-3,4-methylenedioxyphenyl isopropanol in 95 per cent yield and 99.9 per cent enantiomeric excess by *Zygosaccharomyces rouxii.*

Both substrate and product were toxic to the biocatalyst, so polymeric hydrophobic resins such as XAD-7 were used to supply substrate to and remove product from the reaction mixture as it formed. Using the solid adsorbent increased yields from 6 to 40 g/litre, allowing 75 g/day to be produced in a 300-litre-scale reaction.

Practical Application of Biodegradation in Aromatic Desulphuration

Microbial biocatalysts are useful for complete or controlled degradation reactions, in addition to syntheses. As a case in point, *Rhodococcus* sp. strain IGTS8 is able to release inorganic sulphur from dibenzo-thiophene and other sulphur heterocyclic compounds in petroleum using a multienzyme pathway consisting of two monooxygenases and a desulphinase. Expression of the gene cluster coding for these enzymes is regulated by sulphate- and sulphur-containing amino acids.

This organism enzymatically oxidises the sulphur atom of dibenzothiophene to the sulphoxide, then to the sulphone, which hydrolyses to the sulphinate. Cleavage of the sulphur-carbon bond affords 2-hydroxybiophenyl and sulphate. Recombinant strains of this and other organisms are being used to desulphurise fuels.

Catalysis with Purified Enzymes

Commercially available enzymes are useful in preparative biocatalytic reactions. Often, enzyme-catalysed reactions are highly regioselective, stereoselective, or both. The use of an enzyme in a simple yet highly stereoselective synthetic reaction is illustrated by the use of pig liver esterase to produce a chiral monoester enantiomer by selective hydrolysis of the symmetrical diester, 3-methylglutaric acid, dimethyl ester. A 15-gram sample of the diester is suspended in 100 ml of 0.01 M phosphate buffer (pH 8.0), and 1000 U of pig liver esterase (Sigma) is added with vigorous stirring

The pH is kept constant by the addition of 1 N NaOH. After consumption of 1 mol equivalent of base (overnight), the mixture is homogeneous. The pH is adjusted to 9, and the reaction mixture is extracted with ether. Subsequent chemical treatment of the monoacid/monoester by reduction with borane-methyl sulphide complex of the free carboxyl group affords a hydroxyester that yields the R-six-membered lactone (90 per cent ee).

B-12 Synthesis by a Multienzyme Packed Column

The final example we offer illustrates the practical potential of biocatalysis for multistep fine organic synthesis. Roessner and coworkers cloned and expressed 12 separate enzymes used by nature for the biosynthesis of the complex core structure of vitamin B-12. Each enzyme catalyst was immobilised on Sepharose and packed together in a column reactor. A continuous feedstream of a readily available 5-carbon aminolevulinic acid precursor was transformed in 17 consecutive catalytic steps within the column to the 45-carbon 10-chiral-centre B-12 precursor hydrogenobyrnic acid. All reaction chemistries necessary for the synthesis were catalysed under identical, mild conditions on the benchtop, without intermediate purification, in >90 per cent yield per step and 50-mg scale. It must be pointed out that this synthesis was the culmination of about 25 years of development to discover and obtain every enzyme in catalytically active and pure form. However, it clearly illustrates the potential of biocatalysis for clean, efficient, mild, uniform, and selective synthetic processes, especially considering recent, vast improvements in molecular biology.

ENABLEMENT TECHNOLOGIES

Enablement technologies are already starting to make an impact on this promise for future development of biocatalysis. Through advances in molecular biology, new biocatalysts are being produced solely from their DNA and RNA blueprints. Using RNA extracted from environmental samples, many new enzymes have been made available by expressing PCR-amplified sequences in suitable generic microbial hosts. Shotgun cloning and the effort devoted to genomic sequencing are providing many more opportunities to make additional genes, and the encoded biocatalysts, accessible to the synthetic chemist. Building on this, *in vitro* evolution approaches, such as directed evolution and gene shuffling, permit the tailoring of enzymes for broader ranges of operation, higher efficiency, and new synthetic applications.

Additional processes are under development to take greater advantage of the synthetic potential of biocatalysis. Combinatorial biology attempts to engineer biosynthetic pathways within micro-organisms to create modified versions of commercially important natural products. Combinatorial biocatalysis purports to make a general synthetic platform for compound derivatisation by combining enzymatic, microbial, and chemical synthetic techniques.

Chapter 19

Bioremediation: An Advanced Strategy to Restore the Health of Aquaculture Pond Ecosystems

INTRODUCTION

Aquaculture is concerned with 'the propagation and rearing of aquatic organisms under complete human control, involving manipulation of at least one stage of an aquatic organism's life before harvest, in order to increase its production.'

Fish catches from the marine environment have been steadily declining in many parts of the world due to over-exploitation and pollution, making many people turn to aquaculture to improve food production and contribute to economic development. Aquaculture has made encouraging progress in the past two decades producing significant quantities of food, income and employment. Aquaculture, particularly of shrimp like *Penaeus monodon*, *Penaeus japonicus*, *Penaeus vannamei*, prawn like *Macrobrachium rosenbergii*, and various fish species, has been extensively practiced all along major water sources in Asia, the major contributor.

Increased production is being achieved by expansion of culture areas and use of modern methods. This development of aquaculture has led to not only severe disease problems, but also alteration of the quality of our natural habitats through increased effluent discharges from aquaculture systems, which contains high quantities of hitherto non-existent materials of both organic and inorganic forms.

Since recent past, it has been observed that the sustainable development of aquaculture sector can be achieved by adopting eco-friendly aquaculture practices, minimising impact on the surrounding environment. To maintain healthy ecosystem in aquaculture ponds and hatchery tanks, bioremediation is the best biotechnology process. Pathogens, as well as immunity suppressive agents, can be eliminated or minimised through bio-control process and hence can achieve good yield by maximising both survival and growth rates.

During the past 20 years, the aquaculture industry has been growing tremendously, especially that of marine fish, shrimps and bivalves, in addition to freshwater fish and prawn. Penaeid shrimps are among the most important and extensively cultured crustaceans in the world (>60 countries). In 2002, the world's shrimp farmers produced an estimated more than 1.0 MT of whole shrimp and feed mills around the world produced approximately 1.5 MT of shrimp feed.

Shrimp culture all over the world has been frequently affected by viral and bacterial diseases and annual losses due to disease have been estimated to be more than US$5 billion. Pathogenic micro-organisms implicated in these outbreaks were viruses, bacteria, algae, fungi and protozoan parasites. In addition, each year, globally, microbial pathogens cause millions of cases of food-borne disease and result in many hospitalisations and deaths.

Although diseases pose a serious threat to penaeid shrimp aquaculture, the production of these highly valued crustaceans continue to grow. For preventing and controlling diseases, particularly in aquaculture, the best method is improving the health of culture organisms and elimination of pathogens by improving the aquatic environment. In this respect, researchers have proved the use of probiotics in aquaculture to improve water quality by balancing bacterial population in water and reducing pathogenic bacterial load. Researchers are increasingly paying more attention to this new approach (ecological aquaculture), and have made considerable headway.

Competition for survival can be strong, even on a scale invisible to the human eye. Indeed, aquaculture pond bacteria — so small that 10,000 feet on a pinhead — are subject to the same law of evolution as that Darwin documented on the Galapagos, i.e. survival of the fittest or competitive exclusion. Competitive exclusion refers to one species out-competing another in a natural search for habitat dominance. As old as time, competitive exclusion is providing science with a neat new means of addressing health and environmental challenges now. The use of competitive exclusion for improving a specific ecology is called 'probiotics'.

Probiotics therapy intentionally introduces strains of beneficial bacteria in order to replace bad bacteria. The first application of probiotics in aquaculture seems relatively recent, but the interest in such environment-friendly treatments is increasing rapidly.

Aquatic animals are quite different from the land animals for which the probiotic concept was developed, and a preliminary question is the pertinence of probiotic applications to aquaculture. Man and terrestrial livestock undergo embryonic development within an amnion, whereas the larval forms of most fish and shellfish are released in the external environment at an early ontogenetic stage. These larvae are highly exposed to gastro-intestinal microbiota-associated disorders, because they start feeding even through the digestive tract is not yet fully developed, and the immune system is still incomplete. Thus, probiotic treatments are particularly desirable during the larval stages. Moriarty proposed to extend the definition of probiotics to microbial water additives.

1. In 1991, Porubcan reported on two attempts at bacterial treatments to improve water quality and production yield of Penaeus monodon: Pre-inoculated with nitrifying bacteria decreased the amounts of ammonia and nitrite in the rearing water. This treatment increased shrimp survival.

2. The introduction of *Bacillus* spp. in proximity to pond aerators reduced chemical oxygen demand, and increased shrimp harvest.

Moriarty noted an increase of shrimp/prawn survival in ponds where some strains of *Bacillus* spp. were introduced. The actual data of Moriarty showed the inhibitory activity of *Bacillus* spp. against luminous *vibrio* sp. in pond sediment, but the effect on shrimp/prawn survival might be due either to a probiotic effect, or to an indirect effect on animal health. For instance, the degradation of organic matter by *Bacillus* spp. might improve water quality.

The probiotic treatments may be considered as methods of biological control, akin to the limitation or elimination of pests by introduction of adverse organisms, like parasites or specific pathogens. Maeda and others proposed to designate as 'biocontrol' the methods of treatment using 'the antagonism among microbes through which pathogens can be killed or reduced in number in the aquaculture environment.'

Sugita isolated a strain of *Bacillus* sp. that was antagonistic to 63 per cent of the isolates from fish intestine. Pathogenic strains of *Vibrio* or *Aeromonas* have been targeted in most *in vitro* tests. Treatment with *Lactobacillus brevis* and lactic acid reduced the load of *Vibrio alginolyticus* in the Artemia culture water. Some bacteria are antagonistic to viruses and they may be efficient for the biocontrol of viral diseases and some other probiotics are effective in controlling bacterial diseases in fishes.

The resistance caused by probiotics to infections to shrimp, prawn and fish is due to bacterial antagonism, bacterial interference, barrier effect, colonisation resistance and competitive exclusion, in addition to improving biodegradation of waste organic matter through nitrogen cycle.

To best determine, which bacteria make good probiotics for aquaculture production, scientists scoop up quantities of water from healthy habitat in the ocean where species (aquaculture organisms like shrimp) perform at peak capacity. They analyse the water's make-up and culture single or mixed bacteria they find there to use as probiotics. Their culture does not involve any sort of chemicals or toxins. These are fortified with naturally occurring phytoplankton, amino acids, a wide range of vitamins and minerals, an important variety of antioxidants and proteolytic enzymes, as well as an array of nucleic acids. These are the paramount keepers of the code of life, which appears to be in charge of growth and continuous cell repair.

The hypothesis of stimulation of the immune system of aquatic organisms may be also considered. Many immunostimulants have been tested on fish and shellfish, and some of them originated from microbial cell walls, e.g. glucans. It is possible that autochthonous microbiota may stimulate the immune response of aquatic animals to enteric pathogens, as reported in shrimp and in land animals.

BIOREMEDIATION—CONCEPT

The newest attempt being made to improve water quality in aquaculture is the application of probiotics and/or enzymes to the ponds. This type of biotechnology, known as bioremediation, involves manipulation of micro-organisms in ponds to enhance mineralisation of organic matter and get rid of undesirable waste compounds.

Probiotics

The concept of biological disease control, particularly using microbiological modulator for disease prevention, has received widespread attention. The term 'probiotics' was first coined by Parker and originated from two Greek words 'pro' and 'bios' which mean 'for life.' A bacterial supplement of a single or mixed culture of selected non-pathogenic bacterial strains was termed probiotics. Characteristics of various types of probiotics are given in Table 19.1.

Table 19.1. Types of probiotics.

Type	Characteristics
Non-viable probiotics	These are dead
Freeze-dried probiotics	These will die rapidly upon leaving refrigeration
Fermentation probiotics	These are produced through fermentation
Viable probiotics	These are alive with guaranteed shelf life, guaranteed number of organisms, have a protocol for counting, are stable and efficacious

Organisms—be they human, cattle, chicken, fish, prawn or shrimp—require good bacteria to break down nutrients for digestion. Living systems require bacteria to decompose waste. Probiotics generally include bacteria, cyanobacteria, fungi etc. They may be called as 'normal microbiota' or 'effective microbiota'. In literature, probiotic bacteria are generally called bacteria, which can improve the water quality of aquaculture, and (or) inhibit pathogens in water, thereby increasing production. Probiotics, probiont, probiotic bacteria, beneficial bacteria, or friendly bacteria are terms synonymously used for probiotic bacteria.

The theory of ecological prevention and cure in controlling the insect pest of terrestrial higher-grade animals and plants has been in practice for long time, and has achieved remarkable success. The bio-controlling theory has been applied to aquaculture and many researchers attempt to use some kind of probiotics in aquaculture water to regulate the micro flora of aquaculture water, control pathogenic micro-organisms, to enhance decomposition of the undesirable organic substances in aquaculture water, and improve ecological environment of aquaculture. In addition, the use of probiotics can increase the population of food organisms, improve the nutrition level of aquacultural animals and improve immunity of cultured animals to pathogenic micro-organisms.

In aquaculture the mechanism of action of the probiotic bacteria have several aspects.

1. Probiotic bacteria competitively exclude pathogenic bacteria or produce substances that inhibit the growth of the pathogenic bacteria (e.g. Bacitracin and polymyxin produced by *Bacillus* sp.).
2. Provide essential nutrients to enhance the nutrition of cultured animals.
3. Provide digestive enzymes to enhance digestion of cultured animals.
4. Probiotic bacteria directly uptake or decompose organic matter or toxic material in water, improving the quality of water.

Probiotics can decompose the excreta of fish or prawns, remaining food materials, remains of the plankton and other organic materials to CO_2, nitrate and phosphate.

The inorganic salts provide the nutrition for growth of micro algae, while the bacteria grow rapidly and become the dominant group in the water, inhibiting growth of pathogenic micro-organisms. Probiotics and their role in given is Table 19.2.

Table 19.2. Probiotics and their role.

Type	Role
Bacillus sp.	Mineralisation and breakage of proteins
Nitrosomonas sp.	Oxidation of ammonia
Nitrobacter sp.	Oxidation of nitrites
Aerobacter sp.	Reduction of organic matter
Cellulomonas sp.	Breakage of plant material

The photosynthesis of the micro algae provide dissolved oxygen for oxidation and decomposition of organic materials and for the respiration of microbes and cultured animals. This kind of cycle improves the nutrient cycle, and can create a balance between bacteria and micro algae, thus maintaining a good water quality for cultured animals.

Beneficial effects of probiotics may be mediated by:

1. Neutralisation of toxin.
2. Suppression of viable count.
3. Production of antibacterial compounds.
4. Competition for adhesion sites.
5. Alternation of microbial metabolism.
6. Stimulation of immunity in the host.
7. Accelerate sediment decomposition by producing organic acids.
8. Production of hydrogen peroxide.
9. Production of enzymes.

Application of probiotics in aquaculture includes:

1. Regulate the microflora of aquaculture water.
2. Control pathogenic micro-organisms.
3. Enhance decomposition of the undesirable organic substances in aquaculture water and improve ecological environment of aquaculture by minimising toxic gases like ammonia, nitrite, hydrogen sulphide, methane etc.
4. Increase the population of food organisms.
5. Improve the nutrition level of aquaculture animals and improve immunity of cultured animals to pathogenic micro-organisms.
6. Prevent frequent outbreaks of diseases.

Enzymes

Enzymes are organic catalysts formed naturally in living cells. They are compounds, which accelerate the rate at which chemical reactions occur and remain unchanged after the reaction is completed. Thousands of enzymes exist in nature and are responsible for life.

Enzymes work by breaking the chemical bonds that hold compounds together, releasing smaller, more readily absorbed compounds. For example, proteases work on proteins, amylases work on starches, cellulases work on cellulose and lipases work on lipids or fats. Recall that cellulose is the major cell wall material in plants and is therefore quite durable.

Nitrogen Cycle

Ammonia is the principal excretory product of most aquatic organisms. Inputs of ammonia cannot be eliminated from the water body. But ammonia is toxic, acutely and chronically, to fish and invertebrates; thus it is a critical water quality factor. Ammonia levels should be maintained below 0.1 mg/l (total ammonia). The most efficient way to do this is by the establishment of a biological filter.

A biological filter is a collection of naturally occurring bacteria, which oxidise ammonia to nitrite, and other bacteria, which then convert nitrite to nitrate. Nitrite is formed either by the oxidation of ammonia (nitrification) or the reduction of nitrate (denitrification). Nitrite is toxic to fish and some invertebrates and should be maintained below 0.1 mg/l. It is also a critical water quality factor. Nitrate is the end product of nitrification. The vast majority of aquaculture ponds accumulate nitrate as they do not contain a denitrifying filter. In general, nitrate should be maintained below 50 mg/l (measured as NO_3–N), but it is not a critical water quality factor.

The most common ways to reduce nitrate are water changes and growing live plants. More sophisticated systems such as denitrifying filters are also available. A denitrifying filter creates an anaerobic region where anaerobic bacteria can grow and reduce nitrate to nitrogen gas. But they can be complex and easily disturbed, which kills the anaerobic bacteria. A poorly run denitrifying filter does not convert nitrate all the way to nitrogen gas, but instead produces nitrite.

The nitrogen 'cycle' is the oxidation of ammonia to nitrite by bacteria of the genus *Nitrosomonas* and the subsequent oxidation of the nitrite to nitrate by bacteria belonging to the genus *Nitrobacter*. It is easiest to visualise the nitrogen cycle as an endless loop divided into four phases:

1. Fish, prawn and shrimp excrete ammonia as waste from their gills, kidneys and normal respiration. Ammonia also develops from unconsumed feeds, shell moults of prawn and shrimp, dead algae, zooplankton etc. by microbial activity.

2. A species of bacteria called *Nitrosomonas* converts this ammonia into nitrite.

$$2NH_4^+ + 3O_2 \longrightarrow 2NO_2^- + 4H^+ + 2H_2O$$

3. A second species of bacteria called *Nitrobacter* converts this nitrite into nitrate

$$2NO_2^- + O_2 \longrightarrow 2NO_3^-$$

4. Algae and aquatic plants utilise nitrate to produce chlorophyll, which are in turn consumed by zooplankton and then by fish, prawn and shrimp. Thence the cycle repeats.

These bacteria are important to aqua farmers because without them it is difficult to maintain healthy environmental conditions in the aquaculture ponds.

Two enzymes, ammonia monooxygenase (AMO) and hydroxylamine oxidoreductase (HAO) are involved in the oxidation of ammonia to nitrite.

$$NH_3 + O_2 + 2H^+ \xrightarrow{\quad AMO \quad} NH_2 + OH + H_2O$$

$$NH_2OH \xrightarrow{\quad HAO \quad} NO_2^-$$

The biochemical reaction of *Nitrobacter* is a very simple reaction, involving the cytochrome system as follows:

$$NO_2^- \longrightarrow NO_3^-$$

Nitrobacter sp. is facultatively mixotrophic and capable of growing anaerobically with nitrate as electron acceptor, producing nitrite, nitric oxide and nitrous oxide and then to nitrogen gas. Aerobically, it oxidises nitric oxide to nitrite and thence to nitrate. All tricarboxylic acid cycle enzymes are present (e.g. carboxysomes, poly-beta-hydroxybutyrate (PHB) and polyphosphate granules).

The nitrifying bacteria are gramnegative, non acid-fast rods, which may be pleomorphic or coccoid (*Nitrobacter*). They may be motile. The main component of the gram-negative cell wall is lipopoly-saccharide (LPS). Additionally, there is present phospholipid, protein, lipoprotein and a small amount of peptidoglycan. Hence, the component of cell wall of most gram-negative bacteria is associated with endotoxic activity, with which are associated the pyrogenic effects of gram-negative infections like vibriosis. 66 kcal of energy are liberated per gram atom of ammonia oxidised, while 18 kcal of energy is liberated per gram atom of nitrite oxidised.

Nitrification is an obligate aerobic, oxidising process. This means that it can only occur in an environment, which contains oxygen and the process produces electrons. In general, denitrification is a process of bacteria converting nitrate to other substances. It is an anaerobic, reducing process. This means that it occurs in environments without oxygen and the process accepts electrons.

Denitrification is defined as the transformation of nitrate to dinitrogen. Dinitrogen is a gas that is harmless and will bubble out of the system. Between the starting product (nitrate) and the end product (dinitrogen) there are three intermediate products; these are (in the order in which they are produced): nitrite (NO_2^-), nitric oxide (NO) and nitrous oxide (N_2O). Hence, denitrification, like nitrification, is a multi-step process with many intermediate compounds produced before the final product is generated. In most cases these intermediate products are toxic like ammonia and nitrite. Thus, denitrification does proceed to complete its process and to expel dinitrogen gas.

It is worth mentioning that nitrate, which is the end-product of the nitrification process is the major nutrient for growth of primary producers, i.e. phytoplankton, as well as the microbes. Hence, the micro flora and fauna will utilise the nitrate for their growth and limits the process of denitrification.

Another difference between nitrification and denitrification is the type of bacteria, which perform the processes. Nitrification is done by what are called autotrophic bacteria. This term means the bacteria get the carbon they need for cell growth from carbon dioxide. Denitrifying bacteria are heterotrophic bacteria, which get their carbon from organic carbon sources such as methane, sucrose or glucose.

In addition, these probiotics control the formation of toxic hydrogen sulphide by eliminating *Desulfovibrio desulfuricans*, the hydrogen sulphide producing bacteria, through antagonism. The probiotics convert the toxic sulphide to nutritive sulphate.

CONCLUSION

Probiotics can decompose the excreta of shrimp, prawn or fish, remaining food materials, remains of the plankton and other organic materials to CO_2, nitrate and phosphate. These inorganic salts provide the nutrition for the growth of micro algae, while the bacteria grow rapidly and become the dominant group in the water, inhibiting the growth of the pathogenic micro-organisms. The photosynthesis of the micro algae provide dissolved oxygen for oxidation and decomposition of the organic materials and for the respiration of the microbes and cultured animals. This kind of cycle may improve the nutrient cycle, and it can create a balance between bacteria and micro algae, and maintaining a good water quality environment for the cultured animals.

Probiotics reduce the level of infection and mortality in aquaculture organisms. Probiotics compete with the disease-causing bacteria for food. Customarily, ponds have indigenous bad bacteria that leisurely eat on an abundance of undigested food, faecal matter and dead algae. When farmers suddenly introduce a large quantity of probiotics into a pond, the newcomers eliminate the pre-existing bad bacteria out of the nutrient queue. The old bacteria, often-bad bacteria, never having had to compete for food, cannot keep pace with the aggressive probiotics.

Probiotics excretions make the pond medium less inhabitable for bad bacteria. Not only do probiotics bacteria have terrific appetites; they excrete enzymes—exoenzymes—as a natural by-product of their metabolic activity, just as human's sweat.

The enzyme excretions infuse and spread throughout the pond medium, changing its chemistry, resulting destroy of bad bacteria. Hence, probiotics therapy greatly improves pond water quality and reduces the pollution level of effluent before its release into the environment. Probiotics speed the breakdown of organic waste fragments (dissolved proteins and unused feed), thus lessening sludge build-up. If sludge is not removed or does not decompose, dangerous concentrations of sulphide, nitrite, ammonia and various organic acids can occur. While the exo-enzymes of good bacteria go to work on larger waste particles and breaking them down through chemical reaction. As a result, there are fewer harmful chemicals in the medium.

Probiotics balance algae growth through providing nutrients by their biodegradation activity. Probiotics utilises phosphate for their body metabolic activities and hence prevents over growth (heavy blooms) of algae by limiting the phosphate. Dead algae are one of bacteria's favourite foods. Also probiotics diminish nutrients normally consumed by algae and results less slime in the ponds.

Probiotics make better habitat for culture organisms. With less accumulation of organic matter on the pond bottom, more oxygen can penetrate the sediment. For example Prawn and shrimp characteristically burrow in the sediment. By loosening the sediment, probiotics make this burrowing easier. Moreover, they diminish the toxin level in the sediment itself. Probiotics maximise fish, prawn and shrimp nutrition. In addition to consuming the feed administered by farmers, prawn and shrimp graze on tiny zooplankton that is present in the water supply. Zooplankton eats bacteria. Probiotics are another nutrient for existing zooplankton in the pond medium, thus invigorating the zooplankton population, and strengthen up the food supply to culture organisms.

Probiotics optimise the immune systems of culture organisms, increasing their resistance to disease. By upgrading the pond environment, augmenting the food supply, and making habitat more comfortable, probiotics fortify fish, prawn and shrimp immune system. The application of probiotics in aquaculture has shown promise, but further investigations may be expected with propagation of molecular approaches to analyse bacterial communities.

Chapter 20

Biodegradation of Organic Pollutants

INTRODUCTION

It has been said that without micro-organisms and their degradation capabilities, animal life, including human life, on the earth would cease to exist very soon. Whether or not this is an exaggeration as to the time scale, it is true in principle, that we absolutely depend on microbial activities for the renewal of our environment and maintenance of the global carbon cycle. Among the substances that can be degraded or transformed by micro-organisms, are a huge number of synthetic compounds and other chemicals having environmental relevance (e.g. mineral oil components). However, it has to be considered that this statement concerns potential degradability which, in most instances, was estimated in the laboratory by using pure cultures and ideal growth conditions. Under natural conditions in soil and surface waters, the actual degradability of organopollutants is lower, due to a whole range of factors: competition with other micro-organisms, insufficient supply with essential substrates (C, N, P, S sources), unfavourable external conditions (O_2, H_2O, pH, temperature) and low bioavailability of the pollutant that is to be degraded.

Thus, environmental biotechnology has the important assignment of tackling and solving these problems, so as to permit the use of micro-organisms in bioremediation technologies. For this purpose, it is necessary to support the activities of the indigenous micro-organisms in polluted soils and to enhance their degradative potential by bioaugmentation. The former measure particularly applies to bacteria, whereas, bioaugmentation mainly concerns basidiomycetous fungi. In this context, we should point out that neither bacteria nor fungi are 'better' degraders, separately. In nature, both groups of micro-organisms work together and of course, complement one another in their degradative capabilities.

Anaerobic degradation can be applied in technical devices for the treatment of waste material, often leading to CH_4 and CO_2 as products, which can be exploited as an energy source or as a basis for biosynthetic processes. Knowledge of the capacities, strategies, and limits of anaerobic degradation processes is therefore needed to assess the potential risk of synthetic compounds to health or to the environment, no matter whether such synthetics are released intentionally (as with plant protection agents), inadvertently through waste-water treatment, or accidentally through spills.

This overview shows that the degradative potential of anaerobic microbial communities is much greater than assumed only a few years ago: a broad variety of compounds can be subjected to anaerobic degradation, most often down to methane and carbon dioxide as final products. Aliphatic hydrocarbons are degraded if they contain unsaturated bonds, preferentially if these are located terminally, but saturated long-chain aliphatic hydrocarbons are also anaerobically degradable. These processes are slow and can be applied only in long-term incubations, if at all. Ether compounds are degraded anaerobically if they are methyl ethers or if they can be transformed into hemiacetals through, e.g. hydroxyl shift reactions. In the anaerobic degradation of ketones, the primary activation reaction is a carboxylation rather than an oxidation step. Future research will definitely bring better and economically feasible methods for degradation of organopollutants in nature.

Contamination of aquatic ecosystem by different pollutants is a common problem, worldwide, because of the use and discharge of waste-water from domestic and industrial sectors into the surface water. This results in significant changes in the physico-chemical and biological characters of the receiving water body.

Most of the organic matter present in waste-water includes degradable carbohydrates, proteins and lipids of different complexities. A significant part of organic carbon is oils and hydrocarbons, if the waste-water is of industrial origin. The treatment of such waste-water aims at oxidising or degrading the organic compounds so as to decrease the biochemical oxygen demand (BOD) load of the waste-water. Such processes of organic carbon load reduction can be achieved by microbial biodegradation. The degradation can be performed by a single micro-organism or a group of micro-organisms, under aerobic or anaerobic conditions.

AEROBIC VS ANAEROBIC DEGRADATION

Microbial degradation or transformation of organic compounds may involve either of the two processes of aerobic (oxygen dependant) or anaerobic situation, while in some cases it may need both the conditions to detoxify some xenobiotic compounds.

Aerobic Degradation

In the conventional aerobic system, the substrate is used as a source of carbon and energy. It serves as an electron donor resulting in bacterial growth. The extent of degradation is correlated with the rate of O_2 consumption, as also previous acclimation of the organism in the same substrate. Two enzymes primarily involved in the process are di- and mono-oxygenases. The latter enzyme can act on both aromatic and aliphatic compounds, while for the former, only aromatic compounds can act as substrates. Another class of enzymes involved in aerobic condition are peroxidases, which are receiving attention recently for their ability to degrade lignin.

Anaerobic Degradation

This process is of widespread occurrence and relies on the metabolic versatility of mixed microbial populations present in soils or sediments when O_2 supply is limited. Growth yield of anaerobic bacteria is extremely low due to low energy yields. It has drawn attention these years due to the possibility of decomposition of extremely recalcitrant xenobiotics through this process.

Though the anaerobic process is slow, needs long retention time and produces H_2S gas, yet it is more advantageous than the aerobic one due to its non-dependence of O_2 supply. It thus saves the cost of energy for O_2 transfer. Materials like cellulose and fats, which remain unaffected by the aerobic process, breakdown under this situation.

The overall process of anaerobic degradation of complex wastes is shown in Fig. 20.1.

Three temperature ranges are used in anaerobic digestion:

Cold digestion at about 20°C.

Mesophylic digestion at 20°–40°C.

Thermophilic digestion at 40°–55°C.

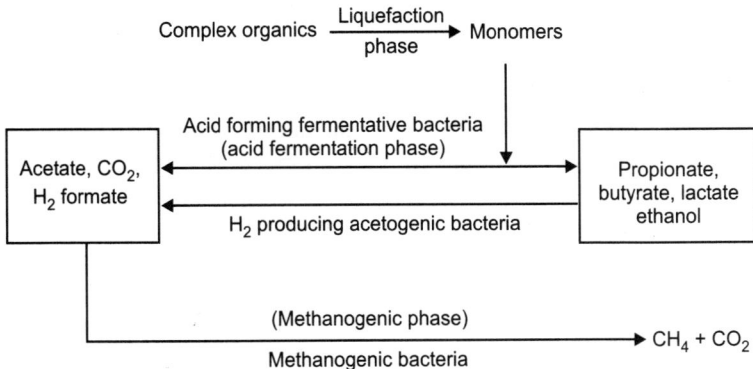

Fig. 20.1. Anaerobic degradation.

Denitrification, sulphate reduction, dehalogenation and fermentation coupled to methanogenesis may occur concurrently in the same soil or sediment as different conditions exist at different microhabitats harbouring consortia of various degrading microbes and their interactions.

Some anaerobic microbial transformation reactions of organic compounds are:

Reaction type	Examples
Hydro-/dehydrogenations	Phenol, catechol, benzoate, fatty acids, unsaturated hydrocarbons
Carboxy-/decarboxylations	Cresol, toluene, benzoate, short hydrocarbons
Reductive dehalogenation	Polychlorinated aromatic compounds
Dechlorination	PCBs, phenols, chlorinated ethylenes
Methylation	Heavy metals

The anaerobic methods of waste-water treatment are considered safe, since few toxic chemicals can be stripped into the ambient air. Chlorinated xenobiotics need to be dehalogenated to make them harmless and biological treatment is an attractive proposition. They mostly need anaerobic situation for dehalogenation by bacterial genera like *Pseudomonas, Arthrobacter, Mycobacterium*, etc. Unlike aerobic condition, in an anaerobic degradation the chlorinated molecule is used as a direct source of electron. This is exemplified by 3-chlorobenzoate reduction.

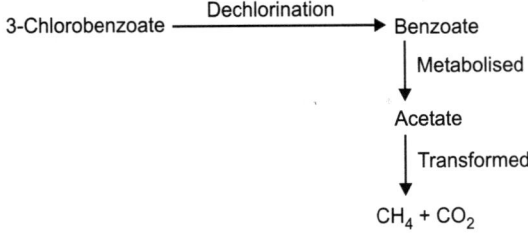

Reductive dechlorination involves successive 'shedding' of chlorine atoms under reduced anaerobic condition and is a common initial step in the biodegradation of chlorinated organics. The process is rather rapid for chemicals having a high number of chlorine substitution, viz. PCBs, hexachlorobenzene, trichloroethane, etc. Initial dechlorination is needed to make the compound less harmful for the microbes working under subsequent aero- and/or anaerobic degradation.

Sequential Degradation

In many cases, both anaerobic and aerobic sequences are combined. This helps in the reduction of toxicity and mineralisation of compounds, which are otherwise recalcitrant. For example, tetrachloroethylene and tetrachloromethane may be mineralised in sequential steps of anaerobic and aerobic conditions, so that initially TCE and chloroform are formed, which, later in aerobic methanogenic stage, are converted into CO_2 and H_2O. In such sequential stages, the BOD reduction is also taken care of, as is being done in case of waste water from pulp and paper industries.

For some xenobiotic chemicals, a single bacterium may transform it to another form, but cannot complete the breakdown. In such a situation a second group of microbe may act in a complementary fashion to have the total breakdown of the compound through a 'team work'. This sort of 'synergistic' action also prevents the build-up of toxic intermediates in the environment.

$$C_{12}H_{25}\text{–⬡} \xrightarrow[\text{rhodochrons}]{\textit{Mycobacterium}} CH_2COOH\text{–⬡} \xrightarrow[\text{species}]{\textit{Arthrobacter}} \text{O=⬡} \xrightarrow{\textit{Arthrobacter}} CO_2 + H_2O$$

Dodecyl-cyclohexane

BIODEGRADABLE ORGANIC POLLUTANTS

Study of the suitability of a bacterium or a bacterial assemblage for the degradation of organic pollutants has greatly aided to the development of strategies for acceleration of the removal of pollutants from the wastes. The stability and metabolism of pollutants in the environment greatly influence their ecotoxicological evaluations. In the aquatic environment the water and sediment biota respond to different organic pollutants through alteration of their growth rate and, if necessary, the physiological activity at the cellular, and/ or organism level. The rate of degradability determines the stability and residence time of the pollutant in the environment. Besides the biotic factors, many other physico-chemical properties of the environment also determine the pollutant's stability.

Determination of Biodegradability

On the basis of degradability, the organic pollutants can be grouped into four types as shown in Table 20.1, viz. (i) very easily degradable, (ii) easily degradable, (iii) potentially degradable, and (iv) very slowly degradable (difficult to degrade).

Table 20.1. The measurement of biodegradability of organic substances in the aquatic ecosystem.

Substance type	Degradation requirement	Residence time (days)
Very easily degradable	Direct uptake and metabolism by bacteria	0–1
Easily degradable	Adaptation of bacteria	7–10
	Exo- and endo-enzyme reaction	10–14
	Bacterial assemblage and biofilm development	
Potentially degradable	Adaptation of bacteria	>7
	Endo- and exo-enzyme reaction at high bacterial biomass	7–21
	Artificial inoculation	
	Bacterial assemblage and biofilm development	

(Contd ...)

Substance type	Degradation requirement	Residence time (days)
Very slowly degradable	Adaptation of bacteria	>7
(difficult to degrade)	Endo- and exo-enzyme reaction at high bacterial biomass	>>21
	Artificial inoculation	
	Bacterial assemblage and biofilm development	>21
	Additional substrate requirement	

Bacterial Succession in the Polluted Environment

The most important factor in the polluted water or sludge is the concentration and type of pollutants which determine the bacterial activity vis-a-vis the rate of degradation. If the pollutants are easily degradable, organic substances that can support bacterial growth and some other parameters, other than the pollutants concentration, determine the rate of degradation. The most important among them are aeration, pH and temperature. Aeration alone not only supplies oxygen for the aerobic oxidation of pollutants, but also stabilises pH through the removal of CO_2 and maintains the temperature (Fig. 20.2).

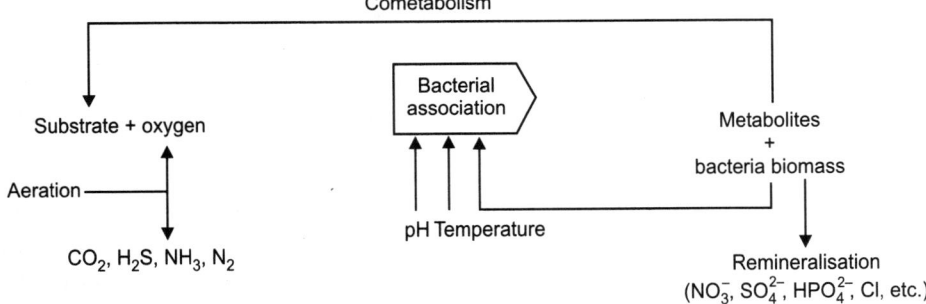

Fig. 20.2. Schematic representation of the bacterial degradation process in water.

After the initiation of the degradation reaction by the adopted strains of microbes, the metabolism may proceed in three different ways, with changes in the diversity of microbes metabolising them (Fig. 20.3).

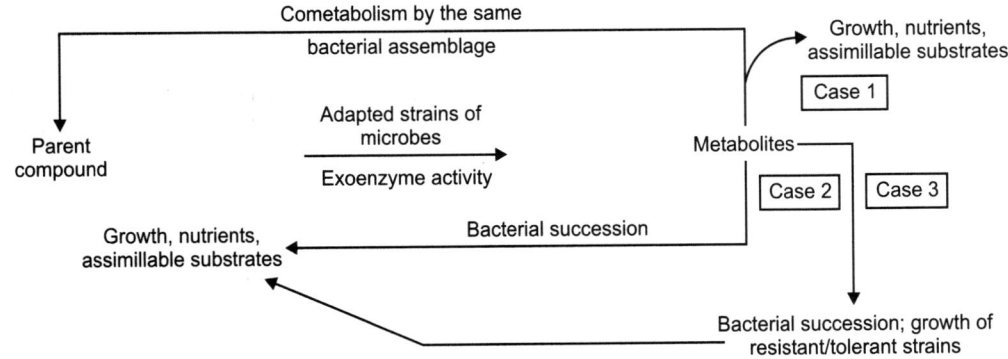

Fig. 20.3. Schematic representation of bacterial succession during degradation reaction of potentially degradable or slowly degradable pollutants.

Case 1: The metabolites are used as substrates for the members of the same microbial assemblage which use the metabolites for their growth. In such a case, there are changes in the diversity of the species assemblage due to elimination of one or more species, caused by competitive elimination.

Case 2: The metabolites of the first degradation reaction do not support growth of the same bacterial assemblage. For example, during degradation of aromatic hydrocarbons, the products of the initial degradation reaction only support selective species, while most of the species of the assemblage do not have the ability to degrade the substrate. In such a case, new species of microbes are encouraged and a new bacterial assemblage is established. Such succession with the process of degradation continues till complete degradation takes place.

Case 3: In such a case, the products of the first few degradation reaction become toxic to the existing bacterial assemblage leading to elimination of a few species from the assemblage; only the tolerant strains survive and metabolise the substrates to a level that becomes non-toxic and then the new species reappear in the assemblage. Such phenomenon is observed during degradation of substances like phenol, PCB, TNT and OC insecticides.

Measurement of Biodegradability

In biological experiments, the metabolic activity of the entire bacterial assemblage is taken to understand the degradation of pollutants. The degradation rate can be estimated directly by measuring the substrate consumption or by many other means like, production of by-products or end products, consumption of O_2, evolution of CO_2, utilisation of DOC and reduction of BOD, etc. The rate of degradation varies with the nature of the substrate, environmental conditions and heterotrophic activity.

TESTING FOR BIODEGRADABILITY

It is usually done in the laboratory conditions, as it is often difficult to conduct the same in the field, though laboratory conditions may not always simulate the field situations. However, a variety of test methods have been developed, depending on the purpose.

Biodegradability of xenobiotic may depend on or be influenced by a host of factors.

1. Chemical structure of the compound and various substitutions.
2. Environmental factors such as the presence or absence of oxygen, pH and temperature of the medium.
3. Whether the substrate can provide carbon and energy for the metabolism and growth of the degrading organism.

So a successful bioremediation of a novel substrate necessitates considerations and attempts from various angles. In many cases, time and efforts may even go waste. So a preliminary idea about the biodegradable potential of the chemical concerned may be obtained through some simple techniques and procedures.

1. If structural features suggests its recalcitrance with respect to a particular microbe, it is advisable to check the need of synergistic effects of microbial community.
2. By comparing the disappearance of the compound from a biologically active or poisoned (with 1 per cent $HgCl_2$) growth medium.
3. Decreased UV absorption at 280 nm may help monitoring the degradation of aromatic compounds.
4. For specific chemical monitoring of certain compounds like aromatic amines and phenols, diazotisation reaction or Folin-Cricalteau reaction may be followed.

5. In certain cases, radiolabelling with C^{14} may indicate the complete mineralisation to $^{14}CO_2$ as an indication of biodegradability.

6. Use of Indicator reagents in the growth media may also help detecting: (i) conversion of anilines to azobenzene by spraying *p*-anisidine, whereby red-brown discolouration of microbial colonies may occur; and (ii) for dechlorination acid-base indicators are used such as eosin-methylene blue or bromo-cresol purple. The change of colour indicates the release of chlorine.

Most non-specific analytical methods monitor one of the three parameters. These are O_2 uptake in an oxidation test (BOD), CO_2 production from complete mineralisation of organics and loss of dissolved organic carbon (DOC). The simplest is the determination of BOD_5 and its comparison with COD. BOD_5 determines the amount of O_2 required for microbial decomposition in a 5-day test at 20°C, while COD indicates the amount of O_2 necessary for chemical oxidation. If BOD/COD is more than 0.6, the organic substance is easily biodegradable; if it is between 0.3 to 0.6, then it points to the possibility of biodegradation, and when the ratio is less than 0.3 it is not bioamenable. Non-specific methods are, however, less sensitive than the chemical specific methods mentioned above.

Test guidelines, primarily for screening, have been suggested by OECD (Organisation for Economic Cooperation and Development) and are generally adopted by EPAs (Environmental Protection Agencies) in different countries.

Surfaces for Biodegradation

Rate of biological oxidation of organic pollutants is determined by the population density and the activity of microbes engaged in the degradation process. The microbial activity is enhanced, when provided a surface. Each of the pollutants, after entry into water, become a potential surface for microbial activity.

When a biodegradable particle is immersed in water, it absorbs some water as per its hydrophilicity and this water may or may not be chemically bound. Ionically active particles are surrounded by different layers of water at room temperature. These structural waters found around all hydrophilic substances (proteins, polysaccharides, colloids, etc.) are called bound waters. The latter are differentiated into two different zones: (i) inner stable and undisturbed zone, and (ii) outer broader, disorganised zone easily penetrable by ions and soluble substances. This zone shows unusually high microbial activity and is termed as the interface. The physico-chemical properties at the interface are completely different from those of either of the phases; solid-liquid; liquid-liquid, or gas-liquid phases. Each of the interfaces provides surfaces for the microbes to assemble, colonise and act. In terms of microbial activity, the interfaces are important as potential nutrient accumulating zones which act as nutrient source and encourage microbial colonisation. The microbial activity is doubted to be surface specific to some extent. Different microbes and even same micro-organism have different rates of activities at different interfaces. The metabolism of substances and heterotrophic breakdown of soluble and particulate pollutants at the same interface are also different at time with changes in environmental conditions and microbial assembalge.

PRINCIPLES OF BACTERIAL DEGRADATION

Decomposition of Organic Pollutants in Ecosystems

Catabolic processes of micro-organisms (bacteria, algae, yeasts, and lower fungi) are the main pathways for total or at least partial mineralisation/decomposition of bioorganic and organic compounds in natural or man-made environments. Most of these materials are derived directly or indirectly from plant or animal biomass. They originate as exudates from carbon dioxide fixation via photosynthesis (plant biomass), from plants that serve as animal feed (detritus), as animal excreta (flaeces, urine, etc.), or from fossil (peat, coal, oil, natural gas, etc.). Even the carbon portion of some xenobiotics can be tracked back to a biological origin, i.e. whether these substances were produced from oil, natural gas, or coal. Only because the mineralisation of carbonaceous material was incomplete, due to decaying plant and animal biomass in nature under anaerobic conditions with shortage of water, did the formation of fossil oil, natural gas, and coal deposition from biomass occur through biological and/or geochemical transformations. The fossil carbon of natural gas, coal, and oil enters the atmospheric CO_2 cycle again as soon as these compounds are incinerated as fuel or used for energy generation in industry or private households.

Key enzymatic reactions of aerobic biodegradation are oxidations, catalysed by oxygenases and peroxidases Oxygenases are oxidoreductases that use O_2 to incorporate oxygen into the substrate. Degradative organisms need oxygen at two metabolic sites-the initial attack on the substrate and the end of the respiratory chain. Certain higher fungi have developed a unique oxidative system for the degradation of lignin, based on extracellular ligninolytic peroxidases and laccases. This enzymatic system possesses increasing significance for the cometabolic degradation of persistent organopollutants.

Under strictly anaerobic conditions, soluble carbon compounds of wastes and waste-water are degraded stepwise, to methane, CO_2, NH_3 and H_2S via a syntropic interaction of fermentative and acetogenic bacteria, with methanogens or sulphate reducers. The complete methanogenic degradation of biopolymers or monomers via hydrolysis/fermentation, acetogenesis, and methanogenesis can proceed only at a low H_2 partial pressure, which is maintained mainly by interspecies hydrogen transfer.

Anaerobic degradation processes are often found useful for the treatment of specific waste-waters rich in phenolic compounds, e.g. from the chemical industry, to avoid the formation of unwanted side products such as condensed polyphenols. In other situations, aerobic treatment may cause technical problems, e.g. by extensive foam formation during aerobic treatment of surface-active compounds such as tensides. Thus, knowledge of the limits and principles of anaerobic degradation processes, under various conditions prevailing in natural habitats, might help to design suitable alternative techniques for the clean up of contaminated soils or for the treatment of specific waste-waters that have so far been applied only insufficiently. On the other hand, in aerobic condition, oxygenases introduce hydroxyl groups into aromatics, and further oxygen may cause the formation of phenol radicals that initiate uncontrolled polymerisation and condensation to polymeric derivatives, similar to humic compounds in soil, which are very difficult to degrade further, whether anaerobically or aerobically.

DEGRADATION OF POLYMERS

Approximately 150 million tonnes of synthetic polymers are produced worldwide each year. Since polymers are extremely stable, their degradation cycles in the biosphere are limited. In Western Europe it is estimated that 7.5 per cent of municipal solid waste is plastic; these plastics are classified as 65 per cent polyethylene (PE)/polypropylene (PP), 15 per cent polystyrene (PS), 10 per cent polyvinyl chloride (PVC), 5 per cent polyester terephthalate (PET), and miscellaneous others. Environmental pollution by synthetic polymers, such as waste plastics and water-soluble synthetic polymers in waste-water, has been recognised as a major problem. Degradation of polymers can be carried out by heat, radiation, or biochemical treatment. The radiant energy may be high-energy radiation from gamma rays, ion beams, and electrons or even low-energy radiation from ultraviolet (UV) light. UV stabilisers added to polymer products reduce the rate of degradation. Chemical degradation results from treatment with chemicals such as acids and alkalis. Biodegradation of polymers results from the use of micro-organisms and enzymes.

Biodegradation

The biodegradability of a compound depends on its molecular weight, molecular form, and crystallinity. Biodegradability decreases with increase in molecular weight, while monomers, dimers, and repeating units degrade easily. Two types of depolymerases are involved in the process, namely, extracellular and intracellular. Microbial exoenzymes first break down the complex polymers in a process called depolymerisation. The resulting short chains are small enough to permeate the cell walls, allowing them to be used as carbon and energy sources. When the end products are carbon dioxide, water, or methane, the process is called mineralisation. Different end-products are formed depends on the degradation pathway (Fig. 20.4).

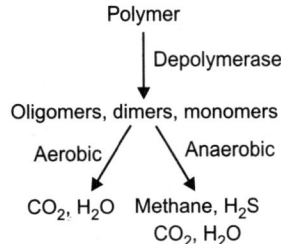

Fig. 20.4. Reaction pathways during polymer biodegradation.

Polyethers

Polyethylene glycols (PEGs), polypropylene glycols (PPGs), and polytetramethylene glycol come under the class of polyethers and are used in pharmaceuticals, cosmetics, lubricants, inks, and surfactants. *Flavobacterium* sp. and *Pseudomonas* sp. together associate and mineralise PEG completely under aerobic conditions. During degradation, PEG molecules are reduced one glycol unit at a time after each oxidation cycle. *Pelobacter venetianus* was found to degrade PEG and ethylene glycol under anaerobic conditions. High molecular weight PEGs (4000 to 20,000) were degraded by *Sphingomonas macrogoltabidus* and *S. terrae*, while PPG was degraded by *Corynebacterium* sp.

Polyesters

Polyesters are polymers in which the component monomers are bonded via ester linkages. Many kinds of esters occur in nature, and the esterases that degrade them are ubiquitous in living organisms. Ester linkages are generally easy to hydrolyse, and hence a number of synthetic polyesters are biodegradable; bacterial polyesters (polyhydroxyalkanoates) have been used to make biodegradable plastics. Hydrolytic cleavage of the ester bond in low molecular weight polyesters by the lipase of *Pseudomonas* sp. has been reported.

Polyhydroxyalkanoates

Polyhydroxybutyrate (PHB) is a naturally occurring polyester that accumulates in bacterial cells as a carbon and energy storage compound. PHB and copolymers containing polyhydroxyalkanoate PHA (e.g. 3-hydroxyvaleratel) are being used for the manufacture of biodegradable plastics. Several PHA and PHB bacterial depolymerases are found to be capable of metabolising PHB and other polyhydroxy-alkanoate (PHA) polymers. The PHA depolymerases are serine, hydrolases, usually having a single substrate-binding domain. Recently a PHB depolymerase with a two substrate-binding domain was reported. PHB depolymerases are able to degrade all-(R) chains, cyclic-(R) oligomers, oligolides, and racemic hydroxybutanoate polymers. The enzymes are generally obtained from micro-organisms like *Alcaligenes faecalis* and *Pseudomonas stutzeri*.

Atactic P(R, S-3HB) (atactic poly(R, S-3-hydroxybutyrate), which does not biodegrade in pure form, can undergo enzymatic hydrolysis in a P(R, S-3HB)/PMMA) polymethacrylatel blend, indicating that the enzymatic degradation can be induced by blending with an amorphous nonbiodegradable polymer. This is possibly because the blend gives P(R-3HB) depolymerase a more stable binding surface than that provided by the rubbery α-P(R,S-3HB). The depolymerase was purified from *Alcaligenes faecalis*. In order to modify their physical properties and retard enzymatic degradation of commercial microbial polyesters like PHA, they are blended with other degradable or nondegradable polymers such as PVA, PMMA, poly(ethylene oxide), PLA, cellulose, PCL, and polystyrene (PS).

Polylcaprolactone (PCL)

Polylcaprolactone (PCL) is a synthetic polyester that can be degraded by micro-organisms and enzymes such as lipases and esterases. *Cutinases*, which are obtained from fungal phytopathogens, degrade cutin (the structural polymer of the plant cuticle) and act as PCL depolymerases. The biodegradability of polycaprolactone in the form of blend sheets (e.g. in polycarbonate-polycaprolactone blend sheets) is much reduced because the packed form of PCL in the blend sheets protects it from enzymatic digestion. However, enzymatic degradation can be promoted by using oxygen plasma treatments to etch the surface. *Penicillium* spp. is known to utilise polyethylene adipate and polycaprolactone as its sole carbon and energy source, respectively.

Poly-L-lactide

Poly-L-lactide (PLLA) is a lactic acid-based aliphatic polyester that is used in medical and packaging applications. It can be degraded both aerobically and anaerobically. Several enzymes, including proteinase K, pronase, and bromelain, can degrade the polymer. Under thermophylic conditions, degradation with bromelain is faster than the others, probably because lactic acid is more favourable for anaerobic micro-organisms than for aerobic organisms. PLLA is also found to degrade completely in 2 weeks in windrow composting.

Polylactic acid (PLA)

Polylactic acid (PLA) is absorbed easily in animals and humans, and hence has been extensively used in medicines. The degradation of the polymer in animals and humans is thought to proceed via nonenzymatic hydrolysis. Several enzymes, including proteinase K, pronase, and bromelain, can degrade the polymer. PLA is also readily degraded in compost to CO_2 (about 90 per cent degradation was achieved in 90 days). A PLA-degrading actinomycete strain reduced 100 mg of PLA film by 60 per cent in the first 14 days in liquid culture at 303K. *Bacillus brevis* is also found to degrade 50 mg of PCL by around 20 per cent in 20 days in liquid culture at 333K.

Poly(p-dioxanone)

Poly(*p*-dioxanone) (PPDO) is known as a poly(etherester) and has good tensile strength and flexibility. It is used for bioabsorbable sutures in clinical applications. PPDO is degraded by strains that belong to the α and β subdivision of the class Proteobacteria and the class Actinobacteria. Degradation leads to the formation of monomeric acids.

Polyurethane (PUR)

Polyurethane (PUR) produced by the diisocyanate polyaddition process is the characteristic chain link of the urethane bond (Fig. 20.5). PUR degradation proceeds in a selective manner, with the amorphous regions being degraded before the crystalline regions. PUR synthesised from polyester polyol is termed 'polyester PUR', and that synthesised from polyether polyol is termed 'polyether PUR'. Although most PUR used at present is polyether PUR, polyester PUR has recently become the focus of attention because of its biodegradability; therefore, it has advantages from the viewpoint of waste treatment. The PUR depolymerases of micro-organisms have not been examined in detail, although because of the presence of the ester linkage, most degradation is carried out by esterases. *Comamonas acidovorans* TB-35 utilises a polyester PUR that contains polydiethyleneglycol adipate as the sole source of carbon but not polyether PUR.

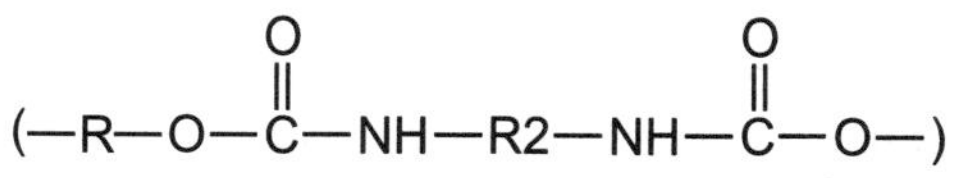

$$(-R-O-\overset{\overset{\displaystyle O}{\|}}{C}-NH-R2-NH-\overset{\overset{\displaystyle O}{\|}}{C}-O-)$$

Fig. 20.5. Structure of PUR.

Phua found that two proteolytic enzymes, papain and urease, degraded medical polyester PUR. Bacteria like *Corynebacterium* sp. and *Pseudomonas aeruginosa* could degrade PUR in the presence of basal media. Several fungi are observed to grow on PUR surfaces, especially *Curvularia senegalensis*, which was observed to have a higher PU-degrading activity. Although cross-linking was considered to inhibit degradation, papain was found to diffuse through the film and break the structural integrity by hydrolysing the urethane and urea linkage, producing free amine and hydroxyl group. Porcine pancreatic elastase degraded polyester PUR 10 times faster than its activity against polyether PUR. Table 20.2 lists the various micro-organisms that degrade PU.

Table 20.2. Polyurethane (PUR) degrading micro-organisms.

Micro-organisms	PUR degraded
Fungi	
Aspergillus niger	PS, PE
A. flavus	PS, PE
A. fumigatus	PE
A. versicolor	PS, PE
Aureobasidium pullulans	PS, PE
Chaetomium globosum	PS, PE
Cladosporium sp.	PS
Curvularia senegalensis	PS
Fusarium solani	PS
Gliocladium roseum	PS
Penicillium citrinum	PS
P. funiculosum	PS, PE
Trichoderma sp.	PS, PE

(Contd ...)

Micro-organisms	PUR degraded
Bacteria	
Comambnas acidovorans	PS
Corynebacterium sp.	PS
Enterobacter agglomerans	PS
Serratia rubidaea	PS
Pseudomonas aeruginosa	PS
Staphylococcus epidermidis	PE

PE, polyether PUR; PS, polyester PUR

Polyvinyl alcohol (PVA)

Polyvinyl alcohol (PVA) is a vinyl polymer joined by only carbon-carbon linkages. The linkage is the same as those of typical plastics such as polyethylene, polypropylene, and polystyrene, and of watersoluble polymers such as polyacrylamide and polyacrylic acid. Among the vinyl polymers produced industrially, PVA is the only one known to be mineralised by micro-organisms. PVA is water soluble and biodegradable; hence it is used to make water-soluble and biodegradable carriers, which may be useful in the manufacture of delivery systems for chemicals such as fertilisers, pesticides, and herbicides.

PVA is completely degraded and utilised by a bacterial strain, *Pseudomonas* O-3, as a sole source of carbon and energy. However, PVA-degrading micro-organisms are not ubiquitous within the environment. Almost all the degrading strains belong to the genus *Pseudomonas*, although some do belong to other genera. Among the PVA-degrading bacteria reported so far, a few strains showed no requirement for pyrroloquinoline quinone (PQQ). From a PVA-utilising mixed culture, *Pseudomonas* sp. VM15C and *P. putida* VM15A were isolated. Their symbiosis is based on a syntrophic interaction. VM15C is a PVA-degrading strain that degrades and metabolises PVA, while VM15A excretes a growth factor that VM15C requires for PVA utilisation.

Nylon

High molecular weight nylon 66 membrane was degraded significantly by lignin-degrading white rot fungi grown under ligninolytic conditions with limited glucose or ammonium tartrate. The characteristics of a nylon-degrading enzyme purified from a culture supernatant of white rot fungal strain IZU-154 were identical to those of manganese peroxidase, but the reaction mechanism for nylon degradation differed significantly from manganese peroxidase. The enzyme could also degrade nylon-6 fibres. The nylon was degraded to soluble oligomers by drastic and regular erosion.

A thermophilic strain capable of degrading nylon 12 was isolated from 100 soil samples by enrichment culture technique at 60°C. At this temperature, the strain not only grew on nylon 12 but also reduced the molecular weight of the polymer. The strain was identified as a neighbouring species to *Bacillus pallidus*. This strain had an optimum growth temperature of around 60°C. It was also found to degrade nylon 6 as well as nylon 12 but not nylon 66.

Polyvinyl chloride

Polyvinyl chloride (PVC) has become a universal polymer with many applications (e.g. for pipes, floor coverings, cable insulation, roofing sheets, packaging foils, bottles, and medical products) because of its low cost and physical, chemical, and weathering properties. PVC degrades at relatively low temperatures (~100°C) in the presence of light to release hydrogen chloride. Hence, to prevent degradation during processing, heat stabilisers are added, part of which are consumed during the processing. Degradation can also be achieved by exposure to molecular oxygen in the presence of alkali at higher temperature. The hydrogen chloride can be used for monomer production. Under regular anaerobic landfill conditions at 50°C, no changes were observed in the PVC, indicating that the polymer matrix is stable and no biodegradation has occurred.

Polyethylene (PE)

Polyethylenes of low density are used widely as films in the packaging industry. They pose a serious problem because of their slow rate of degradation under natural conditions. They pose problems to the environment, freshwater, and animals. Extracellular *Streptomyces* sp. cultures were found to degrade starch blended PE. *Phanerochaete chrysosporium* was also found to degrade starch blended LDPE in soil.

High molecular weight polyethylene is also degraded by lignin-degrading fungi under nitrogen-limited or carbon-limited conditions and by manganese peroxidase. Fungi such as *Mucor rouxii* NRRL 1835 and *Aspergillius flavus* and several strains of *Streptomyces* are capable of degrading polyethylene containing 6 per cent starch. Degradation was monitored by observing changes in mechanical properties such as tensile strength and elongation. The biodegradability of blends of LDPE and rice or potato starch was enhanced when the starch content exceeded 10 per cent (w/w). No micro-organism or bacteria has been found so far that could degrade PE that has no additives.

Polycarbonate (PC)

Bisphenol-A polycarbonate (PC) is widely used because of its excellent physical properties such as transparency, high tensile strength, impact resistance, rigidity, and water resistance. Polycarbonate gets its name from the carbonate groups in its backbone chain. At 300°C in air, a 25 per cent reduction in the molecular weight of PC was observed.

PC is stable to bioorganism attack. PC sheets are known to degrade in lipase AK, but when they are blended with PC they become less biodegradable. Because PC is hydrophobic, it probably suppresses biodegradation. Several authors nave described enzymatic degradation of aliphatic polycarbonate (polyethylene carbonate, PEC). No degradation of PEC with a molecular weight of 300 to 450 kDa in hydrolytic enzymes (including lipase, esterase, lysozyme, chymotrypsin, trypsin, papin, pepsin, collagenase, pronase, and pronase E) was observed. This indicates that hydrolytic mechanisms based on hydrolases or aqueous conditions can be excluded for biodegradation of PEC.

Polyimide

Polyimides find application in the electronic and packaging industries. These polymers possess high strength and resistance to degradation. Fungi such as *Aspergillus versicolor*, *Cladosporium cladosporioides*, and *Chaetomium* sp. were found to degrade this polymer. Bacteria like *Acinetobacter johnsonii*, *Agrobacterium radiobacter*, *Alcaligenes denitricans*, *Comamonas acidovorans*, *Pseudomonas* sp., and *Vibrio anguillarum*, when tested, were not effective in biodegrading this polymer.

Fibre-reinforced polymeric composite

Fibre-reinforced polymeric composite materials (FRPCMs) are materials important in the aerospace and aviation industries. A fungal mixture consisting of *Aspergillus versicolor*, *Cladosporium cladosorioides*, and *Chaetomium* sp. and a mixed culture of bacteria including a sulphate-reducing bacterium were found to grow on this composite material. Only the fungi mixture could cause deterioration detectable over more than 350 days.

Polyacrylamide (PAA)

Polyacrylamides are water-soluble synthetic linear polymers made of acrylamide or the combination of acrylamide and acrylic acid. Polyacrylamide finds applications in pulp and paper production, agriculture, food processing, mining, and as a flocculant in waste-water treatment. Polyacrylamide undergoes thermal degradation at 175° to 300°C and can also undergo photodegradation.

Acrylamide is readily biodegraded under aerobic conditions by micro-organisms in soil and water by deamination to acrylic acid and ammonia, which are utilised as carbon and nitrogen sources. *Pseudomonas stutzeri*, *Rhodococcus* spp., *Xanthomonas* spp., and mixed cultures have demonstrated degrading abilities under aerobic conditions in numerous studies.

Polyamide (PA)

Polyamide-6 (PA-6) is a widely used engineering material. Oxidative degradation of PA-6 membranes was found using lignolytic white rot fungus IZU-154. *Aspergillus niger*-mediated degradation of polyamides based on tartaric acid and hexamethylenediamine and *Corynebacterium aurantiacum*-mediated degradation of ε-caprolactam, as well as its oligomers, have been reported. Lignolytic fungus *Phanerochaete chrysosporium* is also found to degrade PA-6. Degradation of the polymer was observed through a decrease in the average molecular mass (50 per cent after 3 months), as well as in the physical damage to the fibres visible under a scanning electron microscope.

Rubber

Biological attack of natural rubber latex is quite facile, but addition of sulphur and numerous other ingredients reduces biological attack. Straube devulcanised scrap rubber by holding the comminuted scrap rubber in a bacterial suspension of chemolithotropic micro-organisms with a supply of air until elemental sulphur or sulphuric acid was separated. This process can reclaim rubber and sulphur in a simplified manner. The biodegradation of the *cis*-1,4-polyisoprene chain was achieved by bacterium belonging to the genus *Nacardia* and led to considerable weight loss of different soft type NR-vulcanisates. Old tyres with 1.6 per cent sulphur were treated with different species of *Thiobacillus ferrooxidans*, *T. thiooxidans*, and *T. thioparus* in shake flasks and in a laboratory reactor. The best results were obtained with *T. thioparus*— 4.7 per cent of the total sulphur of the rubber powder was oxidised to sulphate within 40 days.

Since most of the polymers are resistant to degradation, research over the past couple of decades has focused on developing biodegradable polymers that are degraded and ultimately catabolised to carbon dioxide and water by bacteria and fungi under natural conditions. During the degradation process, they should not generate any substances that are harmful. These polymers can be classified into three major categories: (i) polyesters produced by micro-organisms, (ii) natural polysaccharides and other biopolymers like starch, and (iii) synthetic polymers like aliphatic polymers (e.g. poly ε-caprolactone, poly L-lactide and poly butylenesuccinate, which are commercially produced).

Another approach toward achieving biodegradability has been through the addition of biodegradable groups into the main chain during the production of industrial polymers prepared by free radical copolymerisation. Two such approaches are the use of ethylene *bis*(mercaptoacetate) as a chain transfer agent during the copolymerisation of styrene and MMA, and the preparation of copolymers of vinylic monomers with cyclic comonomers containing the biodegradable functions such as ketene acetal and cyclic disulphides.

AEROBIC BACTERIAL DEGRADATION OF BIOPOLYMERS

Basic Biology, Mass, and Energy Balance of Aerobic Biopolymer Degradation

In ecosystems in which molecular oxygen is available, plant and animal biomasses are degraded to CO_2 and H_2O, catalysed by either single species of aerobic micro-organisms or the whole population of the ecosystem, in competition for the substrates. A single organism may be able to hydrolyse the polymers and oxidise the monomers to CO_2 and H_2O with oxygen. To make soluble and insoluble biopolymers, mainly carbohydrates, proteins, and lipids, accessible for respiration by bacteria, the macromolecules must be hydrolysed by exoenzymes, which are often produced and excreted only after contact with the respective inducers. The exoenzymes adsorb to the biopolymers and hydrolyse them to monomers or at least, to oligomers. Only soluble, low molecular weight compounds (e.g. sugars, disaccharides, amino acids, oligopeptides, glycerol, fatty acids) can be taken up by micro-organisms and are metabolised for energy production and cell multiplication. The two steps can be represented as:

$$\text{Complex organic compounds} \xrightarrow[\text{action}]{\text{Exoenzyme}} \text{Simple absorbable polymers}$$

$$\text{Simple polymers} \xrightarrow{\text{Respiration}} \text{Basic elements + energy}$$

Once taken up, degradation via glycolysis (sugars, disaccharides, glycerol), hydrolysis and deamination (amino acids, oligopeptides), or hydrolysis and β-oxidation (phospholipids, long-chain fatty acids), proceeds in the cells. Metabolism of almost all organic compounds leads to the formation of acetyl-CoA as the central intermediate, which is used for biosynthesis, excreted as acetate, or oxidised to CO_2 and reducing equivalents in the tricarboxylic acid (TCA) cycle. The reducing equivalents are respired with molecular oxygen in the respiratory chain. The energy of a maximum of only 2 molecules of anhydridic phosphate bonds of ATP is conserved during glycolysis of 1 molecule of glucose, through substrate chain phosphorylation. An additional 2 molecules of ATP are formed during oxidation of 2 molecules of acetate in the TCA cycle, whereas 34 molecules of ATP are formed by electron transport chain, with oxygen as the terminal electron acceptor. During oxygen respiration, reducing equivalents react with molecular oxygen in a controlled combustion reaction.

Growth Associated Degradation of Carbohydrates

Different carbohydrates like starch, polysaccharides, lignin, cellulose and hemicellulose are microbially degraded under aerobic conditions to produce CO_2 and H_2O. The energy released from the degradation is used by the microbes for their growth. The first step in the degradation process is hydrolysis of complex polymers, catalysed by numerous auxiliary enzymes like, cellulase, xylanases, amylases, phosphorylases, etc. Starch and glycogen are converted to D-glucose units by phosphorylases and phosphoglucomutase to gain energy into the glycolytic pathway. Hydrolysis of complex carbohydrates produces many a type of monosaccharides, other than glucose, and also disaccharides like, sucrose, maltose and lactose.

The disaccharides are then hydrolysed to monosaccharides by the enzymes on the cell surface of the microbes, which then gain entry into the cell for aerobic breakdown. The monomers are converted to pyruvate and, subsequently to CO_2 and H_2O in the cell through glycolysis and tricarboxylic acid cycle, respectively. A part of the carbohydrate is also utilised to produce the cell biomass, as well as to be stored in the microbial cells as food reserve.

Growth Associated Degradation of Proteins

The proteins present in the wastes are aerobically degraded by microbes in three successive steps: (i) hydrolysis of proteins to amino acids by proteases and peptidases, (ii) deamination of amino acids by dehydrogenases to produce carboxylic acids, and (iii) oxidative breakdown of the carboxylic acids to CO_2 and H_2O.

Aerobic Degradation of Hydrocarbons

Growth-associated degradation of aliphatics

The aerobic initial attack on aliphatic and cycloaliphatic hydrocarbons requires molecular oxygen. Two types of enzymatic reactions are involved in these processes; a monooxygenase or a dioxygenase reaction, depending on the nature of the substrate and the enzymes possessed by the micro-organisms. The n-alkanes are the main constituents of mineral oil contamination.

A minor pathway proceeds via an epoxide, which is converted to a fatty acid. Branching generally reduces the rate of biodegradation. Methyl side groups do not noticeably decrease the biodegradability, whereas complex branched chains, e.g. the tertiary butyl groups, hinder the action of the degradative enzymes.

The products of hydrocarbon degradation, that are fed into the central tricarboxylic acid cycle, have a dual function: as substrates of energy metabolism and building blocks for the biosynthesis of cell biomass. The cell biomass can be mineralised after the exhaustion of degradable pollutants in a contaminated site.

Biodegradability of aliphatics is also negatively influenced by branching in the hydrocarbon chain. The degree of resistance to biodegradation depends on both the number of branches and the positions of methyl groups in the molecule. Compounds with a quaternary carbon atom (four carbon-carbon bonds).

Alkenes

Alkenes are hydrocarbons that contain one or more double bonds. The majority of alkene biodegradability studies have used 1-alkenes as model compounds. These studies have shown that alkenes and alkanes have comparable biodegradation rates. As illustrated in Fig. 20.7, the initial step in 1-alkens degradation can involve attack at the terminal (1) or a subterminal (2) methyl group as described for alkanes. Alternatively, the initial step can be attack at the double bond, which can yield a primary (3) or secondary alcohol (4) or an epoxide (5). Each of these initial degradation products is further oxidised to a primary fatty acid, which is degraded by β-oxidation as shown in Fig. 20.6 for alkanes.

Halogenated aliphatics

Chlorinated solvents such as trichloroethylene (TCE) have been extensively used as industrial solvents. As a result of improper use and disposal, these solvents are among the most frequently detected types of organic contaminants in groundwater. The need for efficient and cost-effective remediation of solvent-contaminated sites has stimulated interest in the biodegradation of these C_1 and C_2 halogenated aliphatics. Halogenated aliphatics are generally degraded more slowly than aliphatics without halogen substitution. For example, although 1-chloroalkanes ranging from C_1 to C_{12} are degraded as a sole source of carbon and energy in pure culture, they are degraded more slowly than their nonchlorinated counterparts. The presence of two or three chlorines bound to the same carbon atom inhibits aerobic degradation. Further, degradation rates of 1-chloroalkanes, ranging from C_3 to C_{12}, increased with increasing alkyl chain length. These results can be explained by the decreasing electronic effects of the chlorine atom on the enzyme-carbon reaction centre as the alkane chain length increases.

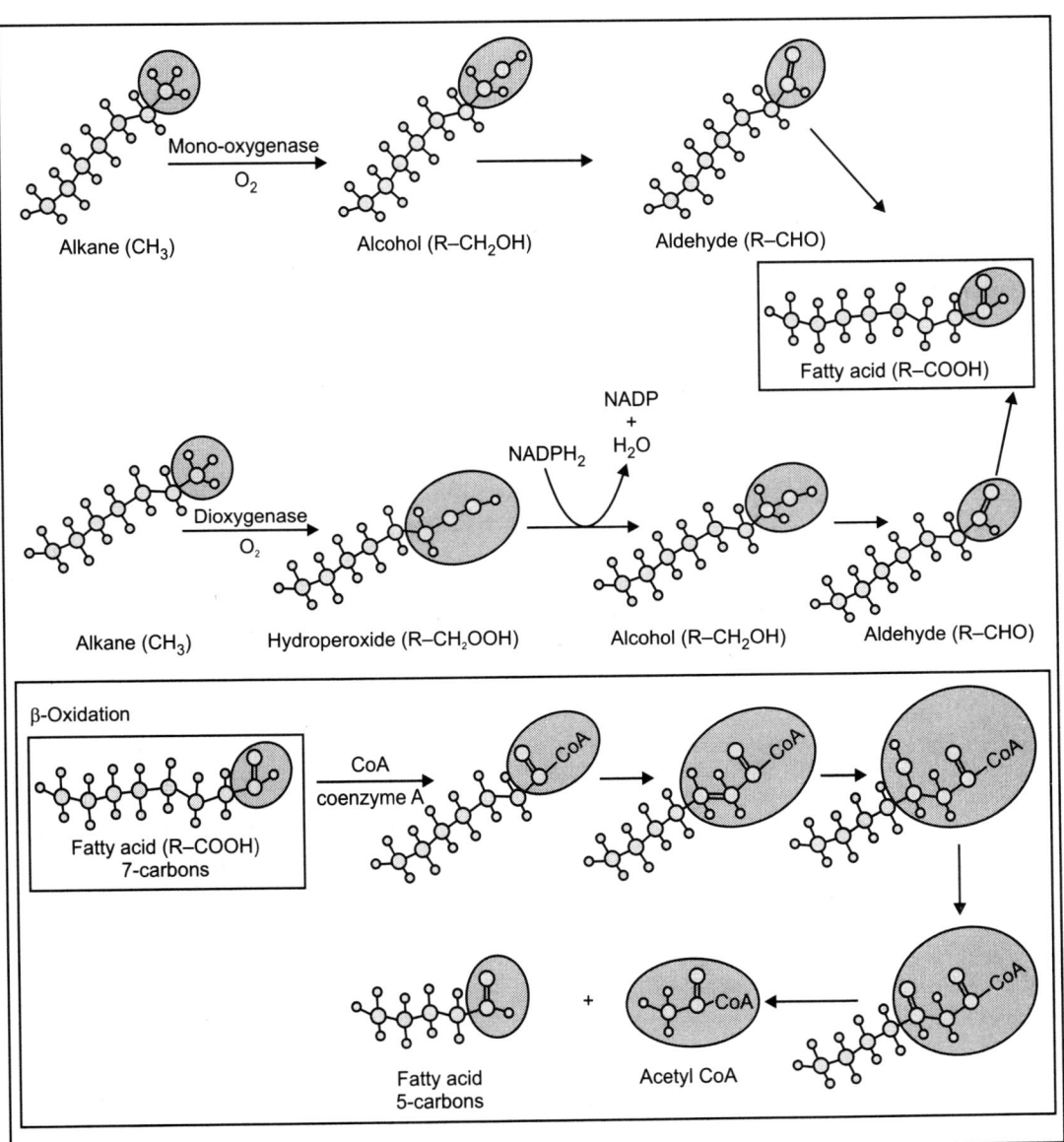

Fig. 20.6. Biodegradation of alkanes.

Biodegradation of halogenated aliphatics occurs by three basic types of reactions. Substitution is a nucleophilic reaction (the reacting species brings an electron pair) in which the halogens on a mono- or dihalogenated compound are substituted by a hydroxy group (Fig. 20.8). Oxidation reactions are catalysed by a select group of monooxygenase and dioxygenase enzymes that have been reported to oxidise highly chlorinated C_1 and C_2 compounds, e.g. TCE.

These mono- and dioxygenase enzymes are produced by bacteria to oxidise a variety of nonchlorinated compounds including methane, ammonia, toluene, and propane. These enzymes do not have exact substrate specificity, and thus they can also participate in the cometabolic degradation of chlorinated aliphatics. Usually, a large ratio of substrate to chlorinated aliphatic is required to achieve cometabolic degradation of the chlorinated aliphatic. Reported examples of oxygenase-substrate systems that cometabolically degrade chlorinated hydrocarbons include methane monooxygenase produced by methanotrophic bacteria during growth on carbon sources such as methane or formate, toluene dioxygenase produced during growth of some bacteria on toluene, ammonia monooxygenase produced by *Nitrosomonas europaea* during growth on ammonia, and propane monooxygenase produced by *Mycobacterium vaccae* during growth on propane. Figure 20.9 shows an example of cometabolic oxidation of a C_1 compound, chloroform (see pathway 1), and a C_2 alkene, TCE (see pathway 2).

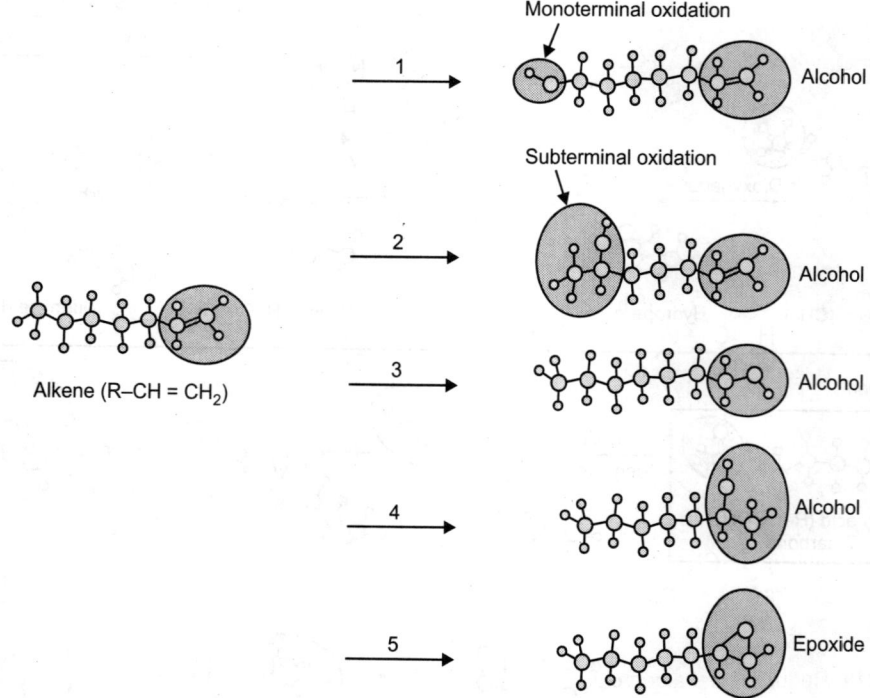

Fig. 20.7. Biodegradation of alkenes.

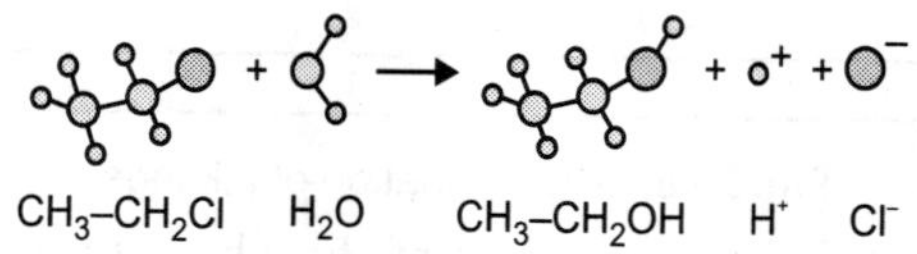

$$CH_3-CH_2Cl \quad H_2O \qquad CH_3-CH_2OH \quad H^+ \quad Cl^-$$

Fig. 20.8. Dechlorination by substitution.

Reductive dehalogenation, the third type of reaction involved in biodegradation of halogenated organics, is mediated by reduced transition metal complexes. Reductive dehalogenation generally occurs in an anaerobic environment. However, the second of the reactions shown in Fig. 20.10, formation of alkenes, can occur aerobically for a limited number of chlorinated compounds that have a higher reducing potential than O_2, e.g. hexachloroethane and dibromoethane. In the first step of reductive dehalogenation, electrons are transferred from the reduced metal to the halogenated aliphatic, resulting in an alkyl radical and free halogen. The alkyl radical can either scavenge a hydrogen atom (1) or lose a second halogen to form an alkene (2).

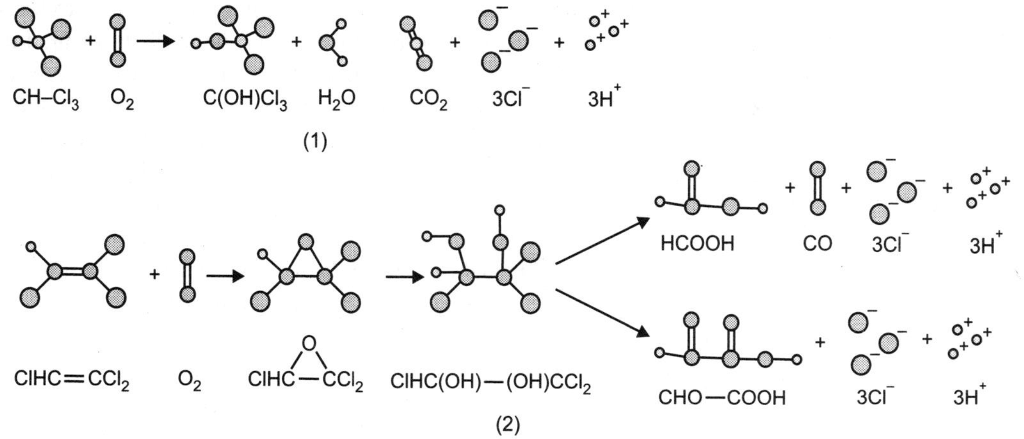

| CH–Cl$_3$ | O$_2$ | | C(OH)Cl$_3$ | H$_2$O | CO$_2$ | 3Cl$^-$ | 3H$^+$ |

(1)

HCOOH   CO   3Cl$^-$ 3H$^+$

| ClHC=CCl$_2$ | O$_2$ | ClHC—CCl$_2$ | ClHC(OH)—(OH)CCl$_2$ |

CHO—COOH   3Cl$^-$ 3H$^+$

(2)

Fig. 20.9. Dehalogenation by oxidation.

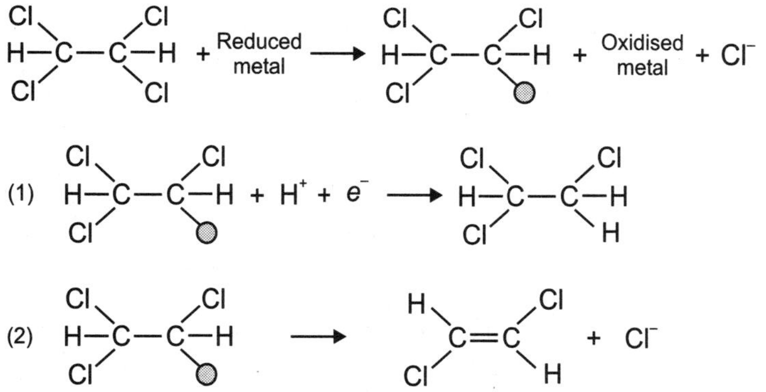

Fig. 20.10. Reductive dehalogenation of tetrachloroethane to trichloroethane (1) or dichloroethylene (2).

Generally, aerobic conditions favour the biodegradation of compounds with fewer halogen substituents, and anaerobic conditions favour the biodegradation of compounds with a high number of halogen substituents. However, complete biodegradation of highly halogenated aliphatics under anaerobic conditions often does not take place. Therefore, some researchers have proposed the use of a sequential anaerobic and aerobic treatment. Initial incubation under anaerobic conditions would be used to decrease the halogen content, and subsequent addition of oxygen would create aerobic conditions to allow complete degradation to proceed aerobically.

One important consideration in the bioremediation of sites containing chlorinated, aliphatics is the potential toxicity of such compounds. For example, the effect of solvent concentration on inhibition of a propylene-grown *Xanthobacter* strain capable of oxidising several chlorinated alkenes, including TCE, was determined. It was found that alkene monooxygenase activity was up to 90 per cent inhibited by chlorinated alkene concentrations between 25 and 330 μM, depending on the compound. Similarly, it was found that toluene used to support the aerobic metabolism of TCE in soil could be inhibitory.

Specifically, increasing the TCE concentration from 1 to 20 μg/ml decreased the numbers of toluene and TCE degraders in the soil and decreased the rate of TCE degradation. Also of concern is that TCE transformations can result in oxidised derivatives more toxic than TCE itself. This toxicity has been attributed to a nonspecific binding of TCE transformation products to cellular proteins. For example, TCE transformation by methane monooxygenase results in a transformation product that can bind to a protein subunit of the mono oxygenase enzyme, resulting in inhibition of enzyme activity. Recovery of oxidising activity is possible by replacement of the enzyme following *de novo* protein synthesis. Similar behaviour was found for **ammonia** monooxygenase. In this experiment, a wide variety of chlorinated aliphatic compounds **were** tested and it was found that ammonia monooxygenase activity was strongly inhibited after the oxidation of some chlorinated ethylenes and compounds containing a dichlorinated carbon. These examples all demonstrate that harnessing cometabolic activity for unusual substrates is a complex process. Not only does one have to understand the cometabolic reaction, one must also consider the potential toxicity of the cometabolic substrate and its metabolites to degrading microbes.

Alicyclics

Alicyclic hydrocarbons are major components of crude oil, 20 to 70 per cent by volume. They are commonly found elsewhere in nature as components of plant oils and paraffins, microbial lipids, and pesticides. The various components can be simple, such as cyclopentane and cyclohexane, or complex, such as trimethylcyclopentane and various cycloparaffins. The use of alicyclic compounds in the chemical industry, and the release of alicyclics to the environment through industrial processes, other than oil processing and utilisation, is more limited than for aliphatics and aromatics. Consequently, the issue of health risks associated with human exposure to alicyclics has not reached the same level of importance as for the other classes of compounds, especially the aromatics. As a result, far less research has focused on the study of alicyclic biodegradation.

It is known that there is no correlation between the ability to utilise *n*-alkanes and the ability to oxidise cycloalkanes fully. Further, it is difficult to isolate pure cultures that degrade alicyclic hydrocarbons using enrichment techniques. Although micro-organisms with complete degradation pathways have been isolated, alicyclic hydrocarbon degradation is thought to occur primarily by commensalistic and cometabolic reactions as shown for cydohexane in Fig. 20.11. In this series of reactions, one organism converts cyclohexane to cyclohexanone via a cyclohexanol (step 1 and step 2), but is unable to lactonise and open the ring. A second organism that is unable to oxidise cyclohexane to cyclohexanone can perform the lactonisation, ring opening, and mineralisation of the remaining aliphatic compound.

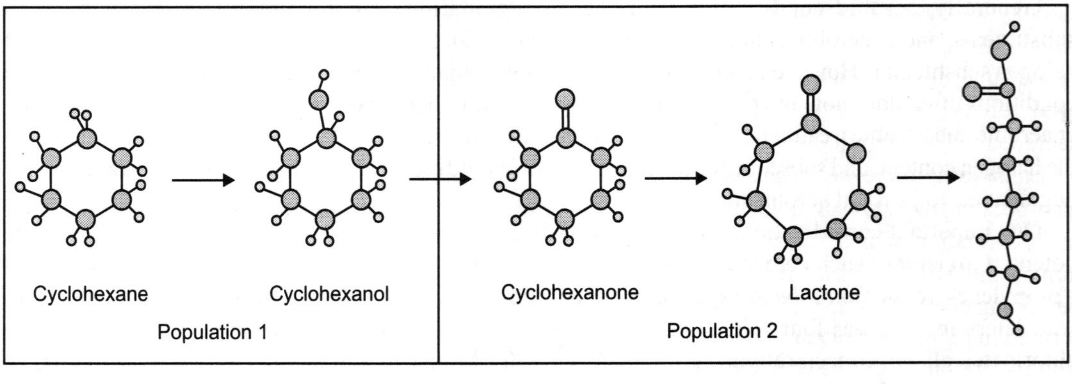

Cyclohexane   Cyclohexanol   Cyclohexanone   Lactone

Population 1   Population 2

Fig. 20.11. Degradation of cyclohexane.

Cyclopentane and cyclohexane derivatives that contain one or two OH, C=O, or COOH groups are readily metabolised, and such degraders are easily isolated from environmental samples. In contrast, degradation of alicyclic derivatives containing one or more CH_3 groups is inhibited. This is reflected in the decreasing rate of biodegradation for the following series of alkyl derivatives of cyclohexanol: cyclohexanol > methylcyclohexanol > dimethylcyclohexanol.

Aromatics

Unsubstituted aromatics

Aromatic compounds contain at least one unsaturated ring system with the general structure C_6R_6, where R is any functional group. Benzene (C_6H_6) is the parent hydrocarbon of this family of unsaturated cyclic compounds. Compounds containing two or more fused benzene rings are called polyaromatic hydrocarbons (PAH). Aromatic hydrocarbons are natural products; they are part of lignin and are formed as organic materials are burned, for example, in forest fires. However, the addition of aromatic compounds to the environment has increased dramatically through activities such as fossil fuel processing and utilisation and burning of wood and coal. The quantity and composition of the aromatic hydrocarbon component in petroleum products are of major concern when evaluating a contaminated site because several components of the aromatic fraction have been shown to be carcinogenic to humans. Aromatic compounds also have demonstrated toxic effects toward micro-organisms. For example, the toxicity of the water-soluble fraction of refined oil is more toxic to the growth of heterotrophic micro-organisms than the water soluble fraction of crude oil. This is attributed to the greater proportion of aromatic compounds, particularly naphthalene and alkylnaphthalenes, present in refined oils compared with crude oils. For example, the total naphthalene concentration of the refined oil was 1800 µg/l, compared with only 45 µg/l in the crude oil tested. Autotrophs are also affected adversely. When the impact of the aliphatic, aromatic, and asphaltic fractions from five petroleum oils on photosynthesis and respiration of a representative cyanobacterium was determined, it was found that growth inhibition was most strongly associated with the aromatic fraction.

Because of the potential human health impacts of aromatic compounds, their biodegradation has been extensively studied. The results of this work showed that a wide variety of bacteria and fungi can carry out aromatic transformations, both partial and complete, under a variety of environmental conditions. Under aerobic conditions, the most common initial transformation is a hydroxylation that involves the incorporation of molecular oxygen. The enzymes involved in these initial transformations are either monoxygenases or dioxygenases. In general; prokaryotic micro-organisms transform aromatics by an initial dioxygenase attack to *cis*-dihydrodiols. The *cis*-dihydrodiol is rearomatised to form a dihydro-xylated intermediate, catechol. The catechol ring is cleaved by a second dioxygenase either between the two hydroxyl groups (ortho pathway) or next to one of the hydroxyl groups (meta pathway) and further degraded to completion.

Eukaryotic micro-organisms initially attack aromatics with a cytochrome P-450 monooxygenase, incorporating one atom of molecular oxygen into the aromatic and reducing the second to water, resulting in the formation of an arene oxide. This is followed by the enzymatic addition of water to yield a *trans*-dihydrodiol (Fig. 20.12). Alternatively, the arene oxide can be isomerised to form phenols, which can be conjugated with sulphate, glucuronic acid, and glutathione. These conjugates are similar to those formed in higher organisms and seem to aid in detoxification and elimination of aromatic compounds. The exception to this is the white-rot fungi which under certain conditions are able to completely mineralise aromatic compounds.

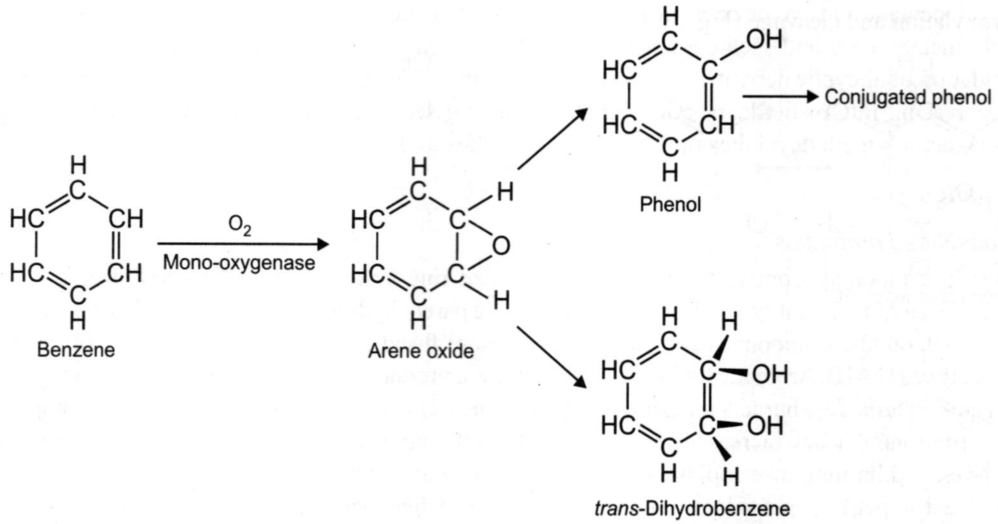

Fig. 20.12. Fungal mono-oxygenase incorporation of oxygen into the aromatic ring.

Thus far, six families of genes responsible for PAH degradation have been identified. Often the capacity for aromatic degradation, especially chlorinated aromatics, is plasmid mediated. Plasmids can carry both individual genes and operons encoding partial or complete biodegradation of an aromatic compound.

In general, aromatics composed of one, two, or three condensed rings are transformed rapidly and often completely mineralised, whereas aromatics containing four or more condensed rings are transformed much more slowly, often as a result of cometabolic attack. This is due to the limited bioavailability of these high-molecular-weight aromatics. Such PAHs have very limited aqueous solubility and sorb strongly to particle surfaces in soil and sediments. However, it has been demonstrated that chronic exposure to aromatic compounds will result in increased transformation rates because of adaptation of an indigenous population to growth on aromatic compounds.

Substituted aromatics

One group of aromatics of special interest is the chlorinated aromatics. These compounds have been used extensively as solvents and fumigants (e.g. dichlorobenzene), and wood preservatives [e.g. pentachlorophenol (PCP)] and are parent compounds for pesticides such as 2,4-dichlorophenoxyacetic acid (2,4-D) and DDT. The difficulty for microbes in the degradation of chlorinated organics is that the carbon-chlorine bond is very strong and requires a large input of energy to break. Second, the common intermediate in aromatic degradation is catechol or dihydroxybenzene. This molecule requires two adjacent unsubstituted carbons so that hydroxyl groups can be added. Chlorine substituents can block these sites. Some strategies for degradation of chlorinated aromatics are shown in Fig. 20.13 for pentachlorophenol and dichlorobenzene.

Methylated aromatic derivatives, such as toluene, constitute another common group of substituted aromatics. These are major components of gasoline and are commonly used as solvents. These compounds can initially be attacked either on the methyl group or directly on the ring as shown in Fig. 20.14. Alkyl derivatives are attacked first at the alkyl chain, which is shortened by β-oxidation to the corresponding benzoic acid or phenylacetic acid, depending on the number of carbon atoms. This is followed by ring hydroxylation and cleavage (Fig. 20.14).

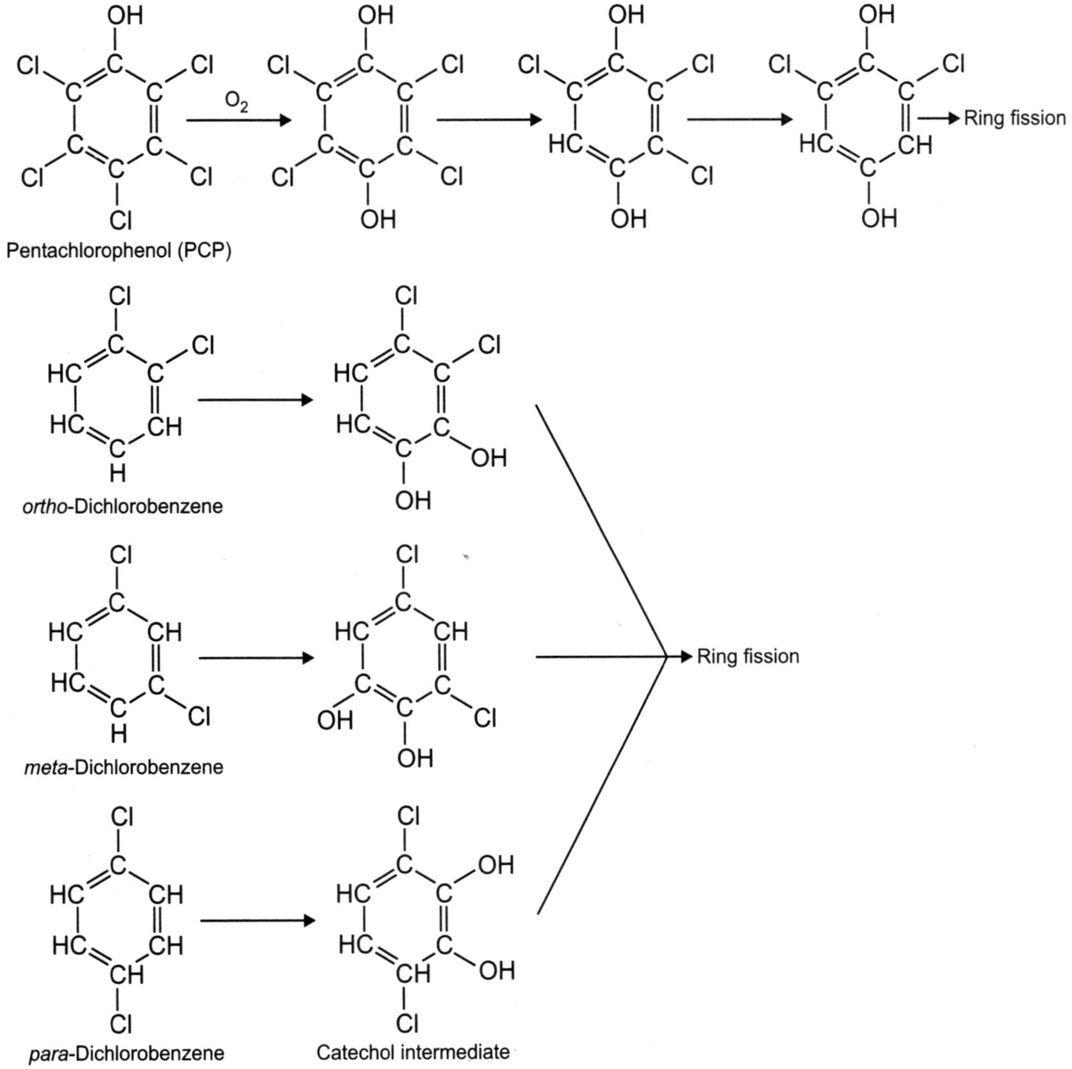

Fig. 20.13. Initial steps in the arobic degradation of pentachlorophenol and three dichlorobenzenes.

Dioxins

Dioxins and dibenzofurans are created during waste incineration and are part of the released smoke stack effluent. Once thought to be one of the most potent carcinogens known, 2,3,7,8-tetrachlorodibenzop-dioxin (TCDD) is associated with the manufacture of 2,4-D and 2,4,5-trichlorophenoxy acetic acid (2,4, 5-T), hexacholorophene, and other pesticides that have 2,4,5-T as a precursor. Current thinking is that TCDD is less dangerous in terms of carcinogenicity and teratogenicity than once thought, but that noncancer risks including diabetes, reduced IQ, and behavioural impacts may be more important.

For example, a mixture of six bacterial strains isolated from TCDD-contaminated soil obtained from Seveso, Italy was able to produce a metabolite presumed to be 1-hydroxy-TCDD. However, less than 1 per cent of the original TCDD was degraded in 12 weeks. In addition, the fungus *Phanerochaete chrysosporium* was only able to mineralise 2 per cent of the parent compound to CO_2. More recent work has focused on the reductive dechlorination of TCDD and more highly chlorinated isomers.

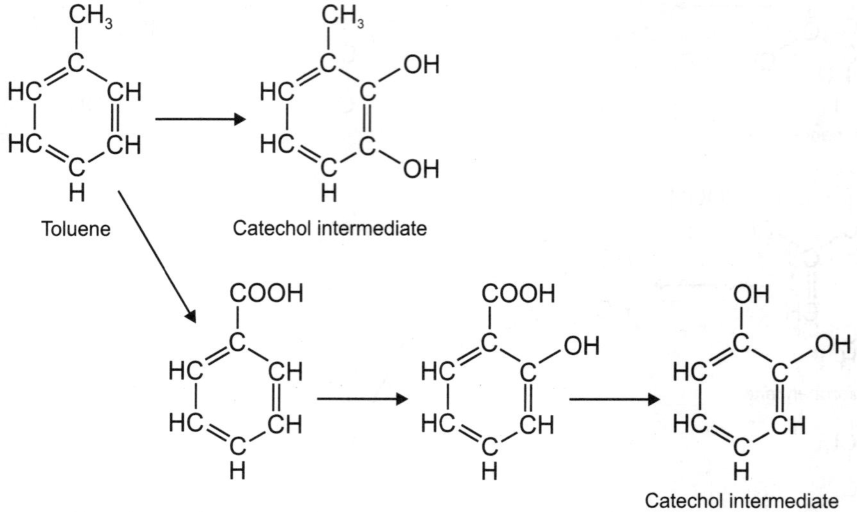

Fig. 20.14. Biodegradation of toluene.

Heterocyclic compounds

Heterocyclics are cyclic compounds containing one or more heteroatoms (nitrogen, sulphur, or oxygen) in addition to carbon atoms. In general, heterocyclic compounds are more difficult to degrade than analogous aromatics that contain only carbon. This is probably due to the higher electronegativity of the nitrogen and oxygen atoms compared with the carbon atom, leading to deactivation of the molecule toward electrophilic substitution. Heterocyclic compounds with five-membered rings and one heteroatom are readily biodegradable, probably because five-membered ring compounds exhibit higher reactivity toward electrophilic agents and are hence more readily biologically hydroxylated. The susceptiblity of heterocyclic compounds to biodegradation decreases with increasing number of heteroatoms in the molecules.

Pesticides

Pesticides are the biggest nonpoint source of chemicals added to the environment. The majority of the currently used organic pesticides are subject to extensive mineralisation within the time of one growing season or less. Synthetic pesticides show a bewildering variety of chemical structures, but most can be traced to relatively simple aliphatic, alicyclic, and aromatic base structures. These base structures bear a variety of halogen, amino, nitro, hydroxyl, carboxyl, and phosphorus substituents. For example, the chlorophenoxyacetates, such as 2,4-D and 2,4,5-T, have been released into the environment as herbicides over the past 50 years. Both of these structures are biodegradable and pathways are presented in Fig. 20.15.

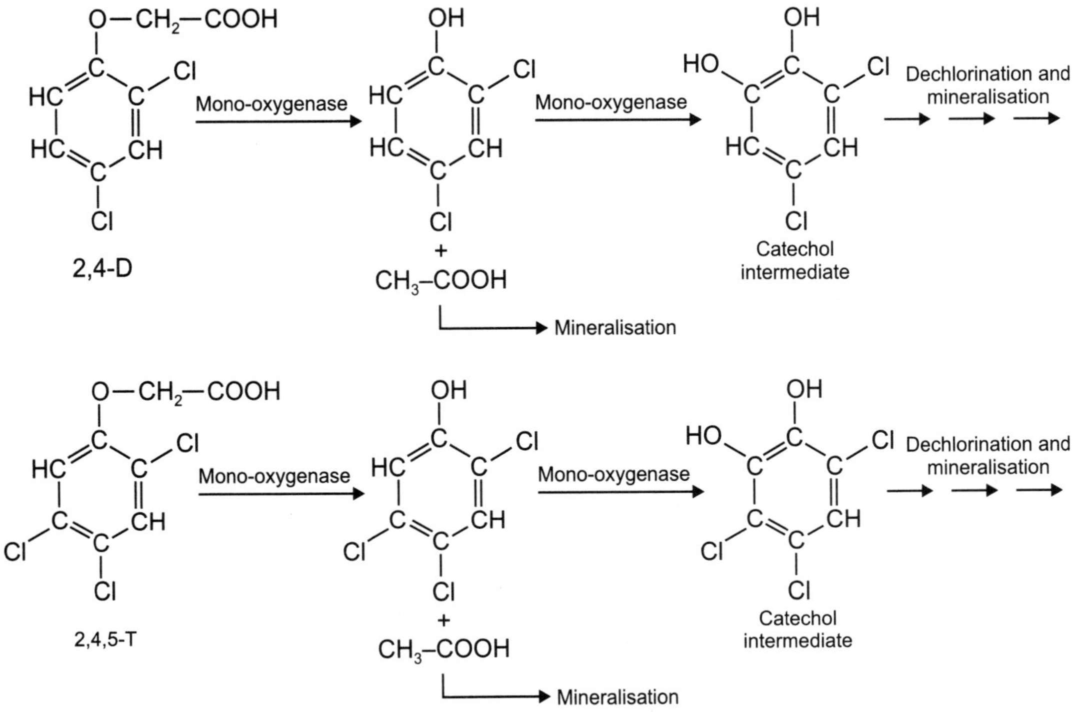

Fig. 20.15. Biodegradation of 2,4-D and 2,4,5-T.

Anaerobic Conditions

Anaerobic conditions are not uncommon in the environment. Most often, such conditions develop in water or saturated sediment environments. But, even in well-aerated soils there are microenvironments with little or no oxygen. In all of these environments, anaerobiosis occurs. Anaerobiosis occurs when the rate of oxygen consumption by micro-organisms is greater than the rate of oxygen diffusion through either air or water. In the absence of oxygen, organic compounds can be mineralised through anaerobic respiration using a terminal electron acceptor other than oxygen. There is a series of alternative terminal electron acceptors in the environment including iron, nitrate, manganese, sulphate, and carbonate. These alternative electron acceptors have been listed in the order of most oxidising to most reducing, and are usually utilised in this order, because the amount of energy generated for growth depends on the oxidation potential of the electron acceptor. Because none of these electron acceptors are as oxidising as oxygen, growth under anaerobic conditions is never as efficient as growth under aerobic conditions.

Aliphatics

Saturated aliphatic hydrocarbons are degraded slowly if at all under anaerobic conditions. This is supported by the fact that hydrocarbons in natural underground reservoirs of oil (which are under anaerobic conditions) are not degraded despite the presence of micro-organisms. However, both unsaturated aliphatics and aliphatics containing oxygen (aliphatic alcohols and ketones) are readily biodegraded anaerobically. The suggested pathway of biodegradation for unsaturated hydrocarbons is hydration of the double bond to an alcohol, with further oxidation to a ketone or aldehyde and, finally, formation of a fatty acid (Fig. 20.16).

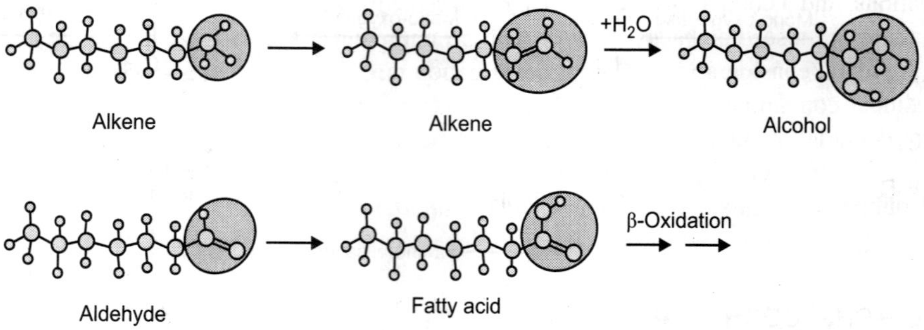

Fig. 20.16. Anaerobic biodegradation of aliphatic compounds.

As previously discussed, halogenated ahphatics can be partially or completely degraded under anaerobic conditions.

Aromatics

Like aliphatic hydrocarbons, aromatic compounds can be completely degraded under anaerobic conditions if the aromatic is oxygenated. There is also evidence that even nonsubstituted aromatics are degraded slowly under anaerobic conditions. Anaerobic mineralisation of aromatics often requires a mixed microbial community that works together even though each of the microbial components requires a different redox potential. For example, mineralisation of benzoate can be achieved by growing an anaerobic benzoate degrader in co-culture with a methanogen and sulphate reducer. The initial transformations in such a system are often carried out fermentatively, and this results in the formation of aromatic acids, which in turn are transformed to methanogenic precursors such as acetate, carbon dioxide, and formate. These small molecules can then be utilised by methanogens (Fig. 20.17). Such a mixed community is called a consortium. It is not known how this consortium solves the problem of requiring different redox potentials in the same vicinity in a soil system. Clearly, higher redox potentials are required for degradation of the more complex substrates such as benzoate, leaving smaller organic acid or alcohol molecules that are degraded at lower redox potentials. To ultimately achieve degradation may require that the organic acids and alcohols formed at higher redox potential be transported by diffusion or by movement with water (advection) to a region of lower redox potential. On the other hand, it may be that biofilms form on the soil surface and that redox gradients are formed within the biofilm allowing complete degradation to take place. Environmental microbiologists are actively exploring how anaerobes operate in the soil and vadose environments. Such an understanding is expected to aid in developing technologies to enhance degradation processes in anaerobic contaminated environments.

BIOREMEDIATION

The objective of bioremediation is to exploit naturally occurring biodegradative processes to cleanup contaminated sites. There are several types of bioremediation. *In situ* bioremediation is the in-place treatment of a contaminated site. *Ex situ* bioremediation may be implemented to treat contaminated soil or water that is removed from a contaminated site. Intrinsic bioremediation or natural attenuation is the indigenous level of contaminant biodegradation that occurs without any stimulation or treatment. All of these types of bioremediation continue to receive increasing attention as viable remediation alternatives for several reasons. These include generally good public acceptance and support, good success rates for some applications, and a comparatively low cost of bioremediation when it is successful. As with any technology, there are also drawbacks. Success can be unpredictable because a biological system is being used. A second consideration is that bioremediation rarely restores an environment completely. Often the residual contamination left after treatment is strongly sorbed and not available to micro-organisms for degradation. Over a long period of time (years), these residuals can be slowly released. There is little research concerning the fate and potential toxicity of such released residuals, and therefore there is both public and regulatory concern about the importance of residual contamination.

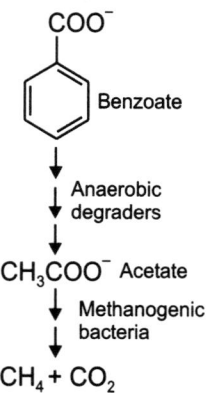

Fig. 20.17. Anaerobic biodegradation of aromatic compounds by a consortium of anaerobic bacteria.

Although it is often not thought of as bioremediation, domestic sewage waste has been treated biologically for many years with resounding success. In application of bioremediation to other environmental problems, it must be kept in mind that biodegradation is dependent on the pollutant structure and bioavailability. Therefore, application of bioremediation to other pollutants depends on the type of pollutant or pollutant mixtures present and the type of micro-organisms present. The first successful application of bioremediation outside sewage treatment was the cleanup of oil spills, and success in this area is now well documented. In the past few years, many new bioremediation technologies have emerged that are being used to address other types of pollutants (Table 20.3).

Several key factors are critical to successful application of bioremediation: environmental conditions, contaminant and nutrient availability, and the presence of degrading micro-organisms. If biodegradation does not occur, the first thing that must be done is to isolate the factor limiting bioremediation, and this can sometimes be a very difficult task. Initial laboratory tests using soil or water from a polluted site can usually determine whether degrading micro-organisms are present and whether there is an obvious environmental factor that limits biodegradation, for example, extremely low or high pH or lack of nitrogen and/or phosphorus. However, sometimes the limiting factor is not easy to identify. Often pollutants are present as mixtures and one component of the pollutant mixture can have toxic effects on the growth and activity of degrading micro-organisms. Low bioavailability due to sorption and ageing is another factor that can limit bioremediation and can be difficult to evaluate in the environment.

Actual application of bioremediation is still limited in practice but is rapidly gaining in popularity. Most of the developed bioremediation technologies are based on two standard practices: addition of oxygen and addition of other nutrients.

Table 20.3. Current status of bioremediation.

Chemical class	Frequency of occurrence	Status of bioremediation	Evidence of future success	Limitations
Hydrocarbons and derivatives				
Gasoline, fuel oil	Very frequent	Established	Aerobically biodegradable under a narrow range of conditions	Forms nonaqueous phase liquid
PAHs	Common	Emerging	Aerobically biodegradable under a narrow range of conditions	Sorbs strongly to subsurface solids
Creosote	Infrequent	Emerging	Readily biodegradable under aerobic conditions	Sorbs strongly to subsurface solids; forms nonaqueous phase liquid
Alcohols, ketones, esters	Common	Established		
Ethers	Common	Emerging	Biodegradable under a narrow range of conditions using aerobic or nitrate reducing microbes	
Halogenated aliphatics				
Highly chlorinated	Very frequent	Emerging	Cometabolised by anaerobic microbes; cometabolised by aerobes in special cases	Forms nonaqueous phase liquid
Less chlorinated	Very frequent	Emerging	Aerobically biodegradable under a narrow range of conditions; cometabolised by anaerobic microbes	Forms nonaqueous phase liquid
Halogenated aromatics				
Highly chlorinated	Common	Emerging	Aerobically biodegradable under a narrow range of conditions; cometabolised by anaerobic microbes	Sorbs strongly to subsurface solids; forms nonaqueous phase either liquid or solid
Less chlorinated	Common	Emerging	Readily biodegradable under aerobic conditions	Forms nonaqueous phase either liquid or solid
Polychlorinated biphenyls				
Highly chlorinated	Infrequent	Emerging	Cometabolised by anaerobic microbes	Sorbs strongly to subsurface solids
Less chlorinated	Infrequent	Emerging	Aerobically biodegradable under a narrow range of conditions	Sorbs strongly to subsurface solids
Nitroaroamatics	Common	Emerging	Aerobically biodegradable; converted to innocuous volatile organic acids under anaerobic conditions	
Metals (Cr, Cu, Ni, Pb, Hg, Cd, Zn, etc.)	Common	Possible	Solubility and reactivity can be changed by a variety of microbial processes	Availability highly variable and controlled by solution and solidphase chemistry

Addition of Oxygen or Other Gases

One of the most common limiting factors in bioremediation is availability of oxygen. Oxygen is an element required for aerobic biodegradation. In addition, oxygen has low solubility in water and a low rate of diffusion (movement) through both air and water. The combination of these three factors makes it easy to understand that inadequate oxygen supplies will slow bioremediation. Several technologies have been developed to overcome a lack of oxygen. A typical bioremediation system used to treat a contaminated aquifer as well as the contaminated zone. This system contains a series of injection wells or galleries and a series of recovery wells that comprise a two-pronged approach to bioremediation. First, the recovery wells remove contaminated groundwater, which is treated above ground, in this case using a bioreactor containing micro-organisms that are acclimated to the contaminant. This would be considered *ex situ* treatment.

Following bioreactor treatment, the clean water is supplied with oxygen and nutrients, and then it is reinjected into the site. The reinjected water provides oxygen and nutrients to stimulate *in situ* biodegradation. In addition, the reinjected water flushes the vadose zone to aid in removal of the contaminant for above-ground bioreactor treatment. This remediation scheme is a very good example of a combination of physical, chemical, and biological treatments being used to maximise the effectiveness of the remediation treatment.

Bioventing is a technique used to add oxygen directly to a site of contamination in the vadose zone (unsaturated zone). Bioventing is a merging of soil vapour extraction technology and bioremediation. To initiate bioventing, a vacuum is drawn on these wells to force accelerated air movement through the contamination zone. This effectively increases the supply of oxygen throughout the site, and thus the rate of contaminant biodegradation. In some cases, depending on the type of pollutant in the site, pollutant volatility becomes an issue, e.g. in gasoline spills. In this case, some of the pollutants will be removed as air is forced through this system. This contaminated air can also be treated biologically by passing the air through above ground soil beds in a process called biofiltration.

In contrast, air sparging is used to add oxygen to the saturated zone. In this process, an air sparger well is used to inject air under pressure below the water table. The injected air displaces water in the soil matrix, creating a temporary air-filled porosity. This causes oxygen levels to increase, resulting in enhanced biodegradation rates. In addition, volatile organics will volatilise into the airstream and be removed by a vapour extraction well.

Methane is another gas that can be added with oxygen in extracted groundwater and reinjected into the saturated zone. Methane is used specifically to stimulate methanotrophic activity and cometabolic degradation of chlorinated solvents. As already discussed, methanotrophic organisms produce the enzyme methane mono-oxygenase to degrade methane, and this enzyme also cometabolically degrades several chlorinated solvents.

Cometabolic degradation of chlorinated solvents is presently being tested in field trials to determine the usefulness of this technology.

Nutrient Addition

Perhaps the second most common bioremediation treatment is the addition of nutrients, in particular nitrogen and phosphorus. Many contaminated sites contain organic wastes that are rich in carbon but contain minimal amounts of nitrogen and phosphorus. Injection of nutrient solutions takes place from an above-ground batch feed system. The goal of nutrient injection is to optimise the ratio of carbon, nitrogen, and phosphorus (C:N:P) in the site to approximately 100:10:1. However, sorption of added nutrients can make it difficult to achieve the optimal ratio accurately.

Stimulation of Anaerobic Degradation Using Alternative Electron Acceptors

Until recently, anaerobic degradation of many organic compounds was not even considered feasible. Now it is being proposed as an alternative bioremediation strategy even though aerobic degradation is generally considered a much more rapid process. This is because it is difficult to establish and maintain aerobic conditions in some groundwater sites. Several alternative electron acceptors have been proposed for use in anaerobic degradation, including nitrate, sulphate, iron (Fe^{3+}), and carbon dioxide.

There has even been a limited number of field trials using nitrate that show promise for this approach. This is a relatively new area in bioremediation that will undoubtedly receive increased attention in the next few years.

Addition of Surfactants

Surfactant addition has been proposed as a technique for increasing the bioavailability and hence biodegradation of contaminants. Surfactants can be synthesised chemically and are also produced by many micro-organisms, in which case they are called biosurfactants. Surfactants work similarly to industrial and household detergents that effectively remove oily residues from machinery, clothing, or dishes. Alternatively, surfactant molecules can coat oil droplets and emulsify them into solution. In addition, biosurfactants seem to enhance the ability of microbes to stick to oil droplets. In laboratory tests, synthetic surfactants and biosurfactants can be used to increase the apparent aqueous solubility of organic contaminants. However, field tests have been attempted only with synthetic surfactants and results have been mixed.

Addition of Micro-organisms or DNA

If appropriate biodegrading micro-organisms are not present in soil or if microbial populations have been reduced because of contaminant toxicity, specific micro-organisms can be added as 'introduced organisms' to enhance the existing populations. This process is known as bioaugmentation. Scientists are now capable of creating 'superbugs', organisms that can degrade pollutants at extremely rapid rates. Such organisms can be developed through successive adaptations under laboratory condition, or can be genetically engineered. In terms of biodegradation, these superbugs are far superior to organisms found in the environment. The problem is that introduction of a micro-organism to a contaminated site may fail for two reasons. First, the introduced microbe often cannot establish a niche in the environment. In fact, these introduced organisms often do not survive in a new environment beyond a few weeks. Second, there are difficulties in delivering the introduced organisms to the site of contamination, because micro-organisms, like contaminants, can be strongly sorbed by solid surfaces.

Currently, very little is known about microbial transport and establishment of environmental niches. These are areas of active research, and in the next few years scientists may gain a further understanding of microbial behaviour in soil ecosystems. However, until we discover how to successfully deliver and establish introduced micro-organisms, their addition to contaminated sites will not be a viable bioremediation option.

One way to take advantage of the superbugs that have been developed is to use them in bioreactor systems under controlled conditions. Extremely efficient biodegradation rates can be achieved in bioreactors that are used in above ground treatment systems.

A second bioaugmentation strategy is to add specific genes that can confer a specific degradation capability to indigenous microbial populations. The addition of degradative genes relies on the delivery and uptake of the genetic material by indigenous microbes. There are two approaches that can be taken in delivery of genes. The first is to use microbial cells to deliver the DNA via conjugation. The second is to add 'naked' DNA to the soil to allow uptake via transformation. This second approach may reduce the difficulty of delivery since DNA alone is much smaller than a whole cell. However, little is known as yet about these two approaches. Di Giovanni demonstrated that gene transfer can occur in soil resulting in 2,4-D degradation activity. However, whether such transfer is common, and conditions that are conducive or inhibitory to such transfer are not yet defined.

SECTION VI

Special Topics

Chapter 21

Environmental Monitoring

INTRODUCTION

To effectively monitor the environment as well as devise pollution abatement methods, it is necessary to know the quality of the environment-quantitatively. It is essential to be aware of the components responsible for environmental pollution and their concentration in waste-water and solid waste. In addition, the environment required for the growth of eco-friendly micro-organisms, which can be utilised to reduce the amount of pollutants in waste, is also required to be evaluated.

The air and water in our environment contain a wide assortment of toxic organic and inorganic pollutants. They enter the environment as emissions into the atmosphere or as discharges to water bodies. These may be either in concentrated point sources, such as from factory smoke, stacks and sewage discharges, or in diffuse forms, such as from automobiles' exhausts and run-off from agricultural land. These pollutants eventually endanger the life of both humans and animals. These pollutants can range from parts per billion (ppb) or below in rural areas to hundreds of parts per million (ppm) or higher in large industrial and urbanised areas.

In recent years, many chemicals previously considered only moderately toxic have been identified very toxic, e.g. potential carcinogens, and thus have been assigned lower threshold limit values (TLVs). In addition, the number of newly identified toxic substances are increasing everyday.

Hence, there is an increasing need for rapid screening and monitoring of toxic substances in air and water to meet the requirements of pollution control authorities.

In order to control the levels of these pollutants in the environment, it is necessary to know their chemical or biochemical route of formation and degradation, the extent of their occurrence in the environment and their ecotoxicity. Analytical chemistry plays the most vital role in determining the extent of their occurrence in the environment while the degree of their ecotoxicity determines the priority of pollutants and the overall sensitivity required for the analytical method to be employed for their measurement.

As the TLVs are lowered, the strain on analytical technology increases, since improved and increased sensitivities are essential in measuring lower concentration of pollutants. Many of the conventional methods are time consuming and do not have adequate sensitivities to measure the lower concentration. Additionally, due to lack of specificities, they often lead to unreliable results.

In the recent past, a great deal of advances have been made in analytical methodology and instrumentation. With the ever-increasing advancement of microprocessor technology, these analytical instruments have become more versatile. These are computer-aided instruments (so called 'intelligent instruments) that offer highly improved detection limits (down to parts per billion (ppb) to parts per trillion (ppt) level), better precision, accuracy and increased specificity.

Thus environmental monitoring must be able, in many cases, to detect with accuracy and consistency contaminants present at very low levels. In the determination of the pollutants present, their fate, and their effect on the environment, biotechnology can be of considerable value, especially as molecular biology techniques are increasingly employed.

Using this information, the level of residual pollutants can be evaluated vis-*a*-vis the prescribed minimum. The results of such analysis are further used for mass and energy balance, design kinetics of biodegradation processes, design of bioreactors and fermenters, etc.

SAMPLING

In order to analyse any component of the environment, samples need to be taken and a number of features need to be considered. These features include consideration of what part of the environment needs to be sampled (e.g. water, soil, or air), how many samples need to be taken to cover the area of interest, and the relevant statistical analysis. Also the timing of sampling can introduce variation and seasonal variations need to be taken into consideration. The part of the environment to be sampled will depend on the questions to be answered about the pollutant(s). For example, a chemical spill may contaminate the soil but depending on conditions it may also reach and contaminate the groundwater or adjacent lakes or rivers. In this case a broad spread of sampling will be required to determine whether this has occurred. Samples will have to be taken from the surface and subsurface soil and from any contaminated water. The number of samples is important as results may vary between samples and this variation needs to be estimated. A high degree of variation would indicate that pollution is localised and that further sampling is needed. The collection of a representative sample from a homogeneous source is no problem, but with soil, air, and water samples this is rarely the case. Often soil contamination may be very localised and waste-stream contamination may be intermittent and poorly mixed.

Land (Site) Sampling

Contaminated sites often require some form of survey, as all the information as to the pollution present cannot be determined from the site history and management. Some directives suggest that 17 samples should be taken for a 5-hectare site, at three different depths, which should be decreased for sites below 0.5 hectares. However, contamination is frequently patchy so that the number of samples taken will depend on how small an area the contamination covers. Table 21.1 gives the probability of locating contamination using random-sampling grids. These grids can be rectangular, square, diamond-shaped, or herringbone-shaped. The drawback of these types of grid is that they can generate a large number of samples, which can be expensive to analyse. Therefore, a site history can be of great use in directing the sampling process, and reducing costs.

Table 21.1. Probability of locating contamination using random-sampling grids.

Contamination as % of total area	Percentage probability (%)		
Number of samples taken ...	10	30	50
1	10	26	39
5	40	79	92
10	65	96	99
25	94	100	100

Water Sampling

Sampling of most waste-water and contaminated water is difficult due to their highly variable nature. To obtain an accurate assessment, samples will have to be taken over a time period, over different sections of the waterway, and at different depths. There are various automatic methods of taking samples that can be used. Some industrial discharges into waterways are intermittent, which will extend the time that sampling must be carried out. Where to sample in the waterway depends on any inflow and outflow of water; stratification and the whole water way may need to be assessed. If groundwater is to be monitored wells will have to be drilled and the very process of drilling can alter or contaminate samples. Contamination can come from the drilling method; the casing material, and the sample process. These types of consideration have to be evaluated when choosing the sampling method and analysing the results.

When a specific organism is to be surveyed in the environment in order to assess contamination, the samples have to be as representative as possible. One example is the sampling of the edible mussel *Mytilus edulis*, which accumulates metals and can, therefore, be used as an indicator of metal pollution. The following points had to be taken into consideration when sampling the mussels:

1. Time of the year; late winter is favoured as metal concentrations are stable at that time.
2. Size or age; dominant size is taken.
3. Position on shore; mussels are taken from rocks to avoid contamination by silt.
4. Sample size; a minimum of 25 samples.

After sampling the mussels would be washed in fresh water, the soft tissue removed, as this is the site of accumulation, and the tissue extracted and assayed. Alternatively, the soft tissue can be stored at −20°C before assay.

Air Sampling

Air sampling has much the same problems as water but is also influenced by wind direction and strength. The purpose of sampling is to obtain a representative sample and in general there are three sampling systems used for air: pumped systems, pre-concentration, and grab samples. In the pumped system the sample is pumped directly from the air into the analyser. In cases where the pollutant is present at very low concentrations pre-concentration is required before analysis. An example of the type of system is the adsorption of the contaminant on to activated charcoal for removal and analysis at a later date. Grab samples involve the capture of samples of air in bottles, syringes, bellows, and bags for analysis later. Under normal conditions the air is well mixed and samples are normally taken at a height of 2 metres, but if boundary layers form then stratification of the air may occur and towers will be required to take samples above 2 metres.

If they cannot be analysed immediately samples taken from soil, water, or air can be stored but care is required, as pollutants can be lost or can change during storage. In a number of cases some form of extraction will be needed to prepare and concentrate the sample for analysis and there are a number of liquid/liquid, solid/liquid systems that can be used. Often the extraction methods will also concentrate the sample, helping analysis.

Analysis

Three parameters need to be known before the analysis can be carried out.

1. The limit of detection of the compound, which will give the minimum concentration that can be detected.

2. The variation found with the method of analysis, which will give an estimate of the variation expected between identical samples.
3. How stable is the compound once the sample has been taken?

The number of methods available for the analysis of environmental pollutants and conditions is very great but can be divided into physical, chemical, and biological. Clearly it is in the biological methods that biotechnology will have the greatest influence.

PHYSICAL ANALYSIS

Physical methods are often used to determine the conditions that the compounds are exposed to as well as the contaminants, and are in general as follows.

1. Gravimetrics: Used to determine suspended solids (SS), total or volatile solids, and sulphate levels.
2. pH: Very acid or alkaline conditions will be corrosive and restrict   biological activity. Easily measured with a pH electrode.
3. Colourimetric: Colour and turbidity are important in water quality. These can be determined using comparison tubes, colour discs, colourimeters, and spectrophotometers.
4. Dissolved oxygen: This can be measured using an oxygen electrode. Oxygen levels are very important in water quality in order to maintain aerobic biological organisms.
5. Ion-specific electrodes: These electrodes can be used to determine the levels of ammonia, nitrate, nitrite, calcium, sodium, and other ions. The determination of nitrate and nitrite is important, as minimum levels have been set for water quality.

The oxygen- and ion-electrode technology allows the possibility of automated analysis, remote sensing, and monitoring. However, many of the newer electrodes suffer from instability and all are prey to fouling and damage.

CHEMICAL ANALYSIS

For proper understanding of our environment, we must have a clear idea of the identities and quantities of pollutants and other chemical species in air, water, soil and biological samples, etc. These may be either in concentrated point source such as from factory smoke, stacks and sewage discharge or in diffused forms, such as from automobile's exhausts and run-off from agricultural land. These pollutants eventually endanger the life of both humans and animals. These pollutants can range from parts per billion (ppb) to hundreds of parts per million (ppm). In order to control the level of these pollutants in the environment, it is necessary to know their chemical or biochemical route of formation and degradation, the extent of their occurrence in the environment and their ecotoxicity. Analytical chemistry plays the most vital role in determining the extent of their occurrence in the environment while the degree of their ecotoxicity determines the priority of pollutants and the overall sensitivity required for analytical methods to be employed for their measurement.

Spectrophotometric Methods

Absorption spectrophotometry

Absorption spectrophotometry of light-absorbing species in solution, historically called colourimetry when visible light is absorbed, is still used for the analysis of many water and some air pollutants. Basically, absorption spectrophotometry consists of measuring the percentage transmittance (%T) of monochromatic light passing through a light-absorbing solution as compared to the amount passing through a blank solution containing everything in the medium but the sought-for constituent (100 per cent). The absorbance (A) is defined as the following:

$$A = \log \frac{\% \, T}{100} \qquad \text{... (21.1)}$$

The relationship between A and the concentration (C) of the absorbing substance is given by Beer's law:

$$A = abC \qquad \text{.... (21.2)}$$

where, A is the absorptivity, a wavelength-dependent parameter characteristic of the absorbing substance, b is the path length of the light through the absorbing solution and C is the concentration of the absorbing substance. A linear relationship between A and C at constant path length indicates adherence to Beer's law. In many cases, analyses may be performed even when Beer's law is not obeyed, if a suitable calibration curve is prepared. A colour-developing step is usually required in which the sought for substance reacts to form a coloured species, and in some cases a coloured species is extracted into a nonaqueous solvent to provide a more intense colour and a more concentrated solution.

A number of solution spectrophotometric methods have been used for the determination of water and air pollutants. Some of these are summarised in Table 21.2.

Table 21.2. Solution spectrophotometric (colourimetric) methods for pollutants.

Pollutant	Reagent and method
Ammonia	Alkaline mercury (II) iodide reacts with ammonia, producing colloidal orange-brown $NH_2Hg_2I_3$, which absorbs light between 400 and 500 nanometres (nm)
Arsenic	Reaction of arsine, AsH_3, with silver diethylthiocarbamate in pyridine, forming a red complex
Boron	Reaction with curcumin, forming red rosocyanine
Bromide	Reaction of hypobromite with phenol red to form bromphenol blue-type indicator
Chlorine	Development of colour with orthotolidine
Cyanide	Formation of a blue dye from reaction of cyanogen chloride, CNCl, with pyridine-pyrazolone reagent, measured at 620 nm
Fluoride	Decolourisation of a zirconium-dye colloidal precipitate ('lake') by formation of colourless zirconium fluoride and free dye
Nitrate and nitrite	Nitrate is reduced to nitrite, which is diazotised with sulphanilamide and coupled with N-(l-naphthyl)-ethylenediamine dihydrochloride to produce a highly coloured azo dye measured at 540 nm
Nitrogen, Kjeldahl phenate method	Digestion in sulphuric acid to NH_4^+ followed by treatment with alkaline phenol reagent and sodium hypochlorite to form blue indophenol measured at 630 nm
Phenols	Reaction with 4-aminoantipyrine at pH 10 in the presence of potassium ferricyanide, forming an antipyrine dye which is extracted into pyridine and measured at 460 nm
Phosphate	Reaction with molybdate ion to form a phosphomolybdate which is selectively reduced to intensely coloured molybdenum blue.
Selenium	Reaction with diaminobenzidine, forming coloured species absorbing at 420 nm
Silica	Formation of molybdosilicic acid with molybdate, followed by reduction to a heteropoly blue measured at 650 nm or 815 nm
Sulphide	Formation of methylene blue
Sulphur dioxide	Collection of SO_2 gas in tetrachloromercurate solution, followed by reaction with formaldehyde and pararosaniline hydrochloride, to form a red-violet dye measured at 548 nm
Surfactants	Reaction with methylene blue to form blue salt
Tannin and lignin	Blue colour from tungstophosphoric and molybdophosphoric acids

Atomic absorption and emission analyses

Atomic absorption analysis has become the method of choice for most metals analysed in environmental samples. This technique is based upon the absorption of monochromatic light by a cloud of atoms of the analyte metal. The monochromatic light is produced by a source composed of the same atoms as those being analysed. The source produces intense electromagnetic radiation, with a wavelength exactly the same as that absorbed by the atoms, resulting in extremely high selectivity. The basic components of an atomic absorption instrument are shown in Fig. 21.1.

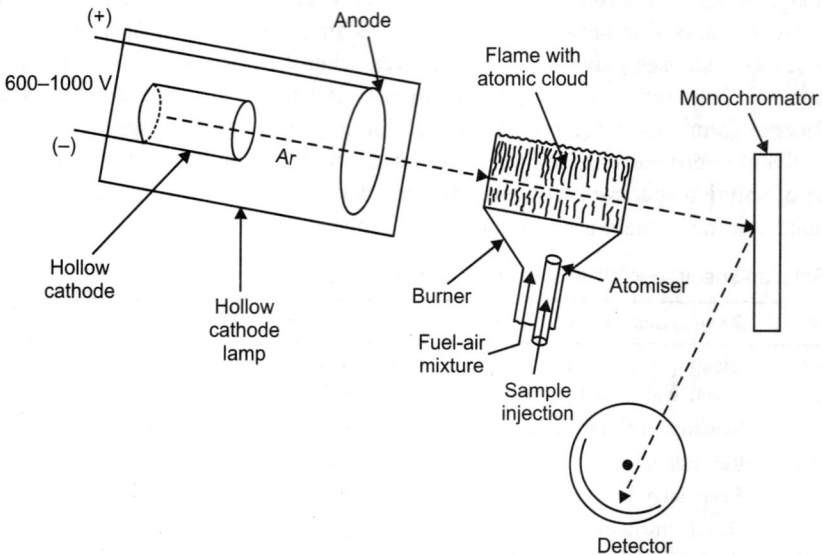

Fig. 21.1. The basic components of an atomic absorption spectrophotometer.

The key element is the hollow cathode lamp, in which atoms of the analyte metal are energised so that they become electronically excited and emit radiation, with a very narrow wavelength band characteristic of the metal. This radiation is guided by the appropriate optics through a flame into which the sample is aspirated. In the flame, most metallic compounds are decomposed and the metal is reduced to the elemental state, forming a cloud of atoms.

These atoms absorb a fraction of radiation in the flame. The fraction of radiation absorbed increases with the concentration of the sought for element in the sample according to the Beer's law relationship (Eq. 21.2.) The attenuated light beam next goes to a monochromator to eliminate extraneous light resulting from the flame and then to a detector.

Atomisers other than a flame can be used. The most common of these is the graphite furnace, which consists of a hollow graphite cylinder placed so that the light beam passes through it. A small sample of up to 100 μL is inserted in the tube through a hole in the top. An electric current is passed through the tube to heat it gently at first to dry the sample, then rapidly to vapourise and excite the metal analyte.

The absorption of metal atoms in the hollow portion of the tube is measured and recorded as a spikeshaped signal. A diagram of a simple graphite furnace with a typical output signal is shown in Fig. 21.2. The major advantage of the graphite furnace is that it gives detection limits up to 1000 times lower than those of conventional flame devices.

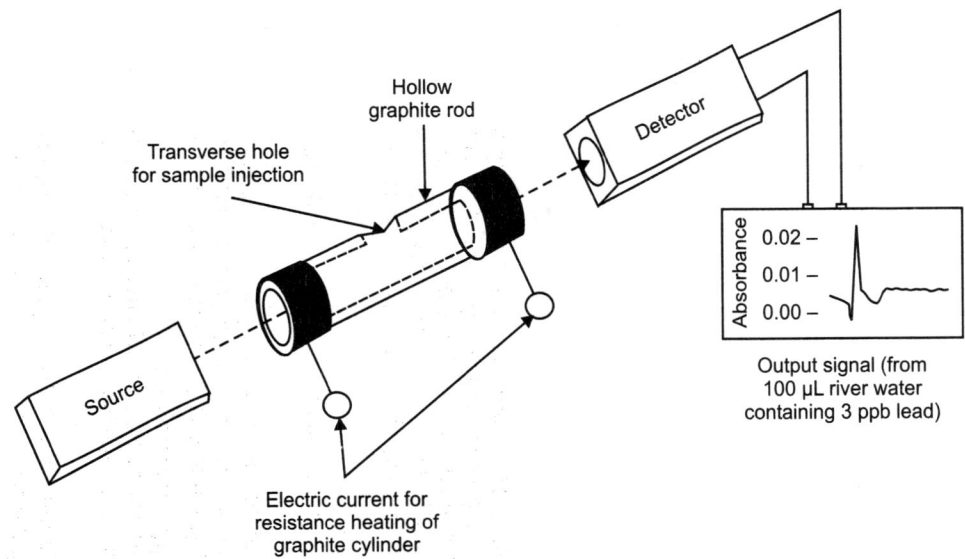

Fig. 21.2. Graphite furnace for atomic absorption analysis and typical output signal.

A special technique for the flameless atomic absorption analysis of mercury involves its room-temperature reduction to the elemental state by tin (II) chloride in solution, followed by sweeping it into an absorption cell with air. Nanogram (10^{-9}g) quantities of mercury can be determined by measuring mercury absorption at 253.7 nm.

Atomic emission techniques

Metals may be determined in water, atmospheric particulate matter, and biological samples very well by observing the spectral lines emitted when they are heated to a very high temperature. An especially useful atomic emission technique is inductively coupled plasma atomic emission spectroscopy. The 'flame' in which analyte atoms are excited in plasma emission consists of an incandescent plasma (ionised gas) of argon heated inductively by radiofrequency energy at 4–50 MHz and 2–5 kW (Fig. 21.3). The energy is transferred to a stream of argon through an induction coil, producing temperatures up to 10,000 K. The sample atoms are subjected to temperatures around 7000 K, twice those of the hottest conventional flames (for example, nitrous oxide-acetylene at 3200 K). Since emission of light increases exponentially with temperature, lower detection limits are obtained. Furthermore, the technique enables emission analysis of some of the environmentally important metalloids such as arsenic, boron and selenium. Interfering chemical reactions and interactions in the plasma are minimised as compared to flames. Of greatest significance, however, is the capability of analysing as many as 30 elements simultaneously, enabling a true multi-element analysis technique. Thus, plasma atomisation combined with mass spectrometric measurement of analyte elements is a relatively new technique that is an especially powerful means for multi-element analysis.

X-ray fluorescence

X-ray fluorescence is another multi-element analysis technique that can be applied to a wide variety of environmental samples. It is especially useful for the characterisation of atmospheric particulate matter, but it can be applied to some water and soil samples as well. This technique is based upon measurement of X-rays emitted when electrons fall back into inner shell vacancies created by bombardment with energetic X-rays, gamma radiation, or protons.

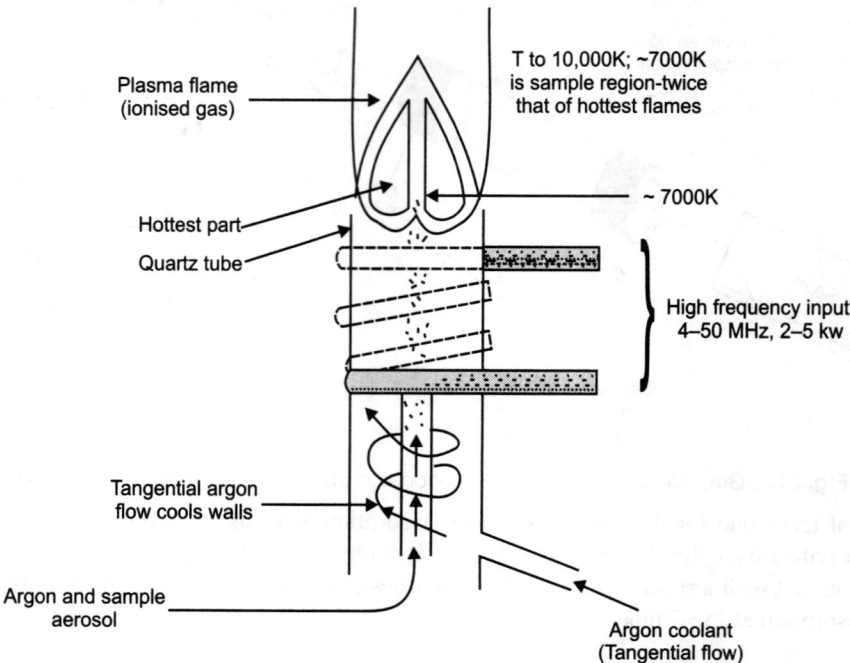

Fig. 21.3 Schematic diagram showing inductively coupled plasma used for optical emission spectroscopy.

The emitted X-rays have an energy characteristic of the particular atom. The wavelength (energy) of the emitted radiation yields a qualitative analysis of the elements and the intensity of radiation from a particular element provides a quantitative analysis. A schematic diagram of a wavelength-dispersive X-ray fluorescence spectrophotometer is shown in Fig. 21.4. An excitation source, normally an X-ray tube emitting 'white' X-rays (a continuum), produces a primary beam of energetic radiation which excites fluorescent X-rays in the sample. A radioactive source emitting gamma rays or protons from an accelerator may also be used for excitation. For best results, the sample should be mounted as a thin layer, which means that segments of air filters containing fine particulate matter make ideal samples.

The fluorescent X-rays are passed through a collimator to select a parallel secondary beam, which is dispersed according to wavelength by diffraction with a crystal monochromator. The monochromatic X-rays in the secondary beam are counted by a detector which rotates at a degree twice that of the crystal to scan the spectrum of emitted radiation.

Energy-selective detectors of the Si(Li) semi-conductor type enable measurement of fluorescent X-rays of different energies without the need for wavelength dispersion. Instead, the energies of a number of lines falling on a detector simultaneously are distinguished electronically. An energy-dispersive X-ray fluorescence spectrum from an atmospheric particulate sample is shown in Fig. 21.5. A significant advantage of X-ray fluorescence multielement analysis is that sensitivities and detection limits do not vary greatly across the periodic table as they do with methods such as neutron activation analysis or atomic absorption. Proton-excited X-ray emission is particularly sensitive.

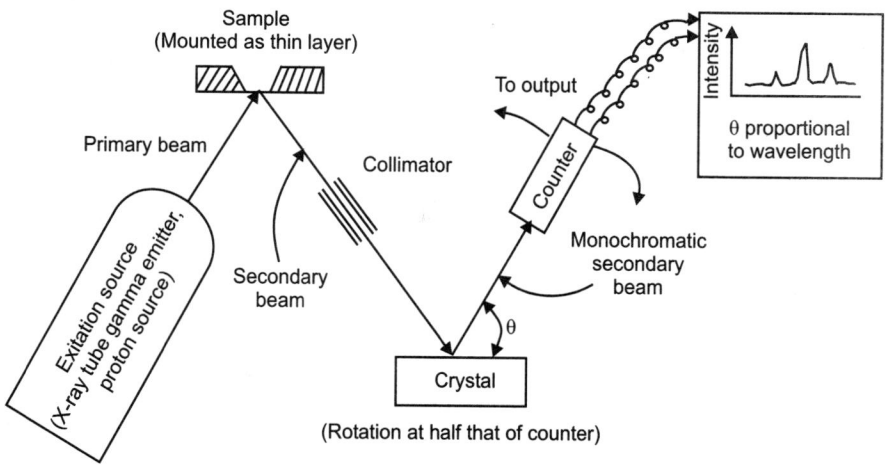

Fig. 21.4. Wavelength-dispersive X-ray fluorescence spectrophotometer.

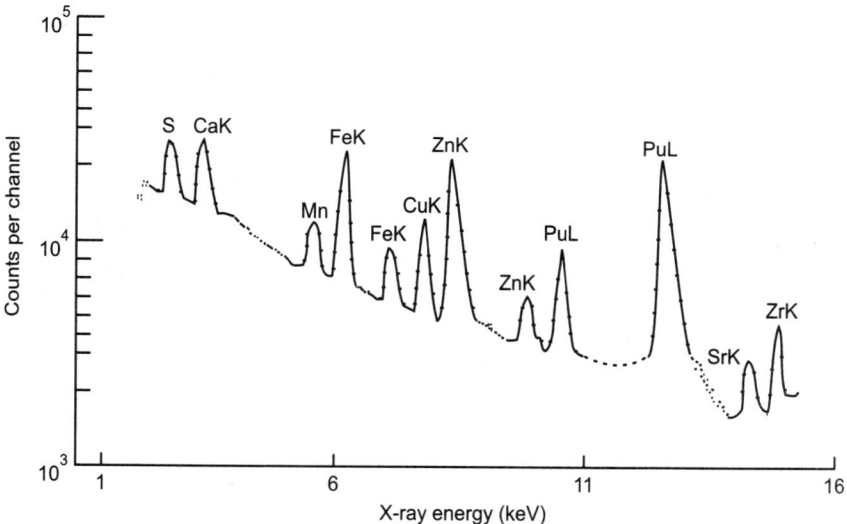

Fig. 21.5. Energy-dispersive X-ray fluorescence spectrum from an atmospheric particle sample.

Electrochemical methods of analysis

Several useful techniques for water analysis utilise electrochemical sensors. These techniques may be potentiometric, voltammetric, or amperometric. Potentiometry is based upon the general principle that the relationship between the potential of a measuring electrode and that of a reference electrode is a function of the log of the activity of an ion in solution. For a measuring electrode responding selectively to a particular ion, this relationship is given by the Nernst equation,

$$E = E° + \frac{2.303\,RT}{zF} \log(a_z) \qquad \qquad \dots (21.3)$$

where, E is the measured potential;

$E°$ = is the standard electrode potential;

R = is the gas constant;

T = is the absolute temperature;

z = is the signed charge (+ for cations, – for anions);

F = is the Faraday constant; and a is the activity of the ion being measured.

At a given temperature, the quantity 2.30 RT/F has a constant value; at 25°C it is 0.0592 volt (59.2 mV). At constant ionic strength, the activity, a, is directly proportional to concentration, and the Nernst equation may be written as the following for electrodes responding to Cd^{2+} and F^-, respectively:

$$E \text{ (in mV)} = E° + \frac{59.2}{2} \log[Cd^{2+}] \qquad \text{... (21.4)}$$

$$E = E° + 59.2 \log[F^-] \qquad \text{... (21.5)}$$

Electrodes that respond more or less selectively to various ions are called ion-selective electrodes. Generally, the potential-developing component is a membrane of some kind that allows for selective exchange of the sought-for ion. The glass electrode used for the measurement of hydrogen-ion activity and pH is the oldest and most widely used ion-selective electrode. The potential is developed in a glass membrane that selectively exchanges hydrogen ion in preference to other cations, giving a Nernstian response to hydrogen ion activity, a_{H^+} :

$$E = E° + 59.2 \log(a_{H^+}) \qquad \text{... (21.6)}$$

Of the ion-selective electrodes other than glass electrodes, the fluoride electrode is the most successful. It is well-behaved, relatively free of interferences and has an adequately low detection limit and a long range of linear response. Like all ion-selective electrodes, its electrical output is in the form of a potential signal that is proportional to the log of concentration. A small error in E leads to a variation in log of concentration, which leads to relatively high concentration errors. Voltammetric techniques, the measurement of current resulting from potential applied to a microelectrode, have found some applications in water analysis. One such technique is differential-pulse polarography, in which the potential is applied to the microelectrode in the form of small pulses, superimposed on a linearly increasing potential. The current is read near the end of the voltage pulse and compared to the current just before the pulse is applied. It has the advantage of minimising the capacitive current from charging the microelectrode surface, which sometimes obscures the current due to the reduction or oxidation of the species being analysed. Anodic-stripping voltammetry involves deposition of metals on an electrode surface over a period of several minutes followed by stripping them off very rapidly using a linear anodic sweep. The electrodeposition concentrates the metals on the electrode surface and increased sensitivity results. An even better technique is to strip the metals off using a differential pulse signal. A differential-pulse anodic-stripping voltammogram of lead, cadmium, and zinc in tap water is shown in Fig. 21.6.

Gas Chromatography

Gas chromatography has played an important role in the analysis of organic materials. Gas chromatography is both a qualitative and quantitative technique; for some analytical applications of environmental importance, it is remarkably sensitive and selective. Gas chromatography is based upon the principle that when a mixture of volatile materials transported by a carrier gas is passed through a column containing an adsorbent solid phase, or, more commonly, an absorbing liquid phase coated on a solid material, each volatile component will be partitioned between the carrier gas and solid or liquid. The length of time required for the volatile component to traverse the column is proportional to the degree to which it is retained by the non-gaseous phase. Since different components may be retained to different degrees, they will emerge from the end of the column at different times. If a suitable detector is available, the time at which the component emerges from the column and the quantity of the component are both measured. A recorder trace of the detector response appears as peaks of different sizes, depending upon the quantity of material producing the detector response. Both quantitative and (within limits) qualitative analyses of the sought-for substances are obtained.

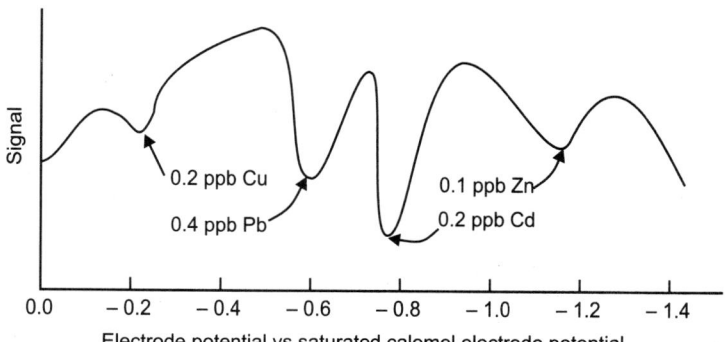

Fig. 21.6. Differential-pulse anodic-stripping voltammogram of tap water at a mercury-plated, wax-impregnated graphite electrode.

The essential features of gas chromatography are shown schematically in Fig. 21.7. The carrier gas generally is argon, helium, hydrogen, or nitrogen. The sample is injected as a single compact plug into the carrier gas stream immediately ahead of the column entrance. If the sample is liquid, the injection chamber is heated to vapourise the liquid rapidly. The separation column may consist of a metal or glass tube packed with an inert solid of high surface area covered with a liquid phase, or it may consist of an active solid, which enables the separation to occur. More commonly now, capillary columns are employed which consist of very small diameter, long tubes in which the liquid phase is coated on the inside of the column.

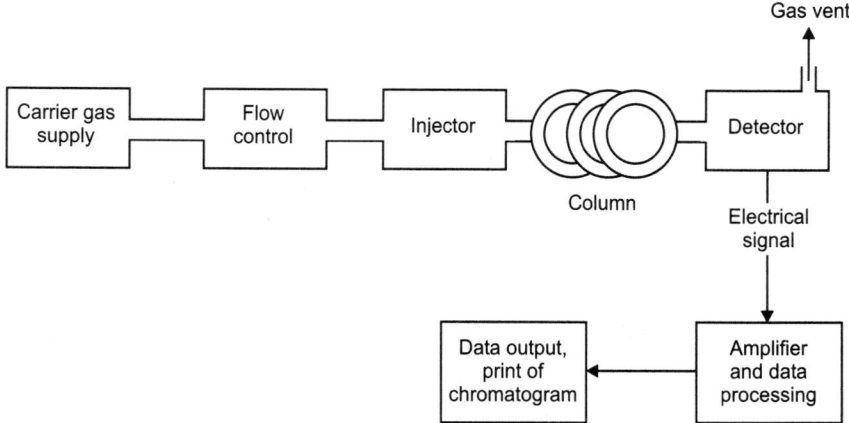

Fig. 21.7. Schematic diagram of the essential features of a gas chromatograph.

The component that primarily determines the sensitivity of gas chromatographic analysis, and for some classes of compounds the selectivity as well, is the detector. One such device is the thermal conductivity detector, which responds to changes in the thermal conductivity of gases passing over it. The electron-capture detector, which is especially useful for halogenated hydrocarbons and phosphorus compounds, operates through the capture of electrons emitted by a beta-particle source. The flame-ionisation gas chromatographic detector is very sensitive for the detection of organic compounds. It is based upon the phenomenon by which organic compounds form highly conducting fragments, such as C^+, in a flame. Application of a potential gradient across the flame results in a small current that may be readily measured. The mass spectrometer may be used as a detector for a gas chromatograph. A combined gas chromatograph/mass spectrometer (GC/MS) instrument is an especially powerful analytical tool for organic compounds. Gas chromatographic analysis requires that a compound exhibit at least a few mm of vapour pressure at the highest temperature at which it is stable. In many cases, organic compounds that cannot be chromatographed directly may be converted into derivatives that are amenable to gas chromatographic analysis. It is seldom possible to analyse organic compounds in water by direct injection of the water into the gas chromatograph; higher concentration is usually required.

Two techniques commonly employed to remove volatile compounds from water and concentrate them are extraction with solvents and purging volatile compounds with a gas, such as helium, concentrating the purged gases on a short column and driving them off by heat into the chromatograph.

High-performance liquid chromatography

A liquid mobile phase used with very small column-packing particles enables high-resolution chromatographic separation of materials in the liquid phase. Very high pressures up to several thousand psi are required to get a reasonable flow rate in such systems. Analysis using such devices is called high performance liquid chromatography (HPLC) and offers an enormous advantage, in that the materials analysed need not be changed to the vapour phase, a step that often requires preparation of a volatile derivative or results in decomposition of the sample. The basic features of a high-performance liquid chromatograph are the same as those of a gas chromatograph, shown in Fig. 21.7, except that a solvent reservoir and high-pressure pump are substituted for the carrier gas source and regulator. An HPLC chromatogram of some water pollutants is shown in Fig. 21.8.

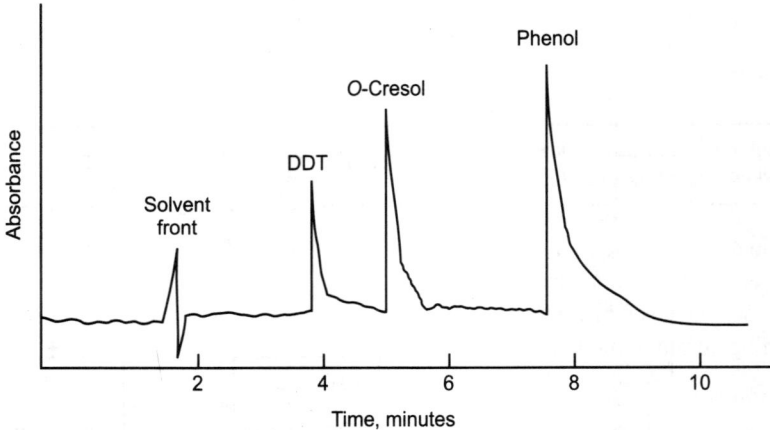

Fig. 21.8. HPLC chromatogram showing separation of some compounds extracted from water contaminated by coal gasification; ultraviolet absorption detection at 272 nm.

Refractive index and ultraviolet detectors are both used for the detection of peaks coming from the liquid chromatograph column. Fluorescence detection can be especially sensitive for some classes of compounds. Mass spectrometric detection of HPLC effluents has led to the development of LC/MS analysis. Somewhat difficult in practice, this technique can be a powerful tool for the determination of analytes that cannot be subjected to gas chromatography. High-performance liquid chromatography has emerged as a very useful technique for the analysis of a number of water pollutants.

Chromatographic analysis of water pollutants

A number of chromatography-based standard methods have also been developed for determining water pollutants. Some of these methods use the purge-and-trap technique, bubbling gas through a column of water to purge volatile organics from the water followed by trapping the organics on solid sorbents, whereas others use solvent extraction to isolate and concentrate the organics. These methods are summarised in Table 21.3.

Table 21.3. Chromatography methods for organic compounds in water.

	Method number			
Class of compounds	*GC*	*GC/MS*	*HPLC*	*Example analytes*
Purgeable halocarbons	601	–	–	Carbon tetrachloride
Purgeable aromatics	602	624, 1624	–	Toluene
Acrolein and acrylonitrile	603	604, 1624	–	Acrolein
Phenols	604	625, 1625	–	Phenol and chlorophenols
Phthalate esters	606	625, 1625	–	*Bis*(2-ethylhexylphthalate)
Nitrosamines	607	625, 1625	–	*N*-Nitroso-*N*-dimethylamine
Organochlorine pesticides and PCBs	608	625	–	Heptachlor, PCB 1016
Nitroaromatics and isophorone	609	625, 1625	–	Nitrobenzene
Polycyclic aromatic hydrocarbons	610	625, 1625	610	Benzo[α]pyrene
Haloethers	611	625, 1625	–	*Bis*(2-chloroethyl) ether
Chlorinated hydrocarbons	612	624, 1624	–	1,3-Dichlorobenzene

Ion chromatography

Liquid chromatographic determination of ions, particularly anions, has enabled the measurement of species that used to be very troublesome for water chemists. This technique is called ion chromatography and its development has been facilitated by special detection techniques using so-called suppressors to enable detection of analyte ions in the chromatographic effluent. Ion chromatography has been developed for the determination of most of the common anions, including arsenate, arsenite, borate, carbonate, chlorate, chlorite, cyanide, the halides, hypochlorite, hypophosphite, nitrate, nitrite, phosphate, phosphite, pyrophosphate, selenate, selenite, sulphate, sulphite, sulphide, trimetaphosphate and tripolyphosphate. Cations, including common metal ions, can also be determined by ion chromatography.

Mass Spectrometry

Mass spectrometry is particularly useful for the identification of specific organic pollutants. It depends upon the production of ions by an electrical discharge or chemical process, followed by separation based on the charge-to-mass ratio and measurement of the ions produced. The output of a mass spectrometer is a mass spectrum, such as the one shown in Fig. 21.9. A mass spectrum is characteristic of a compound and serves to identify it. Computerised data banks for mass spectra have been established and are stored in computers interfaced with mass spectrometers. Identification of a mass spectrum depends upon the purity of the compound from which the spectrum is taken. Prior separation by gas chromatography with continual sampling of the column effluent by a mass spectrometer, commonly called gas chromatography-mass spectrometry (GC/MS), is particularly effective in the analysis of organic pollutants.

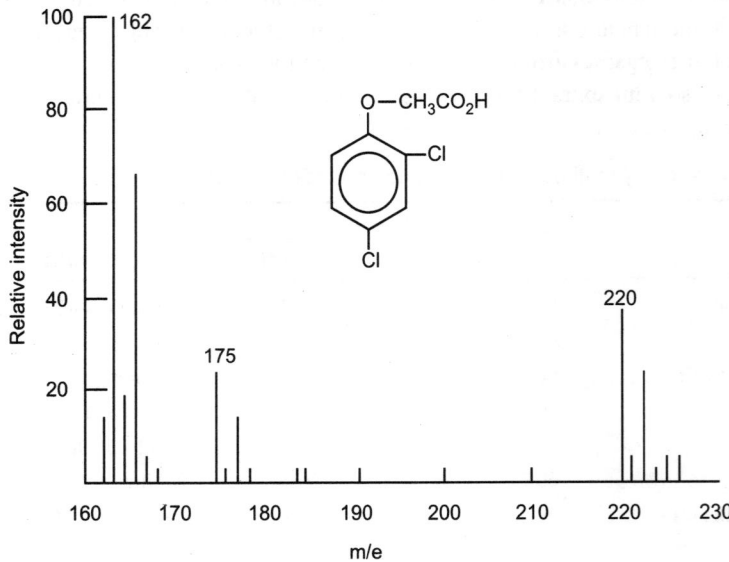

Fig. 21.9. Partial mass spectrum of the herbicide 2,4-dichlorophenoxyacetic acid (2,4-D), a common water pollutant.

Analysis of Water Samples

The major kinds of analysis techniques that are used on water are discussed below:

Physical properties measured in water

The commonly determined physical properties of water are colour, residue (solids), odour, temperature, specific conductance and turbidity. Most of these terms are self-explanatory. All of these properties either influence or reflect the chemistry of the water. Solids, for example, arise from chemical substances, either suspended or dissolved in the water, and are classified physically as total, filterable, non-filterable, or volatile. Specific conductance is a measure of the degree to which water conducts alternating current and reflects, therefore, the total concentration of dissolved ionic material. By necessity, some physical properties must be measured in the water without sampling.

Water sampling

It must be emphasised, however, that the acquisition of meaningful data demands that correct sampling and storage procedures be used. These procedures may be quite different for different species in water. In general, separate samples must be collected for chemical and biological analysis, because the sampling and preservation techniques are quite different. Usually, the shorter the time interval between sample collection and analysis, the more accurate the analysis will be. Indeed, some analyses must be performed in the field within minutes of sample collection. Others, such as the determination of temperature, must be done in the body of water itself. Within a few minutes after collection, water pH may change, dissolved gases (oxygen, carbon dioxide, hydrogen sulphide, chlorine) may be lost, or other gases (oxygen, carbon dioxide) may be absorbed from the atmosphere. Therefore, analyses of temperature, pH, and dissolved gases should always be performed in the field. Furthermore, precipitation of calcium carbonate accompanies changes in the pH-alkalinity-calcium carbonate relationship following sample collection. Analysis of a sample after standing may thus give erroneously low values for calcium and total hardness.

Oxidation-reduction reactions may cause substantial errors in analysis. For example, soluble iron(II) and manganese(II) are oxidised to insoluble iron(III) and manganese(IV) compounds as an anaerobic water sample absorbs atmospheric oxygen.

Microbial activity may decrease phenol or biological oxygen demand (BOD) values, change the nitrate-nitrite-ammonia balance, or alter the relative proportions of sulphate and sulphide. Iodide and cyanide frequently are oxidised. Chromium(VI) in solution may be reduced to insoluble chromium(III). Sodium, silicate, and boron are leached from glass container walls. Acquiring a truly representative sample is as important as sample preservation. A representative single sample of a body of water must be a composite of many samples taken from a number of different locations over a long period of time. Generally, it is much more meaningful to analyse a large number of separate samples taken at different times and different locations than it is to compile and analyse a single representative sample, although this must be balanced against the costs of collecting and analysing large numbers of samples.

Water sample preservation

It is not possible to protect a water sample from changes in composition. However, various additives and treatment techniques can be employed to minimise sample deterioration. These methods are summarised in Table 21.4.

Table 21.4. Preservatives and preservation methods used with water samples.

Preservative or technique used	Effect on sample	Type of samples for which the method is employed
Nitric acid	Keeps metals in solution	Metal-containing samples
Sulphuric acid	Bactericide	Biodegradable samples containing organic carbon, oil, and grease
	Formation of sulphates with volatile bases	Samples containing amines or ammonia
Sodium hydroxide	Formation of sodium salts from volatile acids	Samples containing volatile organic acids or cyanides
Chemical reaction	Fix a particular constituent	Samples to be analysed for dissolved oxygen using the Winkler method

The most general method of sample preservation is refrigeration to 4°C. Freezing normally should be avoided because of physical changes—formation of precipitates and loss of gas—which may adversely affect sample composition. Sample holding times vary, from zero for parameters such as temperature or dissolved oxygen measured by a probe, to six months for metals.

Many different kinds of samples, including those to be analysed for acidity, alkalinity and various forms of nitrogen or phosphorus, should not be held for more than 24 hours. Instructions should be followed for each kind of sample in order to ensure meaningful results.

Total organic carbon in water

Dissolved organic carbon exerts an oxygen demand in water; often this is in the form of toxic substances and is a general indicator of water pollution. Therefore, its measurement is quite important. The measurement of total organic carbon, TOC, is now recognised as the best means of assessing the organic content of a water sample. The measurement of this parameter has been facilitated by the development of methods which, for the most part, totally oxidise the dissolved organic material to produce carbon dioxide. The amount of carbon dioxide evolved is taken as a measure of TOC.

TOC can be determined by a technique that uses a dissolved oxidising agent promoted by ultraviolet light. Potassium peroxydisulphate, $K_2S_2O_8$, is usually chosen as an oxidising agent to be added to the sample. Phosphoric acid is also added to the sample, which is sparged with air or nitrogen to drive off CO_2 formed from HCO_3^- and CO_3^{2-} in solution. After sparging, the sample is pumped to a chamber containing a lamp emitting ultraviolet radiation of 184.9 nm. This radiation produces reactive free radical species, such as the hydroxyl radical, HO. The active species bring about the rapid oxidation of dissolved organic compounds as shown in the following general reaction:

$$\text{Organics} + \text{HO}\bullet \rightarrow CO_2 + H_2O$$

After oxidation is complete, the CO_2 is sparged from the system and measured with a gas chromatographic detector or by absorption in ultrapure water followed by a conductivity measurement. Fig. 21.10 is a schematic of a TOC analyser.

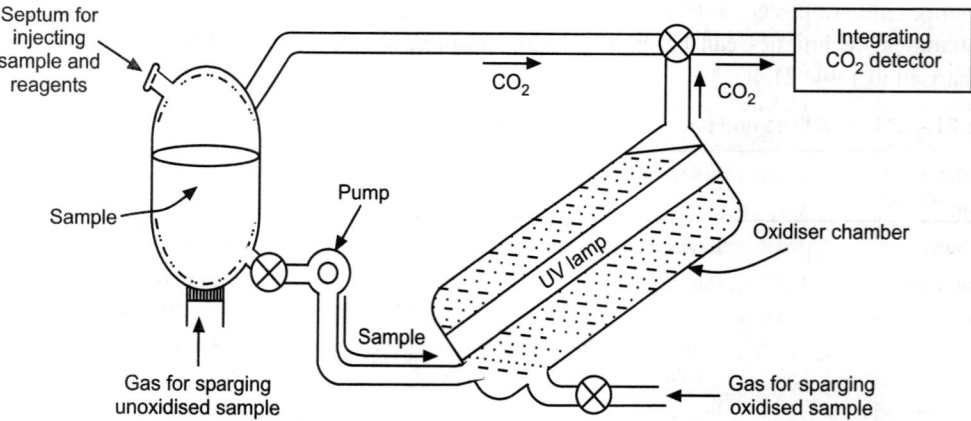

Fig. 21.10. TOC analyser employing UV-promoted sample oxidation.

Measurement of radioactivity in water

There are several potential sources of radioactive materials that may contaminate water. Radioactive contamination of water is normally detected by measurements of gross beta and gross alpha activity, a procedure that is simpler than detecting individual isotopes. The measurement is made from a sample formed by evaporating water to a very thin layer on a small pan, which is then inserted inside an internal proportional counter. This set-up is necessary because beta particles can penetrate only very thin detector windrows, and alpha particles have essentially no penetrating power. More detailed information can be obtained for radio-nuclides that emit gamma rays by the use of gamma spectrum analysis. This technique employs solid state detectors to resolve rather closely-spaced gamma peaks in the sample's spectra. In conjunction with multi-channel spectrometric data analysis, it is possible to determine a number of radio-nuclides in the same sample without chemical separation. The method requires minimal sample preparation.

The main chemical parameters commonly determined in water are summarised in Table 21.5. In addition, a number of other solutes, especially specific organic pollutants, may be determined in connection with specific health hazards or incidents of pollution.

Table 21.5. Chemical parameters commonly determined in water.

Chemical species	Significance in water	Methods of analysis
Acidity	Indicative of industrial pollution or acid mine drainage	Titration
Alkalinity	Water treatment, buffering, algal productivity	Titration
Aluminium	Water treatment, buffering	AA,[a] ICP
Ammonia	Algal productivity, pollutant	Spectrophotometry
Arsenic	Toxic pollutant	Spectrophotometry, AA, ICP
Barium	Toxic pollutant	AA, ICP
Beryllium	Toxic pollutant	AA, ICP, fluorimetry
Boron	Toxic to plants	Spectrophotometry, ICP[b]
Bromide	Seawater intrusion, industrial waste	Spectrophotometry, potentiometry, ion chromatography
Cadmium	Toxic pollutant	AA, ICP
Calcium	Hardness, productivity, treatment	AA, ICP
Carbon dioxide	Bacterial action, corrosion	Titration, calculation
Chloride	Saline water contamination	Titration, electrochemical, ion chromatography
Chlorine	Water treatment	Spectrophotometry
Chromium	Toxic pollutant (hexavalent Cr)	AA, ICP, colourimetry
Copper	Plant growth	AA, ICP
Cyanide	Toxic pollutant	Spectrophotometry, potentiometry, ion chromatography
Fluoride	Water treatment, toxic at high levels	Spectrophotometry, potentiometry, ion chromatography
Hardness	Water quality, water treatment	AA, titration
Iodide	Seawater intrusion, industrial waste	Catalytic effect, potentiometry, ion chromatography
Iron	Water quality, water treatment	AA, ICP, colourimetry
Lead	Toxic pollutant	AA, ICP, voltammetry
Lithium	May indicate some pollution	AA, ICP, flame photometry
Magnesium	Hardness	AA, ICP
Manganese	Water quality (staining)	AA, ICP
Mercury	Toxic pollutant	Flameless atomic absorption

(Contd ...)

Chemical species	Significance in water	Methods of analysis
Methane	Anaerobic bacterial action	Combustible-gas indicator
Nitrate	Algal productivity, toxicity	Spectrophotometry, ion chromatography
Nitrite	Toxic pollutant	Spectrophotometry, ion chromatography
Nitrogen		
(Albuminoid)	Proteinaceous material	Spectrophotometry
(Organic)	Organic pollution indicator	Spectrophotometry
Oil and grease	Industrial pollution	Gravimetry
Organic carbon	Organic pollution indicator	Oxidation CO_2 measurement
Organic contaminants	Organic pollution indicator	Activated carbon adsorption
Oxygen	Water quality	Titration, electrochemical
Oxygen demand	Water quality and pollution	Microbiological-titration
(Biochemical)		
(Chemical)	Water quality and pollution	Chemical oxidation-titration
Ozone	Water treatment	Titration
Pesticides	Water pollution	Gas chromatography
pH	Water quality and pollution	Potentiometry
Phenols	Water pollution	Distillation-colourimetry
Phosphate	Productivity, pollution	Spectrophotometry
Phosphorus		
(hydrolysable)	Water quality and pollution	Spectrophotometry
Potassium	Productivity, pollution	AA, ICP, flame photometry
Selenium	Toxic pollutant	Spectrophotometry, neutron activation
Silica	Water quality	Spectrophotometry, ICP
Silver	Water pollution	AA, ICP
Sodium	Water quality, saltwater intrusion	AA, ICP, flame photometry
Strontium	Water quality	AA, ICP, flame photometry
Sulphate	Water quality, water pollution	Ion chromatography
Sulphide	Water quality, water pollution	Spectrophotometry, titratin, ion chromatography
Sulphite	Water pollution, oxygen scavenger	Titration, ion chromatography
Surfactants	Water pollution	Spectrophotometry
Tannin, Lignin	Water quality, water pollution	Spectrophotometry
Vanadium	Water quality, water pollution	ICP
Zinc	Water quality, water pollution	AA, ICP

[a] AA denotes atomic absorption.

[b] ICP stands for inductively coupled plasma techniques, including atomic emission and detection of plasma-atomised atoms by mass spectrometry.

Atmospheric Monitoring

Good analytical methodology, particularly that applicable to automated analysis and continuous monitoring, is essential for the study and alleviation of air pollution. The atmosphere is a particularly difficult analytical system because of the very low levels of substances to be analysed; sharp variations in pollutant level with time and location; differences in temperature and humidity; and difficulties encountered in reaching desired sampling points, particularly those substantially above the Earth's surface. Furthermore, although improved techniques for the analysis of air pollutants are continually being developed, a need still exists for new analytical methodology and the improvement of existing methodology. Much of the earlier data on air pollutant levels (as well as much of the data currently being taken) were unreliable as a result of inadequate analysis and sampling methods. An atmospheric pollutant analysis method does not have to give the actual value to be useful. One which gives a relative value may still be helpful in establishing trends in pollutant levels, determining pollutant effects and locating pollution sources. Such methods may continue to be used while others are being developed.

Air pollutants measured

Air pollutants generally measured may be placed in several different categories. One such category contains materials for which ambient (surrounding atmosphere) standards have been set by the Environmental Protection Agency. These are sulphur dioxide, carbon monoxide, nitrogen dioxide, non-methane hydrocarbons and particulate matter. The standards are categorised as primary and secondary. Primary standards are those defining the level of air quality necessary to protect public health. Secondary standards are designed to provide protection against known or expected adverse effects of air pollutants, particularly upon materials, vegetation and animals. Another group of air pollutants to be measured consists of those known to be specifically hazardous to human health, such as asbestos, beryllium and mercury. A third category of air pollutants contains those regulated in new installations of selected stationary sources, such as coal-cleaning plants, cotton gins, lime plants and paper mills. Some pollutants in this category are visible emissions, acid (H_2SO_4) mist, particulate matter, nitrogen oxides and sulphur oxides. These substances often must be monitored in the stack to ensure that emission standards are being met. A fourth category consists of the emissions of mobile sources (motor vehicles) — hydrocarbons, CO, and NO_x. A fifth group consists of miscellaneous elements and compounds, such as certain heavy metals, fluoride, chlorine, phosphorus, polycyclic aromatic hydrocarbons (PAH), polychlorinated biphenyls, odourous compounds, reactive organic compounds and radio-nuclides.

For some species, an analytical method is well developed and reasonably satisfactory. For others, no really satisfactory method exists. The development of analytical techniques for air pollutants remains a fertile and challenging area for research.

Levels of air pollutants and other air-quality parameters are expressed in several different kinds of units. These are, for gases and vapours, $\mu g/m^3$ (alternatively, ppm by volume); for weight of particulate matter, $\mu g/m^3$; for particulate matter count, number per cubic metre; for visibility, kilometres; for instantaneous light transmission, percentage of light transmitted; for emission and sampling rates, m^3/min; for pressure, mm Hg; and for temperature, degrees Celsius. Air volumes should be converted to conditions of 10°C and 760 mm Hg (1 atm), assuming ideal gas behaviour.

Sampling

The ideal atmospheric analysis techniques are those that work successfully without sampling, such as long-path laser resonance absorption monitoring. For most analysis, however, various types of sampling are required. In some very sophisticated monitoring systems, samples are collected and analysed automatically, and the results are transmitted to a central receiving station. Often, however, a batch sample is collected for later chemical analysis.

The analytical result from a sample can be only as good as the method employed to obtain that sample. A number of factors enter into obtaining a good sample. The size of the sample required (total volume of air sampled) decreases with increasing concentration of pollutant and increasing sensitivity of the analytical method. Often a sample of 10 or more cubic metre is required. The sampling rate is determined by the equipment used and generally ranges from approximately 0.003 m^3/min. to 3.0 m^3/min. The duration of sampling time influences the result obtained, as shown in Fig. 21.11. The actual concentration of the pollutant is shown by the solid line. A sample collected over an eight-hour period has the concentration shown in the dashed line, whereas samples taken over one-hour intervals exhibit the concentration levels shown by the dotted line. Sampling techniques are discussed briefly for specific kinds of analytes later in this chapter.

The most straightforward technique for the collection of particles is sedimentation. A sedimentation collector may be as simple as a glass jar equipped with a funnel. Liquid is sometimes added to the collector to prevent solids from being blown out. Filtration is the most common technique for sampling particulate matter. Filters composed of fritted (porous) glass, porous ceramics, paper fibres, cellulose fibres, fibreglass, asbestos, mineral wool, or plastic may be used. A special type of filter is the membrane filter, which yields high flow rates with small, moderately uniform pores. Impingers, as the name implies, collect particles from a relatively high-velocity air stream directed at a surface.

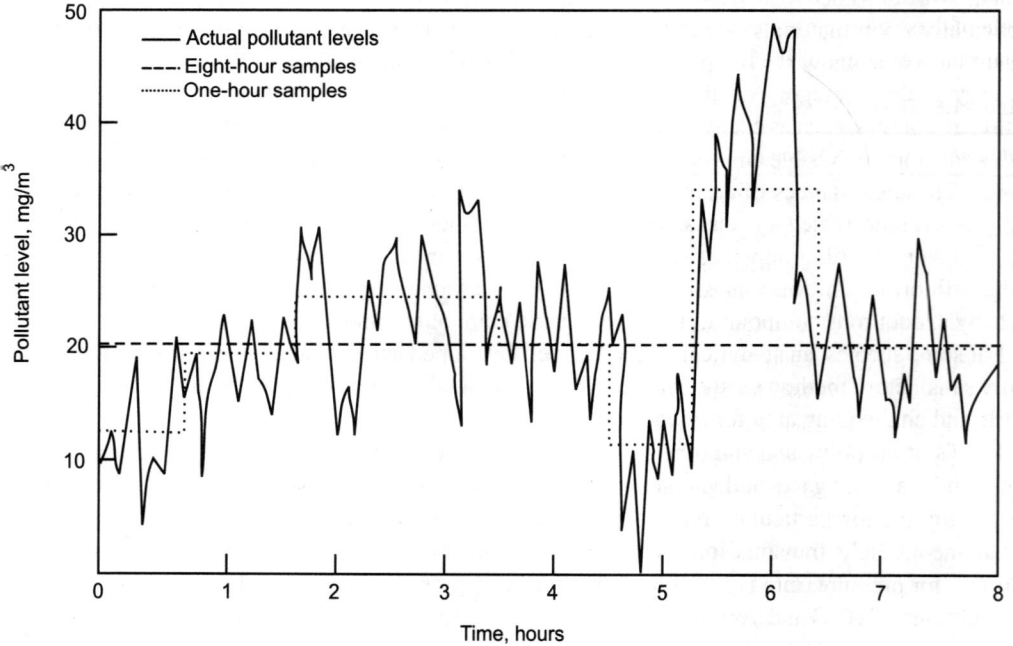

Fig. 21.11. Effect of duration of sampling upon observed values of air pollutants.

Sampling for vapours and gases may range from methods designed to collect only one specific pollutant to those designed to collect all pollutants. Essentially, all pollutants may be removed from an air sample cryogenically by freezing or by liquifying the air in collectors maintained at a low temperature. Absorption in a solvent, such as by bubbling the gas through a liquid, can be used for the collection of gaseous pollutants. Adsorption, in which a gas collects on the surface of a solid, is particularly useful for the collection of samples to be analysed by gas chromatography. Denuders are among the more useful sampling devices for certain kinds of air pollutants. Denuders solve a major sampling problem by enabling collection of gas-phase pollutants free of contamination by particles. Otherwise, for some pollutants such as acids, it is not possible to distinguish relative amounts of analytes in the gas phase from those in the particulate form.

Diffusion denuders run a laminar flow airstream through a tube, the walls of which are covered with a sorptive or reactive collecting medium for the analytes of interest. The diffusion coefficients of small particles are only about 10^{-4} those of gases, so that the particles go through the tube and the gases diffuse to the walls and are collected. Open-bore denuders consist of tubes with coated walls. A more efficient device is the annular denuder composed of concentric tubes separated by 1–2 mm of annular space. Thermodenuders use heat to drive off analytes collected by the device. They can be used for semi-continuous analysis by employing a collection/analysis cycle involving alternate collection and thermal desorption. Diffusion scrubbers are denuders in which walls are composed of membranes so that gas from the sample goes through the wall and is collected in a collecting liquid.

Methods of Analysis

A very large number of different analytical techniques are used for atmospheric pollutant analysis. Some of these whose uses are not confined to atmospheric analysis were discussed earlier in this chapter. A summary of some of the main instrumental techniques for air monitoring is presented in Table 21.6.

Table 21.6. The main techniques used for air pollutant analysis.

Pollutant	Method	Potential interferences
SO_2 (total S)	Flame photometric (FPD)	H_2S, CO
SO_2	Gas chromatography (FPD)	H_2S, CO
SO_2	Spectophotometric (pararosaniline wet chemical)	H_2S, HCl, NH_3, NO_2, O_3
SO_2	Electrochemical	H_2S, HCl, NH_3, NO, NO_2, O_3, C_2H_4
SO_2	Conductivity	HCl, NH_3, NO_2
SO_2	Gas-phase spectrophotometric	NO, NO_2, O_3,
O_3	Chemiluminescent	H_2S
O_3	Electrochemical	NH_3, NO_2, SO_2
O_3	Spectrophotometric (potassium iodide reaction, wet chemical)	NH_3, NO_2, NO, SO_2
O_3	Gas-phase spectrophotometric	NO_2, NO, SO_2
CO	Infrared	CO_2 (at high levels)
CO	Gas chromatography	–
CO	Electrochemical	NO, C_2H_4
CO	Catalytic combustion-thermal detection	NH_3
CO	Infrared fluorescence	–
CO	Mercury replacement ultraviolet photometric	C_2H_4
NO_2	Chemiluminescent	NH_3, NO, NO_2, SO_2

(Contd ...)

Pollutant	Method	Potential interferences
NO_2	Spectrophotometric (azo-dye reaction wet chemical)	NO, SO_2, NO_2, O_3
NO_2	Electrochemical	HCl, NH_3, NO, NO_2, SO_2, O_3, CO
NO_2	Gas-phase spectrophotometric	NH_3, NO, NO_2, SO_2, CO
NO_2	Conductivity	HCl, NH_3, NO, NO_2, SO_2

Analysis of Sulphur Dioxide

The reference method for the analysis of sulphur dioxide is the spectrophotometric pararosaniline method first described by West and Gaeke, and subsequently optimised. It is applicable to the analysis of 0.005–5 ppm SO_2 in ambient air. Figure 21.12 illustrates the various components involved in a sampling train employed to sample the atmosphere for sulphur dioxide to be analysed by the West-Gaeke method. The method makes use of a collecting solution of 0.04 M potassium tetrachloromercurate to collect sulphur dioxide according to the following reaction:

$$HgCl_4^{2-} + SO_2 + H_2O \rightarrow HgCl_2SO_3^{2-} + 2H^+ + 2Cl^- \qquad ... (21.7)$$

Typically, this involves scrubbing 30 litres of air through 10 ml of scrubbing solution with a collection efficiency of around 95 per cent. Sulphur dioxide in the scrubbing medium is reacted with formaldehyde:

$$HCHO + SO_2 + 2H_2O \rightarrow HOCH_2SO_3H \qquad ... (21.8)$$

The adduct formed is then reacted with uncoloured organic pararosaniline hydrochloride to produce a red-violet dye. Although NO_2 at levels above about 2 ppm interferes, the interference may be eliminated by reducing the NO_2 to N_2 gas with sulphamic acid, H_2NSO_3H.

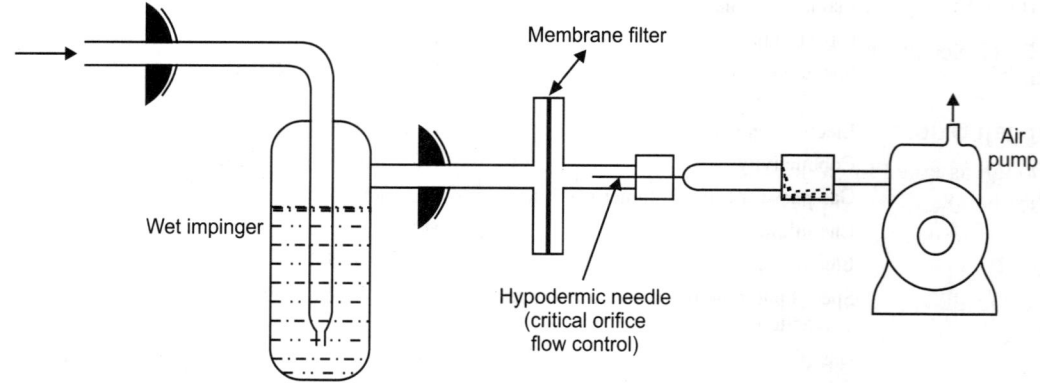

Fig. 21.12. Sampling train for collecting air samples for sulphur dioxide analysis with the West-Gaeke method.

Performed manually, the West-Gaeke method for sulphur dioxide analysis is cumbersome and complicated. However, the method has been refined to the point that it can be done automatically with continuous monitoring equipment. A block diagram of such an analyser is shown in Fig. 21.13.

Generally, sulphur dioxide is collected in a hydrogen peroxide solution and increased conductance of the sulphuric acid solution is measured. Several types of sulphur dioxide monitors are based on amperometry, in which an electrical current is measured that is proportional to the SO_2 in a collecting solution. Sulphur dioxide can be determined by ion chromatography, by bubbling SO_2 through hydrogen peroxide solution to produce SO_4^{2-}, followed by analysis of the sulphate by ion chromatography, a method that separates ions on a chromatography column and detects them very sensitively by conductivity measurement. Flame photometry, sometimes in combination with gas chromatography, is also used for the detection of sulphur dioxide and other gaseous sulphur compounds. The gas is burned in a hydrogen flame and the sulphur emission line at 394 nm is measured. Several direct spectrophotometric methods are used for sulphur dioxide measurement, including non-dispersive infrared absorption, Fourier transform infrared analysis (FTIR), ultraviolet absorption, molecular resonance fluorescence and second-derivative spectrophotometry. The principles of these methods are the same for any gas measured.

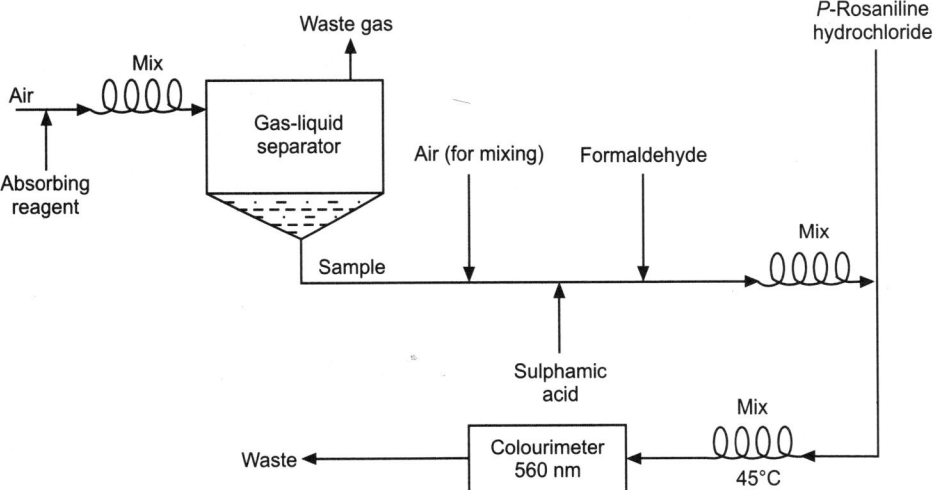

Fig. 21.13. Schematic diagram of an automatic analyser used for sulphur dioxide analysis by the West-Gaeke method.

Nitrogen Oxides

Although as noted in Table 21.6, several methods have been used to determine nitrogen oxides, gas-phase chemiluminescence is the favoured method of NO_x analysis. It results from the emission of light from electronically excited species formed by a chemical reaction. In the case of NO, ozone is reacted with NO to produce NO_2, which loses energy and returns to the ground state through emission of light in the 600–3000 nm range. The emitted light is measured by a photomultiplier; its intensity is proportional to the concentration of NO. A schematic diagram of the device used is shown in Fig. 21.14.

Since the chemiluminescence detector system depends upon the reaction of O_3 with NO, it is necessary to convert NO_2 to NO in the sample prior to analysis. This is accomplished by passing the air sample over a thermal converter. Analysis of such a sample gives NO_x, the sum of NO and NO_2. Chemiluminescence analysis of a sample that has not been passed over the thermal converter gives NO. The difference between these two results is NO_2.

Other nitrogen compounds besides NO and NO_2 undergo chemiluminescence by reacting with O_3, and these may interfere with the analysis if present in an excessive level. Particulate matter also causes interference which may be overcome by employing a membrane filter on the air inlet.

This analysis technique is illustrative of chemiluminescence analysis in general. Chemiluminescence is an inherently desirable technique for the analysis of atmospheric pollutants because it avoids wet chemistry, is basically simple and lends itself well to continuous monitoring and instrumental methods. Another chemiluminescence method, that is employed for the analysis of ozone, is described in the next section.

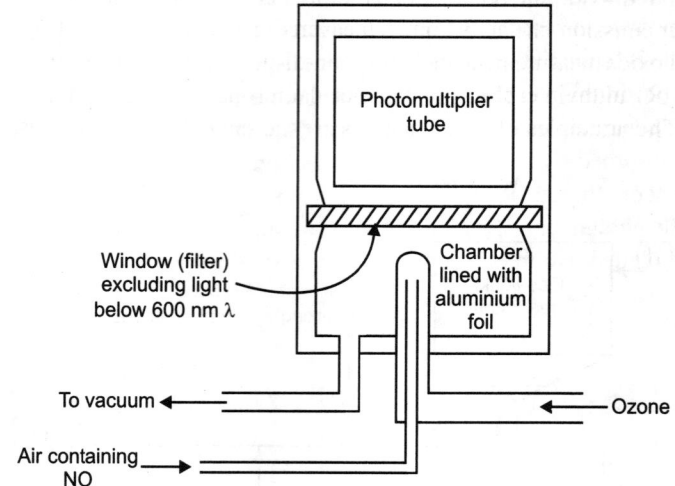

Fig. 21.14. Chemiluminescence detector for NO_x.

Analysis of Oxidants

Atmospheric oxidants that are commonly analysed include ozone, hydrogen peroxide, organic peroxides and chlorine. The classic manual method for the analysis of oxidants is based upon their oxidation of I^- ion followed by spectrophotometric measurement of the product. The sample is collected in 1 per cent KI buffered at pH 6.8. Oxidants react with iodide ion as shown by the following reaction of ozone:

$$O_3 + 2H^+ + 3I^- \rightarrow I_3^- + O_2 + H_2O \qquad \qquad ... (21.9)$$

The absorbance of the coloured I_3^- product is measured spectrophotometrically at 352 nm. Generally, the level of oxidant is expressed in terms of ozone, although it should be noted that not all oxidants— PAN, for example, react with the same efficiency as O_3. Oxidation of I^- may be employed to determine oxidants in a concentration range of several hundreths of a part per million to approximately 10 ppm. Nitrogen dioxide gives a limited response to the method and reducing substances interfere seriously.

Now the favoured method for oxidant analysis uses chemiluminescence. The chemiluminescent reaction is that between ozone and ethylene. Chemiluminescence from this reaction occurs over a range of 300–6000 nm, with a maximum at 435 nm. The intensity of emitted light is directly proportional to the level of ozone. Ozone concentrations ranging from 0.003 to 30 ppm may be measured. Ozone for calibrating the instrument is generated photochemically from the absorption of ultraviolet radiation by oxygen.

Analysis of Carbon Monoxide

Carbon monoxide is analysed in the atmosphere by nondispersive infrared spectrometry. This technique depends upon the fact that carbon monoxide absorbs infrared radiation strongly at certain wavelengths. Therefore, when such radiation is passed through a long (typically 100 cm) cell containing a trace of carbon monoxide levels, more infrared radiant energy is absorbed.

A non-dispersive infrared spectrometer differs from standard infrared spectrometers in that the infrared radiation from the source is not dispersed according to wavelength by a prism or grating. The non-dispersive infrared spectrometer is made very specific for a given compound, or type of compound, by using the sought-for material as part of the detector, or by placing it in a filter cell in the optical path. A diagram of a non-dispersive infrared spectrometer selective for CO is shown in Fig. 21.15. Radiation from an infrared source is 'chopped' by a rotating device, so that it alternately passes through a sample cell and a reference cell. In this particular instrument, both beams of light fall on a detector which is filled with CO gas and separated into two compartments by a flexible diaphragm. The relative amounts of infrared radiation absorbed by the CO in the two sections depend upon level in the sample. The difference in the amount of infrared radiation absorbed in the two compartments causes slight differences in heating, so that the diaphragm bulges slightly toward one side. Very slight movement of the diaphragm can be detected and recorded. By means of this device, carbon monoxide can be measured from 0 to 150 ppm, with a relative accuracy of ±5 per cent in the optimum concentration range.

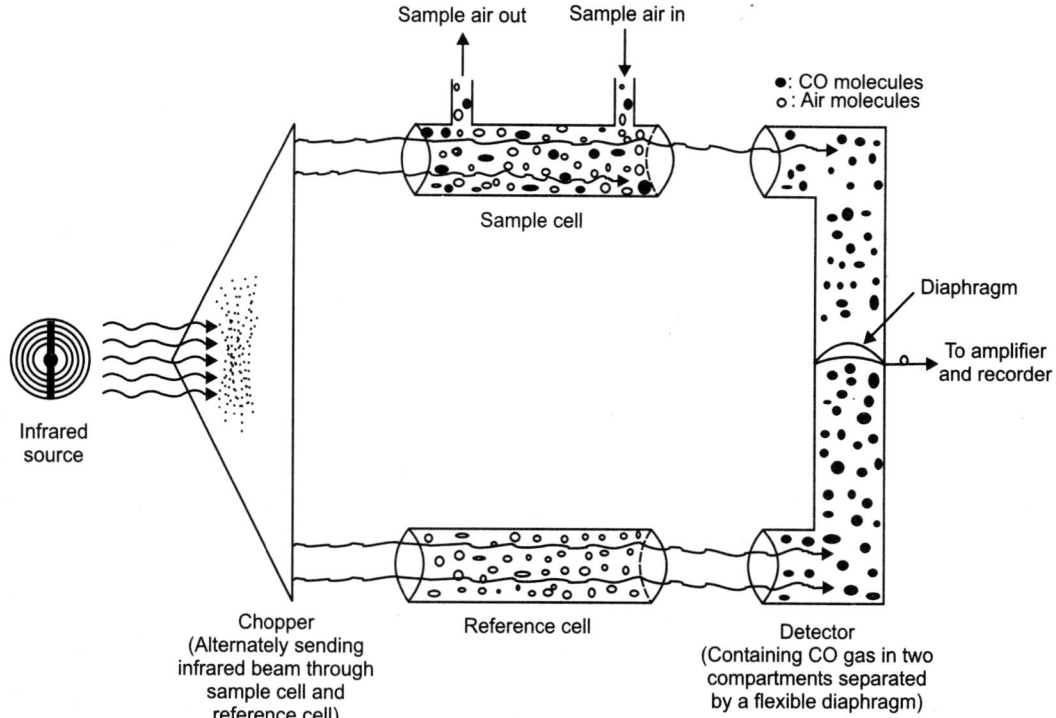

Fig 21.15. Non-dispersive infrared spectrometer for the determination of carbon monoxide in the atmosphere.

Flame-ionisation gas chromatography detection can also be used for the analysis of carbon monoxide. It is selective for hydrocarbons and conversion of CO to methane in the sample is required.

This is accomplished by reaction with hydrogen over a nickel catalyst at 360°C:

$$CO + 3H_2 \rightarrow CH_4 + H_2O \qquad \ldots (21.10)$$

A major advantage of this approach is that the same basic instrumentation may be used to measure hydrocarbons.

Carbon monoxide may also be analysed by measuring the heat produced by its catalytic oxidation to CO_2 over a catalyst consisting of a mixture of MnO_2 and CuO. Differences in temperature between a cell in which the oxidation is occurring and a reference cell through which part of the sample is flowing are measured by thermistors. A vanadium oxide catalyst can be used for the oxidation of hydrocarbons, enabling their simultaneous analysis.

Analysis of Hydrocarbons

Monitoring of hydrocarbons in atmospheric samples takes advantage of the very high sensitivity of the hydrogen flame ionisation detector to measure this class of compounds. Known quantities of air are run through the flame ionisation detector 4 to 12 times per hour to provide a measure of total hydrocarbon content. A separate portion of each sample goes into a stripper column to remove water, carbon dioxide, and non-methane hydrocarbons. Methane and carbon monoxide, which are not retained by the stripper column, are separated by a chromatographic column, passed through a catalytic reduction tube then to a flame ionisation detector. Eluting first, methane is not changed by the reduction tube, and is detected as such by the detector. The carbon monoxide is reduced to methane, as shown by reaction 21.10 in the preceding section, then detected as the methane product by the flame ionisation detector. Concentrations of non-methane hydrocarbons are given by subtracting the methane concentrations from the total hydrocarbons.

Using the method described above, total hydrocarbons can be determined in a range of $0-13$ mg/m^3, corresponding to $0-10$ ppm. Methane can be measured over a range of $0-6.5$ mg/m^3 (0.10 ppm).

Analysis of Particulate Matter

Particles are almost always removed from air or gas (such as exhaust flue gas) prior to analysis. The two main approaches to particle isolation are filtration and removal by methods that cause the gas stream to undergo a sharp bend, so that particles are collected on a surface.

Filtration

The method commonly used for determining the quantity of total suspended particulate matter in the atmosphere draws air over filters that remove the particles. This device, called a Hi-Vol sampler, is essentially a glorified vacuum cleaner that draws air through a filter. The samplers are usually placed under a shelter, which excludes precipitation and particles larger than about 0.1 mm in diameter. These devices efficiently collect particles from a large volume of air, typically 2000 m^3.

The filters used in a Hi-Vol sampler are usually composed of glass fibres and have a collection efficiency of at least 99 per cent for particles with 0.3 μm diameter. Particles with diameters exceeding 100 μm remain on the filter surface, whereas particles with diameters down to approximately 0.1 μm are collected on the glass fibres filters. Efficient collection is achieved by using very small diameter fibres (less than 1 μm) for the filter material.

The technique described here is most useful for determining total levels of particulate matter. Prior to taking the sample, the filter is maintained at 15°–35°C at 50 per cent relative humidity for 24 hours, then weighed. After sampling for 24 hours, the filter is removed and equilibrated for 24 hours under the same conditions used prior to its installation on the sampler. The filter is then weighed and the quantity of particulate matter per unit volume of air is calculated.

The range over which particulate matter can be measured is approximately 2–750 μg/m^3, where volume is expressed at 25°C and 1 atm (760 mm Hg, 101 kPa) pressure. The lower limit is determined by limitations in measuring mass and the upper limit by limited flow rate when the filter becomes clogged.

Size separation of particles can be achieved by filtration through successively smaller filters in a stacked filter unit. Another approach uses the virtual impactor, a combination of an air filter and an impactor. In the virtual impactor, the gas stream being sampled is forced to make a sharp bend. Particles larger than about 2.5 µm do not make the bend and are collected on a filter. The remaining gas stream is then filtered to remove smaller particles.

Results obtained by the analysis of particulate matter collected by the filters should be treated with some caution. A number of reactions may occur on the filter and during the process of removing the sample from the filter. This can cause serious misinterpretation of data.

For example, volatile particulate matter may be lost from the filter. Furthermore, because of chemical reactions on the filter, the material analysed may not be the material that was collected. Artifact particulate matter forms from the oxidation of acid gases on alkaline glass fibres. This phenomenon gives an exaggerated value of particulate matter concentration.

One of the major difficulties in particle analysis is the lack of suitable filter material. Different filter materials serve very well for specific application, but none is satisfactory for all applications. Fibre filters composed of polystyrene are very good for elemental analysis because of the low background levels of inorganic materials.

However, they are not useful for organic analysis. Glass-fibre filters have good weighing qualities and are therefore very useful for determining total particle concentration; however, metals, silicates, sulphates and other species are readily leached from fine glass fibres, introducing error into analysis for inorganic pollutant analysis.

Collection by impactors

Impactors cause a relatively high velocity gas stream to undergo a sharp bend, so that particles are collected on a surface impacted by the stream. The device may be called a dry or wet impactor, depending upon whether collecting surface is dry or wet; wet surfaces aid particle retention. Size segregation can be achieved with an impactor because larger particles are preferentially impacted and smaller particles continue in the gas stream. The cascade impactor, illustrated in Fig. 21.16, accomplishes size separation by directing the gas stream onto a series of collection slides through successively smaller orifices, which yield successively higher gas velocities. Particles may break up into smaller pieces from the impact of impingement; therefore, in some cases impingers yield erroneously high values for levels of smaller particles.

Particle analysis

A number of chemical analysis techniques can be used to characterise atmospheric pollutants. These include atomic absorption, inductively coupled plasma techniques, X-ray fluorescence, neutron activation analysis and ion-selective electrodes for fluoride analysis. Chemical microscopy is an extremely useful technique for the characterisation of atmospheric particles. Either visible or electron microscopy may be employed. Particle morphology and shape tell an experienced microscopist a great deal about the material being examined.

Reflection, refraction, microchemical tests and other techniques may be employed to further characterise the materials being examined. Microscopy may be used for determining the levels of specific kinds of particles and for determining their size.

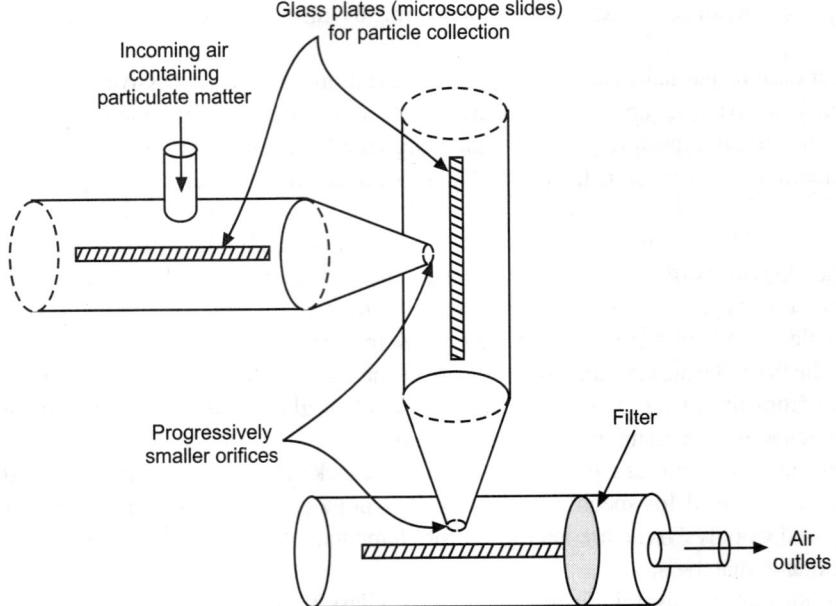

Fig. 21.16. Schematic representation of a cascade impactor for the collection of progressively smaller particles.

Direct Spectrophotometric Analysis of Gaseous Air Pollutants

From the foregoing discussion, it is obvious that measurement techniques that depend upon the use of chemical reagents, particularly liquids, are cumbersome and complicated. It is a tribute to the ingenuity of instrument designers that such techniques are being applied successfully to atmospheric pollutant monitoring. Direct spectrophotometric techniques are more desirable when they are available and when they are capable of accurate analysis at the low levels required. One such technique, non-dispersive infrared spectrophotometry, has been described for the analysis of carbon monoxide. Three other direct spectrophotometric methods are Fourier transform infrared spectroscopy, tunable diode laser spectroscopy and differential optical absorption spectroscopy. These techniques may be used for point air monitoring, in which a sample is monitored at a given point, generally by measurement in a long absorption cell. In-stack monitoring may be performed to measure effluents. A final possibility is the collection of long-line data (sometimes using sunlight as a radiation source), an approach which yields concentrations in units of concentration-length (ppm-metres). If the path length is known, the concentration may be calculated. This approach is particularly useful for measuring concentrations in stack plumes.

Dispersive absorption spectrometers are basically standard spectrometers with a monochromator for selection of the wavelength to be measured. They are used to measure air pollutants by determining absorption at a specified part of the spectrum of the sought-for material. Of course, other gases or particulate matter that absorb or scatter light at the chosen wavelength interfere. These instruments are generally applied to in-stack monitoring. Sensitivity is increased by using long path lengths or by pressurising the cell.

Second-derivative spectroscopy is a useful technique for trace gas analysis. Basically, this technique varies the wavelength by a small value around a specified nominal wavelength. The second derivative of light intensity versus wavelength is obtained. In conventional absorption spectrophotometry, a decrease in light intensity as the light passes through a sample indicates the presence of at least one substance—and possibly many absorbing at that wavelength. Second-derivative spectroscopy, however, provides information regarding the change in intensity with wavelength, thereby indicating the presence of specific absorption lines or bands which may be superimposed on a relatively high background of absorption. Much higher specificity is obtained. The spectra obtained by second-derivative spectrometry in the ultraviolet region show a great deal of structure and are quite characteristic of the compounds being observed.

BIOLOGICAL ANALYSIS

Microbiological Determination of Cell Numbers

Traditional microbiological methods for the detection and estimation of microbial numbers involve a number of techniques both direct and indirect.

The methods used to determine the number or mass of cells present in a sample depends greatly on the nature of the sample and the growth conditions being used. Microbial growth in a simple liquid medium enables a number of direct methods to be used to determine cell numbers or biomass concentrations. Samples from situations where non-microbial solids and cell aggregates are present, such as activated sludge, require more indirect methods to estimate cell numbers or biomass concentration. A rapid, accurate method of estimating cell size and cell number is of great importance in environmental biotechnology. The direct methods are outlined in Fig. 21.17.

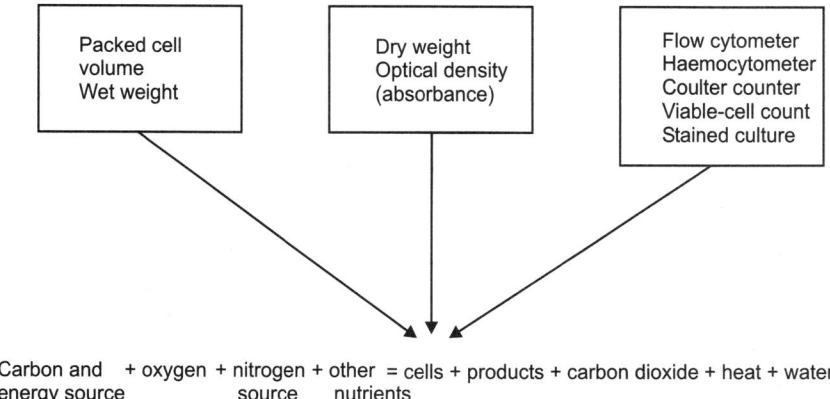

Fig. 21.17. Direct methods of determining the mass or number of microbial cells.

Dry weight

A popular direct method for determining the mass of the cells present is to weigh a sample taken from the culture. The cells can be separated from the medium by centrifugation (10,000 grams × 15 minutes) using preweighed centrifuge tubes and the weight of biomass determined after drying the pellet in an oven. The disadvantage of this method is that it is slow and requires fairly large samples. An alternative is to filter a known volume of culture through a preweighed filter (0.2 μm pore size) and then dry in an oven or under an infrared lamp. Alternatively, the filter can first be weighed wet, and then after drying, thus giving both the wet and dry weights of the biomass. The filter method is faster than centrifugation and can handle smaller samples, although wet-weight determination can be inaccurate.

Cell number

The number of cells in liquid culture can be determined directly by counting the cells. The simplest method is to use a counting chamber (haemocytometer or Petroff-Hausser chamber), which is a special microscope slide, etched with a grid (Fig. 21.18). The grids (normally two) are set 0.1 mm below the level of the slide in a trough cut in the slide. The grid is divided into 400 squares, each $1/400$ mm^2, and as the depth is 0.1 mm the volume of each square is 0.00025 mm^3 or 2.5×10^{-7} ml. A small drop of the culture is placed in the trough and a glass coverslip placed over the trough. To ensure that the depth is correct the coverslip is pressed down until Newton rings are observed. After 20 minutes to allow the cells to settle, the slide is placed under a microscope and the number of organisms per square is counted. To obtain a statistically meaningful result 200–500 cells should be counted in total. The mean value per square is calculated and multiplied by 4×10^6 to give the number of cells/ml.

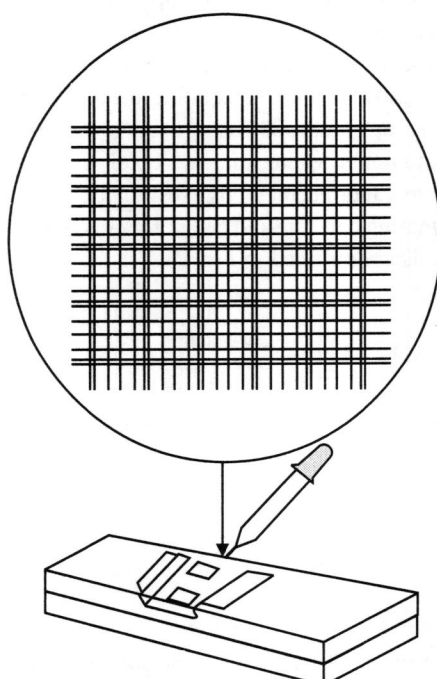

Fig. 21.18. The haemocyrometer slide or Petroff-Hausser chamber used for the counting of microbial cells. The inset shows the grid system at the base of the trough. Each small square is $1/400$ mm^2 and the depth is 0.1 mm, which gives a volume of 2.5×10^{-7} ml. Thus a mean of 20 cells per small square will give a cell density of 8×10^7 cells/ml.

Fluorescent dyes (fluorochromes), such as 4′,6-diamidino-2-phenylindole (DAPI) and propidium iodide (DNA dyes) can be used to stain the cells prior to counting. The organisms are counted in an epifluorescence microscope where ultraviolet (UV) light is shone on to the specimen from above and any visible fluorescence observed in the microscope.

Another direct counting method is to filter a known volume of the sample through a sterile filter with a pore size of 0.2 μm. The micro-organisms collected on the filter can be either counted directly or stained before counting.

There are two mechanical methods of counting cell numbers, which are the Coulter counter and flow cytometer. In the electronic particle counter or Coulter counter the micro-organisms are drawn through a small aperture across which an electric field is applied. A cell passing through the aperture causes a pulse in the field proportional to the cell's size. Thus by passing a fixed volume through the aperture, the number and size distribution of the cells can be determined. The disadvantage of this technique is that the aperture size has to be selected for the cell size expected and the sample has to be diluted sufficiently so that only one cell at a time passes through the aperture. Also, any aggregates in the sample will be counted as one cell or may clog the aperture. In addition, the diluting liquid has to be free of particles as these will give false readings or block the aperture.

The other mechanical method of cell counting is the flow cytometer (cell sorter). In flow cytometry the cell suspension is introduced to a stream of sheath liquid at a slower flow rate, which ensures that drops are formed that contain only one cell or no cells at all. The drops pass a measuring window where a light or laser is shone into the drops, the light is scattered, and the fluorescence of the sample measured. These data can be used to estimate the number of cells, measure their DNA content, and sort the cells. The flow cytometer is rapid, sorting 10,000 cells/s at a volume of 10–100 l/min. The incorporation of a range of stains such as propidium iodide, calcofluor white, and fluorescently labelled antibodies can be used to select cells, determine their viability, and identify micro-organisms. Many of the stains, such as propidium iodide, are specific for DNA and RNA. Antibodies against specific proteins can be made fluorescent by reacting with fluorescein isothiocyanate (FITC). The flow cytometer was initially developed for animal cells and has been used for plant cell suspensions. Sorting bacteria is more difficult as they are considerably smaller, not always spherical, can contain cell aggregates, and autofluorescence can cause problems with this type of cell counting. Other disadvantages are that flow cytometers are complex and expensive machines. However, flow cytometry has been used to determine the number of cells in aqueous samples and bacterioplankton in tropical marine samples.

Viable cell count

One of the main problems with all of the direct counting methods is that they cannot distinguish between viable and nonviable cells. The most commonly used technique for the determination of viable cells is the plate count. Here the sample is serially diluted in a sterile medium (often 0.9 M NaCl) and 0.05–0.2 ml of the diluted suspension spread on to a solid nutrient medium in a Petri dish (Fig. 21.19). The plates are incubated for 24–72 hours at the appropriate temperature. If diluted sufficiently each colony that appears on the medium arises from a single viable cell. If the number of colonies formed is counted and the dilution taken into consideration, the number of viable cells can be found. Here again the number of colonies counted has to be sufficient to give a statistically sound result. The percentage viability can be determined by comparing the total cell count with the viable count. The number of cells that grow and form colonies will depend on using the correct medium and growth conditions, and there may be cells in the sample that are viable but non-culturable.

Variations on the plate technique are the pour-plate method and the Miles and Misra method. In the pour-plate method the liquid sample is mixed with molten agar (at 42°–45°C; low enough not to kill the cells) and poured into a Petri dish where colonies develop within and on the plate. The Miles and Misra method involves dropping a known volume (generally 0.05 ml) of the serial dilutions of the sample around the circumference of a plate (Fig. 21.20). The plate is not spread but each drop will spread out to some extent on the surface as the medium soaks into the agar, and colonies will develop within this area. In this way the number of plates required is considerably reduced.

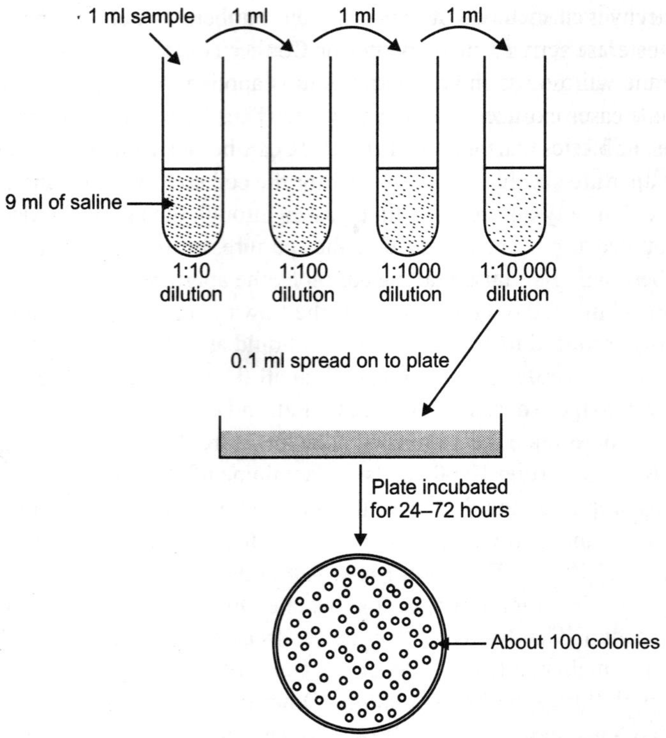

Fig. 21.19. The process for the estimation of viable cells in a sample. The sample is serially diluted in order to obtain about 100 cells in 0.1 ml, which can be spread on to the agar plate. The serial dilution is carried out by placing 1 ml into 9 ml of sterile 0.9 per cent saline, mixing well, and passing on 1 ml to the next step. If the initial cell concentration was 1×10^8 cells/ml then five steps will give a concentration of 1000 cells/ml and 100 cells/0.1 ml. Assuming 100 per cent viability spreading 0.1 ml on the plate will give 100 colonies; 0.1 ml of the diluted culture is dropped on to the agar plate and the liquid spread across the plate using a sterile glass spreader. The plates are incubated at the appropriate conditions and the number of colonies counted after incubation.

If the sample is expected to contain few micro-organisms, too few cells to count accurately, the most probable number (MPN) technique can be used. The sample is diluted progressively using 10-fold dilutions. These dilutions are placed in tubes containing medium and a small inverted tube. If viable cells are present growth will occur and gas will collect in the tube. Normally, five tubes are used for each dilution. The number of cells in the original sample can be estimated from the number of positive tubes at the various dilutions using the most probable table. With dilute samples a large volume of liquid or gas can be filtered through a sterile 0.2 μm filter and the filter placed on the surface of a suitable medium in a Petri dish. Colonies will develop on the surface of the filter and the number of micro-organisms can be determined in relation to the volume filtered. Often these filters will have been marked with a grid to help with the colony count. There are a number of dyes that can be used to distinguish between dead and living cells both under the microscope and in the flow cytometer. The use of these is based on the following parameters.

1. Exclusion of dyes by the cell membrane (*Bac*Light™, Evans Blue, Trypan Blue). Live cells have an intact membrane.

2. Enzyme activity is characteristic of live cells. Dyes that can cross the cell membrane are converted by internal esterase activity into a compound that is coloured or fluorescent. If the cells are dead the membrane will not be intact so that any coloured product formed will diffuse out of the cells. In some cases extracellular enzyme activity has been used as a marker for viability.

3. Addition of antibiotics that will kill or distort any viable cells while leaving head cells untouched (SimPlate™).

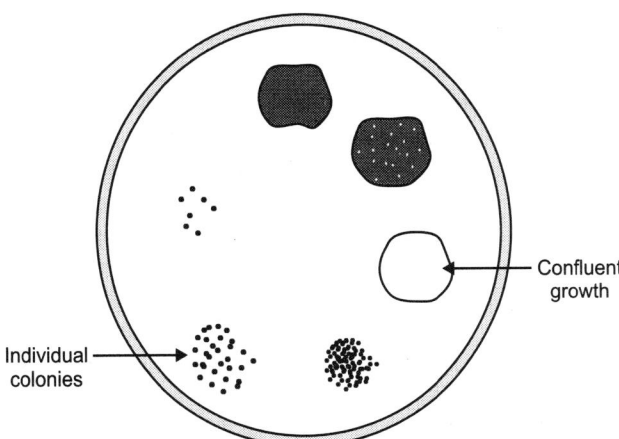

Fig. 21.20. The Miles and Misra variation on the viable count. In this case the 0.5 ml of the diluted culture is dropped around the circumference of a plate. The drops are not mechanically spread out but just allowed to spread out themselves and soak into the agar medium. After incubation at the optimum conditions the pattern of growth obtained will be as shown, when six serial dilutions have been added to the plate. In the more concentrated samples the growth is confluent but at the higher dilutions individual colonies can be seen.

The LIVE *Bac*Light™ stain kit can distinguish between Gram-negative and Gram-positive bacteria using a live culture. Actively growing cells are treated with two dyes, SYTO®, which stains DNA in Gram-negative cells, and hexidium iodide, which stains DNA in Gram-positive cells. Under the epifluorescence microscope hexidium iodide gives an orange colour and SYTO® a green colour. Using a similar technique living and dead cells can be distinguished.

In this case two dyes, SYTO® and propidium iodide, are used. The SYTO® dye will stain the DNA in living and dead cells provided they are Gram-negative, and propidium iodide will only enter dead cells because of their damaged membranes. The propidium iodide is red under blue-light fluorescence, so the dead cells are red and live cells are green.

Dyes like Evans Blue and Trypan Blue only enter cells with damaged membranes, and have also been used with a number of microbial eukaryotes such as algae and fungi to determine viability.

The dyes based on the internal esterase activity of viable cells cleave the dye into a coloured product that can be seen under the epifluorescence microscope. Examples are fluorescein diacetate (FDA) and carboxyfluorescein acetate (CFA), which are converted to fluorescein by esterase enzymes that will be retained by live cells but will leach out of dead cells.

Under an epifluorescence microscope viable cells will appear bright green and dead cells colourless. Other similar stains are ChemChromeB, calcien acetomethyl ester (CalcienAM), and tetrazolium reduction (α-5-cyano-2,3-ditolyltetrazolium chloride).

Direct plate assays incorporating substrates that can be converted into a coloured product have been developed. The SimPlate™ incorporates a compound that on hydrolysis releases 4-methylumbelliferone, which can be seen under UV light (365 nm).

Another direct counting method uses a cocktail of antibiotics (nalidixic acid, piromidic acid, pipemidic acid, cephalexin, and ciprofloxacin) to kill any viable cells that grow. The difference between the number of normal cells on the antibiotic-containing plates and the control gives the number of viable cells. Soil samples stained with DAPI (a DNA stain) after collection on filters did suffer from interference but this was improved with aluminium oxide filters and another DNA stain SYBR Green 1.

The growth techniques used for differentiating between living and dead cells are an important parameter with environmental samples but should be regarded with caution. A cell that does not grow and produce a colony could be regarded as dead, but it may be simply that it has been incubated on the wrong medium or under unsuitable conditions. There are no universal media and conditions suitable for all organisms. This would appear to be particularly true for environmental samples, as they contain such a wide range of micro-organisms. Recent DNA-based analysis has revealed the presence of many more and varied organisms than those detected by growth analysis. It has been estimated that 90–99 per cent of the environmental species were not culturable. Therefore, the growth characteristics of the organisms of interest need to be known before their numbers can be estimated accurately.

An example of the difficulties of estimating microbial populations which use specific substrates or cultural requirements is the estimation of petroleum-degrading organisms. Petroleum-degrading bacteria are abundant in soil and numerous plating techniques have been used for their estimation, including plates containing petroleum, polyaromatic hydrocarbons, and crude oil. However, these have been shown to be difficult to use, as some of the substrates are volatile and the results variable. It has been shown that a medium containing benzoate was better at discriminating petroleum-degrading organisms and could show differences in the microbial populations between clean and petroleum-contaminated soil.

Packed cell volume

The packed cell volume (PCV) can be determined by pelleting the cells by centrifugation in a calibrated centrifuge tube. The volume of the packed cells can be determined from the calibrated tube, giving a value known as the PCV. PCV is a quick method but the results can be inaccurate.

Spectrophotometry

Another direct method is to measure the absorbance of the culture using a spectrophotometer. Micro-organisms in suspension absorb or scatter light and the amount absorbed is proportional to the cell concentration, within limits, but at high absorbance the relationship ceases to be linear. To be able to determine cell number or mass the individual spectrophotometer has to be calibrated for the organism and medium being used. In many cases the samples will have to be diluted before the absorbance can be read. The spectrophotometric method is much more rapid than filtering or centrifugation but is not suitable for media and samples containing particles, coloured materials, and compounds that adsorbate the wavelength used.

Thus, these microbiological methods have limitations with environmental samples. Organisms attached to sediments and particles are difficult to quantify and the results probably grossly underestimate the cell numbers. The viable count methods relies on the premise that each colony formed has been derived from a single cell and by using selective media the number of specific bacteria such as *Salmonella* and coliforms can be estimated. These selective techniques tend to favour the faster-growing species and some of the important slower-growing species can be missed. Pure culture isolation and estimation by viable counts or MPN cannot reproduce conditions found in the environment and the interactions between the micro-organisms, and therefore many cells will not grow. It has been estimated that 90–99 per cent of the environmental species are not culturable. Therefore, the growth characteristics of the organisms of interest need to be known before their numbers can be estimated accurately.

RECOMBINANT DNA TECHNOLOGY

Some of the techniques used in molecular biology and recombinant DNA technology have enabled the study of the environmental microbial population both in the laboratory and *in situ* in considerable detail which was not possible with conventional methods based on the culture of micro-organisms.

The possible methods and the sequence of their use are given in Fig. 21.21, where DNA can be amplified by the polymerase chain reaction (PCR) from extracted DNA or RNA treated with reverse transcriptase. The most frequent primers used in the PCR technique are those that select for the 16 S ribosomal RNA (rRNA) sequences. Denaturing-gradient gel electrophoresis (DGGE) or temperature-gradient gel electrophoresis (TGGE) can separate the product of PCR and the bands obtained can be amplified by PCR and sequenced. Once a sequence has been obtained it can be compared with the database of rDNA sequences to give an identification. The sequence will also allow the design of probes, which can be used in fluorescence *in situ* hybridisation (FISH).

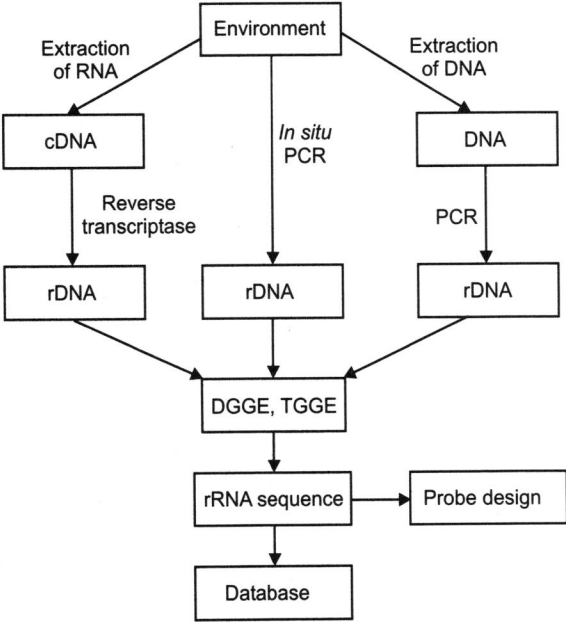

Fig. 21.21. Some of the molecular biology techniques that can be used to determine the microbial population in either environmental samples or *in situ*. Both DNA and RNA can be extracted and the DNA produced amplified by PCR. The PCR products can be analysed by gel fractionation using DGGE or TGGE (denaturing-gradient gel electrophoresis, temperature-gradient gel electrophoresis) giving a number of bands that can be extracted. The extracted DNA can be further amplified by PCR and sequenced. The sequence can be used to identify the micro-organism and to design probes.

If specific primers are chosen these will amplify low-copy or single genes present in the sample, which would not have been detected otherwise.

The use of recombinant DNA techniques for the study of bacterial communities, particularly those in environments difficult to reproduce allows the assessment of bacterial diversity without cultivation. Many of the molecular probes are based on the small-subunit rRNA (ssrRNA). The rRNA genes can then be detected by fractionating the DNA, cloning fragments into the bacteriophage lambda, and screening the clones for rRNA genes. The following are examples of the use of recombinant DNA technology in the study of microbial communities.

1. The microbial ecology of soils and those from extreme habitats such hydrothermal vents.
2. Aerobic and anaerobic sewage systems.
3. Biodiversity.
4. Microbial populations in contaminated groundwater.
5. Bioremediation.
6. Release of genetically manipulated micro-organisms.

An example is the use of whole-cell hybridisation with domain- and kingdom-specific fluorescent-oligonucleotide 16 S-derived probes to study the diversity of the thermophilic micro-organisms in deep-sea hydrothermal vents. Microbial populations in the deep sub-seafloor as far down as 800 m have been shown to be low in culturability although 16 S rRNA techniques have shown a significant biomass. The variation in microbial populations has been investigated by extracting the nucleic acids, amplifying the 16 S rRNA gene by PCR, cloning the fragments, and comparing the gene sequences. The resulting sequences have shown that the majority of micro-organisms in the extreme habitats are unknown and only a small fraction of the microbial diversity had been detected by cultural methods. Quantitative hybridisation can also provide an estimate of the dominance of individuals in populations. Microbial diversity in the natural environment has also been investigated by using variation in the 16 S RNA and a taxonomy based on these data has been adopted.

DNA technology has been used to follow the bacterial population in activated sludge and the population dynamics in a trickle-bed bioreactor. It has been clear that culture techniques are not capable of providing full details of the population in activated sludge and 16 S rRNA probes have shown that the dominant organisms were those of the beta subclass of Proteobacteria, whereas culture methods had shown that the gamma subclass of Proteobacteria was dominant. The trickle-bed study used FISH with 16 and 23 S rRNA probes and gave results different from those obtained by culture methods. The FISH technique showed that there was a very diverse population in the trickle-bed filter.

Recombinant technology can be used to estimate the degree of genetic variation in environmental samples and has been used to detect bioleaching bacteria. In the case of bioleaching PCR was used to amplify the 16 S rRNA obtained from the bacterial population associated with an acidic mining environment. Gene expression can be measured at the protein level (proteomics) or at the messenger RNA (mRNA) level. In the latter case the molecular biology technology of DNA microarrays is being applied to environmental samples. DNA microarrays can be used to examine expression of thousands of genes simultaneously. DNA assays have been used to identify genes that are affected by xenobiotics and metals.

PROTEOMICS

Proteomics is 'the systematic analysis of the protein population in a tissue, cell or subcellular compartment'. The ability to separate and identify proteins from cells allows the study at the protein level of the effects of pollutants and early effects of environmental contamination. Analysis of the protein starts with the one- or two-dimensional separation of the proteins and then the digestion of individual spots or bands (Fig. 21.22). The resulting peptides are extracted and their masses determined by matrix-assisted laser desorption ionisation (MALDI) and electrospray ionisation (ESI) mass spectrometry (MS). Modern machines give accuracy, mass resolution, and sensitivity which allows for the identification of picomolar-femtomolar amounts of proteins and peptides if matching genomic sequences are available. The integration of these new mass-spectrometry methods, data-analysis algorithms, and information databases of protein and gene sequences has enabled the characterisation of the protein profile of an organism.

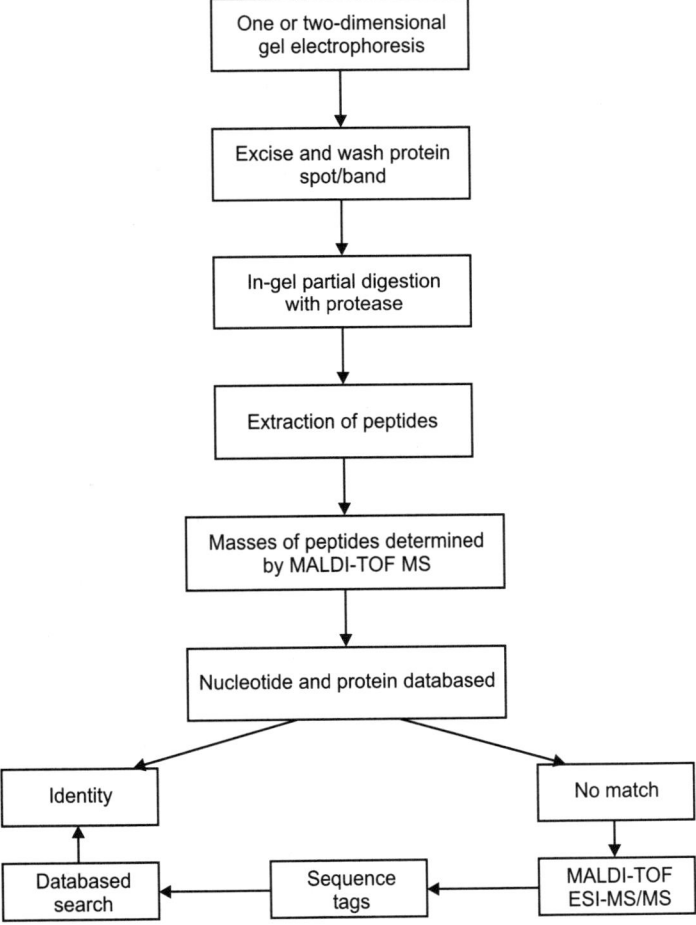

Fig. 21.22. Proteomics, some of the methods used when studying protein expression in micro-organisms. The proteins are separated by one- or two-dimensional electrophoresis and the spots or band are extracted. The extracted proteins are partially digested and the masses of the peptides determined by matrix-assisted laser desorption ionisation-time of flight (MALDI-TOF) mass spectrometry (MS). This may give sufficient information to identify the protein from the databases. If no match is found further analysis using other techniques such as electrospray ionisation (ESI) tandem MS (MS/MS).

DETERMINATION OF BIODEGRADABLE ORGANIC MATERIAL

The biological oxygen demand (BOD) is an important parameter of water quality. It has been a key parameter in the monitoring of water quality and treatment. The BOD is a measure of the oxygen demand in a sample as a result of its metabolisable organic content.

The oxygen demand of waste-waters has been determined traditionally by incubating a sample in a sealed bottle in the dark at 20°C. After 5 days of incubation the oxygen consumed is measured and this is the BOD_5 value. Sometimes the sample is diluted, if necessary, with a volume of activated sludge. Activated sludge is a mixture of aerobic organisms produced by the treatment of waste. The precise test procedure is given in a number of handbooks on water analysis. The test does give reasonable results with normal sewage but the test is biological and will be affected by the time of incubation, temperature, and micro-organisms present. For typical waste this is not a problem but for waste which contains high levels of nitrogenous material longer than 5 days will be required for complete oxidation. If the waste is too strong the oxygen will be depleted before oxidation is complete, and certain compounds require the presence of certain micro-organisms for oxidation and are in fact toxic to many micro-organisms. Variations in the BOD assay are to extend the incubation to 7 days, to oxidise ammonia by addition of allythiourea, and dilution of the sample. Determining BOD is a standard method that requires only simple equipment but although used widely the BOD assay has a number of deficiencies:

1. Slow, taking 5 days before results are obtained.
2. Time-consuming and expensive for a large number of samples.
3. It does not fully represent the natural conditions.
4. Oxidation may not be complete in 5 days.
5. Difficult to interpret with wastes containing high levels of nondegradable organic material.
6. Imprecise, particularly with low levels of organic material.

Due to these concerns alternative methods have been investigated, including absorbance and fluorescence. It was shown that there is a correlation between BOD and absorbance but this is not true for fluorescence. As yet BOD still remains the main indicator of the level of organic material in wastes. BOD is clearly related to the COD; where COD measures all the oxidisable material in the waste, and BOD measures only the biodegradable organic material. Thus, the two values will not be the same for a given sample as some wastes contain organic materials such as lignins which are degraded so slowly as to be regarded as non-biodegradable. The ratio of COD to BOD provides a useful guide to the types of organic material in the waste, but because of the rapidity of obtaining the results TOC is often used to define highly contaminated wastes. In Table 21.7 it can be seen that cattle waste has a COD value considerably higher than the BOD value due to the high levels of fibre, cellulose, and lignin in the waste that degrade only very slowly. This is a feature of ruminant waste whereas with wastes from sugar beet and potato processing the BOD and COD values are much closer.

Table 21.7. Typical BOD_5 and COD values (m/l) for waste streams.

Waste	BOD_5	COD
Sewage	200–400	400–600
Cattle waste	16,000	1,50,000
Pig waste	30,000	70,000
Poultry waste	2400	1,70,000
Whey	45,000	65,000

(Contd ...)

Waste	BOD_5	COD
Brewing	2000	17,000
Sugar beet	2000	3000
Potato processing	2000	3500
Distillery	7000	10,000

MONITORING POLLUTION

The most frequent approach used to determine the effect of pollution on the environment is to determine the concentrations of the pollutants in any environmental situation. To do this, there are a wide range of chemical methods and analyses available. However, this does not determine the real effect of the pollution on the organisms that make up the environment as the effects can be modified by availability, degradation, and transport of the pollutants. Alternatives to the chemical methods are to use a biological system to measure the pollutant or effects *in situ* and include bioindicators, biomarkers, and specific test organisms.

1. The effects of pollutants on whole organisms representative of the environment, known as bioindicators.
2. The effects of pollutants on physiological, biochemical, and molecular characteristics of organisms in the environment, known as biomarkers.
3. The effect of the pollutant on test organisms in the laboratory.

Bioindicators and biomarkers have the advantage that they measure the action of the pollutants in the real and complex environment where there may be many and complex interactions at sublethal levels.

Bioindicators

Bioindicator organisms are those that can be used to identify and quantify the effects of pollutants on the environment and ideally:

1. Are distributed widely.
2. Are abundant and not mobile.
3. Are available all year.
4. Are easy to collect.
5. Have a high concentration factor for the specific pollutant.
6. Are sensitive to the pollutant.

Examples of the types of changes that can be observed are ecological, behavioural, and physiological. Ecological factors involve changes in population density, key species, and species diversity. Behavioural changes can be feeding activities, bacterial mobility, and web spinning. Physiological changes can be the accumulation of heavy metals, carbon dioxide production, BOD, and microbial activity. Some examples of bioindicators are shown in Table 21.8. Lichens are a symbiotic relationship between an alga and fungus and have many of the properties required of a bioindicator. Both lichens and mosses are abundant, not mobile, easy to collect, and lichens are particularly sensitive to air pollutants and have been used widely, used as bioindicators of air quality. Honey bees have been used as a bioindicator for the contamination of the atmosphere by heavy metals (cadmium, chromium, and lead). Honey bees, honey, pollen, and wax were assayed for the presence of the heavy metals and differences were found between reference sites and those in cities.

Table 21.8. Some examples of bioindicators.

Organism	Pollutant	Character
Earthworms (*Eisenia fetida*)	2,4,6-Trinitrotoluene (TNT)	Toxicity and avoidance
Honey bee	Metals	Extracted from bees and honey
Lichens	Air pollution	Physiological parameters
Periphyton*	Acid mine drainage	Chlorophyll content
Mosses	Air pollution	Metal content
Dab (*Limanda limanda*)	DDT	Malformations
Semaphore crab (*Heloecius cordiformis*)	Heavy metals	Extracted from organs
Mussels	Metals	Metal content of soft tissues

*Periphyton is the biomass on surfaces in streams.

Another group of immobile organisms, which are suitable for use as bioindicators, are the bivalve molluscs. The filter-feeding mussels are known to accumulate heavy metals, making them ideal for the monitoring of coastal waters. The Mediterranean mussel *Mytilus galloprovincialis* was used successfully to monitor heavy metal contamination using both metal accumulation and the response of certain enzymes to pollution. Measurements of periphyton chlorophyll content, biomass, and ash-free day weight are commonly used as indicators of pollution. This type of system has been used to assess the impact of acid mine drainage on streams. Marine pollution has been monitored by following increases in malformations in embryos of dab (*Limanda limanda*) in the North Sea, which have been linked to an unusually high input of DDT and polychlorinated biphenyls (PCBs) from the River Elbe.

Behavioural, sublethal, and lethal tests have been applied to concentrations of 2,4,6-trinitrotoluene (TNT) in contaminated soils using earthworms. The semaphore crab (*Heloecius cordiformis*) has been shown to be a good indicator of lead in Australian estuaries.

BIOMARKERS

Biomarkers can be defined as quantitative measures of changes in the biological system that respond to exposure to metals and/or xenobiotic substances that lead to biological effects. The advantages of biomarkers are as follows.

1. The determination can be made over a period of time and not the single sample often used in chemical analysis.
2. They can indicate the risks of exposure to a particular chemical.
3. By determining the effects in various habitats the different routes to exposure can be established.
4. They can provide information on the toxicity of single compounds or mixtures in the real and complex environment at sublethal levels. Biomarkers can be placed into three groups; biochemical, immunochemical, and genetic indicators.

Biochemical Indicators

Biochemical indicators are based on the ability of the pollutant to generate a response at the gene level, inducing or increasing specific enzymes involved with detoxification of contaminants (Fig. 21.23). The extent of this expression serves as a measure of the available concentration of the pollutant. Table 21.9 gives some examples of biochemical indicators used to follow the effect of a number of pollutants. The detoxification of xenobiotics is carried out by the hydrolytic activities of esterase and amidase enzymes but the major reactions are oxidations catalysed by cytochrome P450, which occurs in multiple forms. Exposure to xenobiotics will induce an increase in the enzyme activity. Another process of detoxification found in both mammals and plants is the conjugation with glutathione, catalysed by the enzyme glutathione S-transferase. One of the numerous mechanisms for the detoxification of heavy metals is sequestration by metallothioneins in bacteria and phytochelatins in plants.

These are short cysteine-rich peptides with the general structure (γ-glutamic acid-cysteine)$_n$-glycine, where, $n = 2$–7. These peptides are synthesised from glutathione by the enzyme glutathione synthase. Other enzymes used to measure the effects of pollutants are ethoxyresorufin-o-dethylase (EROD) and aryl hydrocarbon hydroxylase (AHH), which are found to be induced by exposure to hydrocarbons and polyaromatic hydrocarbons (PAHs).

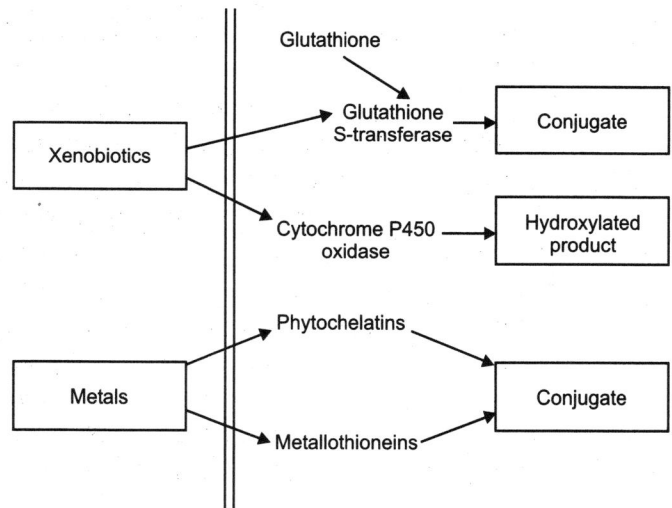

Fig. 21.23. The initial stages of some of the processes for the detoxification of xenobiotics and sequestration of heavy metals. Xenobiotics can be oxidised by the cytochrome P450 complex or conjugated with glutathione. Metals are conjugated with either phytochelatins or metallothioneins.

Table 21.9. Biochemical biomarkers.

Organism	Assay	Pollutant
Oyster (*Crassostrea gigas*)	Metallothioneins	Metals
Mussel (*Mytilus edulis*)	Glutathione	
Plants	EROD*, AHH[†]	Dioxins
Freshwater mussel (*Unio tumidus*)	GSH[‡] enzymes	Copper, thiram
Sea star (*Asterias rubens*)	Cytochrome P450, benzopyrene hydroxylase	PAHs[∥]

* EROD, ethoxyresorufin-o-dethylase.
[†] AHH, aryl hydrocarbon hydroxylase.
[‡] GSH, glutathione.
[∥] SPAH, polyaromatic hydrocarbon.

Immunochemistry

The specific reaction between antigens and antibodies can be used to determine the presence of xenobiotics in environmental samples. Antibodies against PCBs, PCDDs (polychlorinated dibenzo-*p*-dioxins), and PCDFs (polychlorinated dibenzofurans) have been developed and used in an ELISA system to determine PCBs in samples. ELISA has also been used to determine methanogens in samples from an anaerobic digester.

Genetic Indicators

There are a number of molecular techniques that can be used to follow the effect of pollutants in the environment and these include the introduction of genetically engineered indicator organisms, and antibiotic- and heavymetal-resistance genes.

One of the most rapid and sensitive methods of screening for gene expression is to fuse the relevant promoter sequences to those for a product that is easily detected. The detection can be by antibiotic and heavy metal resistance but the best is one where light is produced. A number of examples of these are given in Table 21.10.

Table 21.10. Molecular biology biomarkers.

Selection	Assay
Antibiotic-resistance gene, e.g. *npt*II	Selective plates, resistance to kanamycin
Heavy-metal-resistance gene, e.g. *mer*	Selective plates, e.g. resistance to mercury
Chromogenic marker gene, e.g. *lac*ZY	Plate assay with X-gal converted to a blue-coloured product
Bacterial luciferase gene, e.g. *lux*AB	Bioluminescence with or without luciferin, plate count or luminometry
Eukaryotic luciferase gene, e.g. *luc*	Bioluminescence with plate or luminometry
Green fluorescent gene, e.g. *gfp*	Green fluorescence, flow cytometry, microscopy, and plates

The *gus*A gene product will cleave the colourless substrate X-gal (5-bromo-4-chloro-3-indolyl β-D-galactoside) to give a blue colour and this gene can be fused to a promoter that responds to the pollutant. Another example is the insertion into an *E. coli* strain of a plasmid containing the *lac*Z gene, which codes for the enzyme β-galactosidase, which has been linked to the *ars*R gene that codes for the regulatory protein of the *ars* operon. The *ars* operon is involved in the removal of antimony and arsenic from the cell. Thus when the cells containing the plasmid are exposed to antimony or arsenate the enzyme β-galactosidase is induced and this can be assayed by the addition of *p*-aminophenyl β-D-galacto-pyranoside. The product of the reaction, *p*-aminophenol, can be determined electrochemically. Thus, a bacterial sensing system has been developed that responds to antimony and arsenate.

There is another group of genes where the product does not require substrate addition, as these genes code for light-producing proteins; the luciferase enzyme *lux*AB from prokaryotes and the *luc* gene from eukaryotes, and more recently a green fluorescent protein coded by the *gfp* gene from a jellyfish, *Aequorea victoria*. These types of marker gene have been placed under the control of the promoters of genes associated with a response to toxic compounds. Thus, if the engineered bacteria are exposed to a toxic compound it will trigger light production, which can be detected easily (Fig. 21.24). An example is the construction of an *E. coli* strain which contained a promoter (*alk*B) from *Pseudomonas oleovorans* and the *lux*AB genes of *Vibrio harveyi*.

The cells responded to alkanes by the production of light and were used to detect soil contamination by heating oil. Another *E. coli* construct was used to determine the levels of metals and *Vibrio fischeri* was used to screen the effect of TNT. Bioluminescence was used to track genetically engineered *Xanthomonas campestris* after its release into the environment. *X. campestris* was engineered to contain the *lux* gene, which under the conditions used was constantly bioluminescent. The emission of light was detected using a special camera, which provided real-time measurement of the organisms after release into the field.

Bacterial strains are not the only cell lines used; a recombinant mouse hepatoma cell line containing a luciferase gene under the control of a cytochrome P450 1A1 promoter has been constructed. The cytochrome P450 is induced when the cells are exposed to dioxins, PAHs, and petrochemicals.

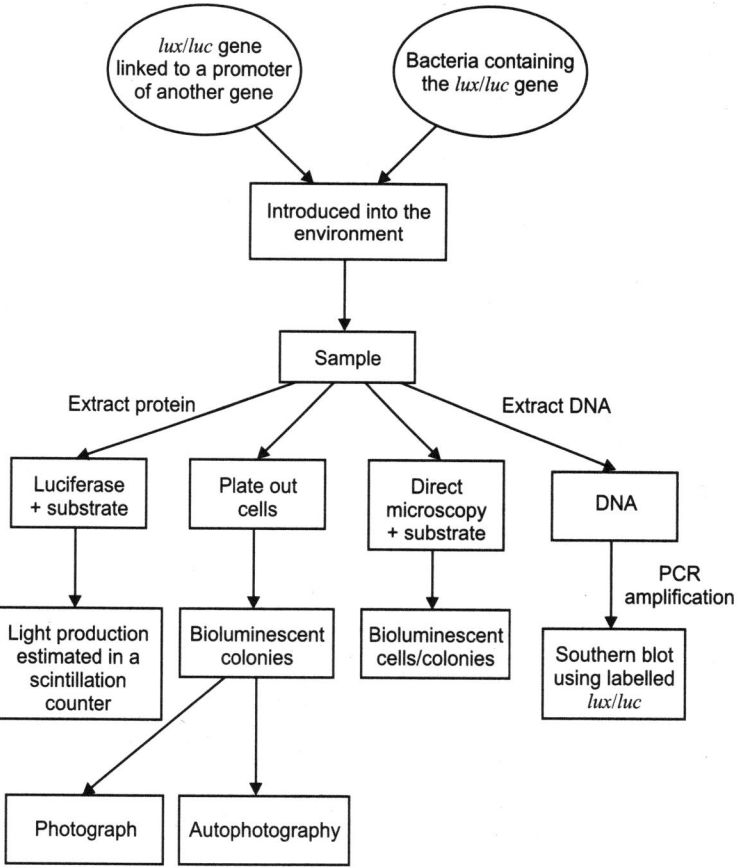

Fig. 21.24. The use of genes coding for protein that can emit light in the detection of effects of pollution in the environment.

TOXICITY TESTING USING BIOLOGICAL MATERIAL

Toxicity bioassays often rely on measurement of the lethal effects of a compound on a specific biological system and this is usually carried out with a single pollutant. Some examples of the use of biological material to detect the effect of a compound on a specific organism are outlined below and examples are given in Table 21.10.

Toxicity Testing Using Plants and Algae

The use of algae for toxicity testing was introduced in 1964 when the alga *Selenastrum capricornutum* (now known as *Pseudokirchneriella subcapitata*) was applied to pollution and is now used for the assessment and evaluation of water quality. Toxicity testing using plants and animals can be represented by a number of trophic levels (Table 21.11). The common freshwater algae *Chlorella vulgaris*, *S. capricornatum*, and *Senendesmus subspicatus* are often used to represent trophic level 1. Toxicity testing with algae has been developed into standard tests with a number of agencies.

Table 21.11. Trophic levels representing toxicity testing.

Trophic level	Type	Example
1	Primary producers	*Chlorella vulgaris, Selenastrum capricarnutum, Senendesus quadricauda, Lemna* spp.
2	Primary consumers	Daphnia water fleas, brine shrimp (*Artemia salina*)
3	Secondary consumers, carnivores	None
4	Tertiary consumers	Fathead minnow, zebra fish, guppy, rainbow trout, blue-gilled sunfish
5	Quaternary consumers, birds of prey	Pigeon, quail, pheasant, kestrel, buzzard

Other aquatic plants have been proposed as alternatives to microalgae, including duckweed (*Lemna* spp.) *Eloidea canadensis*, periphyton, and phytoplankton. Marine algae have also been proposed, including filamentous algae *Ceramium strictum* and *Ceramium tenuicorne*, *Phaedactylum tricornutum*, and *Champia parvula*.

In trophic level 2 the main organism used is the water flea (*Daphnia* spp.), although the brine shrimp (*Artemia salina*) has also been used. The effect of the pollutant is estimated by the number of organisms immobilised after 24 hours of exposure. In trophic level 3 no test organisms exist, possibly due to their similarity in response to level 4 organisms. The tertiary organisms are carnivores such as fish like trout, blue-gilled sunfish, zebra fish, fathead minnow, and guppy. The final group, level 5, represents the top of the food chain and includes a number of bird species.

Luminescent Organisms

MICROTOX™, BIOTOX™, ToxAlert®, and LUMISTox® are systems that use the reduction in light emission by luminous bacteria such as *Photobacterium fisceri* and *Photobacterium phosphoreum* as a measurement of the toxicity of a compound over a 15-minute exposure period.

Ames Test

The Ames test was developed to test substances for their ability to produce mutations in bacteria. The test consists of the treatment of a *Salmonella typhimurium* mutant, which requires the amino acid histidine for growth (*His*⁻), with the test compound along with an extract of rat liver. The rat liver is added because many nontoxic compounds can be converted to mutagens by the enzymes present in the mammalian liver, which are not found in bacteria. If the compound is a mutagen then reverse mutations will occur and colonies will form on a medium lacking histidine. The number of colonies will give a measure of the mutagenic potential.

Molecular Biology Biomarkers

Another development using genetic manipulation of biological material for the estimation of toxicity has been the generation of a transgenic strain of the nematode *Caenorhabditis elegans*. The strain contains the *lacZ* gene from *E. coli* fused to the *hsp*16 gene. The *lacZ* gene codes for the enzyme β-galactosidase and the *hsp*16 is an inducible gene that is induced when the nematode undergoes a heat-shock response. Thus, when the nematode is stressed the enzyme is induced in the worm. The enzyme can be detected by the addition of a substrate such as *o*-nitrophenyl-β-galactopyranoside (ONPG), which will produce a blue colour when cleaved by the enzyme.

Often in the testing of pollutants a combination of many of the tests mentioned are used to determine the effect of the pollutant on the environment. Wild-type and recombinant cell lines have been used to assess aryl hydrocarbon and oestrogen receptor activity of dioxin-like chemicals and the oestrogen receptor activity of a wide range of chemicals. Dioxin-like chemicals are of importance as they cause a range of toxicities and are carcinogenic. The actions of these chemicals are mediated through the aryl receptor (AhR). Compounds that mimic oestrogen activity disrupt normal reproduction and developmental processes, which leads to cancers and reproductive problems. Thus, it is important to monitor these chemicals.

Another example is the range of biomarkers and bioindicators used to study the effect of pentachlorophenol. Pentachlorophenol has been widely used as a wood preservative and because of its highly chlorinated nature is resistant to microbial attack and is toxic, and therefore requires close monitoring.

BIOSENSORS FOR ENVIRONMENTAL MONITORING

Concentrations of environmental pollutants and other chemical compounds that influence biological systems are primarily assessed by chemical procedures. Although, such methods are sensitive indicators of chemical concentrations in environmental samples, they do not assess whether the compounds are present in forms that are biologically available to organisms occupying the natural habitat, and do not provide an accurate assessment of the biological relevance of the chemical to the ecosystem. Thus, it is commonly observed that assessed chemical concentrations do not have the expected effects on biological communities or indicator organisms, creating a need for new methods that can assess biologically meaningful levels of chemical compounds that are present in disturbed or natural ecosystems.

The degree and nature of any pollution must be assessed before it can be treated. It is possible to measure certain indicator parameters by physical, chemical or biological methods. Chemical methods provide information on a particular sample but do not give idea about its subsequent effects. Use of living organisms, to monitor the presence and effects of pollution is more sensible because the ultimate aim is to reduce the possible impact of pollution on the living world. Biomonitoring gives an idea of the pollutant concentration and environmental effects, at the same time. By responding to the 'bioavailable' concentration of a pollutant they measure its impact on the environment more accurately. This is vital to assigning priorities in environmental clean up.

Biodetection methods range from monitoring population biodiversity, and detecting toxin accumulation, to a wide range of methods for assessing the treatability and toxicity of industrial effluents. Using biological indicators to assess effects of pollution may be important in certain circumstances, but the emphasis is now more on using biological indicators (organisms, enzymes or other biomolecules) to detect, measure and thereby possibly prevent pollution.

Methods of Biomonitoring

Biomonitoring methods fall into two basic categories:

1. Prospective biomonitoring carries out biotests with suitable organisms to study possible impact of a pollutant on the ecosystem. These biotests involve biomarkers (test organisms or suborganismic units) in laboratory or enclosed, type experiments with use of appropriate positive and negative controls.

2. Retrospective biomonitoring is carried out to assess what changes have already taken place in ecosystem due to release of particular chemical (pollutant). Retrospective biomonitoring involves the use of bioindicators (plants, animals and micro-organisms) to do *in situ* monitoring.

Need of Biosensors in Environmental Monitoring

Efficiency, accuracy, rapid results, convenience and online monitoring are some of the advantages of use of biosensors over other kinds of biomonitoring. Advanced technologies are becoming necessary for environmental monitoring, efficient pollution prevention and cost-effective industrial process control. In the past few years, important advances have been achieved both in advanced monitoring technologies and their methodologies. These technologies are seeing routine use in a wide spectrum of fields including: industrial process control, environmental monitoring, remedial actions, and environmental regulation. Characterisation of substrate and biomass in biological waste-water treatment system is important. Measurement of microbial activity can give information about:

1. The biodegradability of a substrate.
2. The actual process rates (e.g. nitrification, denitrification, carbon oxidation, etc.).
3. Toxicity of waste stream or a chemical.

This information can be obtained by operating a biosensor. On-line detection of influent toxicity especially of treatment plants receiving industrial waste-water can be carried out. Biosensors are needed to measure biological effects (e.g. genotoxicity, immunotoxicity, biotoxin and endocrine effects) and the concentration of specific analytes which are difficult to detect (e.g. surfactants, chlorinated hydrocarbons, sulphophenyl carboxylates, sulphonated dyes, fluorescent whitening agents, naphthalene-sulphonates, carboxylic acids, dioxins, pesticide metabolites, etc.). In the case of emissions, waste and remediation, the analytes will be dictated by the process in question, but the biosensors proposed should offer improvements over conventional analytical techniques and contribute to greater process efficiency and/or safety.

Many biosensors work on the fact that activity of immobilised enzyme is inhibited in presence of toxic chemical or heavy metal ion. Immobilised on a substrate, properties of enzymes or micro-organisms change in response to some environmental effect in a way that is electronically or optically detectable. It is then possible to make quantitative measurements of pollutants with extreme precision or to very high sensitivities.

The biosensors can be designed to be very selective to measure a single pollutant, or sensitive to a broad range of compounds. For example, a wide range of herbicides can be detected in river water using algae-based biosensors; the stresses inflicted on the organisms being measured as changes in the optical properties of the plant's chlorophyll.

Immunoassays use labelled antibodies and enzymes to measure pollutant levels. If a pollutant is present, the antibody attaches itself to it; the label making it detectable either through colour change, fluorescence or radioactivity. Immunoassays of various types have been developed for the continuous, automated and inexpensive monitoring of pesticides such as dieldrin and parathion. This is possible if antibodies can be developed against the concerned pollutant. Portable biosensors and handy immunoassay kits will make measurement of pollutants in the field convenient.

What are Biosensors?

A biosensor is an analytical tool consisting of biologically active material in close conjunction with a suitable transducer device that will convert a biochemical signal into quantifiable electric signal. Simply put, the aim is for a solid-state device analogue of the canary, a bird that ably serves as a real-live biosensor for oxygen even to this day. The more solid-state the better. Biosensors are composed of a probe and a transducer, the former consisting of a bio-layer made up of:

1. Microbial cells (viable or nonviable).
2. Tissue (e.g. cucumber peels for ascorbate sensors, kidney slices for amino acid sensors).
3. Organelle.
4. Enzymes or multi-enzyme systems.
5. Biological membranes.
6. Antibodies.
7. Nucleic acid.
8. Neurotransmitter molecule.
9. Hormones.

The components of the bio-layer are firmly immobilised on the surface of the biosensor probe by physical or chemical methods, entrapment in a gel, chemical retention in liposomes, or by cross-linking.

$$\text{Analyte} \longrightarrow \text{Biological component} \longrightarrow \text{Transducer} \longrightarrow \text{Electronic device}$$
$$\text{(Sample)} \qquad\qquad \text{(Detector)} \qquad\qquad \text{(Signal)} \qquad\qquad \text{(Output)}$$

The transducer converts the biological event into electronic response that can be displayed directly or can be further processed by microprocessors. The transducer must be amenable to immobilisation of the biological component with which it is in intimate contact.

Different types of transducers are used. These include:

1. Electrochemical (amperometric, potentiometric, conductometric).
2. Optical (photodiodes, waveguide systems, integrated optical sensors).
3. Acoustic (piezoelectric crystals, surface acoustic wave devices).
4. Calorimetric (thermistors, thermopiles).
5. Volume change.

The advantages of biosensors include: rapid analysis at low cost compared to conventional methods, sensitivity, specificity, accuracy, ease of use, and improved stability over a period of time.

Future developments on biosensors for environment monitoring are expected to focus on:

1. Miniaturisation, making the instruments portable and more convenient to use.
2. Integration into multisensor arrays to facilitate analysis via neural networks and chemometrics.
3. Continuous or near-continuous information about rapid and unpredictable fluctuations in the concentration of one or more parameters simultaneously.
4. Measurements of analytes which are otherwise difficult to measure by conventional method.
5. Integration in the process providing enhancing the ability to operate in realistic situations.
6. Development of stable arrays of sensors, possibly combined with other analytical or separation techniques.

The major barrier to the development of a biosensor instrument for environmental measurements is the diversity of the environmental market; no one analyte is large enough to justify the development cost of a biosensor instrument. The project for development of a multianalyte biosensor field screening instrument (MBFI) is going on in US. The MBFI has the potential to reduce the annual cost of environmental analyses in the US alone by more than $20 million and to reduce the analysis turnaround time from approximately 19 days to less than 15 minutes. A common disposable biosensor that is capable of eventually being adapted to dozens of analytes will be developed. Successful completion of this project will result in the development of a battery-operated, hand-held biosensor instrument and a series of disposable biosensors for several applications.

Applications

Biosensors are beginning to move towards field testing and commercialisation in the US, Europe, and Japan. Many research institutes, universities, government agencies and private companies are taking active interest in development of these systems and about 40 biosensor-related patents were filed in the US in 1995, with an equivalent number filed elsewhere in the world. Nevertheless, relatively few biosensors have so far been commercialised. Biosensors have potential for:
1. Continuous and *in situ* applications, such as down-hole or perimeter groundwater surveillance.
2. Use in a variety of matrices including soil extracts groundwater, blood, and urine.
3. Operation in high concentrations of organic solvents (e.g. methanol and acetonitrile).
4. For *in situ* monitoring of contaminated organic media or process streams that contain mixed organic wastes.
5. For continuous monitoring on a site to provide an idea about the progress of bioremediation or other pollution abatement efforts.

They can be constructed from a wide array of immunochemicals and even genetically engineered micro-organisms, and they can be configured to be reversible. Biosensors are compared with existing standard methods in terms of accuracy, sensitivity and reliability, and have been reported to detect phenolics, ammonia, formaldenyde, polyaromatic hydrocarbons, heavy metals, and pesticides.

Other promising applications for environmental biosensors include groundwater monitoring, drinking-water analysis, and the rapid analysis of extracts of soils and sediments at hazardous waste sites.

Rapid BOD measurement is a frequent need of process control operations of waste-water treatment plants. While traditional BOD measurements take five days, biosensors based on immobilised *Trichosporon cutaneum* have been field tested in Japan and Europe, that can be used to measure BOD values in industrial waste-water in as little as 15 minutes.

Enzyme-based biosensors being developed at the US EPA's Las Vegas National Exposure Research Laboratory can give relative percentage of different phenolic compounds in a facile manner.

A bacterial biosensor for benzene, toluene, naphthalene and similar compounds have been constructed, characterised and field tested on contaminated water and soil. Genetically engineered *E. coli* with toluene detecting gene from *Pseudomonas putida* and a gene for luciferase from fruitfly which show luminescence in presence of benzene, toluene, xylene and other similar molecules has been developed. Genetically engineered bacteria have been designed in Oak Ridge and Knoxville to give off a detectable signal, such as light, in the presence of a specific pollutant they like to eat. They may glow in the presence of toluene, and can indicate whether an underground fuel tank is leaking or whether the site of an oil spill has been cleaned up effectively. These informer bacteria are called bioreporters. Bioreporter molecules for naphthalene have also been reported.

The Naval Research Laboratory in the US has developed a fibre-optic biosensor and a continuous-flow immunosensor that can be used to measure explosives in discrete samples or monitor process streams. The fibre-optic system is based on a competitive immunoassay performed on the fibre core of a long optical fibre. The flow system is a displacement immunoassay, with response measured by changes in the fluorescent signal in several minutes. Immunosensors such as these combine the advantages of conventional immunoassay methods with the option of obtaining real-time monitoring measurements with data integration capabilities. Laboratory confirmation is done with high-performance liquid chromatography (Table 21.12).

Table 21.12. Examples of biosensors used for environmental monitoring.

Pollutant	Biosensor	Remark
Herbicides	Algae-toximeter	Blocking of electron transport is measured as fluorescence emitted. As low as 5 ppm of herbicide is detected continuously
Phosphates	Immobilised alkaline	Inhibited by phosphate phosphate electrode
Methanol	Use of alcohol oxidase electrode	Low reactivity with ethanol
Benzopyrene	Cytochrome P-450 metabolism as substrate or antibody binding	
Mercury, cadmium, lead	Yeast alcohol dehydrogenase enzyme	
Fluoride	Urease enzyme or acetylcholine esterase sensor	Urea or acetylcholine is used as substrate, 2 ppm of fluoride is detected
Pesticides	Butyrylcholine esterase	3 ppb of ethylparathion, 4 ppb of malathion is detected
Chlorobenzoate	*Pseudomonas* spp.	
Phenol	*Rhodotorula* spp. or phenol oxidase	Oxygen type electrode; linear relationship; upto 9 ppm
Derivatised aromatic compounds	*Pseudomonas cepacia*	
Lead in fuel combustion		Enzyme inhibition
Organic load (BOD)	*Trichosporon cutaneum*	Results are rapid (within 18 minutes) and yet comparable with conventional method which takes five days
Ammonia	*Nitrosomonas* spp.	Results are comparable with conventional method. Time required is only 12–30 minutes
Nitric oxides (NO), nitrogen dioxide (NO_2)	*Nitrobacter* spp.	
Sulphite and sulphur dioxide in waste-water and atmosphere	Oxidase enzymes from hepatic microsome	

In other biosensor research in France, pesticide detection is being explored. Currently the most promising enzyme based biosensors for the detection of pesticides are those for organophosphates and carbamates and involve the inhibition of cholinesterases. Another European application of environmental biosensors is a series of herbicide sensors developed by researchers at the University of Karlsrue, Germany. These sensors use intact photosynthetic membranes as a source of photosystem II, which is inhibited by triazine and phenylurea herbicides. Researchers in Spain are refining a system, that uses an enzymatic biosensor (confirmed by liquid chromatography) for monitoring organophosphate pesticides. This biosensor system can be used to screen samples of river water for pesticides (organophosphates and their oxometabolites) and as an early warning system.

The Oak Ridge National Laboratory has an ongoing biosensor research and development programme within its Centres for Manufacturing Technology. They have developed antibody-based biosensors (immunosensors) for monitoring benzopyrene, besides a luminescent spectrometer which can be used to detect bacteria and other organisms that may contaminate drinking water. Such organisms release small amounts of adenosine triphosphate (ATP), which, in the presence of oxygen, is converted into light energy by luciferase, which will be added to the assay system to detect the ATP. The luminescence spectrometer would detect and measure the intensity of light emitted by luciferase to determine the concentration of contaminants in water. Immunosensors are available for analysis of explosives like 2,4,6-trinitrotoluene (TNT) and hexahydro-1,3,5-trinitro-1,3,5-triazine, (RDX). Biosensors will be successful in capturing the market if they offer new capabilities or show significant improvements over existing methods. It should not be difficult for biosensors to overcome technical, regulatory and market obstacles to establish competitively with established analytical methods.

Chapter 22

Microbial Biodiversity: Strategies for its Recovery

INTRODUCTION

The microbial world traditionally consists of all organism groups that can be seen only with a microscope, i.e. the fungi, bacteria, archaea, algae, protozoa, and a number of newer and less known lower eucaryotes. If one considers the biodiversity of all these groups, the task is enormous and the subject of many specialised volumes. Several volumes have been devoted to microbial diversity. Hence, this chapter will focus on the bacteria with some comment on the fungi, the two groups of greatest interest in industrial microbiology, and on recovering diversity through retrieving DNA from nature.

MICROBIAL DIVERSITY ON EARTH

Extent of Microbial Diversity on Earth

The extent of bacterial diversity is unknown and without a rationally based extrapolation. This is not the case for fungi. The number of known species is about 72,000. Hawksworth has conservatively estimated the number of fungal species to be about 1.6 million based on an experimentally determined ratio of six unique fungal species per plant species times the 2,70,000 plant species in the world, a reasonably well accepted number. This does not account for species associated with insects and perhaps different ratios of fungal species per plant species in the tropical and polar regions. The case for bacteria is far more primitive. Only about 4200 species have been described. It is widely recognised that this represents, at best, only 0.1 to 1 per cent of the organisms in nature. No rational attempt has been made to extrapolate the global extent of bacterial species as has been done for fungi, because too many coefficients for such an extrapolation are unknown. Several lines of evidence, however, do suggest that the number of bacterial species is much higher than the currently known number of species. First, DNA reannealing studies done by Torsvik on Norwegian forest soil DNA showed that there are 4000 nonhomologous bacterial-sized genomes in a 30-gram sample of soil. If one then factors in the 70 per cent DNA-DNA hybridisation criterion for a species, the unknown relationship of this number to soil sample size as well as a typical species abundance profile, it would not be difficult to reason that a gram of fertile soil could contain several to many thousand species. Second, small subunit ribosomal DNA genes (SSU rDNA) obtained from soil in many studies show extremely high diversity with virtually no resampling of the same clone, even in very large clone libraries. Furthermore, most of the sequences from these clones do not match sequences in the database within 1 to 2 per cent similarity, a rough estimate of species level resolution. This high level of SSU rDNA diversity is consistent with the evidence of high diversity from the DNA reannealing studies. Third, new isolate collections from nature often show that one-third to two-thirds of the strains in the new collection do not match known species with an acceptable level of identity in existing fatty acid methyl ester (FAME), BIOLOG, API, and classical phenotypic databases or descriptions. This indicates that even among the culturable isolates, diversity is much higher than represented by the described species. Fourth, there is no evidence that there is a decline in the reporting of new bacterial taxa, if the annual weight increase in the International Journal of Systematic Bacteriology is any indication.

Furthermore, the new taxa are not simply new species, but often new genera or even families. Some of these taxa would be expected to include species-rich groups. More problematic is the number of very unique organisms that are isolated but die on the shelf because there are few funds to support bacterial systematics, and the effort needed to describe the especially unusual organism can be daunting. We will never know whether these orphans harbour unique physiology, produce valuable pharmaceuticals, or play major roles in biogeochemical cycles.

While the above evidence documents that the extent of bacterial diversity is very high, the absence of information on how different organisms are at different spatial scales and to what degree there are geographic species severely limits our ability to estimate global bacterial diversity. May described a relationship that showed that biodiversity increases as the body length of the organism decreases, at least down to organisms of several millimeters in length. For organisms smaller than this, however, there may not be separate species in different climatic and geographic regions as there are for larger organisms. This is an important issue that remains to be resolved. Furthermore, the above discussion does not consider the variety of different niches known to harbour prokaryotes, e.g. special symbioses, extreme environments (temperature, pH, salt, pressure, and their combinations), and novel energy-generating biochemistry. Procaryotes have been on earth perhaps 3.8 billion years, much longer than higher life forms. Evolution should have created enormous diversity during this extensive period of time. Some extinction would of course have occurred, but the planetary changes during this time are not ones thought to have been particularly lethal to most procaryotes. Hence, this long evolutionary period would also argue for high procaryotic diversity. Given all the above arguments, a global bacterial diversity of 10^5 to 10^6 organisms would not be unreasonable. The global biodiversity assessment uses the estimate of 10^6 for bacteria.

Importance of Microbial Diversity

Microbial diversity has several important values to society and to the earth's ecosystem.

1. Micro-organisms are of critical importance to the sustainability of life on our planet, including recycling elements on which primary productivity depends, producing and consuming gases important to maintaining our climate, and destroying the wastes of human civilisation.
2. Discoveries of microbial biodiversity expand the frontiers of knowledge about the strategies and limits of life, including microbes that live at the extreme conditions known for life and ones that have evolved novel redox couples for capturing energy.
3. Microbial diversity represents the largest untapped reservouir of biodiversity for potential discovery of new biotechnology products, including new pharmaceuticals, new enzymes, new speciality chemicals, or new organisms that carry out novel processes.
4. Microbes often play key roles in conservation of higher organisms and in restoration of degraded ecosystems. Hence, microbial diversity goes hand in hand with goals for maintenance of higher organism diversity.

When many think of industrial interest in microbiology, it is often assumed that biotechnology products are the only focus, but all of the above points are important to industry. Microbial treatment of waste streams is critical to acceptable and economic industrial practice in the modern world; microbes and their enzymes that withstand extreme conditions have obvious potential value for new processes; and restoration of mining, production, and harvesting areas are critical to some industries' existence. These topics are also important to the increasing focus by industry on 'green' chemistries and to life cycle analysis of new products.

Beyond the more global values of biodiversity, there are variants in particular organism traits, i.e. particular phenotypes, that are of interest. Classes of traits for which variation (diversity) may be of value include particular kinetic properties, especially K_m and V_{max} values; tolerances to high or low temperatures, high or low pH, and high solute concentrations, e.g. Na^+, high or low pressure; the ability to attach or to be mobile; the use of particular electron donors or acceptors; and the avoidance of predators, i.e. grazing. Other phenotypic traits of biodiversity that can be of interest are the rates, yields, and efficiencies of production of desired products; enzymes with unique properties such as high temperature or alkaline stability, or high turnover at low temperatures; particular regulatory properties; and genetic stability of strains.

The above phenotypic properties are often why particular strains are sought and why particular strains become a focus in research and production. The range of diversity in these traits in nature, or whether there are evolutionary trade-offs, e.g. between K_m and V_{max}, is usually not known. New genetic combinatorial approaches are now used in an attempt to create diversity in the laboratory since it may be easier to recover diversity there than from nature. But, in principle, given the 3-billion-year time span of evolutionary history of prokaryotes, a high degree of natural diversity in many of these traits can be expected to be extant.

The Problem

Given the probable existence of a huge variety of interesting microbial phenotypes, the challenge is the recovery of those traits for study or use. This entails several challenges, including strategies for site selection and sampling, the major problem of nonculturable microbes, DNA recovery and its expression, and efficient screening. Two major strategies are now used for recovery of microbial biodiversity from nature, and they are the subjects of two sections of this chapter—recovery of culturable organisms and recovery of the genetic blueprint, DNA.

Where is New Diversity to be Found?

Two factors determine where particular organisms reside: their selection, i.e. growth and colonisation in a particular habitat, and the degree of dispersal. Before evaluating these two forces, however, microbiologists have the problem of establishing whether an organism found in a habitat really successfully competes and lives in that habitat versus being a visitor. The latter is problematic because of the great ability of some microbes to survive long periods in environments outside of where they successfully compete. Such transients can be found in many places and do not factor into using ecological principles to evaluate distribution of diversity. As a practical matter, however, any population that is present in high numbers in a particular habitat must be considered a living resident of that habitat, because only with growth could it achieve such dominance.

A key ecological principle is that the most fit organism is the most successful in its niche. Hence, different niches would be expected to harbour different organisms, i.e. biodiversity. Major selective forces for the resulting populations are the energy source, especially the type and amount of carbon; the electron acceptors, especially oxygen or types of alternative electron acceptors used under anaerobic conditions; and stress factors that might demand tolerance features, e.g. resistance to pH or temperature extremes. Most of these factors are chemical; hence, site chemistry would be expected to be a major determinant of diversity. A sampling strategy that is based on different site chemistries should yield higher diversity. Site chemistry could mean a difference in some populations under oak trees versus maple trees versus a particular grass, or a calcareous soil versus a weathered clay soil. Few studies have been done (indeed few have been feasible) to actually define how the level of microbial diversity changes with a gradient of, for example, soil chemistry. As one example, different serogroups of *Bradyrhizobium japonicum* are known to occupy soils of slightly different pH (1 to 1.5 units), an example of a fine level of phenotypic difference dictated by a small change in soil chemistry.

Since the heterotrophic community in soil and water is usually energy starved, the particular carbon resources should be a dominant driving force of selection. An example of the profound influence of vegetation type on microbial community structure is shown in Fig. 22.1. In this case, soil DNA was extracted from two adjacent soils of identical history and chemistry until the native forest was replaced by pasture on a portion of the site approximately 80 years ago. Approximately one-quarter of the soil DNA had a different guanine + cytosine (G+C) composition as a result of the shift to pasture vegetation. Furthermore, some of the DNA of the same G+C composition under the two vegetation types is likely to be from very different organisms with different traits. This is supported by finding different SSU rRNA sequences in soils of the same G+C content under the two different vegetations. Hence, vegetation is a strong driving force in bacterial community selection and should be a primary consideration in schemes to recover new diversity.

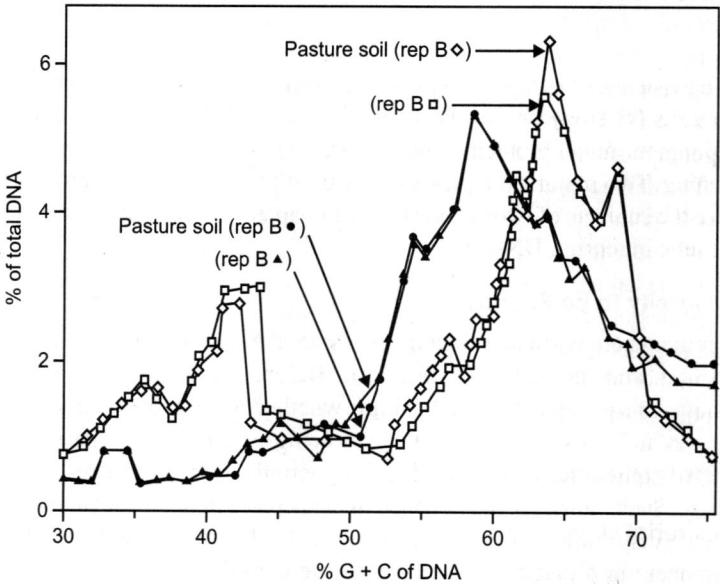

Fig. 22.1. Per cent guanine + cytosine (G + C) profile of DNA extracted from Hawaiian soil of identical parent material, climate, and vegetative cover until one portion was converted to pasture for cattle grazing approximately 80 years ago. Data for two replicate soil samples are shown.

The G + C fractionation method shown in Fig. 22.1 is also a methodology that allows one to recover DNA from more minor members of the community or to target DNA from particular taxonomic groups defined by G + C content. This method is described by Holben and Harris. Briefly, DNA is mixed with *bis*-benzimidazole, which binds to the adenine and thymidine and changes the buoyant density of the DNA in proportion to the G + C content. A gradient of G + C concentrations can then be established by equilibrium density gradient ultracentrifugation. Fractions can be collected with a fraction collector, and the DNA in particular fractions can be amplified by PCR, cloned, hybridised to probes, or analysed as appropriate. The G + C content of each fraction is established by using a standard curve relating G + C content to density measured with a refractometer.

Another type of selective habitat is that provided by a host organism such as a particular part of a plant, insect, animal, or other high organism. Bacterial colonisers of these habitats are often specialists and are not free living. As a result, they may be difficult to cultivate. Nonetheless, such symbionts are thought to be a rich source of microbial diversity. In a few cases where bacterial colonists of invertebrates have been extensively examined, the recovery of novel genera and species has been high, suggesting that the invertebrate hosts are a rich source of novel bacterial diversity. Since there are an estimated 10^8 insect species, this could make insects a very rich source of microbial biodiversity.

The second major factor that determines where new microbial diversity is located is the degree of dispersal of microbial species relative to the local rate of accumulated genetic variation. Another way to evaluate this question is to consider what is the degree of bacterial endemism, i.e. the extent of localised genetic and phenotypic uniqueness. As discussed previously, the answer to the question has a major impact on the extent of microbial diversity on Earth.

The center for microbial ecology has begun to evaluate this question by examining the degree of endemism in organisms that grow on 3-chlorobenzoic acid, a fairly rare trait in nature. Approximately 150 isolates were examined from six continental regions, which included four undisturbed Mediterranean ecosystems (Western Australia, Southwest South Africa, central Chile, and Central California), and two undisturbed boreal forest ecosystems in north central Canada and in northwest Russia. Using repetitive extragenic palindromic PCR (rep-PCR) to indicate genotype, no globally dispersed genotypes were found but several genotypes were regionally endemic. This study suggested a high degree of endemism in this population. The degree of endemism may, however, vary with the type of species. Some species may disperse, survive, colonise, and be more genetically stable, while others may not.

For host-associated organisms, whose hosts are endemic, one would expect some level of endemism. For the nonhost-associated micro-organisms, the degree of bacterial endemism is far from clear. However, cosmopolitan subspecies or ecovars are likely not the rule. Hence, a sampling strategy that considers distinct geographic regions is probably wise in attempts to recover new diversity. Production of the same antibiotic is a trait that is not often conserved in the same species or subspecies, and hence sampling that uses a geographic as well as site chemistry strategy should be beneficial.

BIODIVERSITY OF CULTURABLE BACTERIA

What Level of Bacterial Diversity Matters?

In this sense, level means what level of taxon resolution, e.g. genus, species, subspecies, ecovar (analogous to pathovar), and in a slightly different context, what degree of genetic difference among the organisms. The pragmatic answer is the degree of resolution that is important for the particular problem. If it is a virulent versus a weakly virulent pathogen of the same subspecies, then a fine degree of resolution is critical. If it is a comparison of pine tree and cereal grain rhizosphere populations, a more moderate level of resolution is reasonable, or if it is a comparison of ocean and hydrothermal vent communities, then a coarse level of resolution may be adequate. The pragmatic approach places little emphasis on the species or any other level in a classification hierarchy.

Bacteriologists, however, cannot avoid the need for defining a distinct kind of bacteria, that is, a species, because it is needed to communicate among microbiologists, with other scientists, and in the world of practitioners, e.g. for patents, diagnostics, quality control, quarantine, or international material transport. Hence, we need to continue to evolve the species concept for bacteria. The current recognised bacterial species definition derives from an ad hoc committee on reconciliation of approaches to bacterial systematics. The committee proposed a number of recommendations to combine genotypic and phenotypic data leading to a polyphasic approach, which is the current standard for bacterial taxonomy. This committee proposed 'a bacterial species as a group of strains, including the type strain, sharing 70 per cent or more DNA-DNA relatedness'. Furthermore, phenotypic characteristics should agree with the phylogenetic data, and it was recommended that a genospecies, although distinct, that cannot be differentiated on any known phenotypic grounds cannot be renamed. However, the 70 per cent criterion presents its own technical limitations, including the need for pure cultures, imprecision of the method, lack of suitability for reference databasing, and the virtual impossibility of making all pairwise hybridisation comparisons in a collection. This criterion also lacks a theoretical basis that would explain why two-thirds of the genome should be more highly conserved than some other portion, and it cannot be related to the role of natural selection in determining differential reproductive success that provides the theoretical basis for the species criteria among eucaryotic organisms. It does have the advantage, however, over other species definitions of providing a quantifiable criterion.

Until the relative phylogenetic relevance of any kind of information can be dependably evaluated for bacteria, distinction of one kind of bacterium from all others should be based on every kind of information that can be obtained by the methods available, rather than on one or a few kinds of traits. This has led to some new attempts to define bacterial species. At a biodiversity workshop in 2005, the following definition was proposed. A bacterial species can be defined as 'a group of related organisms that is distinguished from similar groups by a constellation of significant genotypic, phenotypic and ecologic characteristics'. A bacterial species defined in this way is at once a naturally occurring group of like organisms and a taxon sufficiently defined by the collected properties of the group to distinguish the species from closely related groups. With this meaning, a bacterial species should be comparable to eucaryotic species in its adequacy as a unit of diversity in both systematics and ecology. An addition to this definition not present in others is the recognition of ecological characteristics as a determining criterion, which helps bring the microbial criteria in line with reality for higher organisms. Obviously, the particular species definition used is a major factor in any estimate of the global extent of the bacterial species, but it seems reasonable that the definition should have a meaning as similar as possible to that for higher organisms. More recently, DeVoss offered a possible definition of the polyphasic species as 'a group of strains which originated from a common ancestor population in which the steady generation of genetic diversity and recombination after the introduction of foreign DNA, resulted in clones with different degrees of variation but still sharing a significant degree of DNA relatedness and with a common phenotype'. Currently there are a large number of techniques to determine a common phenotype. These include standardised phenotypic tests, such as BIOLOG and API galleries; chemotaxonomic traits such as fatty acid profiles, polyamines, and sodium dodecyl sulphate-polyacrylamide gel electrophoresis patterns of cellular proteins; immunologic data; antibiotic resistance; and morphological characteristics.

For genotypic characterisation there are also a variety of techniques including amplified rDNA restriction analysis; sequencing of the 16S and 23S rRNA gene; ribotyping; rDNA intergeneric spacer region restriction analysis; amplified fragment length polymorphism; rep-PCR using REP, BOX, or ERIC primers; randomly amplified polymorphic DNA analysis; and DNA-DNA hybridisation.

In recent years, SSU rRNA gene sequencing has become an extremely popular method to help identify new isolates as well as nonculturable microbes when their DNA is cloned from microbial communities. The rRNA gene, however, is highly conserved, which makes this methodology alone inadequate tor providing insight into the physiology and ecology of the organism. It cannot be relied on to routinely provide a species-level identification according to any of the above definitions. Figure 22.2, illustrates this point. Some strains with greater than 99 per cent 16S rRNA sequence homology do not meet the greater than 70 per cent DNA-DNA reassociation cirterion. It was found that 'the strength of sequence analysis is to recognise the level at which DNA paring studies need to be performed, which certainly applies to (rRNA) similarities of 97 per cent and higher'. Because of the great current interest in and ease of rRNA analysis, there is a danger that the species-level identification and new description will not be adequately done, leading to misrepresentation of microbial diversity information.

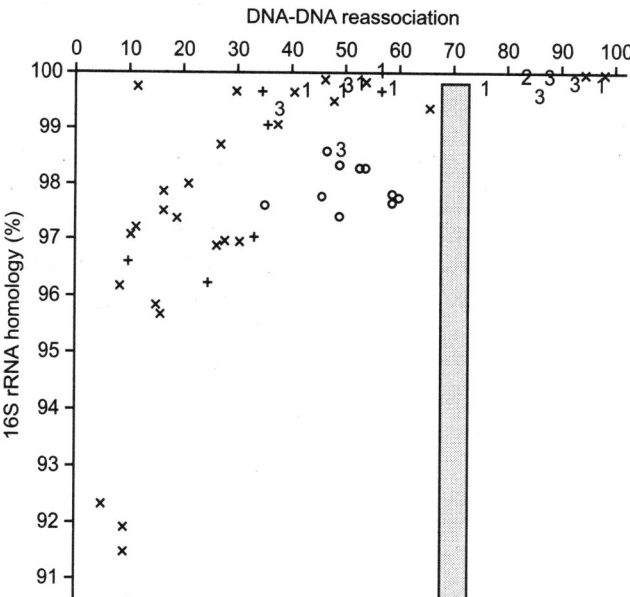

Fig. 22.2. Comparison of 16S rRNA homology and DNA-DNA reassociation values. ×, membrane filter method; #, renaturation rate method; 1, renaturation rate method; 2, renaturation rate method; 3, renaturation rate method; O, S1 nuclease method. The bar indicates the DNA threshold value for species delineation.

Isolation Strategies

Requirements

Skilled microbiologists believe that many nonculturable bacteria will become 'formerly nonculturable' with careful investigation into the physiology and nutrition of the mixed culture, patience, and cleverness. There are many success stories, but all have one thing in common, that it takes considerable time to finally isolate a fastidious nonculturable microbe. Nothing, however, substitutes for the personal skill and insight that some microbiologists have for nurturing difficult-to-grow bacteria, the 'green thumb' of microbiology. The skill of the scientist is the most important strategy.

The ability to track the target population during enrichment is extremely important to gaining insight into what conditions favour or inhibit growth of this organism over the others in the community. Isolation conditions can be constructed from this information. Identification of a means to track the target organism's growth can be challenging without having a pure culture to identify the unique target. Microscopy remains a primary method if there are any morphological clues to distinguish the target organism. Antibodies, oligonucleotide probes, and stains can also aid the recognition in the microscopic field. Non-microscopic molecular methods and chemotaxonomic methods can also be useful if there is a signature to be tracked. Effort spent on identifying a means to track the target population has a good probability of leading to a successful isolation.

One difficulty in isolating nonculturable microbes is that the cell separation step and the cultivation step are usually commingled so that one does not know which is the bottleneck. An ability to resolve those two components to determine which remains the problem helps focus the effort on the real problem preventing isolation.

Mimicking the organism's habitat

The classical enrichment technique was based on mimicking the organism's habitat and using natural selection to enrich the desired population over other members of the community. The technique has been powerful in microbiology, but it can do even more if carried to another level of sophistication. All aspects of mimicking the environment need to be considered. For example, might phosphorus (used as a buffer) be inhibitory, could the atmospheric oxygen concentration be inhibitory, or are the inorganic ions in the medium supplied in inappropriate concentrations or ratios compared to those in the natural habitat? As an example, a very low ionic strength medium was recently found to be necessary to cultivate the formerly nonculturable acidophilic methanotroph; their natural peat bog habitat has an ionic strength much lower than that of conventional mineral media. The carbon content of standard media, such as tryptic soya broth and nutrient broth, has been shown to completely inhibit growth of many important groups of soil bacteria. The RZA medium, originally designed as a relatively low-nutrient medium to recover oligotrophs from waters, has proved much more satisfactory for cultivating a variety of new and diverse types of bacteria from soil and water. A major recommendation in using the mimicry approach is to thoroughly consider all aspects of the targeted population's natural and laboratory environment and to make sure they are as similar as possible.

Rather than trying to construct optimum concentrations of the strain's resources in a defined medium, an alternative is to use gel-stabilised gradients or combinations of gradients. In principle, each of the three spatial dimensions can be used for a gradient to supply different concentrations of resources. The organism is then allowed to find its own optimum for growth within this combination of gradients. Once that combination is identified, those concentrations can be used in a defined medium. Steady-state gradients also more closely mimic the natural condition where the resource pool size is maintained by its natural turnover.

Some bacteria cannot be cultivated because they are members of a tightly interdependent food web. Co-cultures, helper bacteria, and extracts from these bacteria can be used to help cultivate the desired organisms. As an example, isolation of the anaerobic fatty acid-oxidising bacteria was initially successful only because of the use of co-cultures of hydrogen consumers.

Patience

Many of the difficult-to-cultivate organisms from nature seem to be naturally very slow-growing organisms. This is especially true of a number of the obligate anaerobes and some of the aerobic oligotrophs. In the former case, it is not unusual for a skilled microbiologist to take 2 years to isolate a novel anaerobe. Many microbiologists, having grown up with *Escherichia coli* or *Pseudomonas* spp. in laboratory exercises, mistake slow growth for no growth. Hence, patience is needed to determine that growth actually has occurred, and turbidity may never be seen.

Hattori's group has effectively shown how both low-nutrient media and long incubation times (2 months) can be used to recover an order of magnitude higher numbers of bacteria from soil. Furthermore, the physiological and taxonomic features of the bacteria appearing on plates after a 1-month incubation period were very different from those that appeared in the first week of incubation. This cultivation approach shows that the number of CFU can come closer to approximating the number of organisms seen by direct count. The oligotrophic media they use is 1/100-strength nutrient broth. The oligotrophic isolates, which constitute 82 per cent of those colonies found in the second month (Fig. 22.3), do not grow on full-strength complex media. Hence, this method shows that patience for the length of incubation and recognising the appearance of tiny colonies yields a large number of newly culturable strains.

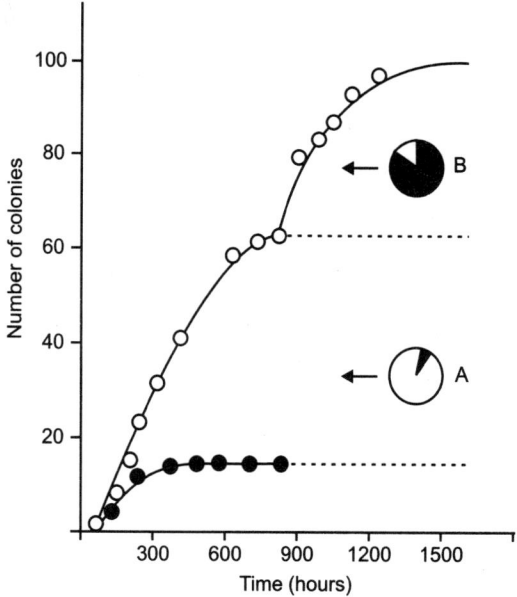

Fig. 22.3. Comparison of the number of colonies on nutrient agar (●) and dilute (1/100) nutrient agar (O). The proportion of oligotrophic isolates at incubation time is shown by the solid portion of the pie chart. (A) 5 per cent of the isolates were oligotrophs; (B) 82 per cent were oligotrophs.

Suppressing weedy bacteria

A major limitation in isolation of new bacterial diversity is fast-growing, nonfastidious bacteria that out-compete slow growers in enrichments or on agar plates. These bacteria, which have the characteristics of weeds, are particularly problematic for isolation of slow-growing bacteria that are present in low numbers. The first strategy to reduce growth of weedy bacteria is to reduce the carbon concentration in the medium, as illustrated in Fig. 22.3. Fast-growing bacteria (high μ_{max}) typically have high K_s values, while slow-growing bacteria have a low K_s. Hence, low substrate concentrations often allow the slow growers to outcompete the fast growers.

Since carbon is the most limiting resource to heterotrophs in nature, it is to be expected that the predominant bacteria in nature are specialised slow growers. A more sophisticated approach to recover low-μ_{max}, low-K_s micro-organisms is by use of a chemostat fed very low concentrations of substrate. This is an effective but labour-intensive isolation strategy.

A second approach to reduce weedy bacteria as well as to impose some selection is to use antibiotics in the enrichment. If one has a means to track the target organism or its activity, appropriate antibiotics can often be identified.

A third approach to reduce weedy bacteria is to omit combined nitrogen from the medium and determine if the desired population fixes N_2. Nitrogen fixation is widespread in bacterial groups, and some slow-growing bacteria can fix nitrogen.

Resuscitation and avoiding the stress of cultivation

Some bacteria are injured in nature, and hence care must be taken for their recovery. Also, some bacteria adapted to natural conditions cannot withstand the conditions of cultivation. Low carbon concentrations in the media, microaerophilic conditions, a supply of critical growth factors, and use of moderate temperatures are means to aid the transition to laboratory cultivation.

Physical separation

Physical separation of target cells from the rest of the community is an alternative to enrichment for the separation phase of isolation. Methods of physical separation include motility to an attractant, micromanipulation more recently by laser tweezers, antibody-linked magnetic beads, and separation by density gradient centrifugation in a nontoxic matrix.

Has the Isolated Strain Been Seen Before?

Once a new isolate has been obtained, the first question is often whether it is novel and, if so, how different it is from what has been seen before. This question can be directed at two levels: is the strain in the collection and hence already counted or screened, or, at a taxonomic level, has it been identified as belonging to an established taxon? To answer these questions, rapid methods are needed so that resources can be focused on discovery of the novel types. This is often termed dereplication by microbiologists in industry. Methods such as FAME and Biolog are automated rapid systems that can be a first-level screen for certain organisms. Recently, the use of genomic fingerprints obtained by PCR amplification using primers binding to randomly interspersed repetitive DNA sequences (rep-PCR) has gained favour. This method is rapid and reproducible, is suitable for a database, and provides the highest level of taxonomic resolution of any current PCR-based method. There are three primer sets that have been found to work in most bacteria; these are known as REP, BOX, and ERIC. Of these, BOX is the most generally useful because it works reliably on new strains and gives the most amplicons and hence a higher degree of resolution among strains. These fingerprints reflect chromosome structure and hence provide resolution at the species-subspecies-ecovar level. Rep-PCR of most bacteria can be done from the cells by using the PCR protocol to lyse enough cells to provide target DNA for the primers. In some cases the DNA must first be extracted, which makes the method more time consuming. The gel images can be digitised, stored in TIFF files, and analysed by software clustering programmes. A complete protocol for use of rep-PCR and GelCompar software for pattern analysis and database construction has been described.

Fungal Biodiversity: Isolation and Identification

Certain fractions of the mycota of temperate soils are reasonably well characterised, and methods for the isolation of these fungi and their identification are available. Other general references that are useful in the identification of soil fungi include von Arx, Farr, and Hawksworth provides a synthesis of the biology, identification, and isolation of a unique subset of soil fungi, the nematode-destroying fungi. The saprotrophic basidiomycetes, in all probability the most important group of fungi in the initial delignification of plant debris entering soil, are poorly represented by methods aimed at isolating soil fungi and are greatly under-represented in discussions of the soil mycota.

New methods for the selective isolation of these and other under-represented groups of soil fungi are presented by Thorn and Bills. Since the saprotrophic basidiomycetes in culture lack sufficient morphological characters or literature for their identification, identification is best attempted using DNA sequencing (e.g. nuclear 18S or 25S rDNA) and placement in a phylogenetic framework of known sequences.

RECOVERING BIODIVERSITY USING ENVIRONMENT DNA

Accessing Uncultivated Microbes

The art and science of cultivating microbial isolates has provided the basis for virtually all of our fundamental knowledge of microbial physiology and diversity. Within the past decade, however, there has been a growing appreciation that the microbes amenable to growth in the dense, monocultural state referred to as 'pure culture' may not be representative of most microbes in the environment. This appreciation has been driven largely by results from the application of molecular techniques on nucleic acids extracted directly from environmental samples. With few exceptions, these studies have shown that the organisms readily cultivated from environmental samples are frequently minor components of the resident microbial population. The percentage of (culturable) microbes varies among environments, with a general theme being that nutrient-poor environments tend to harbour microbes that are more recalcitrant to growth in laboratory culture. There have been many explanations given for this recalcitrance, with most centering on the scrupulous nutritional requirements of the microbes, the lack of appropriate surface attachment materials, or on the difficulty in determining the precise conditions required to revive cells from dormant stages. Perhaps the most encompassing explanation for unculturability is that microbes in natural populations have evolved within the context of a microbial community where the cross-feeding and signalling relationships that have developed among individuals are extremely difficult to duplicate in a laboratory setting.

To circumvent the difficulties of cultivation, several general methods are available to directly describe microbial communities, including microscopic examination, flow cytometric methods, immunological approaches, and the analysis of lipids. Perhaps the most widely used approach, however, is to exploit the information content stored in nucleic acids extracted directly from environmental samples to examine the ecology, phylogeny, and physiology of microbes from natural populations. The great advantage in analysing nucleic acids lies in the fact that a nucleotide sequence represents a high-resolution map to an organism's evolutionary history. Areas on this map can be read and compared among different organisms to derive information on phylogenetic affiliations and physiological potential. In addition, physiological activity, in the form of gene expression, can be determined by examining mRNA extracted from environmental samples.

By far the most extensively applied nucleic acid analysis method for biodiversity studies is the coupling of the PCR with 16S rRNA gene analysis. A cursory key-phrase search on Medline using the term '16S PCR' revealed 1129 citations, a testimony to the broad application and ease of use of this method. The power of this approach comes from the ability to amplify, clone, and analyse homologous regions of 16S rDNA from vanishingly small amounts of sample DNA. This is particularly important when the sample is from environments where DNA is difficult to extract or separate from contaminants, such as in certain soil environments, or when the resident microbial population is present at very low abundance, such as in oligotrophic waters or in deep subsurface environments. Variations of the 16S approach such as denaturing gradient gel electrophoresis or *in situ* hybridisation have been used to examine the complexity and structure of microbial communities, further extending the utility of this approach. Results from these studies have revolutionised our view of microbial diversity and have provided the information required to organise micro- and macro-organisms into the universal tree of life.

Despite the power of this approach, a limitation to using PCR on the 16S or other gene sequence is that prior knowledge of the sequence is required to construct the oligomers used to prime the reaction. Even the so-called 16S 'universal primers', which contain degenerate sites to accommodate base variations in conserved regions, do not match all 16S sequences and will likely vary considerably from a subset of those yet to be discovered. Another drawback is that 16S sequences allow only limited inference of physiological potential. For example, the 16S-based phylogeny of the recently discovered and apparently ubiquitous Group I archaeoplankton suggests that they are hyperthermophiles when in actuality they are most abundant in cold marine environments and possess enzymes adapted to low temperature. Conversely, protein-coding gene sequences amplified from environmental samples can rarely be definitively tied to the 16S sequence of the source organism, making the sequence difficult to place within a broader phylogenetic context. It would thus clearly be advantageous to couple the power of the 16S probing approach with one that could access other portions of an uncultivated organism's genome. This would allow a coupling of phylotype to phenotype that could rapidly expand our knowledge of the phylogeny, physiology, and ecology of uncultivated microbes.

Environmental Genomics

One means to connect phylotype to phenotype in uncultivated organisms is to directly clone DNA from environmental samples, probe the resultant environmental library with labelled 16S oligomers or genes, then sequence the hybridising clones to identify the resident 16S gene along with any protein-coding regions that may provide clues to the organism's physiology. Even though the hybridisation of 16S probes to a library is subject to similar constraints in uncovering novelty as in using PCR, annealing a single probe to a target gene is a less stringent event than PCR priming and may allow the discovery of more 16S variants. The initial report of this approach was by Schmidt, who discovered numerous unique eubacterial phylotypes in an environmental lambda library constructed from marine picoplankton. This study, however, focused on the 16S sequences and did not describe protein-coding regions on the clones carrying the 16S genes. The recent advent of more efficient sequencing methods and robust bioinformatics tools and databases have made practical the rapid analysis of protein-coding regions that are contiguous with the 16S sequence on larger clones. The ends of such large clones can also serve as probes against the library to isolate overlapping clones to identify additional informative sequences. Carrying this approach to its natural end, one can envision that the entire genome of an uncultivated organism could be described given a sufficiently large library. This environmental genomics approach has recently been applied to describe the physiological potential of the group I archaeoplankton that had previously been known only from partial 16S sequences. For this study, an F-factor-based vector, the fosmid, was used to construct a stable 100-million-bp library with an average insert size of approximately 40 kbp per clone. An archaeal-specific probe was used to isolate a clone from this library. Sequence analysis of this clone revealed that it contained the entire 16–23S operon as well as several protein-coding genes, hypothetical proteins and unidentified open reading frames. These sequences were sufficient to provide clues to the physiology of this uncultivated organism. For example, sequence from the end of the rRNA operon showed that the archaeoplankton lack the target sequences for streptomycin and erythromycin, the peptidyl transferase domain of the 23S rRNA, suggesting that they are resistant to these antibiotics. Conversely, a conserved His residue in the elongation factor 2 gene indicated a susceptibility to diphtheria toxin protein. This clone also carried a gene encoding a form of glutamate semialdehyde aminotransferase involved in the synthesis of a precursor of chlorophyll, suggesting that the organism may have the ability to harvest energy from light. In a subsequent study the DNA polymerase gene isolated from another group I archaeal clone (*Cenarccheum symbiosum*) was subcloned and expressed. Analysis of the gene product showed that the polymerase was thermolabile, confirming that the archaeoplankton are not inactive refugees from hydrothermal vent environments but rather are likely to be significant members of many cold marine ecosystems. It is clear from these studies that environmental genomics can offer new insights into the physiological potential of uncultivated microbes and their subsequent role in ecological communities. In addition, this approach can help define the metabolic plasticity of microbes in ways that can help predict responses to environmental stresses or the conditions needed to eventually cultivate these organisms in the laboratory.

The constraints involved in cloning environmental DNA differ considerably from those involved in using PCR. Primary among these is the amount of DNA required. Leaving aside for a moment the inherent biases involved in PCR and cloning, consider that a comprehensive library of 16S molecules can be amplified from as little as 1 ng of DNA from a mixed microbial community. This amount of starting DNA would represent the combined genomes of approximately 10^5 bacteria, the amount in approximately 100 µl of coastal seawater or 1 mg of soil. To construct a comprehensive genomic library, by contrast, requires 10 to 1000 times more DNA depending upon the type of vector/host system used and the quality of the DNA preparation.

Screening Environmental Libraries

By overcoming cloning constraints, the complete microbial diversity of an environmental sample can be made accessible in the form of a recombinant library. In effect, one could propagate uncultivated organisms in the form of genome fragments in surrogate hosts. Given the sheer numbers of microbes in natural samples, screening an environmental library for a particular gene fragment or activity can be challenging. For example, Torsvik estimated that a single 30-gram sample of forest soil contained some 4000 different genomes. Converting this sample to a plasmid library of 5-kbp average insert size would require 20×10^6 clones to have the desired five-fold genome coverage needed to ensure complete representation. Screening a library of this size by standard filter lift hybridisation would require 4000 agar plates containing 5000 clones per plate, a daunting task by any measure. Alternative screening approaches are clearly needed to thoroughly screen environmental libraries. One such approach is to multiplex, i.e. create clone pools that can be screened by hybridisation, expression, or PCR for an initial signal that can be broken out by subsequent screening. The size of the initial pools is determined by the sensitivity of the assay. For example, an initial PCR screen can be used to reduce the clones from the 4000 plates above to 40 pools. A positive signal from one or more of these pools can be followed by screening successively smaller pools. Another approach, which can be used in concert with multiplexing, is to apply high-throughput robotic screening. Such systems are now in place that can screen tens of thousands of clones per day for multiple enzyme activities.

Barriers and Challenges

Even though the concept of diverse, uncharacterised pools of unculturable microbes populating natural environments appears to have been largely accepted, there are key tasks that remain to be addressed in characterising these organisms. First, we have yet to learn sufficient information about an uncultivated organism from sequence data to grow it under laboratory conditions. Laboratory culture still remains an important goal and is still the only way to accurately measure many physiological traits. Second, the complete genome sequence of an uncultivated organisms remains only an intriguing concept. Funding, refinement of bioinformatic tools, and the consensus on which organism to tackle have yet to be resolved. Likely candidates would be symbiont that can be readily separated from its host or a microbe that represents a large fraction of a natural population. A candidate group that meets both of these criteria is the Group I archaea, which are a major fraction of the Antarctic picoplankton and also occur as a specific symbiont of a temperate-water marine sponge. A final goal that would benefit the field of environmental genomics would be to make a prediction of a physiological trait from sequence data and then later confirm expression of this trait with field or laboratory measurements. Several groups are now poised to accomplish this task and in doing so will further increase the interest in examining members of this largely uncharacterised, yet undoubtedly important group of microbes.

Glossary

Activated sludge process	:	Biological waste-water treatment process in which a mixture of the waste-water and activated sludge is aerated in a reactor basin or aeration tank. Active biological solids bio-oxidise the waste matter and the biological solids are removed by secondary clarification or final settling.
Adenosine diphosphate (ADP)	:	Ribonucleoside diphosphate serving as a phosphate group acceptor in the energy cycle of a cell.
Advanced waste treatment	:	The use of physical, chemical and biological means to upgrade the quality of a secondary effluent.
Aerated lagoon	:	Waste-water treatment pond in which mechanical or diffused air aeration is used to supplement oxygen supply.
Aerobes	:	Group of organisms that require air or oxygen for their survival and growth.
Aerobic	:	Presence of free molecular oxygen is required.
Aerobic respiration	:	Respiration that occurs in an oxygen-rich environment.
Aerobic bacteria	:	Bacteria requiring free molecular oxygen for their life processes.
Aerobic digestion	:	Digestion of suspended organic matter by aerobic microbes.
Agar	:	Complex mixture of polysaccharides obtained from marine red algae.
Algae	:	Primitive plant-like organisms, single or multicellular, usually aquatic and capable of utilising food materials through photosynthesis.
Anaerobes	:	Group of organisms that cannot tolerate the presence of air or oxygen, or survive in the absence of air or oxygen.
Anaerobic	:	Without air or oxygen.
Anaerobic bacteria	:	Bacteria that require combined oxygen and the absence of free molecular oxygen.
Anaerobic digestion	:	Digestion of suspended organic matter by anaerobic microbial action.
Anthropogenic	:	Originating in human activity.
Archaebacteria	:	Most primitive type of micro-organism among prokaryotes.
Autotrophic bacteria	:	Bacteria that use inorganic materials for energy and growth.
Available chlorine	:	Measure of the oxidising power of hypochlorous acid and the hypochlorite ion.
Bacilli	:	Rod-shaped or cylindrical bacterial cells.
Bacteria	:	Universally distributed, rigid, essentially unicellular microscopic organisms lacking chlorophyll, usually having a spheroid, or spiral shape. Some use organic matter as a foodstuff, while others use inorganic matter.
Batch operation or process	:	Operating technique that is batch-wise in manner. There are no continuous flows in or out of the operation or process.
Batch reactor	:	A reactor that does not have continuous streams entering or leaving. The reactants are added, reaction occurs, then the products are discharged.

Binary fission	:	The manner in which most bacteria multiply. The parent cell divides, usually into two daughter cells.
Biochemical oxidation	:	Oxidation caused by biological activity resulting in a chemical combination of oxygen with organic matter to produce relatively stable end-products.
Biochemical oxygen demand	:	Oxygen required by microbes in the stabilisation of a decomposable waste under aerobic conditions.
Biochemical pathway	:	Various steps involved in any bioconversion process.
Biodegradation	:	Biological oxidation of natural or synthetic organic materials by soil micro-organisms, either in soils, water bodies, or waste-water treatment plants.
Biogas	:	Gas produced when organic wastes are digested by micro-organisms under anaerobic conditions (in the absence of air or oxygen). The major constituents of biogas are CH_4 and CO_2.
Bioleaching	:	Process of using micro-organisms to recover metals from their ores.
Biological oxidation	:	An oxidation caused by biological activity resulting in a chemical combination of oxygen with organic matter to produce stable end-products known as both biochemical oxidation and bio-oxidation.
Biomarker	:	Biochemical that quantitatively measures the effects of exposure to xenobiotic substances on a biological system.
Biomass	:	Total dry matter of all organisms in a particular sample, population, or area.
Biomining	:	Process of recovering metals from ores using micro-organisms. Biomining is also used for extraction of metallic pollutants from solids or liquid wastes.
Bioreactor	:	Apparatus used to carry out biological reactions or processes, especially on an industrial scale.
Bioremediation	:	Process of using organisms to consume or otherwise help remove pollutants from the environment.
Biosensor	:	Analytical device used to determine the concentration of substances and/or other predefined parameters by converting a biological response into an electrical signal.
Biotechnology	:	Exploitation of biological processes for industrial and other purposes.
BOD_5	:	Five-day biochemical oxygen demand.
BOD_u	:	Ultimate biochemical oxygen demand.
Brackish water	:	Water having a dissolved solids content between freshwater and seawater.
Breakpoint chlorination	:	Addition of chlorine to a water or waste-water until the chlorine demand has been satisfied. Further additions result in a residual that is proportional to the amount added beyond the breakpoint.
Brownian movement	:	Random zig-zag movement of microscopic particles in a gaseous system or suspended in a liquid medium.
Brush aerator	:	A surface aerator consisting of a rotating horizontal axle with protruding steel bristles partially submerged in the still water surface. Oxygen is transferred by air entrainment in the vicinity of the rotating bristles and also by the spray and impingement area.
Buffer action	:	Action of certain ions in solution to oppose a change in pH.
Bulking sludge	:	Activated sludge that settles poorly because of a floc with a low-bulk density.
Carbohydrates	:	Class of carbon-hydrogen-oxygen compounds usually represented chemically by the formula $(CH_2O)_n$, where, $n = 3$.
Carcinogen	:	Cancer-causing agent.

Catabolism	:	Breakdown of complex biological molecules into simpler ones, usually accompanied with the release of energy in the form of ATP.
Chemical coagulation	:	The destabilisation and initial aggregation of colloidal and finely suspended matter by the addition of a floc-forming chemical coagulant.
Chemical oxygen demand (COD)	:	The amount of oxygen required to chemically oxidise the organic and sometimes inorganic matter in water or waste-water. Usually expressed in mg/l. COD test does not measure the oxygen required to convert ammonia to nitrites and nitrites to nitrates. COD is frequently assumed to be equal to the ultimate first-stage biochemical oxygen demand.
Chemical sludge	:	Sludge produced by chemical coagulation or chemical precipitation.
Chemically coagulated raw waste-water	:	Raw waste-water that has been chemically coagulated, settled and filtered.
Chemically conditioned sludge	:	Sludge that has had chemicals added to enhance dewatering characteristics.
Chemically treated secondary effluent	:	Secondary effluent that has been chemically treated, usually by coagulation, along with other processes or operations.
Clarification	:	Removal of settleable suspended solids from water or waste-water by gravity settling in a quiescent tank or basin. Also called sedimentation or settling.
Clarified waste-water	:	Waste-water that has had most of the settleable solids removed by clarification.
Clone	:	Exact genetic replica of a specific gene, cell, or an entire organism.
Cloning	:	Technique involving mitotic division of a progenitor cell to give rise to a population of identical daughter cells.
Coagulant	:	A compound that causes coagulation or a floc-forming agent.
Coagulation	:	In water or waste-water treatment, the destabilisation and initial aggregation of colloidal and finely divided suspended solids by the addition of floc-forming chemicals.
Coliform bacteria	:	A group of bacteria predominately living in the intestines of humans and warm-blooded animals but also found elsewhere, such as in soils. Includes all aerobic and facultative anaerobic, gram-negative, non-spore forming bacilli that ferment lactose with gas production.
Coliphage	:	A virus pathogenic to coliforms.
Complete treatment	:	Waste-water treatment that uses both primary and secondary treatment.
Completely mixed activated sludge	:	An activated sludge process with a completely mixed reactor basin. Usual basin is square, circular, or slightly rectangular in plan view, and the influent, on entering, is almost immediately dispersed throughout the reactor basin.
Completely mixed reactor	:	Reactor where the fluid elements, on entering, are dispersed almost immediately throughout the reactor volume.
Contact stabilisation activated sludge process	:	An activated sludge process with a contact tank where sorption of the organic materials occurs and a sludge stabilisation tank where the sludge bio-oxidises the sorbed organic matter. Same as biosorption.
Continuous-flow process	:	An operating technique that is continuous in manner; that is, there are continuous flows in and out of the operation or process.
Continuous-flow reactor	:	Reactor that has a continuous stream of reactants entering and a continuous stream of products leaving.
Conventional activated sludge process	:	Activated sludge plant with rectangular reactor basin and air diffusers or aerators spaced uniformly along the basin length.

Conventional digester	:	A low-rate anaerobic digester.
Conventional waste-water treatment	:	Use of primary and secondary treatment.
Decomposition of waste-water	:	Breakdown of organic matter in waste-water by microbial action. It may be under aerobic or anaerobic conditions.
Degradation	:	Breakdown of substances by biological oxidation.
Demineralisation	:	Removal of all salts from a water.
Dewatered sludge	:	Sludge that has had some of its water content removed.
Diatomaceous-earth filter	:	A filter usually used in water treatment that utilises a build-up layer of diatomaceous earth as a filter medium.
Diffused air aeration	:	Aeration produced in a liquid by the use of compressed air passed through air diffusers.
Digested sludge	:	Sludge digested by aerobic or anaerobic action to the degree that the volatile content is low enough for the sludge to be stable.
Digester	:	Tank used for sludge digestion.
Dispersed plug-flow activated sludge	:	Activated sludge process with a dispersed plug-flow reactor basin. The basin is rectangular in plan view and has significant longitudinal or axial dispersion of fluid elements throughout its length.
Dispersed plug-flow reactor	:	Reactor that is rectangular in plan view and has significant longitudinal mixing of fluid elements throughout its length.
Dissolved oxygen	:	Oxygen dissolved in a liquid, usually expressed in mg/l. Abbreviated as DO.
Domestic waste-water	:	Waste-water mainly from dwellings, business buildings and institutions.
Dry suspended solids	:	The suspended matter in water and, in particular, waste-water, which is removed by laboratory filtration and is dried for one hour at 103°C.
Effluent	:	Waste-water of other liquid, partially or completely treated, or in its natural state, flowing out of a basin, reservoir, treatment plant, or industrial treatment plant or parts thereof.
Electrophoresis	:	Technique for separating molecules based on the differential mobility in an electric field.
Enteric bacteria	:	Bacteria that inhabit the intestines of humans and animals.
Enzymes	:	Organic catalysts that are proteins and are produced by living cells.
Escherichia coli (E. coli)	:	A species of bacteria in the coliform group. Its presence is considered indicative of fresh fecal contamination.
Eukaryote	:	Organism whose cells have a nucleuse and other membrane-bound organelles.
Excess activated sludge	:	Waste-activated sludge.
Extended aeration activated sludge process	:	Activated sludge process with a detention time long enough to allow the amount of cells synthesised to be endogenously decayed.
Facultative anaerobic bacteria	:	Bacteria that use either free molecular oxygen, if available, or combined oxygen. Also known as facultative bacteria.
Fermentation	:	Biochemical change caused by a ferment, such as yeast enzymes. Biochemical change in organic matter or organic wastes caused by anaerobic biological action.
Fill and draw reactor	:	A batch-operated activated sludge reactor.
Filtration	:	Unit operation that consists of passing a liquid through a granular medium for the removal of suspended and colloidal matter.

Final clarifier	:	Last settling basin or settling tank at a waste-water treatment plant. In the activated sludge process, it separates the biological solids from the final effluent. In the trickling filter process, it separates the trickling filter humus, that is, sloughed growths from the final effluent.
Final effluent	:	Effluent from the final clarifier, final sedimentation basin, or final settling tank at a waste-water treatment plant.
First-stage biochemical oxygen demand	:	That part of the biochemical oxygen demand that results from the biological oxidation of carbonaceous materials, as distinct from nitrogenous materials. Generally, the major portion of carbonaceous materials are bio-oxidised before the bio-oxidation of nitrogenous materials, or the second-stage biochemical oxygen, demand begins.
Five-day biochemical oxygen demand (BOD$_5$)	:	Oxygen required by microbes in the stabilisation of a decomposable waste under aerobic conditions for a period of five days at 20°C and under specified conditions. It represents the breakdown of carbonaceous materials as distinct from nitrogenous materials.
Fixed-bed	:	In carbon adsorption or ion exchange treatments using columns or open beds, this refers to a bed that is stationary in the column or in the structure for the open bed.
Floc	:	The small, gelatinous masses formed in the water by the adding of coagulant. In waste-water treatment, the small, gelatinous biological solids formed at an activated sludge treatment plant.
Flocculation	:	Slow stirring of a coagulated water or waste-water to aggregate the destabilised particles and form a rapid-settling floc. In biological waste-water treatment where a coagulant is not used, aggregation may be accomplished biologically.
Flocculator	:	Basin in which flocculation is done or a mechanical device to enhance the formation of floc in a liquid.
Flotation	:	Raising of suspended matter to the surface of a liquid, where it is removed by skimming.
Fluidised bed	:	Refers to a bed in which the particles are not in continuous contact due to the upward flow of the water or waste-water.
Free chlorine residual	:	Portion of the total residual chlorine remaining in water or waste-water at the end of a specific contact duration, which will react chemically as hypochlorous acid or hypochlorite ion. Same as free available chlorine residual.
Fresh sludge	:	Undigested organic sludge.
Fungi	:	Small, multicellular, non-photosynthetic, plant-like organisms lacking chlorophyll, roots, stems, or leaves that feed on organic matter. Their decomposition after death may cause disagreeable tastes and odours in a water. They are found in water, waste-water, waste-water effluents and soil.
Gene	:	Sequence of nucleotides in the genome of an organism to which a specific function can be attributed.
Glycolysis	:	Metabolic process in which sugars are broken down into smaller compounds along with the release of energy.
Granular medium	:	Granular material, such as sand or crushed anthracite coal, that serves as the filter bed.
Granular-medium filtration	:	Filtration through a bed of granular material.
Gravity filters	:	Filters that have gravity flow of the water through the filter bed.

Gravity thickening	:	Thickening of a sludge using gravity settling in a tank. Pickets, usually mounted on the trusswork for the sludge scrapers, rake through the sludge releasing entrained water. This allows the sludge to subside and concentrate.
Green technology	:	Pollution-free technology, or technology in which pollution is controlled at source, used for manufacturing useful products.
Grit	:	Dense, mineral, suspended matter present in a water or waste-water, such as silt and sand.
Grit chamber	:	A settling chamber to remove grit from organic solids.
Grit removal	:	Removal of heavy suspended mineral matter present in a waste-water, such as sand and silt.
High-rate digester	:	Anaerobic digester with continuous mixing, continuous feeding and digester heating.
High-rate trickling filter	:	Trickling filter with continuous recycle, an organic loading greater than 800 lb BOD_5/ac-ft-day, and hydraulic loading greater than 10 MGD/ac.
Industrial waste-water	:	Liquid wastes from industrial processes.
Infiltration water	:	Water that has migrated from the ground into a sewer system.
Influent	:	Water, waste-water, or other liquid flowing into a reservoir of a treatment plant.
In situ	:	In the natural or original position.
In vitro	:	In a test tube (in glass) or an artificial environment.
In vivo	:	In a living organism.
Isozymes (isoenzymes)	:	Multiple forms of an enzyme that differ in properties such as substrate specificity and maximum activity.
Ligation	:	Formation of a phosphodiester bond to link two adjacent bases separated by a nick in one strand of the double helix of DNA.
Lime recalcination	:	Heat treatment of a sludge resulting from lime coagulation. Converts the calcium carbonate precipitate to calcium oxide.
Lysis	:	Process of cell disintegration or membrane rupturing.
Macromolecules	:	Large molecules, contained within a cell, with molecular weights ranging from a few thousand to hundreds of millions.
Mechanical aeration	:	Transfer of oxygen from the atmosphere into a liquid by the mechanical action of a turbine or other mechanisms. Mixing by mechanical means of the mixed liquor in the reactor basin or aeration tank of an activated sludge treatment plant.
Mesophilic digestion	:	Anaerobic digestion by biological oxidation by anaerobic action at or below 45°C (110°F).
Microbe	:	Micro-organism.
Microbial activity	:	Chemical changes resulting from biochemical action, the metabolism of living organisms.
Micro-organism	:	Minute organisms, some being plant-like or animal-like, visible only by means of a microscope; microbe.
Mixed culture	:	Microbial culture consisting of two or more species.
Mixed liquor suspended solids (MLSS)	:	Suspended solids in the mixed liquor that is, the mixture of waste-water and activated sludge undergoing aeration at an activated sludge waste-water treatment plant.
Mixed liquor volatile suspended solids (MLVSS)	:	Volatile fraction of the mixed liquor suspended solids. The MLVSS is usually considered to be more representative of the active biological solids than the MLSS.

Monosaccharides	:	Chemical building blocks of carbohydrates with the empirical formula $(CH_2O)_n$.
Multimedia filtration	:	Filtration of water or waste-water through a granular bed containing two or more filter media.
Mutagen	:	Chemical or physical agent capable of producing a genetic mutation in a living organism.
Mutant	:	Product of a mutation or heritable genetic change.
Mutation	:	Any change that alters the sequence of nucleotide bases in the DNA of the cell of an organism.
Oligomer	:	Relatively short molecular chain consisting of repeating units.
Organic industrial waste-water	:	Industrial waste-water that has organic compounds as the objectionable constituents.
Organic sludges	:	Sludges that have a high organic content. Usually, these are primary or secondary sludges at a waste-water treatment plant.
Parasitic bacteria	:	Bacteria that require living host organism but do not harm the host.
Pathogenic bacteria	:	Bacteria that require a living host organism and harm the host by causing disease.
Photosynthesis	:	Process in green plants of converting carbon dioxide and water into sugar using light as the source of energy.
Phytoremediation	:	Use of certain plants to remove contaminants or pollutants either from soil or from the environment.
Plain sedimentation	:	Gravity settling of suspended solids in a water or waste-water without the aid of chemical coagulants.
Pollution	:	Condition caused by the presence of harmful or objectional material.
Polymerase chain reaction (PCR)	:	Reaction that uses DNA polymerase to catalyse the amplification of a DNA strand through repeated cycles of DNA synthesis.
Polysaccharide	:	Long chain molecule composed of multiple units of monosaccharides.
Preliminary treatment	:	In a waste-water treatment plant, this refers to unit operations such as screening, comminution, or grit removal that prepare the waste-water for subsequent major operations.
Primary clarifier	:	The first clarifier used. It is for removal of settleable suspended solids. Also called primary settling tank.
Primary treatment	:	Treatment of waste-water by sedimentation to remove a substantial amount of the suspended solids.
Protoplast	:	Part of the cell that includes the cell membrane and all intracellular components, except the cell wall.
Prokaryotes	:	Primitive type of micro-organisms.
Pure oxygen activated sludge process	:	Activated sludge process that uses pure molecular oxygen for microbial respiration instead of atmospheric oxygen.
Reactor basin	:	Aeration tank at an activated sludge plant.
Recarbonation	:	Diffusion of carbon dioxide in water or waste-water after lime coagulation to lower the pH.
Recombinant	:	Cell formed by a recombination of genes.
Recombinant DNA	:	Technology of cutting and recombining DNA fragments from different sources.
Recombination	:	Formation of new gene combinations by joining different genes, sets of genes, or parts of genes.

Rotary biological filter	:	Biological filter consisting of circular discs mounted on a horizontal rotating axle. Fixed biological growths are on the discs and the discs are partially submerged in a vat containing the waste-water. As the discs rotate, the fixed biological growths absorb the organic matter and bio-oxidise the materials. Oxygen is supplied by absorption from the atmosphere as the discs are partially exposed during their rotation.
Sanitary landfill	:	Landfill for disposing of solid wastes.
Sanitary waste-water	:	Domestic waste-water without storm and surface runoff. Waste-water from the sanitary conveniences in dwellings, office buildings, industrial plants and institutions. Water supply of a community after it has been used and discharged to a sewer.
Secondary effluent	:	Effluent leaving the secondary or final clarifier at a waste-water treatment plant.
Secondary sludge	:	Sludge from the final clarifier at waste-water treatment plant. For the activated sludge process, it is the sludge to be recycled. For the trickling filter process, it is the trickle filter growths that have sloughed off-that is, the trickling filter humus.
Secondary treatment	:	Treatment of waste-water by biological oxidation after primary treatment by sedimentation.
Second-stage biochemical oxygen demand	:	Part of the biochemical oxygen demand that results from the biological oxidation of nitrogenous materials. Includes the bio-oxidation of ammonia to nitrites and nitrites to nitrates. Oxidation of nitrogenous materials usually does not begin until a significant portion of the carbonaceous material has been bio-oxidised in the first stage.
Sedimentation	:	Removal of settleable suspended solids from water or waste-water by gravity settling in a quiescent tank or basin. Also called clarification or settling.
Sedimentation basin	:	Basin or tank through which water or waste-water is passed to remove settleable suspended solids by gravity settling. Also called sedimentation tank, settling tank, settling basin, or clarifier.
Settled waste-water	:	Waste-water that has been treated by sedimentation. Also called clarified waste-water.
Sludge collector	:	Mechanical device for scraping the sludge along the bottom of a settling tank to a hopper where it can be withdrawn.
Sludge conditioning	:	Treatment of sludge, usually by chemical means, to enhance its dewatering characteristics.
Sludge dewatering	:	Removal of part of the water in a sludge by any method such as centrifugation, filter pressing, vacuum filtration, or passing through a belt press.
Sludge digestion	:	Biological oxidation of organic or volatile matter in sludges to produce more stable substances.
Sludge digestion tank	:	Tank used for the anaerobic digestion of organic sludges.
Sludge gas utilisation	:	Use of digester gas from anaerobic digesters for beneficial purposes such as heating and fuelling engines.
Sludge thickening	:	To increase the solids content of a sludge.
Sludge treatment	:	Processing of waste-water sludges to render them innocuous. Common methods are anaerobic or aerobic digestion followed by sludge dewatering.
Standard-rate trickling filter	:	Low-rate trickling filter.
Stoichiometry	:	Science of balancing the material and energy involved in a chemical or biological conversion process.

Surface water	:	Water that appears on the surface of the earth, as distinguished from groundwater.
Suspended matter	:	Solids in suspension in water or waste-water that can be removed by laboratory filtration techniques, such as membrane filtration.
Tapered aeration activated sludge process	:	Activated sludge plant with a rectangular reactor basin and air diffusers or aerators spaced along the reactor length in accordance to the oxygen demand.
Tertiary treatment	:	Use of physical, chemical, or biological means to upgrade a secondary effluent.
Theoretical oxygen demand (TOD)	:	The amount of oxygen stoichiometrically required to convert organic matter to stabilised substances such as CO_2, H_2O, NO_3^{-1}, and so on.
Transformation	:	Process of transferring a foreign piece of DNA into a cell.
Trickling filter	:	Biological filter consisting of a bed of coarse material, such as stone, over which waste-water is distributed by a spray from a moving distributor or other device. The waste-water trickles through the bed to the underdrains, giving the microbial slimes an opportunity to absorbed the organic material and clarify the waste-water.
Trickling filter media	:	Packing in trickling filter.
Turbidity	:	Suspended matter in water or waste-water that causes the scattering or absorption of light rays.
USW	:	Unprocessed solid waste. USW is solid waste that has not been processed to isolate organic constituents from inorganic constituents or subjected to any size reduction before being dumped into an incinerator or any other treatment system.
Waste activated sludge	:	Excess activated sludge produced by the microbial solids in an activated sludge plant. This amount has to be wasted from the system at the rate it is produced. Same as excess activated sludge.
Waste stabilisation	:	Process of reducing the BOD or COD of organic wastes to render them harmless.
Waste-water analysis	:	The determination of the physical, chemical, and biological characteristics of a waste-water or treatment plant effluent.
Waste-water treatment	:	Operation or process that removes objectionable constituents from a waste-water and renders it less offensive or dangerous.
Water-borne disease	:	Disease caused by organisms or toxic materials transported by water. The most common water-borne diseases are typhoid fever, cholera, dysentery and other intestinal disturbances.
Water treatment	:	Treatment of water by operations and processes to make it acceptable for a specific use.
Xenobiotic	:	Group of chemicals unfamiliar or foreign to micro-organisms and thus not easily degradable by them.
Zooglea	:	The gelatinous material resulting from the attrition of bacterial slime layers. An important constituent of activated sludge floc and trickling filter growths.

References

Allard, T.K., *Trends in Biotechnology*, Applied Science Publishers, London.

Bailey, J.E., *Environmental Analysis*, McGraw-Hills, New York.

Bekken, T., *Environmental Pollution*, Marcel Dekker, New York.

Benedik, S., *Biodeterioration and Biodegradation*, Prentice-Hall Inc., Englewood Cliffs, USA.

Burtis, M., *Fundamentals of Biotechnology*, McGraw Hill, Columbus, Ohio, USA.

Cainey, K., *Environmental Toxicology*, Cambridge University Press, Cambridge.

Davey, K., *Environmental Science and Biotechnology*, Peragam, Oxford.

Denizen, M.J. and Evans, J., *Handbook of Biotechnology*, Humana Press Inc., New Jersey.

Eichler, A., *Microbial Biotechnology*, Progress Publishers, Moscow.

Eklun, R., *Biotechnology of Waste Treatment*, Academic Press, London.

Fox, A., *Applied Environmental Biotechnology*, John Wiley & Sons, New York.

Frische, B., *Waste-water Engineering*, Marcel Dekker Inc., New York.

Garbisu, C.C., *Aquatic Pollution*, University of Wisconsin Press, Madison.

Haki, M.N., *Principles of Environmental Sampling*, Humana Press Inc., New Jersey.

Jetten, N.S., *Microbial Biotechnology*, McGraw Hill, Columbus, Ohio, USA.

Keith, V., *Environmental Monitoring and Assessment*, Pergamon Press, Oxford, New York.

Kemp, J., *Introduction to Environmental Engineering*, Cold Spring Harbour Press, UK.

Lessen, D., *Biochemical Engineering*, Science Publishers, New York.

Liebier, F., *Anaerobic Biological Treatment Processes*, Tata McGraw Hill, New York.

Machacon, L., *Biomass Bioenergy*, Oxford University Press, Oxford.

Ndon, D., *Biomethanation of Waste Biomass*, Reston Publishing Co., Reston, Virginia.

Reeve, O.M., *Chemistry and Ecotoxicology of Pollution*, Prentice-Hall of India Pvt. Ltd., New Delhi.

Stephens, W.D., *Encyclopaedia of Bioprocess Technology*, John Wiley & Sons, New York.

Saano, B., *Microbial Fundamentals of Biotechnology*, Pearson Education, Singapore.

Tellez, P.K., *Integrated Solid Waste Management*, Affiliated East-West Press, Pvt. Ltd.

Umetsu, P., *Biology and Biotechnology*, Plenum Publishing Corporation, London.

Watson, K.C., *Biohazards*, Routledge, New York.

Wuebbles, M., *Fundamentals of Ecology*, John Wiley & Sons, New York.

Wrobel, A., *Pollution Prevention*, Ellis Harwood, New York.

Zeikus, J.G., *Environmental Biotechnology*, Marcel Dekker Inc., New York.

Index